Endosonography

Endosonography

THIRD EDITION

ROBERT H. HAWES, MD

Medical Director
Florida Hospital Institute for Minimally Invasive Therapy
Professor of Internal Medicine
University of Central Florida College of Medicine
Orlando, Florida

PAUL FOCKENS, MD, PhD

Professor and Chairman
Department of Gastroenterology and Hepatology
Academic Medical Center
University of Amsterdam
The Netherlands

SHYAM VARADARAJULU, MD

Medical Director
Florida Hospital Center for Interventional Endoscopy
Professor of Internal Medicine
University of Central Florida College of Medicine
Orlando, Florida

ELSEVIER
SAUNDERS

1600 John F. Kennedy Blvd.
Ste 1800
Philadelphia, PA 19103-2899

ENDOSONOGRAPHY, Third Edition   ISBN: 978-0-323-22151-1
Copyright © 2015 by Saunders, an imprint of Elsevier Inc.

Library of Congress Cataloging-in-Publication Data

Endosonography (Hawes)
  Endosonography / [edited by] Robert H. Hawes, Paul Fockens, Shyam Varadarajulu.—Third edition.
    p. ; cm.
  Includes bibliographical references and index.
  ISBN 978-0-323-22151-1 (hardcover : alk. paper)
  I. Hawes, Robert H., editor.   II. Fockens, Paul, editor.   III. Varadarajulu, Shyam, editor.   IV. Title.
  [DNLM: 1. Endosonography—methods.   2. Gastrointestinal Neoplasms—ultrasonography.   WN 208]
  RC78.7.E48
  616.07′543—dc23
                                                                        2014008832

Senior Content Strategist: Suzanne Toppy
Content Development Specialist: Lauren Boyle
Publishing Services Manager: Patricia Tannian
Senior Project Manager: Sharon Corell
Senior Book Designer: Ellen Zanolle

Printed in China.

Last digit is the print number: 9   8   7   6   5   4   3   2   1

Working together
to grow libraries in
developing countries

www.elsevier.com • www.bookaid.org

For Chris, Grant, and Taylor
RH
For Marischka, Matthijs, and Kiki
PF
For Deepa, Archith, and Raksha
SV

Contributors

Mohammad Al-Haddad, MD, MSc, FASGE
Associate Professor of Medicine
Division of Gastroenterology and Hepatology
Indiana University School of Medicine
Indianapolis, Indiana

Tiing Leong Ang, MD, FRCP
Chief, Department of Gastroenterology
Changi General Hospital
Adjunct Associate Professor
Yong Loo Lin School of Medicine
National University of Singapore
Singapore

Jouke T. Annema, MD, PhD
Pulmonologist
Professor of Pulmonary Endoscopy
Department of Respiratory Medicine
Academic Medical Center
University of Amsterdam
The Netherlands

William R. Brugge, MD
Professor of Medicine, HMS
Director, Pancreas Biliary Center
Medicine and Gastrointestinal Unit
Massachusetts General Hospital
Boston, Massachusetts

John DeWitt, MD, FACG, FACP, FASGE
Associate Professor of Medicine
Director of Endoscopic Ultrasound
Division of Gastroenterology and Hepatology
Indiana University Medical Center
Indianapolis, Indiana

Mohamad A. Eloubeidi, MD, MHS, FACG, FACP, FASGE, AGAF
Professor of Medicine
Division of Gastroenterology and Hepatology
American University of Beirut
Beirut, Lebanon

Douglas O. Faigel, MD, FACG, FASGE, AGAF
Professor of Medicine
Division of Gastroenterology and Hepatology
Mayo Clinic
Scottsdale, Arizona

Paul Fockens, MD
Professor and Chairman
Department of Gastroenterology and Hepatology
Academic Medical Center
University of Amsterdam
The Netherlands

Larissa L. Fujii, MD
Instructor of Medicine
Division of Gastroenterology and Hepatology
Mayo Clinic College of Medicine
Rochester, Minnesota

Ferga C. Gleeson, MD, FASGE, FACG
Associate Professor of Medicine
Division of Gastroenterology and Hepatology
Mayo Clinic College of Medicine
Rochester, Minnesota

Steve Halligan, MD, FRCP, FRCR
Professor of Gastrointestinal Radiology
Centre for Medical Imaging
Division of Medicine
University College London
London, England

Robert H. Hawes, MD
Medical Director
Florida Hospital Institute for Minimally Invasive Therapy
Professor of Internal Medicine
University of Central Florida College of Medicine
Orlando, Florida

Bronte Holt, MBBS, BMedSc, FRACP
Advanced Endoscopy Fellow
Florida Hospital Center for Interventional Endoscopy
Orlando, Florida

Joo Ha Hwang, MD, PhD
Chief, Gastroenterology Section
Harborview Medical Center
Associate Professor of Medicine
Adjunct Associate Professor of Bioengineering and Radiology
University of Washington
Seattle, Washington

Takao Itoi, MD, PhD, FASGE
Department of Gastroenterology and Hepatology
Tokyo Medical University
Tokyo, Japan

Darshana Jhala, MD, B MUS
Interim Chief of Pathology and Laboratory Medicine
Services
Director of Anatomic Pathology
Department of Pathology and Laboratory Services
Philadelphia VA Medical Center
Associate Professor of Pathology
Department of Pathology and Laboratory Medicine
Hospital of the University of Pennsylvania
Philadelphia, Pennsylvania

Nirag Jhala, MD
Director of Cytopathology
Perelman Center for Advanced Medicine
Surgical Pathologist
GI Subspecialty
Professor of Pathology and Laboratory Medicine
Hospital of the University of Pennsylvania
Philadelphia, Pennsylvania

Abdurrahman Kadayifci, MD
Pancreas Biliary Center
Medicine and Gastrointestinal Unit
Massachusetts General Hospital
Boston, Massachusetts
Professor of Medicine
Division of Gastroenterology
University of Gaziantep
Turkey

Tatiana D. Khokhlova, PhD
Acting Instructor
Department of Medicine
Division of Gastroenterology
University of Washington
Seattle, Washington

Eun Young (Ann) Kim, MD, PhD
Professor of Internal Medicine
Division of Gastroenterology
Catholic University of Daegu School of Medicine
Daegu, Republic of Korea

Michael B. Kimmey, MD
Clinical Professor of Medicine
University of Washington
Franciscan Digestive Care Associates
Tacoma, Washington

Alberto Larghi, MD, PhD
Digestive Endoscopy Unit
Catholic University
Rome, Italy

Anne Marie Lennon, MD, PhD, FRCPI
Director of the Pancreatic Cyst Clinic
Assistant Professor of Medicine
Department of Gastroenterology
The Johns Hopkins Hospital
Baltimore, Maryland

Michael J. Levy, MD
Professor of Medicine
Division of Gastroenterology and Hepatology
Mayo Clinic College of Medicine
Rochester, Minnesota

Leticia Perondi Luz, MD
Assistant Professor of Medicine
Division of Gastroenterology and Hepatology
Indiana University Medical Center
Director, Endoscopic Ultrasound
Roudebush Veterans Affairs Medical Center
Indianapolis, Indiana

John Meenan, MD, PhD, FRCPI, FRCP
Consultant Gastroenterologist
Guy's and St. Thomas' Hospital
London, England

Faris M. Murad, MD
Assistant Professor of Medicine
Division of Gastroenterology and Hepatology
Department of Internal Medicine
Washington University
St. Louis, Missouri

Nikola Panić, MD
Digestive Endoscopy Unit
Catholic University
Rome, Italy

Sarto C. Paquin, MD, FRCPC
Assistant Professor of Medicine
Division of Gastroenterology
Centre Hospitalier de l'Université de Montréal
Hôpital Saint-Luc
Montréal, Canada

Ian D. Penman, BSc, MD, FRCP Edin
Consultant Gastroenterologist
Centre for Liver and Digestive Disorders
Royal Infirmary of Edinburgh
Part-Time Senior Lecturer
University of Edinburgh
Edinburgh, Great Britain

Shajan Peter, MD
Assistant Professor of Medicine,
Gastroenterology/Hepatology
University of Alabama at Birmingham
Birmingham, Alabama

Joseph Romagnuolo, MD, MSc (Epid), FRCPC, FASGE, FACG, AGAF, FACP
Professor of Medicine
Director, Advanced Endoscopy Fellowship (AEF) Program
Director, Clinical Research
Divisions of Gastroenterology and Hepatology
Departments of Medicine, Public Health Sciences
Medical University of South Carolina
Charleston, South Carolina

Thomas Rösch, MD
Professor of Medicine
Department of Interdisciplinary Endoscopy
Hamburg Eppendorf University Hospital
Hamburg, Germany

Adrian Săftoiu, MD, PhD, MSc, FASGE
Visiting Clinical Professor
Gastrointestinal Unit
Copenhagen University Hospital
Herlev, Denmark
Professor of Diagnostic and Therapeutic Techniques in
Gastroenterology
Research Center of Gastroenterology and Hepatology
University of Medicine and Pharmacy
Craiova, Romania

Anand V. Sahai, MD, MSc (Epid), FRCPC
Professor of Medicine
Chief, Division of Gastroenterology
Centre Hospitalier de l'Université de Montréal
Hôpital Saint-Luc
Montréal, Canada

Wajeeh Salah, MD
Advanced Therapeutic Endoscopy Fellow
Department of Gastroenterology and Hepatology
Mayo Clinic
Scottsdale, Arizona

Thomas J. Savides, MD
Professor of Clinical Medicine
Division of Gastroenterology
University of California San Diego
La Jolla, California

Stefan Seewald, MD, FASGE
Professor of Medicine
Center of Gastroenterology
Klinik Hirslanden,
Zurich, Switzerland

Mark Topazian, MD
Professor of Medicine
Division of Gastroenterology and Hepatology
Mayo Clinic College of Medicine
Rochester, Minnesota

Shyam Varadarajulu, MD
Medical Director
Florida Hospital Center for Interventional Endoscopy
Professor of Internal Medicine
University of Central Florida College of Medicine
Orlando, Florida

Peter Vilmann, MD, DSc, HC, FASGE
Professor of Endoscopy at Faculty of Health Sciences
Copenhagen University
GastroUnit, Herlev Hospital
Herlev, Denmark

Charles Vu, MD, FRACP
Consultant Gastroenterologist
Tan Tock Seng Hospital
Singapore

Preface

It is with great pleasure that we present the third edition of *Endosonography*. The first edition was a project that we embraced enthusiastically (albeit somewhat naively, not realizing how much work goes into a first-edition textbook) because we believed there was a need for a comprehensive resource that could serve as a reference for those wishing to learn about endoscopic ultrasonography (EUS). At that time, EUS had matured in Japan, Europe, and the United States and was routinely taught in gastroenterology fellowships. To address the learning needs of the time, we selected expert endosonographers to write chapters that comprehensively covered all clinically relevant topics within the discipline of EUS while at the same time developing "how to" sections and a DVD that provided text and videos to teach the actual technique of EUS. The first edition was extremely well received, and we are grateful that the hard work by the authors and Elsevier has resulted in moving EUS forward.

Time marches on, and medicine is a constantly evolving discipline. Gastrointestinal endoscopy has undergone significant advances, and so has EUS. As we observed the progress in EUS and particularly the explosion of interest in Asia (especially in China and India), Eastern Europe, and the Middle East, it became apparent that it was time to develop a second edition. The publishing landscape had changed, more and more people (young and old) have "gone digital," and we needed to analyze the needs of the current generation of EUS trainees. We also wanted this edition to maintain its relevance for a longer time. We added an on-line component, distributed e-mail updates from the editors, switched from a DVD to putting the videos on-line, and focused more on linear EUS with FNA (fine-needle aspiration) and EUS-guided interventions. Some of these new features were a success and some were not. Whereas putting the videos on-line obviated the need to carry the DVD, our readers' access to the videos was not seamless.

In part to improve access to videos, we developed the EUS App. It is a free download to an iPhone, Android, and iPad. Over 10,000 unique users from 75 countries have downloaded the App, which can now serve as a readily available tool to aid in the mastery of EUS.

It is imperative that we keep *Endosonography* relevant and useful and fill it with the latest trends. It is for this reason that we were advised that it was time to bring out a new edition. We applied the same rigorous due diligence to determining how to improve this product as we did with earlier editions. In this third edition, improvements have included the following:

1. **On-line version:** The field of endosonography is constantly evolving, and the EUS landscape had undergone a great transformation with time. Consequently, published information sometimes becomes outdated and irrelevant. To overcome this, the third edition of *Endosonography* will continue to have an on-line component.

2. **New chapters:** Due to the emerging interest in core biopsies and the use of contrast-enhanced EUS and elastography, we have included additional chapters in these areas authored by international experts.

3. **Frequent e-mail updates from editors:** When one registers online for the electronic version of the textbook, frequent e-mails, which will provide updates on new contributions to the EUS literature, will be sent by the editorial team. The editors will regularly review the most recent literature and will keep readers informed on how these articles influence the practice of endosonography. Thus we strongly encourage all readers to register on-line for the third edition of this textbook.

4. **Interventional EUS:** More comprehensive coverage of EUS includes significant modifications to existing chapters and the introduction of new chapters, especially in the area of interventional EUS. All procedural techniques have been carefully detailed in a stepwise fashion with accompanying videos (narratives included).

5. **"How to" sections:** Learning EUS remains a challenge for the beginner. Hence, the "how to" sections were revised, and clearer correlations were made among the text, illustrations, and videos (with narration). These sections provide a better teaching system for those learning how to perform EUS.

6. **Video component:** The videos for the third edition will continue to be exclusively available on the *Endosonography* Expert Consult website. This will allow frequent updating of the videos and will prevent the problems of losing or damaging the DVD. New videos have been added to coincide with the release of the third edition.

We remain steadfastly committed to advancing EUS through education and training. We feel that the third edition of *Endosonography* can play an important role in enabling one to achieve excellence in EUS and that a more widespread practice of quality endoscopic ultrasound will ultimately improve patient care around the world. It is our sincere hope that *Endosonography* will play a key role in allowing you to master the discipline of EUS.

Robert H. Hawes

Paul Fockens

Shyam Varadarajulu

Acknowledgments

It seems incredible that we are releasing the third edition of *Endosonography*. This event is a cause for me to reflect on my EUS journey. My introduction to EUS occurred in 1985 when I began my advanced endoscopy fellowship year at the Middlesex Hospital in London. Due to Peter Cotton's influence, Olympus placed early prototypes at Middlesex that were actually used by Bill Lees, an outstanding radiologist with incredible knowledge and experience in abdominal ultrasound of the pancreas. I returned to a faculty position at Indiana University (IU) in 1986 and was convinced that EUS would become an important tool in endoscopy. Through the encouragement and support of Glen Lehman, we established an EUS program at IU in 1987. Our program attracted young superstars like Mike Kochman, Amitabh Chak, Yang Chen, Tom Savides, and Frank Gress, to whom I am forever grateful for establishing IU as one of the early meccas for learning EUS. This IU tradition has continued to this day. In 1994, I moved south rejoining Peter Cotton to help establish a new Digestive Disease Center at the Medical University of South Carolina. I was very fortunate that Brenda Hoffman had established an EUS program before I arrived. This began a 17-year relationship with Brenda that saw the MUSC EUS program grow and receive national and international recognition and attracted the best and brightest from around the world to continue the legacy of advanced training in EUS. Manoop Bhutani, Ian Penman, David Williams, Anand Sahai, and Mike Wallace are only a few whose EUS careers began at MUSC as advanced EUS fellows. Perhaps the most important advanced fellow, however, was Shyam Varadarajulu. Shyam spent 2 years at MUSC (ERCP and EUS) and then established himself as one of the brightest stars in EUS during a 9-year tenure at the University of Alabama at Birmingham. I have now been doubly blessed—first, to have Shyam officially join Paul and me as the third editor for *Endosonography* and, second, to have him as my partner, along with Muhammad Hasan, at Florida Hospital Orlando. Our goal and expectation are to continue to play a significant role in advancing EUS around the world. I hope that our latest edition of *Endosonography* will be a useful resource to help readers master the art of EUS. I am incredibly grateful to all the nurses, GI fellows, advanced fellows, and faculty colleagues throughout my career who have contributed so significantly to teaching EUS and caring for our patients. I have been truly blessed to have the opportunity to work with such dedicated and talented people, and I am very grateful. This book is a reflection of a strong commitment of many to care for patients while advancing EUS.

Robert H. Hawes

This third edition is dedicated to my EUS partners at the Academic Medical Center of the University of Amsterdam: Jeanin van Hooft, Sheila Krishnadath, Barbara Bastiaansen, Manon van der Vlugt, and Jacques Bergman. Together we evaluate approximately 1000 patients for EUS per year, conduct EUS-related research, and train our advanced endoscopy fellows, who increasingly appreciate the value of EUS in combination with ERCP for tertiary pancreatobiliary care. It has been our pleasure to receive many visitors from all over the world who spend anywhere from 2 hours to 2 months at the Academic Medical Center observing EUS procedures. And finally, over the past 17 years we have organized an annual EUS conference in Amsterdam in June, which attracts between 150 and 200 participants, several of whom are avid readers of our textbook.

I am grateful to our nursing staff for providing expert support for all our procedures. We are also excellently supported by our anesthesiology team, who provide deep sedation for our EUS patients, especially when these examinations are interventional. Finally, I am deeply grateful to my three pillars in life: my wife, Marischka, and my two children, Matthijs and Kiki, who are now in medical school. The future is bright and I am curious to see where it will take us.

Paul Fockens

I wish to thank my endoscopy partners Robert Hawes and Muhammad Hasan at Florida Hospital for their unstinting support and enthusiasm toward this project. I am indebted to my pathologist Shantel Hébert-Magee, research coordinator Amy Logue, and nurse manager Rochelle Nogamos for their support and infinite patience. These are the core members of my team and a vital part of my academic career at Florida Hospital. I am also very thankful to my nursing and technical staff for supporting the nearly 2000 EUS procedures that are performed annually at Florida Hospital. They have helped me tremendously with recording videos for this textbook and efficiently conducting my clinical trials. I owe a special thanks to my former colleagues at the University of Alabama at Birmingham, Mel Wilcox, Shajan Peter, and Ji Bang, for their perennial encouragement and support of my academic and personal endeavors.

Many visitors from around the world, and particularly from my home country of India, have visited Florida Hospital to learn EUS. Their presence at our center is a great source of inspiration for me and I hope to have the pleasure of seeing some of the *Endosonography* readers in our unit in the near future.

I wish to thank Rob and Paul for the once-in-a-lifetime opportunity to be a co-editor of the third edition of this textbook. They gave me a free hand and offered all the support I needed to make this venture a success. I really wish and hope that in my second birth they would remain my mentors!

My parents and family are my motivation to whom I owe my existence and every success in life—thank you to Mom, Dad, Deepa, Archith, and Raksha.

Shyam Varadarajulu

Contents

Endosonography

SECTION I

Basics of EUS

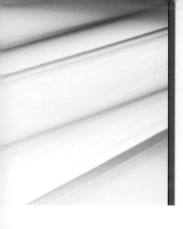

1

Principles of Ultrasound

Joo Ha Hwang • Tatiana D. Khokhlova • Michael B. Kimmey

Key Points

- Ultrasound is mechanical energy in the form of vibrations that propagate through a medium such as tissue.
- Ultrasound interacts with tissue by undergoing absorption, reflection, refraction, and scattering and produces an image representative of tissue structure.
- Imaging artifacts can be recognized and understood based on a knowledge of the principles of ultrasound.

A basic understanding of the principles of ultrasound is requisite for an endosonographer's understanding of how to obtain and accurately interpret ultrasound images. In this chapter, the basic principles of ultrasound physics and instrumentation are presented, followed by illustrations of how these principles are applied to ultrasound imaging and Doppler ultrasound and explanations of some common artifacts seen on endosonography. Knowledge of the basic principles of ultrasound will help the endosonographer to understand the capabilities of ultrasound imaging, as well as its limitations.

Basic Ultrasound Physics

Sound is mechanical energy in the form of vibrations that propagate through a medium such as air, water, or tissue.[1] The frequency of audible sound ranges from 20 to 20,000 Hz (cycles per second). Ultrasound involves a frequency spectrum that is greater than 20,000 Hz. Medical applications use frequencies in the range of 1,000,000 to 50,000,000 Hz (1 to 50 MHz). The propagation of ultrasound results from the displacement and oscillation of molecules from their average position and the subsequent displacement and oscillations of molecules along the direction of propagation of the ultrasound wave.

Ultrasound waves can be described using the common properties of waves. Figure 1-1 is an illustration of a sinusoidal wave with the pressure amplitude along the y-axis and the time or distance along the x-axis. Figure 1-1 is referred to in the following sections to introduce the basic properties of waves.

Wavelength, Frequency, and Velocity

The *wavelength* is the distance in the propagating medium that includes one complete cycle (see Figure 1-1). The wavelength (λ) is dependent on the frequency (f) of the oscillations and the velocity (c) of propagation in the medium. The relationship of wavelength, frequency, and velocity is given in Equation 1.1.

$$c = f\lambda \tag{1.1}$$

The *frequency* of a wave is the number of oscillations per unit of time. Typically in ultrasound, this is stated in terms of cycles per second or Hertz (1 c/s = 1 Hz). The *period* of a wave (τ) is the inverse of the frequency and represents the time required to complete one cycle. The relationship between frequency and period is given in Equation 1.2.

$$c = \frac{1}{\tau} \tag{1.2}$$

The *velocity* of propagation depends on the physical properties of the medium in which the wave is propagating. The primary physical properties governing the velocity of propagation are the density and compressibility of the medium.

Density, Compressibility, and Bulk Modulus

The *density* (ρ) of a medium is the mass per unit volume of that medium (kg/m^3 in SI units). The *compressibility* (K) of a medium is a property that reflects the relationship between the fractional decrease in volume and the pressure applied to a medium. For example, air has high compressibility (a small amount of pressure applied to a volume of air will result in a large fractional decrease in volume), whereas bone has relatively low compressibility (a large amount of pressure applied to a volume of bone will result in a small fractional decrease in volume). Finally, the *bulk modulus* (β), which is the inverse of the compressibility, is the negative ratio of pressure applied to a medium and the fractional change in volume of the medium and reflects the stiffness of the medium.

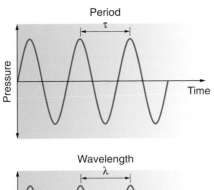

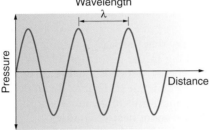

FIGURE 1-1 Sinusoidal wave depicted on the time axis and distance axis. The time to complete one cycle is the period (τ). The distance to complete one cycle is the wavelength (λ).

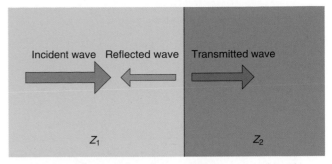

FIGURE 1-2 Reflection of an ultrasound wave at normal incidence to an interface between two media with different acoustic impedances (Z).

The acoustic velocity (c) of a medium can be determined once the density (ρ) and the compressibility (K), or bulk modulus (β), are known. Equation 1.3 demonstrates the relationship of the three physical properties.

Density, compressibility, and bulk modulus are not independent of one another. Typically, as density increases, compressibility decreases and bulk modulus increases. However, compressibility and bulk modulus typically vary more rapidly than does density, and they dominate in Equation 1.3.

$$c = \frac{1}{\sqrt{K\rho}} = \frac{\sqrt{\beta}}{\sqrt{\rho}} \qquad (1.3)$$

The acoustic velocity in different media can be determined by applying the equations to practice. For example, water at 30°C has a density of 996 kg/m³ and a bulk modulus of 2.27×10^9 N/m².[2] Inserting these values into Equation 1.3 yields an acoustic velocity of 1509 m/s in water. Values for density and bulk modulus have been characterized extensively and can be found in the literature.[2] A summary of relevant tissue properties is given in Table 1-1. The acoustic velocity is not dependent on the frequency of the propagating wave (i.e., acoustic waves of different frequencies all propagate with the same acoustic velocity within the same medium).[3]

Ultrasound Interactions in Tissue

Ultrasound imaging of tissue is achieved by transmitting short pulses of ultrasound energy into tissue and receiving reflected signals. The reflected signals that return to the transducer represent the interactions of a propagating ultrasound wave with tissue. A propagating ultrasound wave can interact with tissue, and the results are *reflection*, *refraction*, *scattering*, and *absorption*.

Reflection

Specular reflections of ultrasound occur at relative large interfaces (greater than one wavelength) between two media of differing acoustical impedances. At this point, it is important to introduce the concept of *acoustic impedance*. The acoustic impedance (Z) of a medium represents the resistance to sound propagating through the medium and is the product of the *density* (ρ) and the *velocity* (c):

$$Z = \rho c \qquad (1.4)$$

Sound will continue to propagate through a medium until an interface is reached where the acoustic impedance of the medium in which the sound is propagating differs from the medium that it encounters. At an interface where an acoustic impedance difference is encountered, a proportion of the ultrasound wave will be reflected back toward the transducer, and the rest will be transmitted into the second medium. The simplest case of reflection and transmission occurs when the propagating ultrasound wave is perpendicular (90 degrees) to the interface (Figure 1-2). In this case, the percentage of the incident beam that is reflected is as follows:

$$\%\mathrm{reflected} = \left(\frac{Z_2 - Z_1}{Z_2 + Z_1}\right)^2 \times 100 \qquad (1.5)$$

The percentage of the incident beam that is transmitted is as follows:

$$\%\mathrm{transmitted} = 100 - \%\mathrm{reflected} \qquad (1.6)$$

Refraction

When the incident beam arrives at the interface at an angle other than 90 degrees, the transmitted beam path diverges from the incident beam path because of refraction

TABLE 1-1

PHYSICAL PROPERTIES OF TISSUE

Tissue or Fluid	Density (kg/m³)	Bulk Modulus (×10⁹ N/m²)	Acoustic Velocity (m/s)
Water (30°C)	996	2.27	1509
Blood	1050-1075	2.65	1590
Pancreas (pig)	1040-1050	2.63	1591
Liver	1050-1070	2.62	1578
Bone, cortical	1063-2017	28.13	3760

Adapted from Duck FA. Physical Properties of Tissue. *London: Academic Press; 1990.*

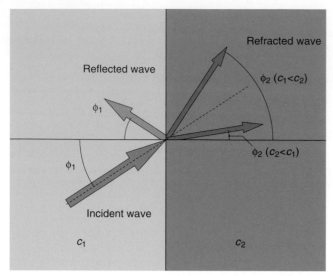

FIGURE 1-3 Refraction and reflection of an incident wave that is not normal to the interface between media with different acoustic velocities (*c*). The angle of reflection is identical to the angle of incidence. The angle of the refracted wave is dependent on the acoustic velocities of the two media and can be determined by applying Snell's law (see text).

(Figure 1-3). The angle at which the transmitted beam propagates is determined by Snell's law:

$$\frac{\sin \varphi_1}{\sin \varphi_2} = \frac{c_1}{c_2} \qquad (1.7)$$

The angle of *refraction* is determined by the *acoustic velocities* in the incident (c_1) and transmitted (c_2) media. There are three possible scenarios for a refracted beam, depending on the relative speeds of sound between the two media: (1) if $c_1 > c_2$, the angle of refraction will be bent toward normal ($\phi_1 > \phi_2$); (2) if $c_1 = c_2$, the angle of refraction will be identical to the angle of incidence, and the beam will continue to propagate without diverging from its path; (3) if $c_1 < c_2$, the angle of refraction will be bent away from normal ($\phi_1 < \phi_2$). Refraction of the ultrasound beam can lead to imaging artifacts that are discussed later in the chapter.

Scattering

Scattering, also termed *nonspecular reflection*, occurs when a propagating ultrasound wave interacts with different components in tissue that are smaller than the wavelength and have different impedance values than the propagating medium.[4] Examples of scatterers in tissue include individual cells, fat globules, and collagen. When an ultrasound wave interacts with a scatterer, only a small portion of the acoustic intensity that reflects off of the scatterer is reflected back to the transducer (Figure 1-4). In addition, a signal that has undergone scattering by a single scatterer will usually undergo multiple scattering events before returning to the transducer. Scattering occurs in heterogeneous media, such as tissue, and is responsible for the different echotextures of organs such as the liver, pancreas, and spleen. Tissue containing fat or collagen scatters ultrasound to a greater degree than do other tissues, and this is why lipomas and the submucosal layer of the gastrointestinal tract appear hyperechoic (bright) on ultrasound imaging.[4]

Multiple reflections from nonspecular reflectors within the tissue returning to the transducer result in a characteristic acoustic speckle pattern, or echotexture, for that tissue.[4] Because speckle originates from multiple reflections and does not represent the actual location of a structure, moving the transducer will change the location of the speckle echoes while maintaining a similar speckle pattern. In addition, the noise resulting from acoustic speckle increases with increasing depth as a result of the greater number of signals that have undergone multiple reflections from nonspecular reflectors returning to the transducer.

Absorption

Ultrasound energy that propagates through a medium can be absorbed, resulting in the generation of heat. The *absorption* of ultrasound energy depends on tissue properties and is highly frequency dependent. Higher frequencies cause more tissue vibration and result in greater absorption of the ultrasound energy and more heat generation.

Ultrasound Intensity

The *intensity* of the ultrasound signal is a parameter that describes the power of the ultrasound signal over a cross-sectional area. As ultrasound waves propagate through tissue, the intensity of the wave becomes attenuated. Attenuation is the result of effects of both scattering and absorption of the ultrasound wave.[1] The *attenuation coefficient* (*a*) is a function of frequency that can be determined experimentally, and it increases with increasing frequency. The frequency of the ultrasound pulse affects both the depth of penetration of the

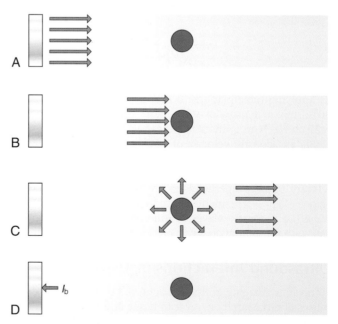

FIGURE 1-4 Schematic representation of single scattering. Scattering occurs from an interface that is smaller than the wavelength of the propagating ultrasound signal. The transducer is responsible for sending and receiving the signal. I_b is the back-scattered intensity that will propagate back to the transducer. **A**, The ultrasound signal is transmitted by the transducer and propagates toward the scatterer. **B**, The pulse reaches the scatterer. **C**, The incident acoustic intensity is scattered in different directions. **D**, The back-scattered energy received by the transducer is only a small fraction of the incident acoustic intensity that is scattered.

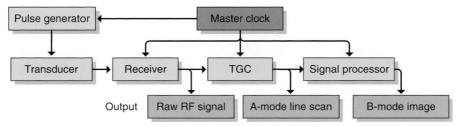

FIGURE 1-5 Ultrasound instrumentation schematic. The overall system is synchronized by a master clock. A pulse generator sends an electrical signal to the transducer, and the result is a transmitted ultrasound pulse. The transducer then receives the back-reflected signal resulting from the transmitted pulse. This signal is then passed on to the receiver, which amplifies the entire signal. The output from the receiver is the raw radiofrequency (RF) signal. The signal can then undergo time gain compensation (TGC), and the subsequent output will be the A-mode line scan. After TGC, the signal is further processed, including demodulation and registration, to yield a B-mode image.

pulse and the obtainable resolution. In general, as the frequency is increased, the depth of penetration decreases, owing to attenuation of the ultrasound intensity, and axial resolution improves, as discussed later in this chapter.

The intensity of the propagating ultrasound energy decreases exponentially as a function of depth and is given by the following equation:

$$I_x = I_0 e^{-2ax} \qquad (1.8)$$

where I_0 is the initial intensity of the ultrasound pulse and I_x is the intensity of the ultrasound pulse after it has passed a distance x through tissue with an attenuation coefficient a in Neper/cm (Np/cm). As the attenuation coefficient increases with frequency, intensity also decreases exponentially as frequency increases. This equation partially explains the limitation on the depth of imaging because the returning ultrasound pulse from the tissue must be of sufficient intensity to be detected by the ultrasound transducer.

Basics of Ultrasound Instrumentation

The key component of an ultrasound system is the transducer. A *transducer* is a device that converts one form of energy to another. In the case of ultrasound transducers, electrical energy is converted to mechanical energy, resulting in the transmission of an ultrasound pulse. When an ultrasound signal is then received by the ultrasound transducer, the received mechanical signal is converted back to an electrical signal that is then processed and digitized by the ultrasound processor to yield a real-time image of the tissue being interrogated by the ultrasound transducer (Figure 1-5).

Transducers

The active element of an ultrasound transducer, responsible for generating and receiving acoustic signals, is made typically from a piezoelectric ceramic. Piezoelectric ceramics are composed of polar crystals that are aligned in a particular orientation such that when an electric field is applied, the material changes shape.[3] Therefore if an alternating electrical field is applied to the material at a particular frequency, the material will vibrate mechanically at that frequency, similar to an audio speaker. In addition, if the piezoelectric material is deformed by sufficient mechanical pressure (e.g., a reflected ultrasound wave), a detectable voltage will be measured across the

material with a magnitude proportional to the applied pressure. The magnitude of the voltage then determines how brightly that signal is represented in B-mode imaging (this is explained in the later section on B-mode imaging).

Single-Element Transducers

The single-element transducer represents the most basic form of ultrasound transducer and the easiest to understand, owing to its geometric symmetry. Therefore single-element disk transducers are explained in some detail, to illustrate the basic principles of ultrasound transducers. Single-element transducers can be of any shape or size, and they can be focused or unfocused. Figure 1-6 illustrates variations of a single-element disk transducer.

The beam width originating from a flat circular disk transducer in a nonattenuating medium is shown in Figure 1-7. Beam width is an important concept to understand because this parameter determines the lateral resolution (further discussed in the later section on imaging principles). The two distinct regions of the ultrasound field are termed the *near-field* and the *far-field*. The near-field/far-field transition is the location where the flat circular disk transducer has a natural focus, with the focal diameter equal to one-half of the diameter (or equal to the radius) of the transducer. The distance from the transducer at which this occurs is given by the following equation:

$$D = \frac{r^2}{\lambda} \qquad (1.9)$$

where D is the near-field/far-field transition distance or focal length, r is the radius of the transducer, and λ is the

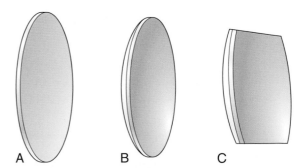

FIGURE 1-6 Potential configurations of single-element transducers. **A,** Flat circular disk. **B,** Spherically curved disk. **C,** Truncated, spherically curved disk.

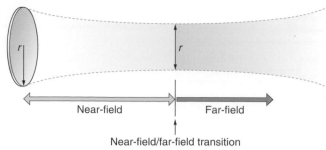

FIGURE 1-7 Single-element unfocused disk transducer. In a nonattenuating medium, an unfocused transducer has a self-focusing effect with the diameter of the ultrasound beam at the focus equal to the radius of the transducer (*r*). The location of the beam waist occurs at the near-field/far-field transition.

wavelength of ultrasound in the propagating medium. Equation 1.9 demonstrates that, as the radius of the transducer decreases, the focal length is reduced if the frequency remains constant. In addition, for a constant radius, increasing the wavelength (i.e., decreasing the frequency) also reduces the focal length. However, in attenuating media such as tissue, this self-focusing effect is not seen, and the beam width in the near-field is approximately equal to the diameter of the transducer (Figure 1-8). The beam width then rapidly diverges in the far-field.

Focusing. A single-element transducer can be focused by fabricating the transducer with a concave curvature (spherically curved) or by placing a lens over a flat disk transducer. Focusing is used to improve the lateral resolution and results in a narrow beam width at the focal length (distance from the transducer to the location of the beam width that is most narrow). However, the degree of focusing affects the depth of focus (the range where the image is in focus) and the focal length. For weak focusing, the focal length is long, as is the depth of focus. Conversely, for a beam that is highly focused, the focal length is short, as is the depth of focus (Figure 1-9).

Arrays. Multiple single-element transducers can be combined in several different configurations. The linear array configuration is the most widely employed clinically. The array is composed of multiple identical crystals that are controlled electronically (Figure 1-10). They can be fired individually in sequence or in groups, depending on the imaging algorithm.

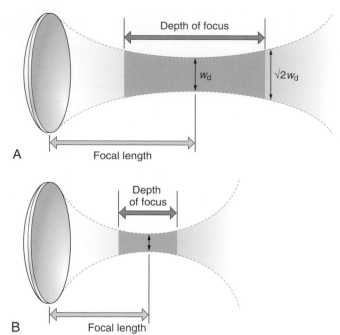

FIGURE 1-9 Effect of focusing. Focusing increases lateral resolution by decreasing the beam waist in the focal region *(highlighted in blue)*. The depth of focus is the distance between where the diameter of the beam is equal to $\sqrt{2}w_d$, where w_d is the diameter of the beam at the waist or focus. The degree of focusing influences the focal length, as well as the depth of focus. This figure compares two transducers of equal diameters with different degrees of focusing. The transducer in (**A**) exhibits weak focusing, whereas that in (**B**) exhibits strong focusing. The diameter of the waist at the focus is narrower with strong focusing, and this leads to improved lateral resolution in the focal region. However, the trade-off is a decrease in the depth of focus with rapid divergence of the beam beyond the focus. In addition, the focal length is much shorter (i.e., the focus is closer to the transducer) for the highly focused transducer.

This configuration allows for electronic focusing at different depths based on the timing of the excitation of the individual transducer crystals.

Processors

Figure 1-5 is a block diagram of the components of an ultrasound imaging system. The main components are the ultrasound transducer, processor, and display. Within the processor

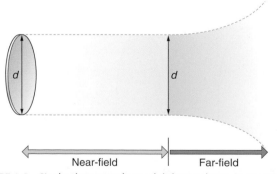

FIGURE 1-8 Single-element unfocused disk transducer. In an attenuating medium, the beam width of an unfocused transducer is approximately equal to the diameter of the transducer (*d*) until the near-field/far-field transition. The beam then rapidly diverges in the far-field.

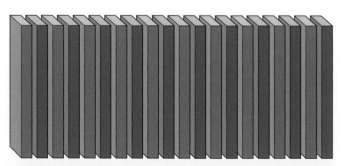

FIGURE 1-10 Configuration of a linear array transducer. This configuration consists of several rectangular elements, which are controlled individually. The sequence and timing of excitation of each individual element dictate the beam pattern that is transmitted from the array.

are electronic components that are responsible for controlling the excitation of the transducer, amplification of the received signal, time gain compensation (TGC), and signal processing resulting in an output signal to the display.

Transmit/Receive

As described earlier, the ultrasound transducer is responsible for transmitting the ultrasound pulse and receiving reflected pulses. The time interval between the transmission of a pulse and the detection of the reflected pulse gives information about the distance from the interface or nonspecular reflector where the reflection occurred. The distance, or depth, of the interface from the transducer is given by the following equation:

$$D = \frac{v \times t}{2} \qquad (1.10)$$

where D is the distance from the transducer, v is the velocity of ultrasound in tissue (assumed to be uniform [1540 m/s] by most ultrasound processors), and t is the time between the transmitted and received pulses. The product of v and t is divided by 2 because the pulse travels twice the distance (to the reflector and back). In addition, the strength of the received signal gives information regarding the impedance mismatch at the interface where the reflection occurred.

System Gain and Time Gain Compensation

The amplification of the output can be adjusted by the operator in two ways. One is to increase the overall gain of the system, an approach that uniformly increases the amplitude of all echoes received by the transducer. This can improve the detection of weak echoes; however, it generally comes at the expense of overall resolution.

TGC is used to compensate for the decreased intensity of echoes that originate from structures further from the transducer. As described earlier, the intensity of the ultrasound signal diminishes exponentially with distance (see Equation 1.8); therefore reflections from interfaces further from the transducer have significantly decreased intensities. The TGC function of ultrasound processors allows selective amplification of echoes from deeper structures. Current EUS processors allow the operator to vary the gain by depth.

Signal Processor

After TGC of the signal has occurred, additional signal processing is performed. The algorithms for signal processing performed differ among ultrasound processors and are closely held proprietary information. In general, some form of demodulation of the radiofrequency (RF) signal is performed to obtain an envelope of the RF signal, which is used to produce a B-mode image. In addition, processing can include threshold suppression to eliminate signals that are below an operator-specified threshold. Leading edge detection, peak detection, and differentiation are additional methods that can be employed by processors to improve image quality.[1]

Imaging Principles

Now that the basic principles of ultrasound physics and instrumentation have been introduced, an overview of imaging principles can be described.

Resolution

In ultrasound imaging, three different aspects of resolution must be considered: axial, lateral, and elevation or azimuthal resolution.

Axial Resolution

Axial resolution refers to the smallest separation distance between two objects along the beam path that can be detected by the imaging system. Axial resolution is determined by the ultrasound frequency and the spatial pulse length (SPL) of the transmitted ultrasound pulse.[5] The SPL can be determined by the following equation:

$$SPL = \frac{c}{f} \times n \qquad (1.11)$$

where c is the speed of sound in tissue, f is the center frequency of the transmitted ultrasound pulse, and n is the number of cycles per pulse (typically four to seven cycles). The limit of axial resolution is equal to SPL/2. This equation demonstrates why using higher frequencies results in greater axial resolution (assuming that pulses have the same number of cycles per pulse). To illustrate this concept, two different ultrasound pulses with qualitatively different center frequencies and SPL are shown in Figure 1-11. Axial resolution is the most important property in imaging the layered structures of the gastrointestinal tract wall.

Lateral Resolution

The *lateral resolution* of an imaging system represents the ability to discriminate between two points that are in a plane perpendicular to the ultrasound beam. The beam width of the transducer determines the achievable lateral resolution and is a function of transducer size, shape, frequency, and focusing. Figure 1-12 illustrates the concept of lateral resolution.

Elevation Resolution

Elevation, or *azimuthal, resolution* relates to the fact that, although the image displayed is two dimensional, the actual interrogated plane has a thickness associated with it. The factors governing elevation resolution are similar to those for lateral resolution. In fact, the elevation resolution for a focused, circular disk transducer (as used in the Olympus GF-UM series) is the same as for lateral resolution because of its circular symmetry. For the linear array transducers, the elevation resolution is determined by the beam width characteristics along the plane of imaging.

A-Mode Scanning

A-mode, or amplitude mode, scanning is obtained by the transmit/receive process described previously with an output yielding an RF line scan of the echoes detected along the axis of a stationary transducer after a pulse of ultrasound has been transmitted. The received signal by the transducer is amplified, yielding the A-mode signal (Figure 1-13). This form of scanning, rarely used by the clinician, is the basis for all other modes of scanning including B-mode scanning. In addition, RF signal analysis is an important aspect of research in the area of advanced imaging techniques.

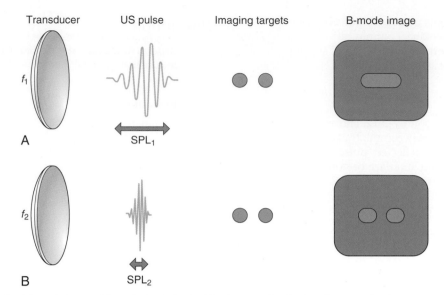

FIGURE 1-11   Concept of axial resolution. Axial resolution is limited by the spatial pulse length (SPL). This figure compares the axial resolution of two different ultrasound pulses with different frequencies ($f_1 < f_2$) and identical pulse lengths; therefore $SPL_1 > SPL_2$. In **A**, the distance between the imaging targets is less than $SPL_1/2$, thus resulting in a B-mode image that is not able resolve the two discrete targets. In **B**, the distance between the imaging targets is greater than $SPL_2/2$, thus resulting in the ability to resolve the two discrete targets.

B-Mode Imaging

B-mode, or brightness mode, scanning results in additional signal processing and movement of the transducer either mechanically or electronically. A B-mode image is created by processing a series of A-mode signals (see Figure 1-13). For each line in the B-mode image (corresponding to a single A-mode line scan), the digitized RF signal is demodulated, yielding an envelope of the RF signal. The amplitude of the demodulated signal is then used to determine the brightness of the dot corresponding to its location in the B-mode image. As the axis of the transducer output is translated (either mechanically or electronically), additional A-mode signals are obtained and processed, eventually yielding a compound B-mode image (see Figure 1-13). EUS imaging systems generate a compound B-mode image.

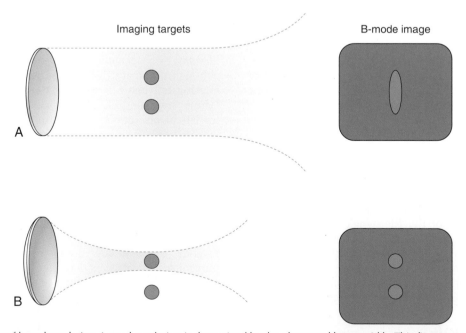

FIGURE 1-12   Concept of lateral resolution. Lateral resolution is determined by the ultrasound beam width. This figure compares the lateral resolution of an unfocused transducer (**A**) and a focused transducer (**B**) with apertures of the same diameter. The beam width of the unfocused transducer in (**A**) cannot resolve the two imaging targets; therefore the two targets are displayed as one target on B-mode imaging. The beam width of the focused transducer in (**B**) is sufficiently narrow to resolve the two imaging targets. If the imaging targets were beyond the focus of the transducer in (**B**), the broadened beam width would not be able to resolve the two objects, and the B-mode image would be similar to that in (**A**).

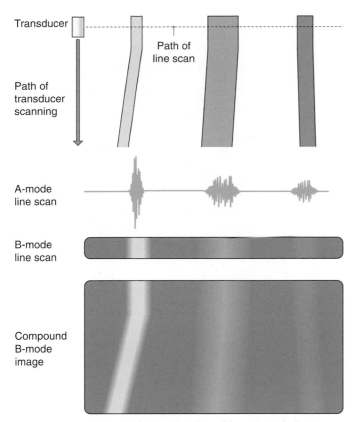

FIGURE 1-13 Conceptual representation of how A-mode line scans, B-mode line scans, and compound B-mode images are obtained. The transducer output is directed into the tissue determining the path of the line scan. An A-mode line scan is obtained after amplification of the received signals by the transducer. The B-mode line scan is obtained after demodulation and additional signal processing of the A-mode signal. The compound B-mode image is produced by obtaining multiple line scans by translating the path of the line scan. This can be accomplished either by mechanically scanning the transducer or by electronically steering a linear array transducer.

Doppler

The Doppler effect is used in ultrasound applications to identify objects that are in motion relative to the transducer. In biologic applications, the reflective objects in motion are red blood cells. Doppler ultrasound is used in endoscopic ultrasonography (EUS) examinations to identify blood flow in vessels. The fundamental basis for the Doppler effect in ultrasound is that an object in motion relative to the source transducer will reflect an ultrasound wave at a different frequency relative to the frequency transmitted by the source transducer; this is termed the *Doppler shift*. The difference between the transmitted frequency and the shifted frequency is dictated by the velocity (*v*) of the object in motion relative to the transducer. The Doppler shift can be determined by the following equation:

$$f_D = \frac{2vf_t \cos\theta}{c} \qquad (1.12)$$

where f_D is the Doppler shift frequency, which is the difference between the transmitted and reflected frequencies; v is the velocity of the object in motion (red blood cells); f_t is the transmitted frequency; θ is the angle at which the object in

motion is traveling relative to the direction of the source beam (Figure 1-14); and *c* is the speed of sound in tissue (1540 m/s). This equation illustrates why a Doppler shift is not detected if the transducer is aimed perpendicular (90 degrees) to a blood vessel. At an angle of 90 degrees, Equation 1.12 demonstrates that $f_D = 0$, as cos 90 degrees = 0. Therefore interrogation of a blood vessel should be at an angle other than 90 degrees, with the greatest Doppler shift detected when the object in motion is moving along the axis of the transmitted ultrasound wave (cos 0 degrees = 1 and cos 180 degrees = −1).

The different implementations of Doppler ultrasound include continuous-wave, pulsed-wave, color, and power Doppler.

Continuous-Wave Doppler

Continuous-wave Doppler represents the simplest configuration of Doppler ultrasound and requires two different transducers: a transmitting and a receiving transducer. The transmitting transducer produces a continuous output of ultrasound at a fixed frequency. The receiving transducer then receives the continuous signal. The transmitted and received signals are added, resulting in a waveform that contains a beat frequency that is equivalent to the Doppler shift frequency. Continuous-wave Doppler does not give any information regarding the depth at which the motion causing the Doppler shift is occurring.

Pulsed-Wave Doppler

Pulsed-wave Doppler was developed to obtain depth information regarding the location of the motion causing the Doppler shift. In addition, a pulsed-wave Doppler system required only a single transducer to transmit and receive ultrasound signals. The pulse length used for pulsed-wave Doppler is substantially longer than pulses used for imaging. Using electronic gating to time the interval between transmitting and receiving a pulse, this method allows the operator to interrogate a specific location along the axis of the transmitted ultrasound beam for motion. The output from pulsed-wave Doppler is usually in the form of an audible signal. The combination of pulsed-wave Doppler with B-mode imaging, termed *duplex scanning*, allows the operator to interrogate a specific location within a B-mode image.

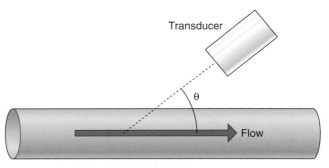

FIGURE 1-14 Conceptual image of Doppler measurements. The angle θ determines the strength of the Doppler signal. If θ is 90 degrees, then no Doppler signal can be detected.

Color Doppler

Color Doppler is a method of visually detecting motion or blood flow using a color map that is incorporated into a standard B-mode image. The principles of color Doppler are similar to those of pulsed-wave Doppler. However, a larger region can be interrogated, and detected blood flow is assigned a color, typically blue or red, depending on whether the flow is moving toward or away from the transducer. Frequency shifts are estimated at each point at which motion is detected within an interrogated region, thus yielding information on direction of motion and velocity. Shades of blue or red are used to reflect the relative velocities of the blood flow. All stationary objects are represented on a gray scale, as in B-mode imaging. The benefit of color Doppler is that information on the direction and relative velocity of blood flow can be obtained. Color Doppler is limited by its dependence on the relative angle of the transducer to the blood flow.

Power Doppler

Power Doppler is the most sensitive Doppler method for detecting blood flow. Again, the basis for power Doppler is similar to that for pulsed-wave and color Doppler. However, in processing the Doppler signal, instead of estimating the frequency shift as in color Doppler, the integral of the power spectrum of the Doppler signal is estimated. This method essentially determines the strength of the Doppler signal and discards any information on velocity or direction of motion. This method is the most sensitive for detecting blood flow and should be used to identify blood vessels when information on direction of flow and velocity is not needed.

Imaging Artifacts

Image artifacts are findings on ultrasound imaging that do not accurately represent the tissue being interrogated. An understanding of the principles of ultrasound can be used to explain image artifacts. It is important to identify and to understand the basis for image artifacts, to interpret ultrasound images correctly. Some common ultrasound imaging artifacts are discussed.

Reverberation

Reverberations occur when a single transmitted pulse undergoes multiple reflections from a strong reflector over the time of a single line scan. The transmitted pulse first is reflected by the reflector back to the transducer. The reflected pulse then is reflected off the transducer back toward the reflector. This sequence is repeated, and each time a reflection returns to the transducer a signal is generated, until the signal has been attenuated to the point where it is not detected by the transducer or the line scan has been completed (Figure 1-15). The duration of the line scan depends on the depth of imaging. A reverberation artifact can be identified by the equal spacing between hyperechoic (bright) bands, with decreasing intensity as the distance from the transducer increases. Reverberation artifact from a mechanical radial scanning ultrasound probe is demonstrated in Figure 1-16. This particular reverberation artifact is also called the *ring artifact*.[6] The reflections are from the housing of the ultrasound transducer.

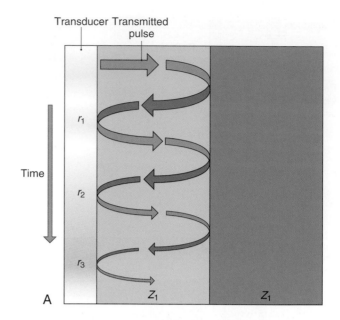

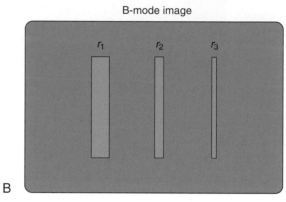

FIGURE 1-15   Reverberation artifacts result from strong reflections of a transmitted pulse from an interface with a large impedance mismatch (e.g., air-water interface). **A,** Depiction of how a transmitted signal is reflected by an interface with a large impedance mismatch. The reflected signal is detected by the transducer and is redirected back into the medium. This sequence can be repeated multiple times, depending on the depth of imaging. The reflected signal is progressively attenuated. **B,** The corresponding B-mode image from the reverberation depicted in (**A**). The reflected signals (r_1, r_2, and r_3) are spaced equally.

Reverberation artifacts are also seen with air-water interfaces, such as bubbles (Figure 1-17).

Reflection (Mirror Image)

The *reflection,* or *mirror image, artifact* occurs when imaging near an air-water interface such as a lumen filled partially with water.[7] In this situation, transmitted ultrasound pulses reflect off the air-water interface (because of the significant impedance mismatch). The result is the creation of multiple reflections that are eventually received by the transducer and lead to production of a mirror image opposite the air-water interface (Figures 1-18 and 1-19). This artifact is easily identified and can be avoided by removing air and adding more water into the lumen.

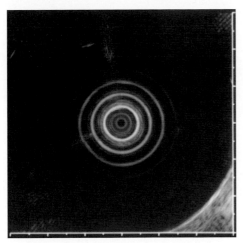

FIGURE 1-16 EUS image of reverberation artifact resulting from multiple reflections from the transducer housing. The concentric rings are equally spaced, with the intensity of the rings decreasing as the distance from the transducer increases.

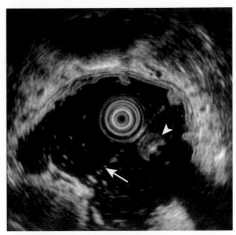

FIGURE 1-18 Reflection or mirror image artifact. A mirror image of the transducer *(arrowhead)* and gastric wall is produced by the reflection of the ultrasound signal from the interface between water and air *(arrow)* within the gastric lumen.

Acoustic Shadowing

Acoustic shadowing is a form of a reflection artifact that occurs when a large impedance mismatch is encountered. When such a mismatch is encountered, a majority of the transmitted pulse is reflected with minimal transmission. This results in a hyperechoic signal at the interface with no echo signal detected beyond the interface, thus producing a shadow effect. This finding is useful in diagnosing calcifications in the pancreas (Figure 1-20) and gallstones in the gallbladder (Figure 1-21).

Acoustic shadowing can also result from refraction occurring at a boundary between tissues with different acoustic velocities, especially if the boundary is curved (e.g., tumor or cyst). As discussed earlier, refraction of an ultrasound beam occurs when the angle of incidence is not normal to the boundary between tissues with different acoustic velocities,

with resulting bending of the ultrasound beam. Because the ultrasound beam is redirected at this boundary, some regions of the tissue are not interrogated by the ultrasound beam, and the result is an acoustic shadow (Figure 1-22).[8]

Through Transmission

Through transmission is the enhancement of a structure beyond a fluid-filled structure such as a cyst. The structure beyond a fluid-filled structure demonstrates increased enhancement because the intensity of transmitted ultrasound undergoes less attenuation as it propagates through the cyst and as the reflected signal returns to the transducer. This finding is useful in diagnosing fluid-filled structures such as a cyst or blood vessel (Figure 1-23).

Tangential Scanning

If the thickness of a structure is being measured, it is important that the ultrasound beam is perpendicular to the structure. If the transducer is at an angle other than 90 degrees to the structure, the thickness will be overestimated.[9] This is particularly important when assessing the thickness of the layers of the gastrointestinal (GI) tract wall and in staging tumors of the GI tract. On radial scanning examination of the GI tract, this artifact can be identified because the thicknesses of the wall layers will not be uniform throughout the image (Figure 1-24). When staging tumors involving the GI tract wall, tangential imaging can result in overstaging of the tumor. To avoid this artifact, the endoscope tip should be maneuvered to maintain the proper orientation such that the plane of imaging is normal (at 90 degrees) to the structure being imaged.

Side Lobe Artifacts

Side lobes are off-axis secondary projections of the ultrasound beam (Figure 1-25).[3] The side lobes have reduced intensities compared with the main on-axis projection; however, they can produce image artifacts. Usually, on-axis reflections are greater in intensity than side lobe reflections and thereby

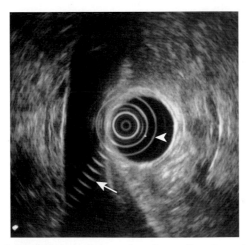

FIGURE 1-17 EUS image of reverberation artifact *(arrow)* resulting from multiple reflections from an air bubble in the water-filled balloon. The intensity of the artifact does not decrease as rapidly as the reverberation artifact *(arrowhead)* from the transducer housing. This is because the impedance mismatch of the air-water interface is much greater than the transducer housing interface, with resulting reflected signals of greater intensity.

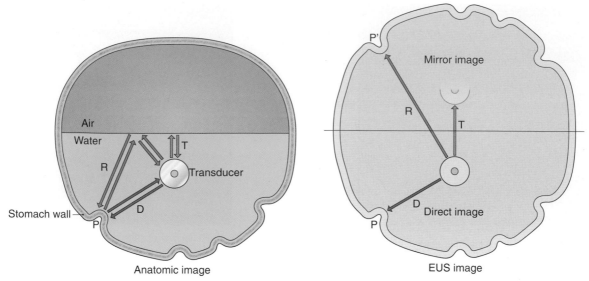

Anatomic image   EUS image

FIGURE 1-19 Reflection from an air-water interface produces a mirror image artifact. Because of the large impedance mismatch between water and air, an ultrasound signal that interacts with an air-water interface is reflected almost completely. The figure on the *left* is an illustration of an ultrasound probe imaging the gastric wall with an air-water interface. The path denoted by D directly images location P along the gastric wall. The path denoted by R images location P because of a reflection from the air-water interface. The path T images the transducer because of a reflection from the air-water interface. The figure on the *right* is an illustration of the resulting ultrasound image. The ultrasound processor registers the location of the image by the direction of the transmitted pulse and the time it receives the reflected signal. The processor accurately registers point P, resulting from the reflected signal from path D; however, the signal from path R is incorrectly registered as point P', with a resulting mirror image appearance. In addition, the reflected signal from path T results in shadowing artifact in the mirror image.

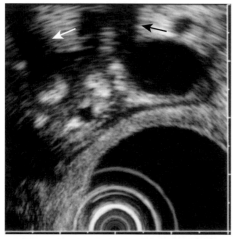

FIGURE 1-20 Shadowing artifact *(arrows)* resulting from calcifications in the pancreas.

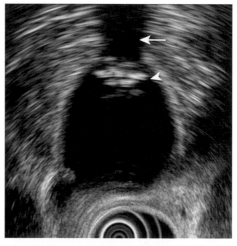

FIGURE 1-21 Shadowing artifact *(arrow)* resulting from gallstones *(arrowhead)*.

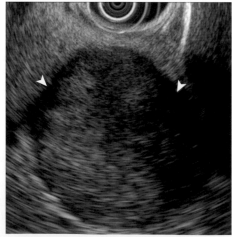

FIGURE 1-22 Acoustic shadowing *(arrowheads)* resulting from refraction from an interface between normal tissue and tumor.

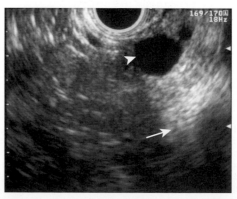

FIGURE 1-23 Anechoic cystic lesion *(arrowhead)* demonstrating enhancement beyond the cyst relative to other structures *(white arrow)* that are of similar distance from the transducer. This artifact is also called *through transmission.*

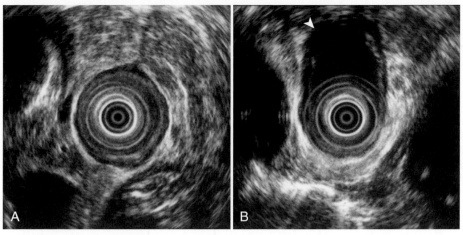

FIGURE 1-24 Tangential imaging artifact. **A,** Normal imaging of a hypertrophic lower esophageal sphincter in a patient with achalasia. **B,** Tangential imaging of the same lower esophageal sphincter (note that the balloon was not inflated during acquisition of this image). The gastrointestinal (GI) tract wall layers are distorted and are not uniformly thick circumferentially, a finding suggesting that the transducer is not imaging a normal GI tract wall. As a result, areas of abnormal thickening are noted on imaging and can give the incorrect appearance of a tumor in the GI tract wall *(arrowhead).*

obscure any side lobe reflections. However, during imaging of an anechoic structure, the reflected ultrasound energy from a side lobe can be of sufficient intensity to yield a detected signal that is then interpreted by the processor as an on-axis reflection.[10] A side lobe artifact is recognized when the hyperechoic signal does not maintain its position within an anechoic structure such as a cyst or the gallbladder. It may be misinterpreted as sludge in the gallbladder or a mass within a cyst.[6] Figure 1-26 is an image of a side lobe artifact within the gallbladder. Repositioning of the transducer causes the artifact to disappear.

Endoscopic Ultrasound Elastography

Elastography is an ultrasound-based method for evaluation of tissue "hardness," that is, the change in tissue dimensions (strain) arising from an applied force. This concept is closely related to palpation, which physicians have used for centuries to detect pathology associated with higher tissue "stiffness." There are multiple parameters describing tissue elastic properties, including bulk modulus (Equation 1.3, Table 1-1), which describes the change in *volume* of the material in response to external stress. As seen from Table 1-1, bulk

modulus only varies by no more than 15% among different tissue types. However, palpation elicits different elasticity parameters—Young's modulus and/or shear modulus, which represent the ratio of tissue *displacement* (or strain) in a certain direction (longitudinal or transverse) to the applied stress. The elastic moduli of normal soft tissues are known to vary as much as four orders of magnitude and are elevated by the pathologic changes, such as fibrosis, by up to two orders of magnitude, with benign tumors being generally softer than malignant tumors.[11]

In elastography, stress is applied to tissue either externally (e.g., vibration, manual pressure, or balloon inflation in the case of transluminal examination) or internally (e.g., by vascular pulsations and respiratory motion). The resulting strain is measured using ultrasound as illustrated in Figure 1-27, showing B-mode images are recorded before and after the application of stress. Each of the B-mode line scans recorded before and after compression is then analyzed using cross-correlation techniques to extract the in-depth strain distribution. These strain line scans are then combined into a

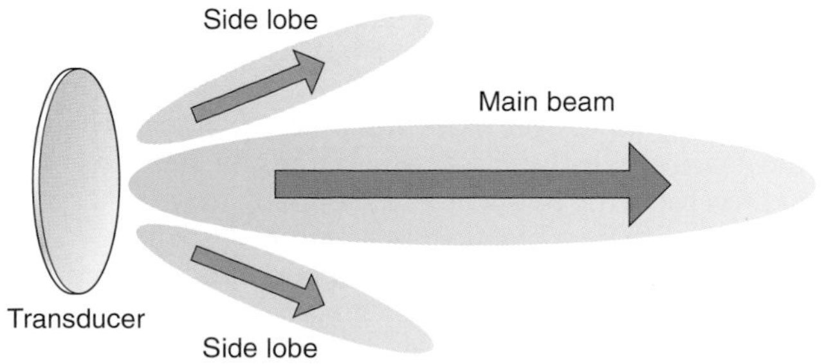

FIGURE 1-25 Side lobes represent secondary projections off-axis from the main beam. Side lobes have lower intensities than the main beam, but they can still produce back-reflected signals from the tissue of sufficient intensity to be detected by the transducer. However, the transducer assumes that all back-reflections originate from the main lobe. Therefore image artifacts can result from side lobe projections.

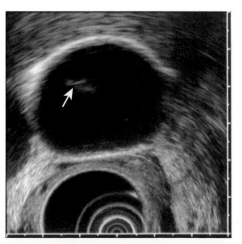

FIGURE 1-26 Side lobe artifact identified in the gallbladder *(arrow).* Repositioning of the transducer results in disappearance of this signal.

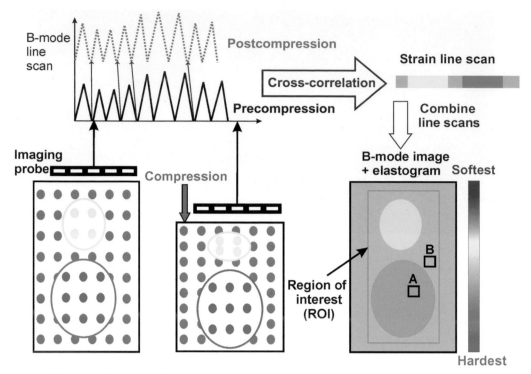

FIGURE 1-27 Conceptual diagram of ultrasound elastography. Two B-mode images are acquired, before and after tissue compression. Tissue displacement within hard inclusions (*blue*), which are often associated with pathologic changes, is smaller than the displacement of surrounding tissue (*gray*) or soft inclusions (*yellow*). B-mode line scans from each of the array elements obtained before and after tissue compression are then compared using cross-correlation techniques to reconstruct the in-depth tissue displacement distribution. The line scans are then combined into a two-dimensional color image representing tissue softness, with a hue diagram range of 1 to 255. This image is only calculated within the region of interest defined by the user to include the lesion of interest and some of the surrounding tissue. Although this qualitative information is often helpful, quantitative measurements of tissue elasticity are more reliable and can be obtained, for example, as follows. Two areas (A and B) are selected on the elastogram, in the lesion of interest and in the fat or connective tissue, and the ratio of the mean strain within these areas is measured.

two-dimensional elastogram, which is superimposed in semitransparent color onto the B-mode image. To indicate tissue softness, the system uses hue color map (on a scale of 1 to 255) where the hardest tissue appears as dark blue and the softest tissue as red. A region of interest (ROI) in which the elasticity information is calculated is selected manually to include the targeted lesion and some of the surrounding tissue. It is worth noting here that the displayed elasticity map is, strictly speaking, not a direct representation of tissue elastic modulus distribution in absolute units, but rather relative tissue displacement distribution within the ROI (because the stress is unknown). Moreover, the diagnosis made based solely on color (blue means malignant) is subject to strong bias and is operator dependent. This approach is called qualitative elastography.[12] Recently, second-generation EUS elastography allows for quantitative analysis of tissue stiffness.[13] Two different areas (A and B) from the region of interest are selected for quantitative elastographic analysis, so that area A includes the mass of interest and area B refers to a soft peripancreatic reference area outside the tumor. The parameter B/A (strain ratio) is considered as the measure of the elastographic evaluation.

Contrast-Enhanced Harmonic Imaging

Contrast enhancement in ultrasound imaging is based on the backscatter of the ultrasound waves from the ultrasound contrast agents (UCAs) that are administered intravenously. UCAs are usually gas bodies or bubbles of 2-6 mm diameter surrounded by a shell and are stable in the circulation and restricted to the inside of the blood vessels until they are eliminated in the expired air. The way UCAs interact with and scatter the incident ultrasound waves with frequency *f* depends primarily on the ultrasound pressure amplitude, as illustrated in Figure 1-28. At low ultrasound pressure levels, the bubble expands and contracts synchronously with the incident pressure wave, and these oscillations are small compared to the bubble radius. The frequency of the scattered ultrasound wave in this case is also *f*, and the bubble simply plays the role of an efficient reflector. At larger ultrasound wave amplitudes, bubble oscillations become unstable and include periods of slower growth and subsequent rapid collapse. These collapses lead to the generation of secondary ultrasound waves, or harmonics, with a frequency higher than the fundamental frequency by an integer factor multiple: 2*f*, 3*f*, etc. Therefore if the imaging transducer is tuned to transmit at the frequency *f* and receive at the frequency 2*f*, then only the areas containing bubbles, that is, blood vessels, will be visualized.

The process described above is commonly referred to as contrast-enhanced harmonic imaging and has been increasingly used in the past years for characterization of microvasculature and perfusion inside the lesion of interest with the aim of improved differential diagnosis, as well as longitudinal monitoring of the effects of chemotherapy and/or antiangiogenic therapy in advanced digestive cancers. The movement of UCAs through the circulation can be monitored by

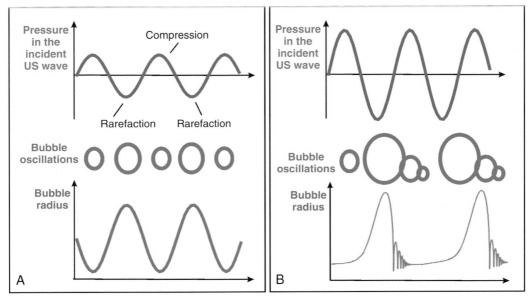

FIGURE 1-28   Scenarios of the response of an ultrasound contrast agent—2-6 μm gas bubble covered by a thin shell—to an incident ultrasound wave. **A**, Low amplitude ultrasound wave. The bubble oscillations are spherically symmetric and small compared to the bubble's initial radius. The compression and expansion of the bubble are synchronized with the compression and rarefaction phases in the ultrasound wave. **B**, Higher amplitude ultrasound wave. The bubble oscillations become unstable, with a slow growth phase followed by a rapid collapse and several rebounds. The frequency of bubble collapses is higher than the frequency of the incident ultrasound wave.

harmonic imaging in real time, which allows measurement of a number of useful quantitative parameters that correlate with the microvascular blood flow such as wash-in and wash-out time, and mean transit time.[13]

Summary

The basic principles of ultrasound physics and instrumentation are reviewed in this chapter. In addition, common imaging artifacts are presented and explained by applying the basic principles of ultrasound. These principles should provide an understanding of the capabilities and limitations of ultrasound and how ultrasound images are formed. Understanding these principles will aid the endosonographer in obtaining accurate, high-quality images.

REFERENCES

1. Hedrick WR, Hykes DL, Starchman DE. *Ultrasound Physics and Instrumentation*. 3rd ed. St. Louis: Mosby; 1995.
2. Duck FA. *Physical Properties of Tissue*. London: Academic Press; 1990.
3. Christensen DA. *Ultrasonic Bioinstrumentation*. New York: John Wiley; 1988.
4. Shung KK, Thieme GA. *Ultrasonic Scattering in Biological Tissues*. Boca Raton, FL: CRC Press; 2000.
5. Harris RA, Follett DH, Halliwell M, et al. Ultimate limits in ultrasonic imaging resolution. *Ultrasound Med Biol*. 1991;17:547-558.
6. Kimmey MB. Basic principles and fundamentals of endoscopic ultrasound imaging. In: Gress F, Bhattacharya I, eds. *Endoscopic Ultrasonography*. Malden: Blackwell Science; 2001:4-14.
7. Grech P. Mirror-image artifact with endoscopic ultrasonography and reappraisal of the fluid-air interface. *Gastrointest Endosc*. 1993;39:700-703.
8. Steel R, Poepping TL, Thompson RS, et al. Origins of the edge shadowing artifact in medical ultrasound imaging. *Ultrasound Med Biol*. 2004;30:1153-1162.
9. Kimmey MB, Martin RW. Fundamentals of endosonography. *Gastrointest Endosc Clin N Am*. 1992;2:557-573.
10. Laing FC, Kurtz AB. The importance of ultrasonic side-lobe artifacts. *Radiology*. 1982;145:763-768.
11. Greenleaf JF, Fatemi M, Insana M. Selected methods for imaging elastic properties of biological tissues. *Annu Rev Biomed Eng*. 2003;5:57-78.
12. Iglesias-Garcia J, Dominguez-Munos JE. Endoscopic ultrasound image enhancement elastography. *Clin N Am*. 2012;22:333-348.
13. Gheonea D-I, Saftoiu A. Beyond conventional endoscopic ultrasound: elastography, contrast enhancement and hybrid techniques. *Curr Opin Gastroenterol*. 2011;27:423-429.

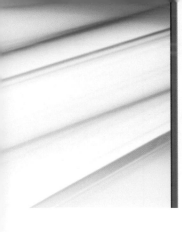

2

Equipment

John Meenan • Charles Vu

Key Points

- The choice of equipment is informed by the case-mix. The choice of equipment should be based on what types of cases realistically will be performed regularly not what one would prefer to do.
- If resources are limited, focus on linear equipment.
- The operating characteristics of scopes and FNA needles differ between manufacturers; it is important to try out several makes in order to determine which one is the most compatible with how you perform EUS.
- Archiving and video editing are important features of practicing EUS. Give some thought as to how this will be achieved.

Introduction

Delivering an endoscopic ultrasonography (EUS) service of quality that is consistently reliable for referrers and patients alike is demanding and takes concentrated planning. Endoscopic ultrasound equipment, furthermore, is expensive to both purchase and maintain; there is no second chance for making the wrong decisions. For these pressing reasons a lot of honest, focused, and objective thought must go into developing such a service—it is not just a bolt-on to endoscopic retrograde cholangiopancreatography (ERCP) and cannot be a rushed process.

Before embarking on establishing a EUS service you must know why you want to do it and where the true demand lies. Although there may be a large degree of equivalence across the equipment offerings of the main endoscopy manufacturers, subtle differences in specification can have a large impact on utility in certain pathologies.

Establishing an EUS Service

The idiosyncrasies of various health care systems are legion and impossible to cater for in a book such as this. Differences in coding principles and national recommendations for manpower will certainly inform your business case for establishing an EUS unit, but that is not what we will discuss here. This chapter describes how a service is best configured, managed, and developed.

Many of those who are setting up a EUS service, hopefully, will be coming from an established facility where they have trained. Such services did not appear out of the blue, nor do they exist because of good luck. It takes thought and attention to detail to found and sustain a new service. Honesty, neurosis, and perseverance are helpful qualities to have in equal amounts.

Several principles hold true across the globe for the founding of an EUS service. The single most important question to be answered is: "What is the true demand for EUS here?" Do not confuse a personal wish for a local imperative.

There is a broad range of standard indications for EUS, from the staging of esophageal cancer to defining pancreaticobiliary pathology. Therefore some questions will need to be answered: (1) If you work with upper esophageal/gastric surgeons, what might they want from an EUS—just a description of T stage and putative N staging, or node biopsy? (2) How many patients undergo magnetic resonance imaging (MRI) for possible choledocholithiasis? (3) How many mature pancreatic pseudocysts do you see in a year? (4) Do you have the backup to allow you to attempt and fail at complex biliary or pancreatic duct drainage? Talk to your colleagues, search whatever databases are available, and talk with potential referrers rather than guessing. Remember to talk also with thoracic colleagues as plans to introduce endobronchial ultrasound will potentially lower costs through a shared ultrasound platform. Equally, there may be some shared ground with endoanal services or more broadly with the imaging unit.

The numbers can tell you certain things—for example, what the key pathologies to be serviced are. Through their analysis, a measure of likely financial implication can be reached. There are many published papers on the cost effectiveness of EUS in certain settings, but the results of such work may not translate well to other units or regions, so do your own math. Talk with colleagues and local professional organizations about how they approach coding to maximize returns, as there are often tricks that can change entirely the landscape of the possible. The numbers can also tell you what type of equipment you should be considering.

Who is to perform EUS? In most countries EUS falls to the remit of gastroenterologists, but both surgeons and radiologists also perform this procedure. No particular professional background has been shown to confer any advantage in proficiency and, indeed, in the United Kingdom, some centers have developed nurse-led services. Importantly, the presence of an ultrasound machine in the room does not mean that a radiologist must be present.

Disseminating knowledge is the life blood of any service. That is not the same as blowing your own trumpet. It is possible, of course, to talk up the benefits of any new service and garner test referrals, but be wary and be sensible. In talking about the strengths of EUS, you must give equal focus to the weaknesses, such as performance of EUS fine-needle aspiration (FNA) with chronic pancreatitis or the exclusion of small cholangiocarcinomas.

Using case studies can be a good way of conveying messages and preempting failures when they are sure to happen. You need to keep repeating these messages because other physicians may want you to resolve their problems and often turn a deaf ear to the subtleties or limitations of a new procedure. It is important to realize that, whereas the weaknesses of computed tomography (CT) are largely ignored, those of a new EUS service are not. Remember that, even in the best of times, EUS pancreatic cancer is incorrectly staged in one of five cases. That CT might have an equally prominent Achilles heel provides no protection against an unfavorable reputation.

Establishing an EUS service is not just about the numbers of cases that might be performed, revenues generated, or personal wishes; the facilities available, endoscopy staff, local cytopathology skills, and interacts with referring physicians will all have a dramatic impact on the success of the endeavor.

The training of endoscopy room staff is central to reducing running costs (returns for repairs are expensive and likely to halt services) and ensuring that procedures are optimized (a simple FNA procedure can easily be made useless through poor teamwork). The responsibility for some of this training will fall on both the practitioner and the scope manufacturer at the time of equipment purchase. Talk with both nursing and technical staff to find out what their training needs might be.

You should be familiar with the space required and the physical layout of the endoscopy room from your first experiences performing EUS. It is important when trialing equipment from different manufacturers to make sure that sufficient room is allowed for FNA specimens to be prepared comfortably. Equipment is discussed later in this chapter, but bear in mind that space-saving ultrasound processors are usually inferior to free-standing standard machines.

An EUS service will attract cases from surgical departments at other institutions, and you will need to determine your role. Is it just to perform a procedure and forward results, or are you to proffer a management opinion? These questions are important to answer because giving opinions can confuse and upset patients and irritate the referrer. If you are to offer an opinion, you will need to see the patient in consultation first and allow time to review investigation results. Usually, an opinion on how to manage less common lesions, such as subepithelial lesions, will be noncontentious, but opinions may differ, for example, on the need for surgery for pancreatic cysts or epithelial high grade dysplasia. Tread carefully!

The difficult issue of cytopathology support must be grasped from the start, particularly because all EUS services should offer FNA. The days of "look but don't touch" EUS are gone.

You can get very good cytopathological results by preparing samples yourself for later evaluation, but the literature indicates that results are better if a cytotechnician (not necessarily a cytopathologist) is present. His or her role is to prepare good specimens and comment on cellularity (i.e., adequacy) so that you know when to stop the procedure, not to give immediate results. A rushed diagnosis does no one any favors.

Talk to your local pathology service and see what experience the staff has, what they can provide, and if it's feasible or cost effective. Transenteric FNA is not the same as other forms of cytology because of the mucus present, so there will be a learning curve (approximately 60 cases) before they stop diagnosing everyone as having a well-differentiated mucus-secreting tumor. If a technician cannot attend your procedures, go to him or her and learn the optimal way of spreading slides and how he or she wants samples preserved (e.g., in fixative or in buffered saline). Discuss with the cytopathologist if you are going to use a Cook ProCore needle because it provides samples that are halfway between cytology and pathology and so may need slightly different handling.

No matter how good and well intentioned you and your staff are, bad administration with regard to ease of booking, reliability of contact, and lack of any degree of flexibility will have a negative impact. Your responsibility is not confined to the time that the procedure might take.

Poor communication can kill a service. It is important that the referring physician appreciates what you need to know: degree of dysphagia, exact site/size of the lesion, unexpected findings on CT and other imaging methods, use of anticoagulants/platelet agents, and, most importantly, if an FNA is to be done. When talking to the referring physician, emphasize points such as these, along with the risks of seeding (now perceived to be very low). Equally important, be precise in writing your report by giving exact sizes, numbers, and positions. Unfortunately, there are no good reporting systems widely available for EUS, so you will most likely have to adapt a module within a generic reporting system. E-mail or fax reports to the referring physician, and ensure that all pathology results are forwarded in a timely fashion. Provide the contact details for the laboratory on the report, and ask for reports to be automatically copied to the referring physician. Do not make yourself the only conduit of all reports. If the result is particularly time sensitive, you should phone or text (SMS) the referring physician. Again, be very careful in discussing results and their implications with the patient at the time of discharge if he or she is coming from another service.

The scheduling of EUS cases will be affected by factors such as the number of scopes available, level of skill, likely presence of a trainee, and type of sedation used. In general terms, an EUS with FNA can be scheduled for every 30 minutes, allowing 60 to 90 minutes for recovery to discharge with the use of midazolam/opiate. If you are training fellows in EUS, fewer cases are better than too many (time and quality of teaching outweigh the quantity of cases). When scheduling cases, give an indication of which scope is likely to be used to allow for good list planning. Scheduling patients for EUS followed by ERCP at the same sitting can be ideal for cancer cases but is wasteful of time slots when looking for common bile duct stones.

Equipment

Equipment for EUS is not kind to endoscopists; it is expensive, lacks versatility, and, when not bulky and fragile, is just small and exquisitely fragile.

The purchasing of equipment usually comes at the end of a long process of justifying a local need in order to obtain a once-off access to limited funds. It is ironic that, more often than not, this project is led either by someone who has not found their endosonographic feet or by someone that sees a need and can make things happen but will not be actually involved in the service itself.

There is no right or wrong EUS equipment because the products of the main manufacturers are comparable. There is, however, right and wrong equipment to meet your needs.

It is perfectly feasible to run EUS equipment from one manufacturer in a room where the standard scopes are provided by another. Mixing EUS equipment from different manufacturers, however, does not work.

General

Echoendoscopes fall broadly into two categories: radial (or "sector") and linear (or "convex array") with both electronic and mechanical (the latter now largely superseded) formats available in each. Specialty probes with specific clinical needs in mind are available and provide bespoke tools to investigate subepithelial masses and pancreatobiliary ductal pathology (mini-probes), esophageal and proximal gastric cancer (use of an endobronchial scope replaces the now discontinued Olympus "slimprobe" [MH908]), the colon proximal to the rectum (mini-probes), and the anal canal (rigid probes).

The coupling of electronic echoendoscopes to mid- and upper-range standard ultrasound processors has now brought to EUS the added dimensions of Doppler/Powerflow, three-dimensional rendering, tissue elastography, an ability to use newer contrast agents (e.g., SonaVue), and indeed any future development in mainstream ultrasonography. It also brings many more illuminated buttons, most of which will be ignored. The key features to look for remain: how good the image is and how the scope handles in your hands.

Radial echoendoscopes provide circumferential views at right angles to the shaft of the scope, similar to those provided by CT scans. This similarity to generally appreciated views of the gastrointestinal tract makes this format attractive to the majority of trainees and endosonographers in general.

The linear format of EUS yields views more analogous to those obtained with transabdominal ultrasound. Because the view is in the same line or plane as the scope shaft, images are blinkered and orientation is more difficult. It is very easy to get lost when landmarks are not seen. This perception of difficulty, fueled by a general lack of exposure to transabdominal ultrasound by most clinicians, historically has relegated linear EUS for many practitioners to being merely an interventional tool. It is uncomfortable with its use beyond an unduly narrow range of indications.

EUS, however, has moved resolutely in the direction of linear scopes. No one has ever shown that learning linear rather than radial EUS is more difficult or that performing linear studies takes longer. The bottom line is that if you are buying EUS equipment, you need a good reason for it not to be linear.

Radial Echoendoscopes

The three major manufacturers (Olympus, Hitachi-Pentax, and Fujinon) all offer electronic radial scopes with 360° fields of view that will operate from an ultrasound platform common to that manufacturer's linear scopes. The scopes handle differently, some being more flexible than others, so pay attention to how the scope meets the challenges of passing into the second part of the duodenum when trialing equipment. Just because a scope is forward viewing does not mean it is necessarily easier to use.

Look carefully at the shape of the scope as measurements given for distal tip diameter maybe misleading. Some scopes have a large bulge immediately behind the tip that cannot pass by a stricture. Also, each manufacturer has a different way of controlling the distal water-filled balloon—for example, a two-step button (Olympus) or separate syringe channel (Pentax) with a knob directing water flow from bowel lumen to balloon. In practice, such differences make little difference in ease of use.

Olympus offers both an electronic radial scope (Olympus GF-UE160-AL5; Figure 2-1A; scans at 5, 6, 7.5, and 10 MHz) and the mechanical GF-UM2000 (scans at 5, 7.5, 12, and 20 MHz; lighter model as the motor is in the shaft, not on the top of the scope). All these scopes are luminally oblique viewing scopes, so they cannot be relied on to fully substitute for a standard gastroscope. Balloon filling and emptying are achieved through ergonomically helpful dual-step suck/blow buttons. Again, both have a small accessory channel (2.2 mm) capable of taking "blue-handled" bronchoscopy-size mucosal biopsies; an elevator lifts the forceps into view.

The continuing sale of mechanical scopes in an electronic age requires some explanation. They provide images as good as their electronic successor and generally tend to be cheaper, but they do not support Doppler and have, until recently, required a stand-alone ultrasound processor that cannot be used for linear scopes. This Achilles heel has been addressed by the introduction of the "multi-compatible" format EU-ME1 processor (see later discussion).

Although robust and capable of a long clinical life, the dual requirement for a drive shaft and an exposed oil bath housing might be perceived to be inherent weaknesses. In practice, the mechanical nature of these scopes does not carry any greater susceptibility to break down. Care must be exercised, however, when placing or removing the balloon that the oil bath is not crushed or dislocated, which is a potentially significant problem in units with many trainees. The development of a bubble and resulting diffuse degradation in the quality of the ultrasound image is a sign that the oil bath requires topping-up; this may occur once or twice a year.

Olympus scopes have two identification numbers: The more common "100" versions, available in most countries, are scopes with color CCD chips, whereas the "200" series (mainly Japan and UK) scopes have black and white chips that permit narrow-band imaging.

Pentax was the first company to market an electronic radial instrument. The initial scope was limited by an incomplete field of ultrasound view (270°; Pentax-Hitachi EG-3630UR). This has long been replaced by a full 360° viewer, which scans at 5, 7.5, and 10 MHz (Pentax-Hitachi EG-367OURK; Figure 2-1B). Endoscopically, it is a forward viewing scope (140°), but this advantage is offset by an inability to fully retroflex.

FIGURE 2-1 Radial echoendoscopes. **A,** Olympus GF-UE160 (Olympus America Inc., Center Valley, CA). **B,** Pentax EG-3670URK (Pentax Medical Company, Montvale, NJ). **C,** Fujinon EG-53OUR (Fujinon Inc., Wayne, NJ).

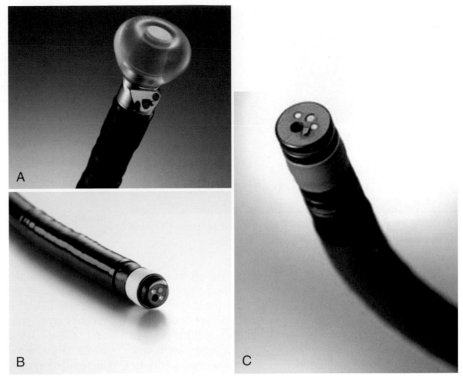

Again, it will not reliably replace a standard gastroscope for complete luminal inspection. There is a biopsy channel that can take standard size mucosal biopsy forceps.

Fujinon offers the slimmest (11.5 mm) and most endoscopically flexible electronic radial echoendoscope (EG-530UR2; 5, 7.5, 10 and 12 MHz; Figure 2-1C) that has forward luminal views and also permits 360° ultrasound scanning.

Linear Scopes

The Pentax FG-32, launched in 1991, was the standard linear echoendoscope for many years. The EUS transducer sited distal to the viewing lens is gently curved, similar in shape to those used for transabdominal studies, giving a 120° field of ultrasonic view. This shape gives very nice, stable views of the celiac axis and aortopulmonary window for neurolysis and node sampling.

The standard Pentax linear scope is the EG-3870UTK (Figure 2-2A). It has an elevator for needle guidance and has a 3.8 mm accessory channel. Although this may be only 0.1 mm wider than the Olympus offering, it does allow slightly freer manipulation of stents. A slightly slimmer scope is the newer EG-3270UK, but this only has a 2.8 mm channel and so is used for FNA only, which is quite limiting for a marginal benefit in handling.

The Fujinon EG-530UT2 (Figure 2-2B) linear scope again has a 3.8 mm working channel and an elevator.

The Olympus linear echoendoscopes have a pea-like tip transducer allowing for a 180° scanning plane. There are three models, the newest being the GF-UCT180 (UK/Japan UCT 260) that allows for contrast-enhanced EUS (3.7 mm accessory channel and detachable cable [MAJ 1587] for easier insertion into washing machines). The two older models are differentiated only by accessory channel size: 2.8 mm (GF-UCT140P-AL5) and the larger (and so more versatile)

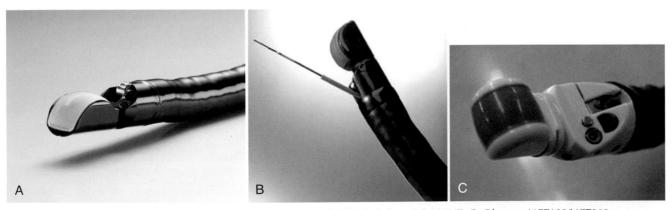

FIGURE 2-2 Linear echoendoscopes. **A,** Pentax EG-3870UTK. **B,** Fujinon EG-530UT. **C,** Olympus UCT180/UCT260.

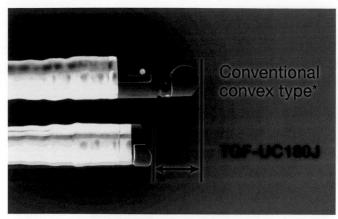

FIGURE 2-3 The Olympus TGF-UC180J, forward ultrasound viewing scope for pancreatic cyst puncture.

3.7 mm (GF-UCT140-AL5). Both scopes have elevators to assist needle guidance. The latter scope is said to be capable of deploying a 10 Fr stent; however, any angulation of the scope tip required to obtain appropriate views lessens the functional diameter of the accessory channel, making passage of large bore stents difficult. It might be conjectured that performing FNA with the larger channel scope could be more problematic due to the needle wobbling within the channel; in practice, this does not occur. Equally, as with the Pentax-Hitachi scopes, there is no difference in actual scope size between the limited FNA versions and the larger bore version.

Olympus is scheduled to launch a snub-nosed forward ultrasound viewing scope (Figure 2-3), designed especially for therapeutic procedures such as pseudocyst drainage. The 100 series has the label TGF-UC180 J (there is no sequential RGB 200 series [UK/Japan] equivalent as yet). There is no information on how the shape of this scope will cope with the demands of pancreatic tumor staging where comprehensive views, including of the uncinate process, are essential. This scope has no elevator, but its field of view makes it more "needle friendly" than standard scopes. One should not presume that this scope would be a better all-rounder than the current linear scopes, so trial it well for your purposes before purchasing.

Toshiba has discontinued offering an echoendoscope with development devolved to Fujinon.

EUS Processors

There has always been little to truly separate the various offerings available from the major companies, but this is even truer now that Hitachi (Pentax platform) has taken over Aloka (Olympus platform). It is said that the two streams will continue to work independently. Olympus discontinued their cooperation with Philips some time ago.

Compatibility between radial, linear, and endobrachial EUS (EBUS) systems is the standard. Both Olympus and Pentax run their scopes from physically separate free-standing "standard" ultrasound machines (Aloka and Hitachi, respectively), and Fujinon uses a proprietary machine (Fujinon Sonart SU-8000). This is not necessarily an issue of concern, but do pay attention to the image quality when trialing.

An additional processor, importantly, may be required to allow for the use of some specialty probes. This differs depending on manufacturer. Olympus sees choice as a virtue, but some practitioners may find the choice confusing. Perhaps the best way to cut this Gordian knot is to abandon radial EUS and dive resolutely into the world of linear ultrasound.

As mentioned above, Olympus has a broad range of radial scopes. If money is not (too much of) an issue and if you want to use a radial scope (presuming that you do not have old mechanical scopes that you need to keep in use), then purchase an electronic radial scope that will allow you platform compatibility with a linear scope (Hitachi-Aloka F75 or the now obsolescent but good Aloka Prosound Alpha 10 or the "compact" Aloka 7). The Alpha 5, which had poorer image quality, is now defunct for the purpose of EUS.

The approach above will not allow you to run Olympus mini-probes, as they require the UM-ME1 processor, which can also run the newer Olympus linear and radial scopes at the cost of an inferior processor. Such an approach is perhaps a case of the tail wagging the dog. If you want to have mini-probes and a high-end Olympus radial/linear service, it would be best to have both an F75 and the UM-ME1.

A new EU-ME2 processor (Figure 2-4) has been developed recently by Olympus. The updated processor is very compact and allows for a broad range of available frequencies (5-20 MHz), good focus (to a range of 1 cm), good image manipulation including instant video replay, and, with appropriate software, mini-probe three-dimensional rendering. The unique ability of this processor is that it facilitates the use of contrast imaging and elastography. The processor has tissue harmonic echo capability with penetration (THE-P) and resolution (THE-R) modes, pulse-wave Doppler, and high-resolution flow mode.

Fujinon radial and linear scopes run off the SU-8000 ultrasound processor. This is the smallest processor available and will fit easily into a standard endoscopy stack.

Hitachi processors run Pentax scopes. There is a broad range that allows for EUS/EBUS. Most are now several years old, but they are very good and offer the ability to perform tissue elastography and contrast-enhanced procedures, as well as endoscopy/EUS image "picture-in-picture" on the one screen. They include EUB-5500 HV, EUB-7000 HV, EUB-7500 HV, HI VISION 900, and the newer HI VISION Preirus (compact), as well as the top-end HI VISION Ascendus. Have

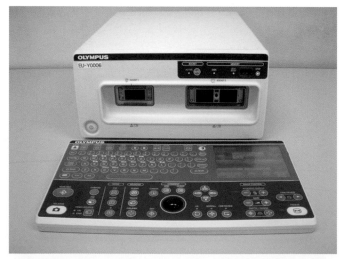

FIGURE 2-4 The new Olympus EU-ME2 (termed EU-Y0006 at development phase) processor that is compatible with use of contrast agents also facilitates elastography.

a detailed list of what you want to achieve with your EUS and then see which machine meets your needs; the key factor being image quality.

Specialty Probes

A variety of probes are available for specific clinical situations. Whereas such instruments may be used only relatively infrequently, the advantages of their use must be considered in planning for departmental needs.

Esophagus and Stomach

The Olympus MH908 slim (esophago) probe has now been withdrawn from the market, because an endobronchial scope can be used in its place to traverse strictures without the need for prior dilatation. This approach can certainly work and allows for tissue sampling down to the celiac axis, but scope control is not always perfect.

The ability to add an unplanned EUS examination to a gastroscopy is an ever present ambition. The Fujinon PL2226B-7.5 is a torpedo-shaped mechanical radial probe (7.5 MHz; head diameter, 7.3 mm) that may be back loaded through a large channel gastroscope in a fashion analogous to the loading of a variceal band cartridge. This clever design is offset by a resultant diminishment in endoscopic luminal view, which is problematic with strictures. The probe is driven by the SP702 processor. This processor also permits easy switching between radial and linear formats ("bi-planar" ultrasound) when using Fujinon mini-probes.

Mini-Probes

Catheter probes range in size between 1.4-2.6 mm, are mostly mechanical radial, and require an additional, small motor-drive unit intervening between the probe and the ultrasound processor (important to remember when budget planning). In length, all probes will reach to the duodenum and terminal ileum (through a colonoscopy), but Fujinon offer a 2700 mm length probe that can be deployed through a balloon enteroscope. They are usually of high frequency (12-30 MHz, most 20 MHz and above) with a shallow depth of view and a resulting reduction in useful application. Whereas such probes are particularly good at inspecting small mucosal/subepithelial lesions and for intraductal use, they are not good for the regular staging of esophageal tumors or larger colonic polyps as their penetration is rapidly attenuated, particularly with colonic polyps.

Another drawback with catheter probes is the difficulty of excluding air from the site of mucosal contact. Proprietary balloon sheaths are available, but these require the use of scopes with large caliber accessory channels. There have been many reports of other methods to provide a water interface, including use of (nonlubricated) condoms and water-flooding of the esophagus with prior cuffed intubation.

Mini-probes are said to have a useful life of 50 to 100 procedures. With care, the longevity of catheter probes can be extended considerably beyond this time frame. In particular, storing probes in a hanging position, rather than coiled flat, prolongs life span. When in use, the transducer should never be rotating when the probe is passed or withdrawn through the scope and the elevator should never be touched when a probe is in place. Although several probes are advertised as having the capacity to be used within the biliary tree, this is not feasible unless they are wire guided (very few are),

as the acute angulation needed for ampullary cannulation snaps the motor wires. Both Olympus and Fujinon offer a wide range of mini-probes.

Fujinon mini-probes include the 2.6-mm wide (so it is possible to pass through the accessory channel of a standard 2.8 mm gastroscope) 25 MHz (P2625M), 20 MHz (P2620M), 15 MHz (P2615M), and 12 MHz (P2612M) models. Of interest may be the extra-long probes (2700 mm) that allow passage through a balloon enteroscope (P2620L, P2615L, and P2612L—20, 15, and 12 MHz, respectively).

The probe range from Olympus is huge and confusing. The main ones fall into two broad categories: (1) those for general use (UM-2R [12 MHz], UM-3R [20 MHz], and UM-S30-25R [30 MHz]), all of which can be used down a standard gastroscope (2.8 mm) channel (a sheath [MH246R] is available but is not required as it adds little); and (2) those for intraductal ultrasound studies (IDUS), the key one being the UM-G20-29R (20 MHz) as it is wire guided. Other variations on the same theme, while not necessarily ideal for EUS are small enough to pass through a bronchoscope channel (2.2 mm), so permit non-FNA EBUS of the peripheral lung (e.g., UM-S20-20R; UM-S30-20R and the very fine 1.4 mm UM-S20-17S used with a 2 mm sheath [K-201 or K-202]).

The "spiraling" probes (UM-DP12-25R [12 MHz], UM-DP-20-25R [20 MHz] probes; Figure 2-5A and B) offer the added capacity to permit dual-plane ("three-dimensional") rendering when used off the EU-ME1 processor, provided that the appropriate software has been loaded. In principle, both these probes will give a three-dimensional reconstruction of, for example, an esophageal stricture/tumor, ultrasound signal penetration allowing. A wire-guide version for use in the biliary tree is the UM-DG20-31R. The MAJ-935 driver connector is required to run these probes because they will not plug directly into the ultrasound console.

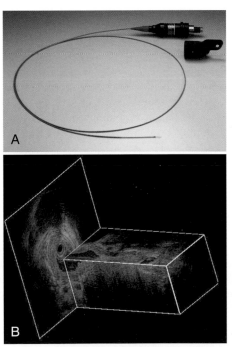

FIGURE 2-5 The Olympus UM-DP range of mechanical probes "spiral" within the catheter (**A**) to yield dual-plane, or, three-dimensional images (**B**).

Colon and Anorectum

The Olympus rigid rectal probes (RU-12M-R1 and RU-75M-R1, 12 and 7.5 MHz, respectively) work off the EU-ME1 compact, cut-down "universal" processor.

The Olympus dedicated EUS-colonoscopy is now no longer available. However, standard length mini-probes will easily pass down through a standard colonoscope. Their use is limited though by the tendency of colorectal polyps to markedly attenuate the ultrasound signal.

Accessories

Needles for FNA

Needles for FNA remain expensive and less than ideal. Needle sizes range from 19 G to 25 G. Additionally, specialized needles for specific tasks, such as pancreatic sampling, celiac axis neurolysis, core biopsy, and pancreatic cyst drainage are available (availability subject to national licensing). There have been refinements to the attached suction syringes, permitting variable degrees of negative pressure to suit a specific clinical situation. The tips of all needles are specially treated to allow for good EUS visualization.

Much tedious work has been performed in an attempt to define the best needle size and appropriate amount of negative pressure for a given task (whether it is by syringe suction or stepped withdrawal of the stylet). These factors are covered elsewhere in this book, but, in general, the basic principle is that the larger the needle, the more bloody the sample and the less happy the cytopathologist.

The 22-G needle has been the standard size for many years, but equivalent results can be obtained using the 25-G format, the latter being as useful for pancreatic sampling as it is for lymph nodes. The use of negative pressure is to be avoided for soft lesions (lymph nodes, neuroendocrine tumors, and gastrointestinal stromal tumors [GISTs]) and may be of questionable value for sampling other solid pancreatic lesions. A 22-G needle is the standard size to puncture small- or medium-sized cystic lesions. If the needle tip is in a good position (i.e., away from the wall/septation) and the tap seemingly dry, it is worthwhile changing to a 19-G needle because the lesion may be mucoid. A capacity to fix the syringe plunger in different positions and to vary the degree of negative pressure is an advantage for any needle format.

The larger, stiffer, and more awkward 19-G needle is often required for larger cyst drainage becuase it will allow for a quicker procedure, the aspiration of viscous contents, and, where needed, the passage of a 0.035-inch guidewire. Core samples of nodes and lesions such as GISTs may be obtained using this large needle, without resorting to the Tru-Cut model.

Two newer variations on sampling needles are: (1) the "ProCore" series from Cook that has a sharp edged "carve-out" near the needle tip, which in principle can obtain a tissue fragment as well as cytology; and (2) the Beacon FNA needle that allows the endoscopist to use a "delivery system" that remains in place while the needle can be taken out for processing and another one (even of different size) used during that time.

Cook

Cook produces a broad, multipurpose range of fully disposable EUS FNA needles (Echotip; 19 G, 22 G, and 25 G). They have a one-piece, sturdy, comfortable/ergonomic handle, easily adaptable to the length of scope. Furthermore, the green-sheathed, slippery-coated EUSN-3 22 G needle can be passed with great ease, even under conditions of marked scope torque. Both the 25-G and 19-G needles retain the older, less slippery EUSN-1 blue sheath. The 19-G needle is difficult to advance when the scope is beyond the pylorus. The three needle sizes come with a two-step, double-trigger (5 mL/10 mL) suction syringe.

The EUSN-1 range comes with a stylet with a tip beveled to the needle tip, whereas a protruding ball-tip stylet accompanies the EUSN-3 needles. The ball-tip version might protect the scope channel should the needle be deployed accidentally. In general use, the ball-tip stylet must be withdrawn a centimeter or so before puncture in order to "sharpen" the needle. Immediately following puncture and before sampling, the stylet is pushed in to extrude any plugs of extraneous tissue. If you have a small channel "puncture" scope from Olympus or Hitachi-Pentax, check whether the needle will pass before ordering.

A 19-G Tru-Cut needle (Figure 2-6) will yield core samples. The Cook "Quick-Core" needle, however, is often neither quick to use nor does it always produce a core. The stiffness inherent to 19-G needles lessens the effectiveness of this instrument. While it can be deployed successfully in the mediastinum and stomach, transduodenal sampling is often impossible. The range of sites that can be sampled using the Tru-Cut is subject to local licensing.

Both 19-G and 22-G needles can be used for celiac axis neurolysis. A specially styled 20-G "spray" needle is available for this task from Cook (EUSN-20-CPN; certain geographic regions only). The needle has a solid, sharp, cone-tip with proximal side holes, in order to allow for a bilateral spray effect.

Pancreatic pseudocyst drainage with placement of a transgastric or duodenal stent is achieved using a combination of 19-G needle, guidewire, biliary dilatation balloon, and biliary endoprosthesis. Cook, however, produces a single-step, 8.5-Fr stent-loaded needle wire for this purpose (Giovannini needle wire; NWOA-8.5; certain geographic regions only). A 10-Fr cystotome delivering a 5-Fr catheter with 0.038-inch needle knife is also available (Cook CST-10; certain geographic regions only).

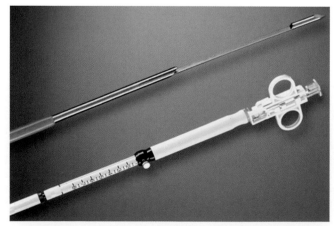

FIGURE 2-6 The Cook 19-G Tru-Cut needle ("Quick-core").

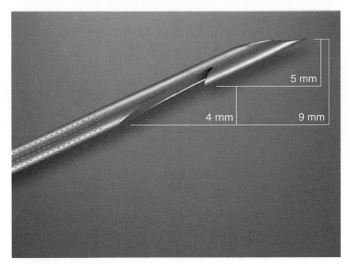

FIGURE 2-7 The Cook ProCore needle with cutting edge cut-out for obtaining tissue fragments.

Cystic, potentially neoplastic lesions of the pancreas present a specific problem for obtaining representative epithelial cell samples because standard aspirates are generally acellular. In order to address this difficulty, a dedicated EUS cytological brush (Echobrush) is available, but results are mixed. There are different ways to use this brush; one is to aspirate half the volume of the cyst (send for biochemistry; sample 1), pass the brush and sweep vigorously with the cytology brush (sample 2), and then aspirate the rest of the hopefully now cell-enriched fluid (sample 3). The occurrence of significant bleeding and a death have been reported for this tool.

The ProCore series of needles (19 G, 22 G, 25 G; Figure 2-7) carry a price premium and should allow a small tissue sample to be obtained. This though is far from a certain outcome.

Boston Scientific

Boston Scientific offers standard needles of sizes 19 G, 22 G and 25 G. The 19 G needle is worth mentioning as it is more flexible than the Cook equivalent and so, in theory, easier to deploy.

Olympus

Olympus produces both disposable and partially disposable FNA needles, as well as a spring-loaded device designed for hard lesions.

The single-sized (22 G), fully disposable FNA needle (EZ-Shot; NA-200H-8022) comes with a 20-mL suction syringe that will allow for variable degrees of negative pressure by twisting and locking the plunger in place. The brown-colored needle sheath is not as slippery as that of the Cook 22-G needle, making it slightly more difficult to deploy in the duodenum. Olympus also produces a reusable handle/sheath apparatus with a disposable needle piece (NA-10J-1).

The Olympus "Power-Shot" apparatus is a reusable, spring-loaded device that fires a disposable needle (22 G) into a lesion, to a defined depth (NA-11J-1). This instrument has been designed with pancreatic tumors in mind. It must be pointed out, however, that the majority of such tumors are in fact quite soft and that the sensation of "hardness" comes from poor scope positioning or the needle being gripped by the scope's elevator.

Mediglobe

The Mediglobe needles were perhaps the first dedicated EUS FNA needles to be developed. The disposable Sonotip Pro Control range (19 G, 22 G, and 25 G) have a similar "double-handle" structure to those from Boston Scientific and Cook, but it is a simple twist-lock, rather than a screw. The shape of the handle has been altered so that it is larger and easier to grip than in its previous incarnation. The stylet is of Nitinol and comes with both rounded (19 G, 22 G, and 25 G) and beveled (22 G) tips. Mediglobe offers two "thicknesses" of needle sheath, on the basis that needles might wobble in large channel scopes. In reality, as mentioned before, this is not a real clinical problem. The aspiration syringe allows for a fixed negative-pressure volume.

Beacon

Beacon needles are the biggest change from standard needles in that they allow for the needle "insert" itself to be removed fully for sample processing ("bnx system"; Figure 2-8). This allows the endoscopist to carry on taking further samples, even with a different caliber needle. There are various safety mechanisms in place to prevent needle-stick injuries and an aerosol effect. The delivery system comes with 19-G, 22-G, or 25-G needles, and additional needles come in packs of five. The 22-G and 25-G sizes can be bought in the format of a single delivery system with two needles, thus encouraging the use of two needles during a procedure.

Balloons

Proprietary balloons are offered by the major echoendoscope manufacturers but usually at exorbitant prices. International Medical Products (Zutphen, The Netherlands) offers cheaper, reliable balloons for the Olympus radial EUS scopes. Whereas regulatory bodies allow such generic substitution, it is always worthwhile asking colleagues from other centers in your region whether such products can be sourced.

As most EUS balloons contain latex (though US Endoscopy offer a latex-free version), standard echoendoscopy with a balloon should not be used in patients with latex sensitivity. Linear scopes can be used perfectly well without a balloon, or it may be possible, depending on the pathology in question, to use a mini-probe. Mini-probes from Olympus are latex free.

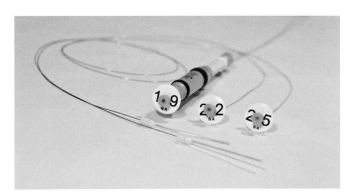

FIGURE 2-8 The Beacon delivery system with exchangeable needle inserts.

Water Pump

The UWS-1 water-instilling pump is available from Olympus in certain geographic regions. This pump permits the rapid instillation of water into the bowel lumen to allow for improved imaging of small, epithelial lesions. Care must be exercised when water is used in the esophagus without prior intubation. Furthermore, it is important to change a sterile connecting tube between each patient. It is always worth considering that sterile 50-mL syringes are universally available and cheap.

Reporting Systems

There is no good, universally available reporting system. Modules are offered by several sources including Endosoft, Unisoft, Fujinon (ADAM), and Olympus (EndoWorks, USA, and EndoBase, continental Europe). The major drawback with these and other programs is that they require a tremendous amount of work to "bed" them in for local use.

Archiving

Modern, "full-size" processors from all the major manufacturers have built-in image/video capture units including local hard disks, USB ports, or SD card slots. Potential to store images in a DICOM format to digital archives (as in radiology department PACS system) is common to current mid- and upper-range ultrasound processors. However, such software options may not be included in the "package" offered for EUS users and so must be discussed at the time of tender. If linking to a PACS system is possible, consider whether it will be for still images only and/or video images, because there will likely be storage capacity issues for anything other than short runs of video footage.

Lengthy paper streamers of photographs from a simple "hot" black and white printer are always satisfying to see after an examination. Such images are a good option for most cases and will not fade even after many years, although folded paper may stick together. Sending hard transparent copies to a laser printer is another, albeit more expensive, option.

Hard copy photographs can be scanned easily. If there is ever a chance that they might be used for publication, it is worthwhile scanning them as gray-scale images at a resolution of at least 300 dpi but preferably 500 dpi (most scanners have a default setting of 200 dpi).

Video image capture is a mainstay of EUS teaching. Whereas high-specification digital recorders are available, these are an expensive option. The best option is obviously to store to a USB stick, but other options are a standard laptop connected to an internally fixed video-out cable, or from the monitor or attached to the line-out connector of the printer.

Editing of captured video is simple using generally available programs such as those from Pinnacle or Nero. High-specification, very expensive video-editing software (e.g., Adobe) is not necessary.

Downloaded procedure videos may be prepared in a format called DICOM. There are several "converting" programs available for free on the internet that will convert DICOM to MPEG or the better quality .avi format files. The images from the .avi file type are of very high quality but, consequently, of very large size.

Video-editing programs offer to convert the snippets of movie into a range of formats including MPEG1, MPEG2, and avi. Choosing MPEG1-type movies is a compromise in terms of quality, but they are widely playable on most computers (this is important if you are going to use them for talks in many different places). Furthermore, most projectors used to show such videos cannot handle higher-quality file types. The MPEG2 format is superior to that of MPEG1 but will not play on many computers unless the appropriate piece of software (a "codec") has been installed. One minute of an MPEG1 movie will use approximately 11 MB of memory. Single, still frames can be captured from downloaded videos using Pinnacle, but the quality does not compare with that from "true" single-shot images taken at the time of the procedure.

When the EUS examination has been recorded, downloaded, edited, and put into a movie format, the next problem is how to show it. The easiest way is to double-click on the icon and allow a universal program like Windows Media Player (WMP) to show it. This approach gives the advantage of control. The buttons of WMP allow freezing, fast forwarding, and other features. Another approach is to "insert" the movie into PowerPoint. This will permit annotation and the incorporation of stills. PowerPoint, however, is not very good at handling video, and MPEG2 files are particularly problematic. Current smart phones are capable of storing large amounts of video and displaying them with good fidelity, even when only placed on the platform of a video-type X-ray viewing box/projector.

Patient confidentiality is a problem with videos because masking names with a black box will not work in PowerPoint; this program automatically puts any video in front of anything else on that page. Video-editing programs will allow one to place a mask, but it can be tedious to work this out. In general, it is much easier not to put the patient's name/details on the EUS screen at all.

Choosing Equipment

The equipment for endoscopic ultrasound is expensive and, consequently, compromise is an ever-present reality. It is worth restating several points that ought to be addressed in drafting a call for tenders.

The single most important question to be answered is this: What is the equipment for? It is too easy to find a need for every type of equipment, but such loose thinking makes for an unfocussed business plan.

Small lesions, celiac neurolysis, and pancreatic pseudocyst drainage are niche areas. The cornerstone of most EUS practice is cancer staging, supported possibly by benign work to extend equipment usage further (e.g., the substitution of EUS for MRI in the investigation of possible choledocholithiasis). Another consideration is that not all centers will manage all types of cancer.

If the staging of non–small-cell lung cancer will be a significant source of referrals, a linear system capable of FNA is an absolute requirement. The information yielded by radial EUS is of little value. The situation is less clear for both esophageal and pancreatic cancer staging and is heavily influenced by local practice.

In the United Kingdom, all operable esophageal cancers undergo neoadjuvant chemotherapy. Consequently, linear EUS is not an absolute requirement for initial staging. The clinical significance of involved local nodes after chemotherapy (to operate or administer further chemotherapy) is unknown, so does a positive nonceliac node FNA redirect management?

Pancreatic cancer can present an equally opaque decision process. If the lesion is operable, what is the role of FNA, and does it add any useful information? If the lesion is inoperable, can a percutaneous biopsy not be performed? Perhaps a radial scan is all that is required.

The point of these preceding few paragraphs is to highlight the importance of detailing exactly how EUS is to be used and where it might fit in a local care pathway algorithm. This will help to prioritize equipment need.

Once the decision has been made about what the equipment is for, the next issue to tackle is which system to buy. Taking linear systems, is there a difference in the performance characteristics between the linear echoendoscopes? Could the shape of the different transducers translate into better or worse endosonographic views? In essence, the answers are "no" and "no."

Outside regions where nonradiologists routinely perform transabdominal ultrasound, discussions with radiologic colleagues will often yield preferences for one manufacturer over another, but it must be remembered that a significant amount of the capability of these processors is redundant to EUS.

There is little advantage in buying a top-end processor over a more modest one, providing that the quality of screen image is adequate. Most processors are ergonomically similar to use.

The case for a high-specification processor might come from audiology and endoscopy sharing the unit. If this is the case, it ought to be considered that moving a complex electronic machine around an institution exposes it to risk, not to mention the inevitable aggravation of both parties needing it at the same time.

Cost is very much, like beauty, in the eye of the beholder. There are regional differences between how companies compete. In some areas, cost is the paramount issue, whereas in others a perception of quality carries a premium. The final price will be a balance between how much the unit is willing to pay and how much the company needs the business or the badge of a recognized, "trophy" name.

When choosing EUS equipment, the costs go beyond those of the initial setup alone. The equipment is delicate, and pressure to train fellows exposes it to significant wear and tear. Support packages that include the availability of replacement echoendoscopes is of great importance. The devil here is in the detail, as cheaper scopes may come with very expensive and/or weak service support. When obtaining bids for new scopes ask for full, "no question" running costs over 5 years to be included in the price offered.

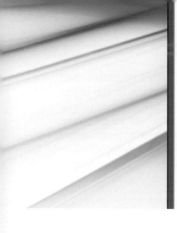

3

Training and Simulators

Wajeeh Salah • Douglas O. Faigel

Key Points

- EUS is an advanced endoscopic procedure that requires a level of training exceeding that of general endoscopy. Acquisition of the skills necessary to perform EUS competently often requires training beyond the scope of a traditional gastroenterology fellowship program.
- Competence in routine endoscopic procedures should be documented because it provides a vital foundation for EUS training.
- Competence in EUS requires both cognitive and technical skills, including an understanding of the appropriate indications for EUS, performance of appropriate preprocedure and postprocedure evaluations, and management of procedure-related complications.
- A variety of tools are available to gauge and assess competency in EUS as well as assist in the training process. These include newly developed survey tools that can be combined with digital video recordings of EUS cases.
- EUS simulators, both computer based and porcine explant based, continue to be developed and refined. As new generations of simulators continue to improve they may have a role as an adjunct to the training process at select institutions.
- On successful completion of EUS training, the trainee must be able to integrate EUS into the overall clinical evaluation of the patient as well as communicate the EUS findings to both the patient and the multidisciplinary team.
- An important part of training in EUS should include training in gastrointestinal tumor staging and the TNM classification system. At the completion of EUS training, the trainee should be able to demonstrate accuracy and competency in the staging of gastrointestinal tumors.
- A general consensus of expert endosonographers suggests that luminal endosonography requires at least 3 to 6 months of intensive training to establish competency and that pancreatobiliary EUS and fine-needle aspiration may require up to 1 year.
- Each program that teaches EUS should be able to provide sufficient numbers of procedures that will substantially surpass those required for minimal competence.
- The threshold number of EUS FNA cases needed to achieve competence has not been studied. However, it is generally agreed that FNA of pancreatic lesions is more complex and carries a higher risk than EUS FNA at other anatomic sites.

Over the two past decades, endoscopic ultrasound (EUS) has emerged as a valuable endoscopic resource for the diagnosis and treatment of a variety of gastrointestinal disorders including, but not limited to, pancreatic cysts, mucosal and submucosal tumors, chronic pancreatitis, and various gastrointestinal malignancies. The diagnosis, staging, and treatment of gastrointestinal cancers have evolved into a multidisciplinary approach often utilizing endosonography as a central tool for both diagnosis and staging. Multiple studies have demonstrated the superiority of EUS compared to conventional abdominal computed tomography (CT) in the staging of esophageal, gastric, and pancreatic cancers.[1–4] Furthermore, the advent of endoscopic ultrasound-guided fine-needle aspiration (EUS FNA) provides an alternative approach to traditional percutaneous biopsies obtained under CT or ultrasound guidance. Moreover, compared to other modalities, EUS FNA results from pancreatic masses are superior with sensitivities ranging between 85% to 90% and a specificity of 100%.[5,6] Recently, therapeutic applications of EUS have been developed to gain access to the bile and pancreatic ducts, drain fluid collections, treat bleeding, and inject tumor suppressing agents.[7] The introduction of endoscopic ultrasound into clinical practice has revolutionized the field of gastroenterology, in particular gastrointestinal oncology, with potential applications continuing to evolve.

As the applications for EUS have become increasingly recognized by other clinical practitioners, the demand for well-trained endosonographers has increased.[8] The limited availability of EUS is largely due to a lack of skilled endosonographers. Additional barriers include equipment cost, ease of use, and reimbursement costs. A relative lack of training centers combined with the extensive commitment required by the trainee has limited the growth of EUS and its availability in community practices. Ensuring adequate training of practicing endosonographers has become a priority for the American Society for Gastrointestinal Endoscopy (ASGE), evidenced by the guidelines and core curriculum set forth on advanced training in EUS.[9] EUS is an advanced endoscopic procedure that requires a level of training exceeding that of general endoscopy. Acquisition of the skills necessary for conducting and understanding EUS often requires training beyond the scope of a traditional gastroenterology fellowship program. Additional training often involves a 1-year fellowship following completion of an accredited gastroenterology training program. Although a minority of gastroenterology training programs provide adequate exposure to EUS during a traditional 3-year fellowship, providing only a brief exposure to EUS and allowing independent practice by inadequately trained fellows is unacceptable. While clinical workshops with hands-on training may provide an understanding for the indications and complications of EUS, they are not a substitute for formal fellowship training. This chapter covers the guidelines for individual trainees, training programs, and credentialing in EUS. Although computer-based training simulators are in their infancy in the field of endosonography, they represent an exciting adjunct to formal training and will also be discussed.

Guidelines for Training

Guidelines for training in advanced endoscopy have previously been published by the American Society for Gastrointestinal Endoscopy.[10] Although many gastroenterology training programs have incorporated advanced endoscopy training into the second and third year curriculum, the majority of programs are now requiring an additional fourth year of training for advanced procedures (i.e., endoscopic retrograde cholangiopancreatography [ERCP], EUS). EUS training is available at relatively few academic centers in the United States Currently, there are more than 50 recognized programs in the United States offering a fourth year fellowship in EUS (American Society for Gastrointestinal Endoscopy [ASGE] website: www.asge.org). Many of these programs provide dual training in both ERCP and EUS, while others separate the training into either EUS or ERCP. Although these programs may vary in the design of their training experience, two critical components are necessary for a qualified training program: large patient volume and recognized faculty expertise.

In certain unusual circumstances, a trainee may acquire the necessary skills for EUS in a standard 3-year fellowship provided that an adequate patient volume is available, and the trainee can demonstrate the necessary aptitude and skills required for advanced endoscopy. However, given the complexity of these procedures and necessary volume of cases required to achieve competency, it seems less likely that an individual would be adequately trained in a traditional 3-year program. A survey by Azad and colleagues found that the majority of gastroenterology fellowship programs in the United States have established the necessary EUS volume to annually train at least one EUS fellow.[11] However, most 3-year and many advanced fellows receive insufficient EUS training according to ASGE guidelines.[11] For 3-year GI fellows, 55% received less than 3 months of training with 43% not receiving actual "hands-on" experience, and 61% not learning EUS-guided FNA. Programs offering advanced training in EUS had a median advanced-trainee EUS volume of 200 procedures (range 50-1100). Of the advanced fellows, 20% failed to receive hands-on training and 52% performed less than 200 procedures. Although there are limitations to this study, the findings highlight some of the inadequacies in training for EUS and demonstrate areas for improvement.

Competency is defined as the minimum level of skill, knowledge, and/or expertise acquired through training and experience, required to safely and proficiently perform a task or procedure.[12] Unfortunately, there have been few published reports regarding training of individuals in EUS or the number of procedures required to attain competence.[13-20] A common goal for all gastroenterology training programs is the production of knowledgeable, experienced, and competent endoscopists. Recognizing this goal and understanding the limitations of a 3-year curriculum has been the major impetus for establishing fourth year fellowships in EUS.

Although the demand for qualified endosonographers is increasing, not all trainees should pursue such advanced training due to both variations in individual skill level and regional manpower needs. Similarly, not all training programs should offer EUS training due to restraints on patient volume and faculty interests. Individuals wishing to pursue further training in EUS must have completed at least 24 months of a standard GI fellowship or demonstrate equivalent training. Moreover, competence in routine endoscopic procedures should be documented as it provides a vital foundation for advanced endoscopic training. Obviously, trainees in endoscopy develop skills at widely varying rates that can be evaluated objectively by experienced endoscopists. However, the use of an absolute or threshold number of procedures may be misleading and should therefore be employed with caution in the evaluation of individual trainees. The minimum number of procedures required to achieve competency in EUS will vary based on the individual's skill level, understanding of ultrasound principles, and quality of the training experience. Performing an arbitrary number of procedures does not necessarily guarantee competency. Although the Standards of Practice Committee of the ASGE published a minimum number of procedures necessary to perform before assessing competency (Table 3-1), these numbers simply represent a minimum requirement and should serve only as a guide for evaluating individual trainees. These numbers are derived from studies on training in EUS, published expert opinion, and consensus of the Ad Hoc EUS and Standards of Practice committees of the ASGE. Many, if not most, trainees will require procedure numbers in excess of these minimum requirements. A prospective multicenter study of five advanced endoscopy trainees, without any previous EUS experience, evaluated the variation in learning curves for EUS.[16] This study showed a substantial variability in achieving

MINIMUM NUMBER OF EUS PROCEDURES REQUIRED BEFORE COMPETENCY CAN BE ASSESSED

Site/Lesion	Number of Cases Required
Mucosal tumors (cancers of the esophagus, stomach, and rectum)	75
Submucosal abnormalities	40
Pancreaticobiliary	75
EUS-guided FNA	50 (25 of which are pancreatic FNA)
Nonpancreatic	25
Pancreatic	25
Comprehensive competence	150[a]

[a]Including at least 75 pancreaticobiliary and 50 FNA procedures.
ASGE 2001 Guidelines for credentialing and granting privileges for endoscopic ultrasound. *Gastrointest Endosc.* 2001;54:811-814. Reviewed and reapproved 11/08.

competency and that some trainees may require nearly double (or more in some cases) the minimum number of procedures required to achieve competency. Ideally, competency should be gauged on objective criteria and direct observation by an experienced endosonographer.

A variety of tools and techniques have been proposed to gauge and assess competency in EUS. A recent study utilized a combination of a newly developed survey assessment tool designed to measure competence in EUS FNA for mediastinal staging of non–small-cell lung cancer (NSCLC), in addition to direct expert observation and video-based performance review.[20] In this study, three advanced endoscopy trainees and three experienced endosonographers performed EUS-guided FNA on a total of 30 patients with proven or suspected NSCLC. They received evaluation by direct observation by three experienced endosonographers. Digital video recordings of these procedures were made and reviewed by the expert endosonographers in a blinded fashion 2 months later. Experienced endosonographers then completed a scoring sheet called the Endoscopic Ultrasound Assessment Tool (EUSAT). The EUSAT is a scoring sheet that was specifically created for the standardized assessment of EUS-guided FNA in mediastinal staging of NSCLC. The assessment consisted of 12 items related to the techniques of endoscope insertion, identification, and presentation of anatomic landmarks, and biopsy sampling. The results showed that there was good intrarater reliability based on direct observation and blinded video recording, and that the assessment tool was able to provide an objective discrimination between trainees and expert physicians. This suggests that objective assessment tools can be combined with direct supervision and video-based feedback to create a high-quality EUS training experience.

Competence in EUS requires both cognitive and technical skills,[21] including an understanding of the appropriate indications for endoscopic ultrasound, conducting appropriate preprocedure and postprocedure evaluations, and managing procedure-related complications. Trainees must be able to perform the procedure in a safe and efficient manner while also recognizing and understanding the ultrasound images. Furthermore, understanding the implications for EUS in

staging gastrointestinal malignancies must be appreciated for integration of the endosonographic findings into the treatment plan for each patient (i.e., surgical versus medical and/or radiation oncology referrals). Formal supervised EUS training should also include reviews of cross-sectional anatomy, atlases of endoscopic or abdominal ultrasonography, video recordings of teaching cases, and didactic courses in EUS. A combination of well-supervised EUS procedures and didactic teaching will aid in assuring an adequate training experience as well as an overall understanding of endoscopic ultrasonography.

A crucial component to any EUS training program is focused on gastrointestinal tumor staging. When available, EUS has become the standard of care in staging several gastrointestinal malignancies, including esophageal, gastric, rectal, and pancreatic cancers. Determining the accuracy of tumor staging by a trainee is an important aspect of training by allowing the differentiation between potentially curable early stage tumors and unresectable late-stage tumors. Studies in endosonographic staging of esophageal cancer suggested that at least 75 to 100 procedures were required before an acceptable level of accuracy was achieved.[14,15] Ideally, the accuracy of EUS staging should be compared to a gold standard such as surgical histopathology; however, surgical specimens are not always readily available and patients may have received preoperative radiation and chemotherapy that may affect staging. In these circumstances, staging by a trainee should be compared to that of a skilled and competent endosonographer. Appropriate documentation of all EUS procedures in a training log, along with review of surgical pathology results, will further assist in determining both the quantity and accuracy of tumor staging cases.

Upon successful completion of EUS training, the trainee must be able to integrate EUS into the overall clinical evaluation of the patient. A thorough understanding of the indications, contraindications, individual risk factors, and benefit-risk considerations for individual patients must be demonstrated. Being able to clearly and accurately describe the procedure and obtain informed consent is a necessary requirement. A knowledge of the gastrointestinal anatomy and surrounding anatomic structures as imaged by EUS and of the technical features of the equipment, workstation, and accessories is vital for future independent practice. The trainee must be able to safely intubate the esophagus, pylorus, and duodenum to acquire the necessary images. Moreover, accurately identifying and interpreting the EUS images and recognizing normal and abnormal findings must be demonstrated and assessed by the mentor. The trainee should be able to achieve an accuracy in tumor staging comparable to that within the medical literature (Table 3-2).[9] It is also essential that the trainee understand the basic principles through which ultrasound waves create an image through various mediums as well as the principles of Doppler imaging and how it is used to identify and differentiate vascular structures.[9] The trainee must be able to document and communicate the EUS findings with referring physicians and understand the implications of these findings in formulating treatment plans for patient care. Adhering to these training requirements for EUS will further assist in assuring the production of skilled endosonographers.

Lastly, it is important for the trainee to understand and be able to document quality measures of endosonography such

TABLE 3-2

REPORTED ACCURACY OF EUS COMPARED TO HISTOPATHOLOGY FOR THE LOCAL STAGING OF ESOPHAGEAL CARCINOMA, GASTRIC CANCER, AMPULLARY CARCINOMA, AND RECTAL CANCER

Indication	Number of Procedures	T Stage	N Stage
Esophageal cancer	739	85%	79%
Gastric cancer	1163	78%	73%
Pancreatic cancer	155	90%	—
Ampullary carcinoma	94	86%	72%
Rectal cancer	19	84%	84%

ASGE. Guidelines for Training in Endoscopic Ultrasound. *Gastrointest Endosc.* 1999;49:829-833.

as the proper indication for performing EUS as well as visualization and description of the anatomic structures of interest relevant to the procedure's indication.[22] Evaluating quality measures such as the use of prophylactic antibiotics prior to FNA of a cystic lesion and the appropriate use of EUS-guided FNA is a necessary part of EUS training. Also, keeping a record of complication rates of EUS procedures (i.e., the incidence of pancreatitis, infection, or bleeding after FNA) is an essential part of EUS training and quality improvement.

Training Program Requirements

Although several institutions across the U.S., Canada, and Europe offer brief training courses in endoscopic ultrasound, these programs provide only limited exposure and arguably do not adequately train individuals as independent endosonographers. While formal, supervised training is the most accepted mode of training, experience may be gained in other settings, such as hands-on short courses, use of animal models, EUS teaching video recordings, and computer-based training simulators. However, these teaching methods simply represent useful adjuncts to formal training and should not be used in lieu of a more formal supervised training experience. One retrospective study showed that endosonographers with a formal supervised training experience in pancreaticobiliary EUS achieved a significantly higher sensitivity when using EUS FNA for the diagnosis of pancreatic malignancy as compared to those without formal FNA training.[17] A general consensus by expert endosonographers suggests that luminal endosonography requires at least 3 to 6 months of intensive training to establish competency whereas pancreaticobiliary EUS and FNA may require up to 1year.[23] In fact, one study demonstrated a learning curve for EUS-guided FNA of solid pancreatic masses following third-tier EUS training, suggesting that the learning curve continues to develop after fellowship training because more procedures are needed to gain proficiency and efficiency with EUS-guided FNA.[24] Although short courses and computer-based learning are useful, this form of training without direct supervision may result in an inadequate understanding and appreciation for the technical challenges and complexity of EUS.

When considering advanced training in endoscopic ultrasound, a trainee should investigate all aspects of the training program. Arguably, the most important aspect to a training program is the reputation and expertise of the endosonographer. Programs should have a minimum of one skilled endosonographer who is acknowledged as an expert by his/her peers and is committed to teaching EUS. Unfortunately, the majority of EUS programs across the United States have limited, if any, extramural funding and may require additional clinical responsibilities to help support the trainee's salary. While understanding the financial limitations of most institutions, training programs should strive to limit the clinical responsibilities unrelated to EUS when developing their core curriculum. Ideally, programs should provide protected research time and encourage academic pursuits such as designing research protocols, preparing manuscripts, writing grant proposals, and attending EUS courses. Creating an environment emphasizing endoscopic research and clinical investigation should be a fundamental goal for each training program. Trainees should be provided with the protected time and necessary funds to attend at least one scientific meeting during the course of their training, preferably one related to endosonography. A common goal for all committed trainees should be presenting their endoscopic research at either a national or international meeting. Exposure to endoscopy unit management including scheduling, staffing, equipment maintenance, and management skills is also a valuable asset to any training program. Many trainees in EUS may pursue future academic positions, and these are invaluable skills to acquire early in an academic career. Although a common goal for most training programs is the development of future academic endosonographers, some trainees may express different career interests that conflict with the goals of the training program. Understanding and recognizing the program's expectations and trainee's career interests is crucial to an enjoyable and successful training experience.

Each program in EUS should have the ability to provide sufficient numbers of procedures that will substantially surpass those required for minimal competence (Table 3-1). Although a large procedure volume does not necessarily guarantee competence, it is highly unlikely that a low volume of cases will provide sufficient exposure to these highly complicated and technically challenging procedures to allow adequate assessment of competency. Requiring a large volume of cases is not an elitist attempt by tertiary centers to exclude others from potential training opportunities, but rather an attempt at guaranteeing the delivery of skilled endosonographers into the workforce and answering the demand for endoscopic ultrasound. For these reasons, training in EUS has largely been limited to academic tertiary centers with highly skilled endosonographers conducting a large volume of cases, thus ensuring retention of the necessary skills to train individuals interested in learning EUS.

Equally important to the technical training of endosonography is the cognitive training. This curriculum should focus on a thorough understanding of the relevant anatomic and clinical aspects of EUS (Box 3-1). These include knowledge of the cross-sectional anatomy of the human body and understanding the principles of ultrasonography. EUS will be used to stage malignancies, and the trainee must understand not only TNM staging but also how these stages will be used to guide therapy. The trainee must be able to describe the indications and risks of EUS, understand the alternatives to EUS and their strengths and limitations, understand and use EUS terminology so as to effectively and accurately report EUS findings, and demonstrate interpersonal and communication skills. In cases where EUS is used in the diagnosis of cancers, the trainee must be able to communicate EUS findings in a compassionate and sensitive manner to the patient. Also, the trainee must be able to effectively communicate with the multidisciplinary team and participate in the coordination of patient care.

Credentialing in EUS

Credentialing is the process of assessing and validating the qualifications of a licensed independent practitioner to provide patient care. Determining qualifications for credentialing is based upon an assessment of the individual's current medical license, knowledge base, training and/or experience, current competence, and ability to independently perform the procedure or patient care requested. The ASGE has provided guidelines for credentialing and granting hospital privileges to perform routine gastrointestinal endoscopy.[25] Furthermore, the ASGE has also established guidelines for credentialing and granting privileges in advanced endoscopic procedures, including endoscopic ultrasound.[26] Credentialing for EUS should be determined separately from other endoscopic procedures such as sigmoidoscopy, colonoscopy, esophagogastroduodenoscopy, ERCP, or any other endoscopic procedure. Determining competency and qualifications for credentialing can be somewhat challenging, because trained individuals possess varying degrees of skill in EUS along with recognized limitations. Nevertheless, providing a minimum number of procedures necessary prior to assessing competency (Table 3-1) creates objective criteria for assessment in the credentialing process. As with credentialing in general gastrointestinal endoscopy, competency is ultimately assessed by the training director or other independent proctor.

EUS is performed in a variety of anatomic locations for various indications.[27] These locations include evaluation and staging of mucosally based neoplasms (esophagus, stomach, colon, and rectum), evaluation of subepithelial abnormalities,

assessment of the pancreas and pancreaticobiliary ducts, and performance of EUS-guided FNA. An endoscopist may be competent in one or more of these areas depending on his/her level of training and interest. Privileging in one or more of these areas may be considered separately, but training must be considered adequate in the areas for which privileging is requested.

Mucosal Tumors

Safe intubation of the esophagus, pylorus, and duodenum is essential when evaluating mucosal tumors in the esophagus, stomach, and duodenum. Accurate imaging of the lesion and recognition of surrounding lymphadenopathy, in particular the celiac axis region for upper tract cancers, is critical to the diagnosis and correct staging of mucosally based tumors. Evaluation of rectal cancers should include intubation of the sigmoid colon and identification of the iliac vessels. A prospective study reported competent intubation of the esophagus, stomach, and duodenum was achieved in 1 to 23 procedures (median 1-2), with visualization of the gastric or esophageal wall in 1 to 47 procedures (median 10-15).[13] Adequate evaluation of the celiac axis region required 8 to 36 procedures (median 10-15). Unfortunately, there are limited studies addressing the learning curve for evaluating mucosal tumors of the gastrointestinal tract. Only two studies have addressed the learning curve in staging esophageal cancers. Fockens and colleagues reported that adequate staging accuracy was achieved only after 100 examinations, while Schlick and colleagues reported an 89.5% T stage accuracy after a minimum of 75 cases.[14,15] A survey of the American Endosonography Club in 1995 suggested an average 43 cases for esophageal imaging, 44 for gastric, and 37 for the rectum.[28] Once competence is achieved in one anatomic location, the threshold number of procedures for other anatomic locations may be reduced depending on the skill and training of the endosonographer. The ASGE currently recommends a minimum of 75 supervised cases, with at least two thirds in the upper gastrointestinal tract, before competency for evaluating mucosal tumors can be assessed.[26]

Subepithelial Abnormalities

Evaluation of subepithelial lesions has become a common indication for EUS. Discriminating between neoplasms, varices, enlarged gastric folds, and extrinsic compression from extramural masses can be performed with traditional echoendoscopes or catheter-based ultrasound probes. With the advent of the catheter-based probes, some practitioners have developed competency in subepithelial abnormalities without achieving competence in other indications for EUS. Although no studies are available for determining the threshold number of cases required to accurately assess subepithelial abnormalities, the ASGE Standards or Practice Committee currently recommends a minimum of 40 to 50 supervised cases.[29]

Pancreaticobiliary Imaging

Most endosonographers will agree that accurate imaging and interpretation of images of the pancreaticobiliary system including the gallbladder, bile duct, pancreatic duct, and ampulla are more technically challenging than evaluating mucosal and submucosal lesions. For this reason, a larger volume of supervised pancreaticobiliary cases is required before competence can be adequately assessed. A multicenter, 3-year prospective study reported that adequate imaging of the pancreatic and bile ducts required 13 to 135 cases (median 55), whereas imaging of the pancreatic parenchyma required 15 to 74 cases (median 34).[13] Adequate assessment of the ampulla required 13 to 134 cases (median 54). Although technical competence in pancreaticobiliary imaging may be achieved in less than 100 cases, a survey from the American Endosonography Club suggests that interpretive competence of pancreatic images may require additional procedures (120 cases).[28] Other expert opinion suggests a higher threshold of 150 cases before assessing interpretative competence.[21] Currently, the ASGE Standards of Practice Committee recommends a minimum of 75 pancreaticobiliary cases before competency can be assessed.[26]

EUS-Guided FNA

EUS-guided FNA has emerged as an important diagnostic tool for obtaining tissue from intramural lesions, perigastrointestinal adenopathy, pancreatic lesions, and others.[30] Training in EUS-guided FNA requires knowledge of basic endoscopic ultrasound principles along with mastery of the skills necessary for obtaining and interpreting EUS images. Understanding and appreciating the complexity and risk that EUS-guided FNA add to the procedure is critical for successful training. Unfortunately, the threshold number of FNA cases needed to achieve competence has not been studied. However, it is generally agreed that EUS-guided FNA of pancreatic lesions carries a higher complexity and risk for potential complications than other anatomic sites. Therefore the number of cases required for FNA of pancreatic lesions is considered separately from other anatomic locations. For nonpancreatic lesions (i.e., intramural lesions, lymph nodes, ascites), it is recommended that a trainee be competent in nonpancreatic EUS and conduct at least 25 supervised FNA cases before competency can be assessed.[26] Competence in EUS-guided FNA of pancreatic lesions requires demonstration of competence in pancreaticobiliary EUS (at least 75 cases) in addition to 25 supervised FNA procedures of pancreatic lesions.[26] A recent study has suggested that introducing training in EUS-guided FNA from the onset of training is a safe and feasible way to help maximize exposure to FNA during training.[19] This is the first reported study looking at the safety and diagnostic yield of EUS FNA by attending supervised advanced endoscopy trainees. It found similar diagnostic yield between attending versus fellow FNA passes when the trainee is supervised. Due to the absence of literature supporting a threshold number for EUS-guided FNA, these threshold numbers were adopted from the guidelines set forth for therapeutic ERCP. The current recommendation suggests that a minimum of 50 EUS-guided FNA procedures be performed during training.[9] The similarities between EUS and ERCP, such as side viewing instruments and combined endoscopic and radiologic imaging, led to these recommendations. Larger clinical studies addressing this question for EUS-guided FNA of pancreatic and nonpancreatic lesions are needed to further assess the validity of these recommendations.

One of the problems facing EUS trainees is the absence of an appropriate model for teaching EUS-guided FNA. Practicing EUS-guided FNA on a model prior to performing on a patient may potentially avoid safety and credentialing issues that would ordinarily limit the trainee endosonographer. Recently, Parupudi and colleagues developed a porcine model for EUS-guided FNA.[31] The authors injected autologous blood admixed with carbon particles into the mediastinal lymph nodes of female pigs. After two weeks, the pigs were re-examined with EUS demonstrating significant lymph node enlargement, thereby allowing EUS-guided FNA of lymph nodes in various locations within the mediastinum. A small study using this porcine model was recently conducted to evaluate its effect on trainees' performance on EUS-guided FNA of simulated lymph nodes.[18] This study showed that animal training with this porcine model led to improved trainee performance in the accuracy, speed, and adequacy of sampling. This represents an interesting in vivo hands-on porcine model for future training in EUS-guided FNA.

Advanced and Interventional EUS

In addition to the standard techniques used in EUS, there have been a number of newly described advanced EUS diagnostic and therapeutic procedures.[9] EUS elastography has been used to analyze the tissue stiffness of solid pancreatic masses and may be useful in differentiating between benign and malignant lesions.[32] In cases when ERCP is unsuccessful, the use of EUS in establishing biliary and pancreatic ductal access has been described as an alternative to percutaneous transhepatic cholangiography or surgery.[33] The use of EUS as part of a less invasive treatment approach for the drainage of symptomatic pancreatic fluid collections[34] and for pain relief by celiac plexus neurolysis and block[35] has also been described. EUS may also have a role in providing vascular access and therapy for conditions such as gastric variceal hemorrhage.[36] It is important to realize that many of these applications are still being developed and that there are no currently accepted training guidelines or competency criteria to allow for their evaluation during EUS training.

Comprehensive EUS Competence

Some practitioners may be interested in acquiring competence in only one or two areas of EUS and can therefore focus their efforts on specific anatomic locations as outlined above. However, for those practitioners interested in achieving competence in multiple areas of EUS, training must include exposure to a variety of procedures with differing clinical pathology. It is generally recognized that once competence in one area of EUS has been established, the number of cases required to achieve competence in other areas may be reduced. For trainees interested in only mucosal and submucosal lesions, it is generally recommended that a minimum of 100 supervised cases be performed. Consideration for comprehensive EUS competence, including pancreaticobiliary imaging and FNA, requires a minimum of 150 cases, including 50 EUS-guided FNAs and at least 75 pancreaticobiliary cases.[26]

Recredentialing and Renewal of EUS Privileges

Over the course of time, physicians who have received appropriate privileges to perform EUS may change the scope of their clinical practice and subsequently reduce the frequency of performing one or more endoscopic ultrasound procedures. It has been suggested that ongoing experience in advanced endoscopy is necessary to retain the technical skills required to safely and adequately perform these technically challenging procedures.[37,38] The goal of recredentialing is to assure continued clinical competence while promoting continuous quality improvement and maintaining patient safety. If ongoing experience is not maintained at some objective level, the quality of care provided to the patient may diminish, potentially leading to adverse events.

The ASGE has provided useful guidelines for renewing endoscopic privileges and assuring continued clinical competence in EUS.[39] However, it is the responsibility of each institution to develop and maintain individual guidelines for granting and renewing privileges. The threshold number of procedures necessary for recredentialing may vary between institutions; however, this threshold must be commensurate with the technical and cognitive skills required for advanced procedures such as EUS. Individual institutions must establish a frequency for the renewal process along with contingency plans when minimal competence cannot be assured. The Joint Commission has mandated that renewal of clinical endoscopic privileges be made for a period of no more than two years.[40] Endosonographers seeking renewal of privileges must document an adequate case load over a set period of time in order to maintain the necessary skills required for EUS. This documentation may include procedure log books or patient records, and should focus on objective measures such as number of cases, success rates, and complications. It is also important that endosonographers keep qualitative records of EUS, which may include indications for the EUS procedure as well as any complications from FNA. Ongoing quality improvement efforts may be assessed as part of the recredentialing process and may include measurement of specific quality metrics and diagnostic yield of EUS-guided FNA.[22] Continued cognitive training through participation in educational activities should also be a prerequisite for the renewal of privileges. New EUS procedures and clinical applications continue to emerge, requiring a commitment to continued medical education within this specialized field.

Simulators in Endoscopic Ultrasound

Endoscopic simulators have been developed for training in flexible sigmoidoscopy, esophagogastroduodenoscopy, colonoscopy, ERCP, and most recently EUS.[41] Since development of the first endoscopic mannequin simulator in the late 1960s,[42] considerable technological advances have been made in the development of endoscopic simulators. A variety of simulators are available today, ranging from animal-based simulators (Erlangen Endo-Trainer; Erlangen Germany) to the computer-based simulators manufactured by CAE Healthcare (Endo VR Simulator; Montreal, Quebec, Canada) and Simbionix Corp. (GI-Mentor II; Cleveland, OH).[43] Validation studies and small, prospective, clinical trials assessing the utility of endoscopic

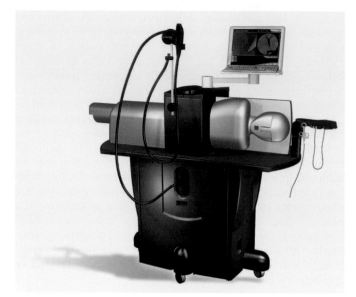

FIGURE 3-1 Simbionix GI-Mentor Simulator. *(Courtesy of Symbionix Corporation USA, Cleveland, OH.)*

simulators have been conducted for upper endoscopy, flexible sigmoidoscopy, and colonoscopy;[44-50] however, the benefits of simulator training have not been clearly demonstrated, emphasizing the need for further investigation with large, prospective trials. Nevertheless, this technology represents an exciting and potentially useful adjunct to formal endoscopic training.

Simbionix Corp. (www.simbionix.com) developed the first computer-based EUS simulator providing a platform for hands-on training and practice of EUS procedures (Figure 3-1).[43] The computer-based simulator generates ultrasound images in real-time from three-dimensional anatomic models constructed from CT and MRI images from real patients. The trainee inserts a customized echoendoscope into the specially designed GI-Mentor mannequin and simultaneously receives visual feedback from the monitor along with tactile sensation from scope maneuvering during the procedure. A highly sensitive tracking system translates position and direction of the camera into realistic computer-generated images. The EUS module allows the trainee to switch from endoscopic to ultrasound images in real time and also provides training in both radial and linear ultrasound probes. Split-screen capability provides ultrasound images alongside of three-dimensional anatomic maps further assisting in the interpretation and understanding of generated EUS images. The module also allows trainees to practice keyboard functions such as labeling of organs, magnifying images, changing frequencies, and measuring with calipers. Following completion of the examination, the computer software permits performance evaluation by reviewing all saved images (up to 50 frozen images per procedure) and indicating anatomy and landmarks that were improperly identified by the user.

Although the Simbionix GI-Mentor II EUS training module presents an exciting approach to training in EUS, there are currently no published validation studies or clinical trials assessing EUS simulators. A small study was published on learning EUS using the new Erlangen Active Simulator for Interventional Endoscopy (EASIE-R) (ENDOSIM, LLC, Nahant, MA).[51] This simulator consists of a complete porcine gastrointestinal tract explant with surrounding structures including the bile duct and pancreas, all embedded in an ultrasound gel. EASIE-R was used by 11 participants (five beginners and six experts) during a 1-day EUS course. Overall, the simulator was thought to be easy to use and useful for teaching both basic and advanced EUS techniques. More recently, data were presented from a study looking at the use of the EASIE-R simulator during three EUS hands-on courses. A total of 59 gastroenterologists who used the simulator completed a survey designed to assess the ease of use of the simulator and provide initial evaluation data.[52] More than half of the gastroenterologists surveyed had less than 1 year of experience with EUS. In this larger series, the simulator was again thought to be realistic, easy to use, and useful in the teaching of EUS skills. Although simulators represent useful educational tools, further studies are needed in a randomized controlled trial to determine their validity for EUS training. Unfortunately, these simulators are not readily available at most training institutions due to cost restraints and regional needs. However, at select institutions, there may be 1- to 2-week workshops in EUS allowing exposure to this technology.

Summary

EUS has become an important imaging tool for the evaluation of a variety of gastrointestinal disorders. It is a challenging endoscopic procedure requiring both cognitive and technical skills beyond the general scope of traditional gastroenterology fellowship training. As the demand for skilled endosonographers continues to increase, the guidelines for training must be critically analyzed to assure the production of well-trained and competent future endosonographers. Although guidelines have been established for credentialing and granting privileges in EUS, additional studies of threshold numbers necessary to achieve competence are needed to fill existing gaps in the current literature. Endoscopists interested in learning EUS must recognize and appreciate the complexity of these procedures and risks for potential complications. Clearly, a 1- to 2-week course in EUS is considered inadequate training and may potentially expose patients to unnecessary risks and poor quality of care. For those truly interested in mastering the skills required for EUS, a formal supervised training program is far superior to hands-on workshops, teaching video recordings, simulators, and inadequate exposure during a standard GI fellowship.

Simulators for training in EUS represent an exciting and useful adjunct to supervised instruction. Although clinical trials investigating the efficacy of simulators in EUS training are lacking, the potential applications for this technology are promising. Unfortunately, these simulators are not readily available at most institutions because of cost restraints and regional needs. Further studies are necessary to determine the role of endoscopic simulators in EUS training.

REFERENCES

1. Botet JF, Lightdale CJ, Zauber AG, et al. Preoperative staging of esophageal cancer: comparison of endoscopic US and dynamic CT. *Radiology.* 1991;181:419-425.

2. Ziegler K, Sanft C, Friedrich M, et al. Evaluation of computed tomography, endosonography, and intraoperative assessment in TN staging of gastric carcinoma. *Gut.* 1993;34:604-610.

3. Palazzo L, Roseau G, Gayet B, et al. Endoscopic ultrasonography in the diagnosis and staging of pancreatic adenocarcinoma: results of a prospective study with comparison to ultrasonography and CT scan. *Endoscopy.* 1993;25:143-150.

4. Muller MF, Meyenberger C, Bertschinger P, et al. Pancreatic tumors: evaluation with endoscopic US, CT and MR Imaging. *Radiology.* 1994;190:745-751.

5. Wiersema MJ, Vilmann P, Giovannini M, et al. Endosonography-guided fine needle aspiration biopsy: diagnostic accuracy and complication assessment. *Gastroenterology.* 1997;112:1087-1095.

6. Gress FG, Hawes RH, Savides TJ, et al. Endoscopic ultrasound-guided fine-needle aspiration biopsy using linear array and radial scanning endosonography. *Gastrointest Endosc.* 1997;45:243-250.

7. Hecht JR, Farrell JJ, Senzer N, et al. EUS or percutaneously guided intratumoral TNFerade biologic with 5-fluorouracil and radiotherapy for first-line treatment of locally advanced pancreatic cancer: a phase I/II study. *Gastrointest Endosc.* 2012;75(2):332-338.

8. Parada KS, Peng R, Erickson RA, et al. A resource utilization projection study of EUS. *Gastrointest Endosc.* 2002;55:328-334.

9. ASGE. EUS core curriculum. *Gastrointest Endosc.* 2012;76:476-481.

10. ASGE. Guidelines for advanced endoscopic training. *Gastrointest Endosc.* 2001;53:846-848.

11. Azad JS, Verma D, Kapadia AS, et al. GI fellowship programs meet American Society for Gastrointestinal Endoscopy recommendations for training in EUS? A survey of U.S. GI fellowship program directors. *Gastrointest Endosc.* 2006;64:235-241.

12. ASGE. Methods of granting hospital privileges to perform gastrointestinal endoscopy. *Gastrointest Endosc.* 2002;55:780-783.

13. Hoffman B, Wallace MB, Eloubeidi MA, et al. How many supervised procedures does it take to become competent in EUS? Results of a multicenter three year study. *Gastrointest Endosc.* 2000;51:AB139.

14. Fockens P, Van den Brande JHM, van Dullemen HM, et al. Endosonographic T-staging of esophageal carcinoma: a learning curve. *Gastrointest Endosc.* 1996;44:58-62.

15. Schlick T, Heintz A, Junginger T. The examiner's learning effect and its influence on the quality of endoscopic ultrasonography in carcinoma of the esophagus and gastric cardia. *Surg Endosc.* 1999;13:894-898.

16. Wani S, Coté GA, Keswani R, et al. Learning curves for EUS by using cumulative sum analysis: implications for American Society for Gastrointestinal Endoscopy recommendations for training. *Gastrointest Endosc.* 2013;77(4):558-565.

17. Nayar M, Joy D, Wadehra V, et al. Effect of dedicated and supervised training on achieving competence in EUS-FNA of solid pancreatic lesions. *Scand J Gastroenterol.* 2011;46(7-8):997-1003.

18. Fritscher-Ravens A, Cuming T, Dhar S, et al. Endoscopic ultrasound-guided fine needle aspiration training: evaluation of a new porcine lymphadenopathy model for in vivo hands-on teaching and training, and review of the literature. *Endoscopy.* 2013;45(2):114-120.

19. Coté GA, Hovis CE, Kohlmeier C, et al. Training in EUS-guided fine needle aspiration: safety and diagnostic yield of attending supervised, trainee-directed FNA from the onset of training. *Diagn Ther Endosc.* 2011;2011.

20. Konge L, Vilmann P, Clementsen P, et al. Reliable and valid assessment of competence in endoscopic ultrasonography and fine-needle aspiration for mediastinal staging of non–small-cell lung cancer. *Endoscopy.* 2012;44(10):928-933.

21. Boyce HW. Training in endoscopic ultrasonography. *Gastrointest Endosc.* 1996;43:S12-S15.

22. Gromski MA, Matthes K. Simulation in advanced endoscopy: state of the art and the next generation. *Tech Gastrointest Endosc.* 2011;13:203-208.

23. ASGE. Role of endoscopic ultrasonography. *Gastrointest Endosc.* 2000;52:852-859.

24. Eloubeidi MA, Tamhane A. EUS-guided FNA of solid pancreatic masses: a learning curve with 300 consecutive procedures. *Gastrointest Endosc.* 2005;61:700-708.

25. Methods of granting hospital privileges to perform gastrointestinal endoscopy. *Gastrointest Endosc.* 2002;55:780-783. Reviewed and reapproved 11/08.

26. ASGE. Guidelines for credentialing and granting privileges for endoscopic ultrasound. *Gastrointest Endosc.* 2001;54:811-814.

27. Chak A, Cooper GS. Procedure-specific outcomes assessment for endoscopic ultrasonography. *Gastrointest Endosc Clin North Am.* 1999;9:649-656.

28. Hoffman BJ, Hawes RH. Endoscopic ultrasound and clinical competence. *Gastrointest Endosc Clin North Am.* 1995;5:879-884.

29. ASGE. Principles of training in gastrointestinal endoscopy. *Gastrointest Endosc.* 2012;75:231-235.

30. ASGE. Tissue sampling during endosonography. *Gastrointest Endosc.* 1998;47:576-578.

31. Parupudi A, Holland C, Milla P, et al. Development of porcine lymphadenopathy model for in vivo hands-on teaching and training of EUS-FNA. *Endoscopy.* 2009;41(Suppl 1):A55.

32. Shami VM, Kahaleh M. Endoscopic ultrasonography (EUS)-guided access and therapy of pancreatico-biliary disorders: EUS-guided cholangio and pancreatic drainage. *Gastrointest Endosc Clin N Am.* 2007;17(3):581-593.

33. Seewald S, Ang TL, Teng KC, et al. EUS-guided drainage of pancreatic pseudocysts, abscesses and infected necrosis. *Dig Endosc.* 2009; 21(suppl 1):S61-S65.

34. Levy MJ, Topazian MD, Wiersema MJ, et al. Initial evaluation of the efficacy and safety of endoscopic ultrasound-guided direct ganglia neurolysis and block. *Am J Gastroenterol.* 2008;103(1):98-103.

35. Romero-Castro R, Pellicer-Bautista FJ, Jimenez-Saenz M, et al. EUS-guided injection of cyanoacrylate in perforating feeding veins in gastric varices: results in 5 cases. *Gastrointest Endosc.* 2007;66(2):402-407.

36. Measuring the quality of endoscopy. *Gastrointest Endosc.* 2006;58: S1-S38.

37. Cass OW. Objective evalutation of competence: technical skills in gastrointestinal endoscopy. *Endoscopy.* 1995;27:86-89.

38. Jowell PS. Quantitative assessment of procedural competence: a prospective study of training in ERCP. *Ann Int Med.* 1996;125:937-939.

39. ASGE. Renewal of and proctoring for endoscopic privileges. *Gastrointest Endosc.* 2008;67:10-16.

40. Joint Commission Comprehensive Accreditation Manual for Hospital 1997.

41. ASGE. Endoscopic simulators. *Gastrointest Endosc.* 2011;73:861-867.

42. Markman HD. A new system for teaching proctosigmoidoscopic morphology. *Am J Gastroenterol.* 1969;52:65-69.

43. Gerson LB. Evidence-based assessment of endoscopic simulators for training. *Gastrointest Endosc Clin N Am.* 2006;16(3):489-509.

44. Verdaasdonk EG, Stassen LP, Monteny LJ, et al. Validation of a new basic virtual reality simulator for training of basic endoscopic skills: the SIMENDO. *Surg Endosc.* 2006;20(3):511-518.

45. Hochberger J, Maiss J. Currently available simulators: ex vivo models. *Gastrointest Endosc Clin N Am.* 2006;16(3):435-449.

46. MacDonald J, Ketchum J, Williams RG, et al. A lay person versus a trained endoscopist: can the preop endoscopy simulator detect a difference? *Surg Endosc.* 2003;17:896-898.

47. Sedlack RE, Kolars JC, Alexander JA. Computer simulation training enhances patient comfort during endoscopy. *Clin Gastroenterol Hepatol.* 2004;2:348-352.

48. Sedlack RE. The state of simulation in endoscopy education: continuing to advance toward our goals. *Gastroenterology.* 2013;144(1):9-12.

49. Pawa R, Chuttani R. Benefits and limitations of simulation in endoscopic training. *Tech Gastrointest Endosc.* 2011;13:191-198.

50. Gromski MA, Brugge W, Chuttani R, et al. Development and Evaluation of a Novel Endoscopic Ultrasound (EUS) Simulator. *Gastrointest Endosc.* 2010;71:286 (abstract).

51. Yusuf TE, Matthes K, Lee Y, et al. Evaluation of the EASIE-R simulator for the training of basic and advanced EUS. *Gastrointest Endosc.* 2009;69:S264.

52. Savides TJ, Donohue M, Hunt G, et al. EUS-guided FNA diagnostic yield of malignancy in solid pancreatic masses: a benchmark for quality performance measurement. *Gastrointest Endosc.* 2007;66:277-282.

4

Indications, Preparation, and Adverse Effects

Faris M. Murad • Mark Topazian

Key Points

- The primary indications for EUS are cancer staging when there is potential additive value after noninvasive imaging has been performed, assessment (usually combined with EUS fine-needle aspiration) of lymph node status, and evaluation of pancreatic disease and subepithelial lesions of the gastrointestinal tract.
- Prophylactic antibiotics are recommended for EUS FNA of cystic lesions.
- Few data are available regarding EUS FNA in patients with increased risk of bleeding. In the absence of data, the following are reasonable guidelines:
  - International normalized ratio (INR) ≤1.5
  - Platelet count ≥50,000
  - Use of a 22- to 25-G needle
  - Performance of as few passes as possible (cytopathologist in room).
- The risk of perforation is probably higher with EUS than for standard endoscopy. Caution should be exercised when intubating the patient, traversing stenotic tumors, and passing the instrument past the apex of the duodenal bulb, because these are all situations in which the long, rigid tip increases the difficulty of passing the instrument.

Indications

Endoscopic ultrasonography (EUS) continues to evolve as a diagnostic and therapeutic modality. EUS should be performed when it has the potential to affect patient management,[1] such as when establishing a diagnosis, performing locoregional tumor staging, or providing therapeutic interventions. Since the introduction of EUS in 1980, its indications and role have continued to expand. This overview of indications and risks is supplemented by the detailed discussions of specific indications that can be found in relevant chapters throughout this book.

Diagnostic Imaging

The endosonographic appearance alone may provide a confident diagnosis for certain lesions including gut duplication cysts, lipomas, bile duct stones, and some branch duct intraductal papillary mucinous neoplasias. In other situations, however, EUS imaging alone may not provide a confident diagnosis. As a result, EUS-guided fine-needle aspiration (FNA) or core biopsy is often indicated to allow for cytologic or histologic diagnosis. Follow-up imaging may be indicated when EUS demonstrates a benign-appearing lesion to identify interval growth or other signs suggestive of malignancy.

Tumor Staging

Initial evaluation of patients with gastrointestinal (GI) cancers includes assessment of operative risk and determination of tumor stage. Accurate staging is necessary to determine prognosis, to guide administration of chemoradiation, and to select the ideal means and extent of resection when appropriate. Staging usually begins with noninvasive imaging such as computed tomography (CT), magnetic resonance imaging (MRI), or positron emission tomography (PET), which are generally superior to EUS for excluding distant metastases. In the absence of metastases, EUS is often performed for T (tumor) and N (nodal) staging because it provides an accuracy of about 85% for GI luminal cancers.[2-11] Prior radiation therapy substantially decreases the T-staging accuracy of EUS.

EUS provides important nodal staging information in patients with lung, esophageal, and rectal cancer. Use of sonographic features of lymph nodes is at best 75% accurate for predicting malignancy. The typical EUS characteristics of malignant lymph nodes in esophageal cancer are echo-poor appearance, round shape, smooth border, and size greater than 1 cm in the short axis.[12-17] Overlap in appearance between benign and malignant lymph nodes makes nodal staging problematic, and the aforementioned criteria are less useful in lung cancer, rectal cancer, and cholangiocarcinoma.[18,19]

Overstaging may result from enlarged reactive lymph nodes that are deemed malignant on the basis of their EUS appearance alone. The addition of FNA improves nodal staging accuracy, but it also introduces the possibility of false-positive results, particularly when luminal cancer is present.[20] When performing biopsy of lymph nodes, one should avoid traversing the primary tumor to minimize the risk of a false-positive cytologic finding and tumor seeding.

EUS has a limited role in establishing the presence or absence of distant metastasis (M stage). Occasionally, a suspicious lesion is best approached for aspiration through EUS, or a previously unsuspected metastasis is diagnosed during EUS performed for local staging (e.g., a liver lesion in a patient with pancreatic cancer). In these cases, EUS FNA appears reasonably safe when sampling the liver and the adrenal glands.[21-29]

EUS has been compared with PET in staging of esophageal cancer. PET has the ability to identify distant nonnodal metastatic disease more accurately than EUS and CT.[30,31] Imaging with PET upstages patients who were previously considered to have local or locally advanced disease and may exclude the possibility of curative R0 surgical resection. However, PET has limited accuracy in staging local and regional disease, and EUS remains superior to PET or CT for this indication.[32,33] It appears that PET and EUS are complementary for optimal staging. It is uncertain whether PET should be performed first, to allow patients with previously undetected metastases to avoid the cost and discomfort of EUS, or whether EUS should be performed first, with PET reserved for patients with locally advanced disease or incomplete EUS examinations resulting from esophageal obstruction.[34]

The role of EUS in pancreatic cancer staging has been debated. In patients whose tumor is visible on CT, EUS and CT provide comparable accuracy with regard to vascular involvement and nodal involvement. However, EUS retains a key role in the evaluation of pancreatic masses for two reasons: its ability to detect abnormalities missed by CT and the capability to obtain tissue specimens during the examination. Studies have shown that EUS can identify small metastatic lesions that were not identified on CT, including left lobe liver metastases, perivascular cuffing by tumor, and malignant involvement of celiac ganglia.[35-37] The ability to obtain tissue specimens from these sites or from the primary pancreatic mass is increasingly important. Pancreatic mass lesions may be adenocarcinoma, other neoplasms such as neuroendocrine tumors or metastases, or benign conditions such as autoimmune pancreatitis, and these lesions cannot always be differentiated by clinical findings, imaging, and laboratory tests. EUS FNA and core biopsy allow efficient diagnosis in many such cases. Finally, EUS remains superior to CT for detection of small pancreatic cancers that are most likely to be resectable. For this reason, EUS should be performed if clinical or CT findings raise the question of a small pancreatic cancer not visualized by CT.

EUS has a role in lung cancer staging. Noninvasive methods for staging non–small-cell lung cancer (NSCLC) include CT and PET. These modalities have low sensitivity and specificity for the detection of mediastinal lymph node metastasis. Patients with negative CT results for mediastinal adenopathy have up to a 35% prevalence of mediastinal adenopathy.[38] To limit false-positive and false-negative diagnoses of nodal stage, lymph node tissue sampling is advocated when it will change the management strategy (typically when a visualized lymph node is contralateral to the primary tumor). Sampling of all relevant nodal stations has traditionally required surgical mediastinoscopy. However, one study showed that a combination of EUS and endobronchial ultrasound (EBUS) for staging in NSCLC had a negative predictive value of 97% in the evaluation of mediastinal lymph nodes.[39] It appears that the combination of EUS and EBUS is comparable to mediastinoscopy for nodal staging. EUS and EBUS are complementary, given that neither test visualizes all relevant mediastinal lymph node stations.[40] EUS also allows evaluation of the left adrenal gland for previously undetected distant metastases.[41]

Tissue Acquisition

The development of linear EUS technology in the early 1990s allowed for EUS FNA and core biopsy of lesions within and extrinsic to the GI tract wall.[42] Common indications for FNA include biopsy of pancreatic mass lesions and nodal staging of esophageal, pancreatic, and rectal cancers. EUS often provides the least invasive and most successful route to obtaining tissue specimens.

Less invasive approaches for establishing a tissue diagnosis include transabdominal ultrasound or CT-guided biopsy. The accuracy and safety of these methods are well established and support their use for initial attempts at diagnosis when these techniques are likely to provide the needed material (e.g., in patients with liver metastases). However, these methods may be limited by their poor sensitivity in the diagnosis of small lesions or by concern for potential tumor seeding of the biopsy needle tract. EUS may be favored in these situations, as well as when EUS is indicated for other reasons such as for locoregional staging or celiac plexus/ganglia neurolysis. In such settings, FNA can be performed during the same examination, thereby offering a cost-effective approach and simplified patient care. This is in contrast to percutaneous approaches for biopsy that are routinely performed as a separate procedure. Although the diagnostic accuracy of EUS FNA for pancreatic cancer and nodal metastases is generally greater than 85%, this method is less accurate in other settings, including diagnosis of pancreatic cystic lesions, stromal tumors, and autoimmune pancreatitis, as a result of limitations associated with cytologic evaluation. A variety of EUS-guided core biopsy devices are available.[43-45] EUS Tru-Cut biopsy (TCB) safely improves the diagnostic accuracy of EUS in selected settings.[46,47]

Therapy

The ability to pass a hollow needle under ultrasound guidance has expanded the applications of EUS. The needle is essentially a conduit that allows for the passage or placement of materials with therapeutic intent. The first such therapy to be developed was EUS-guided celiac plexus/ganglia neurolysis or block,[48,49] followed by EUS-guided pseudocyst drainage.[50] Both of these interventions are now commonly performed under EUS guidance. EUS fine-needle injection (EUS FNI) was introduced as a means to deliver novel, potentially therapeutic agents into solid pancreatic cancers,[51,52] as well as for treatment of pancreatic cystic neoplasms. However, limited data are available to judge the safety and efficacy of EUS FNI for these indications. Other EUS-guided therapeutic interventions have been described, including drainage of otherwise inaccessible biliary and pancreatic ducts,[53,54] coil embolization of bleeding varices,[55] treatment of bleeding pancreatic pseudoaneurysm,[56,57] placement of fiducials to guide radiation therapy,[58] recovery of migrated stents, and transduodenal gallbladder drainage.[59] Insufficient data are available to judge the safety, efficacy, and ultimate clinical role of many of these procedures, some of which are discussed in more detail in other chapters.

Contraindications

Absolute contraindications to EUS are few and include unacceptable sedation risks. EUS FNA is generally contraindicated in the presence of coagulopathy (international normalized ratio [INR] > 1.5), thrombocytopenia (platelets < 50,000), or intervening structures prohibiting biopsy. Relative contraindications to EUS include: (1) newly diagnosed cancer in a patient who has not undergone appropriate initial evaluation; (2) altered anatomy prohibiting access; and (3) mild coagulopathy or thrombocytopenia. Mild coagulopathy is unlikely to cause clinically significant bleeding, but it may increase blood in the aspirates that can decrease diagnostic sensitivity. Limited data suggest that EUS FNA may be relatively safe in patients with portal hypertension.

Patient Preparation

General Measures

Although EUS is typically performed in an ambulatory setting, it is also performed in hospitalized patients, and practices are increasingly allowing open-access referrals. As a result, the setting of the preprocedure evaluation can vary, as may the extent of the evaluation. At a minimum, an initial evaluation including a history, physical examination, and review of the medical records must be conducted to identify factors that influence the need, risks, benefits, alternatives, and timing of EUS and to document acquisition of informed consent (Box 4-1).[60–62] Because emergency EUS is uncommon, involved parties should generally have the necessary time for adequate evaluation, for discussion of patient and family concerns, and for answering questions. A professional and unhurried demeanor facilitates open communication and helps patients and their families develop trust and a bond with the physician.

Initial planning and preparation for EUS of the upper GI (UGI) and lower GI (LGI) tract are similar to those for routine endoscopy and colonoscopy.[63] Efforts are undertaken to help ensure a proficient and accurate EUS examination while maintaining the patient's comfort and safety. Before the procedure, patients are instructed on their preparation responsibilities, the use of other medications, and the need to avoid alcohol and other sedatives. Patients are advised of the use of conscious sedation and resulting restrictions on postprocedure activities and the need for transportation. The potential signs and symptoms of adverse outcomes, as well as contact persons and phone numbers, are given in the event of procedure-related complications. These instructions are reviewed after the procedure with the patient and accompanying adult.

Deeper sedation may be required for EUS than for routine endoscopic procedures because of the longer examination

---

BOX 4-1   Factors That May Affect the Performance of EUS

Severity and urgency of EUS examination
Prior endoscopic examinations (findings and complications)
Other imaging studies (findings and results of tissue sampling)
Administrations of chemoradiation (and timing relative to EUS)
Comorbid illnesses
    Cardiopulmonary disease
    Hepatic disease
    Hematologic disease
        Bleeding diathesis
    Altered anatomy
Medications
    Antihypertensives
    Antithrombotics
    Antiepileptics
    Aspirin and other nonsteroidal anti-inflammatory agents
    Cardiac
    Hypoglycemic agents
    Monoamine oxidase (MAO) inhibitors
    Oral birth control pills
    Pulmonary
    Psychiatric
Drug allergies
Ability to give informed consent
Available transportation

---

time and the need to minimize movement of the patient. As for all patient-sedated endoscopic procedures, careful monitoring is required throughout the procedure and recovery period. Administration of supplemental oxygen to all patients receiving sedation is recommended. Although conscious sedation or monitored anesthesia care (MAC) is routinely given for UGI EUS, it is optional for rectal EUS.

UGI EUS is ideally performed following an overnight fast. At a minimum, patients should avoid solid foods for 6 hours and liquids (except sips of water to ingest medications) for 4 hours before the procedure. When there is concern for incomplete gastric emptying as a result of dysmotility or obstruction, a 1- to 2-day diet of clear liquids may be advised. Retained gastric contents increase the risk of aspiration and may compromise acoustic coupling, produce image artifacts, and impair the overall examination quality.

Although some endosonographers perform rectal EUS after administering enemas alone, a full colon preparation is preferred to optimize acoustic coupling, minimize image artifacts, and potentially reduce infectious complications associated with FNA by decreasing intraluminal contents. More intense or prolonged efforts at cleansing the colon may be required in patients with chronic constipation or a recent barium examination.

Laboratory Studies

The need for and benefits of routine laboratory evaluation have not been formally studied in patients undergoing endoscopic procedures. Current recommendations are based on extrapolation of surgical data. Surgical series have consistently demonstrated a lack of utility of routine preoperative studies such as hemoglobin level, blood crossmatching, routine chemistry studies, coagulation parameters, urinalysis, chest radiograph, and electrocardiogram for patients without evidence of relevant underlying disorders.[64] Routine preoperative testing in healthy patients rarely identifies abnormal findings and does not predict or correlate with patient outcomes. Therefore routine screening in asymptomatic patients is discouraged. Instead, endoscopists are advised to order preprocedure testing selectively, based on clinical suspicion arising from the initial evaluation, including a history of bleeding diathesis. This more focused approach greatly enhances the yield of preoperative testing without compromising patient outcomes.[65]

An exception may be women of childbearing age in whom pregnancy is possible. Although pregnancy is not a contraindication to endoscopic procedures or conscious sedation, in some situations it is important to know whether a woman is pregnant because of the impact on certain procedural aspects. Such circumstances include administration of general anesthesia (in patients who are difficult to sedate) or use of fluoroscopy (when performing EUS as part of a rendezvous procedure following failed endoscopic retrograde cholangiopancreatography [ERCP]).[66] When possible, it is advisable to avoid or delay EUS until after delivery. When EUS cannot be delayed, appropriate measures should be undertaken to lessen the risk to the unborn child.

Medications

Daily Medications

In the absence of controlled trials to guide management, patients are instructed to continue their cardiac, antihypertensive, pulmonary, antiepileptic, psychiatric, and contraceptive medications. These medications are ingested with sips of water early on the day of the procedure. Diabetic patients are advised to take half of their morning insulin dose at the usual time and the remaining dose with a postprocedure meal. Oral hypoglycemic agents are withheld the morning of the procedure and until resumption of a normal diet.

Prophylactic Antibiotics

There is minimal risk (0% to 6%) of developing bacteremia after "routine" procedures such as esophagogastroduodenoscopy (EGD), flexible sigmoidoscopy, and colonoscopy.[67] The risk of bacteremia is not increased as a result of mucosal biopsy, polypectomy, endoscopic mucosal resection, and sphincterotomy.[68,69] However, an increased rate of bacteremia or local infection is reported following other endoscopic procedures including esophageal sclerotherapy, esophageal stricture dilation, ERCP with biliary obstruction,[70] endoscopic drainage of a pancreatic pseudocyst,[71] and endoscopic placement of feeding tubes.[72] Although the risk of developing endocarditis or other infectious complication as a result of endoscopic procedures is low, the resulting morbidity and mortality are high. These findings led the American Heart Association,[73] American Society for Gastrointestinal Endoscopy (ASGE), and other societies and interest groups[74] to recommend antibiotic prophylaxis for high-risk patients undergoing procedures with a high risk of associated bacteremia.

Risk of Bacteremia and Antibiotic Recommendations for Other Endoscopic Procedures. Bacterial endocarditis usually develops in patients with high-risk congenital or acquired cardiac lesions who develop bacteremia with microorganisms commonly associated with endocarditis.[71,75] Cardiac abnormalities are stratified as high risk, moderate risk, and low or negligible risk on the basis of the relative risk of developing endocarditis and the potential outcome if endocarditis develops (Table 4-1). In most patients, with or without underlying risk factors, the resulting transient bacteremia is limited

TABLE 4-1	
CARDIOVASCULAR RISK FACTORS FOR ENDOCARDITIS	
Risk	**Condition**
High	Prosthetic heart valve (bioprosthetic and homograft)
	History of bacterial endocarditis
	Complex cyanotic congenital heart conditions
	Single ventricle states
	Transposition of the great arteries
	Tetralogy of Fallot
	Surgically constructed systemic-pulmonary shunt or conduits
	Synthetic vascular graft (<1 year old)
Moderate	Most other congenital cardiac malformations (other than above and below)
	Acquired valve dysfunction (e.g., rheumatic heart disease)
	Hypertrophic cardiomyopathy (with latent or resting obstruction)
	Mitral valve prolapse with murmur and/or valve regurgitation and/or thickened leaflets and/or emergency need for procedure
Negligible[a]	Isolated secundum atrial septal defect
	Surgical repair (without residua beyond 6 months)
	Atrial septal defect
	Ventricular septal defect
	Patent ductus arteriosus
	CABG (prior)
	Mitral valve prolapse (without valve regurgitation)
	Physiologic, functional, or innocent heart murmurs
	Prior Kawasaki's disease (without valve dysfunction)
	Prior rheumatic heart disease (without valve dysfunction)
	Pacemaker (intravascular and epicardial)
	Implanted defibrillators

CABG, coronary artery bypass graft.
[a]Same risk as the general population.
Adapted from Dajani AS, Taubert KA, Wilson W, et al. Prevention of bacterial endocarditis: recommendations by the American Heart Association. Clin Infect Dis. 1997;25:1448-1458; and Wilson W, Taubert KA, Gewitz M, et al. Prevention of infective endocarditis: guidelines from the American Heart Association Rheumatic Fever, Endocarditis, and Kawasaki Disease Committee, Council on Cardiovascular Disease in the Young, and the Council on Clinical Cardiology, Council on Cardiovascular Surgery and Anesthesia, and the Quality of Care and Outcomes Research Interdisciplinary Working Group. Circulation. 2007; 116(15):1736-1754.

in duration (<15 minutes) and of no clinical significance.[76] Rarely, bacteria may lodge on damaged or abnormal heart valves and result in bacterial endocarditis.

Most cases of bacterial endocarditis (60% to 75%) develop in the absence of a procedure or intervention typically associated with bacteremia. However, certain endoscopic procedures are associated with a high frequency of bacteremia caused by microorganisms commonly associated with endocarditis. The reported rate of bacteremia following particular endoscopic procedures varied greatly among studies. These trials were mostly small and uncontrolled. The discrepancy in results can partly be explained by widely varying differences in methodology. Studies varied in regard to technical aspects of the procedures and in the timing, number, and volume of blood cultures. However, the general consensus is that several endoscopic procedures place patients at higher risk for developing bacteremia. High-risk procedures include esophageal stricture dilation and variceal sclerotherapy and are associated with bacteremia in approximately 30% of patients. Other high-risk procedures include endoscopic retrograde cholangiography with biliary obstruction and endoscopic drainage of a pancreatic pseudocyst. Although endocarditis rarely develops following these endoscopic procedures, antibiotic prophylaxis is recommended in properly selected patients because of the high morbidity and mortality associated with endocarditis (Table 4-2).

EUS Studies. The data regarding the risk of infectious complications following EUS with or without FNA show a frequency of bacteremia in a range similar to that for diagnostic UGI endoscopy. Barawi and colleagues[77] prospectively evaluated the risk of bacteremia and other infectious complications associated with EUS FNA. One hundred patients underwent EUS FNA for a total of 107 lesions. EUS FNA was performed for a variety of UGI indications. Contaminated blood cultures occurred in six patients, but none of the patients in this study developed bacteremia or any infectious complication. The absence of true bacteremia may be partly explained by the minimal quantity (10 mL) of blood collected and the delayed timing (30 minutes after EUS FNA) of the first blood culture, both of which are associated with lower rates of positive blood cultures.[74,78,79]

In a subsequent report of 52 patients who underwent EUS FNA of 74 sites from solid lesions of the UGI tract, with a mean of five needle passes, coagulase-negative *Staphylococcus* grew in three patients (5.8%; 95% confidence interval [CI], 1% to 15%) and was considered a contaminant. Three patients (5.8%; 95% CI, 1% to 15%) developed bacteremia as the result of viridans group *Streptococcus* ($n = 2$) and an unidentified gram-negative bacillus ($n = 1$).[80] This rate is similar to that for routine endoscopy. None of the patients developed signs or symptoms of infection. Janssen and colleagues[81] prospectively studied 100 patients undergoing diagnostic EUS (group A) along with 50 patients who underwent UGI EUS FNA (group B). Excluding contaminants, bacteremia developed in four patients overall, two from each group. These investigators concluded that the rate of bacteremia after EUS of UGI tract lesions with and without FNA is low and that routine administration of antibiotics is not warranted. It appears that EUS FNA of solid UGI tract lesions should be considered a low-risk procedure for infectious complications and does not warrant antibiotic prophylaxis for bacterial endocarditis.

TABLE 4-2

AMERICAN SOCIETY FOR GASTROINTESTINAL ENDOSCOPY RECOMMENDATIONS FOR ANTIBIOTIC PROPHYLAXIS

Patient Condition	Procedure	Antibiotic Prophylaxis
High-risk cardiac lesion	High risk	Yes
	Low risk	±
Moderate-risk cardiac lesion	High risk	±
	Low risk	No
Low-risk cardiac lesion	High risk	No
	Low risk	No
Cirrhosis (with acute GI bleeding)	Any	Yes
Ascites, immunocompromised	High risk	±
Cirrhosis (without acute GI bleeding)	Low risk	No
Biliary obstruction	ERCP	Yes
Pancreatic cystic lesion	ERCP	Yes
	EUS FNA	Yes
All patients	PEG	Yes
Prosthetic joint	Any	No
Solid UGI lesions	EUS FNA	No
Solid LGI lesions	EUS FNA	No
Nonpancreatic cystic lesions	EUS FNA	Yes

ERCP, endoscopic retrograde cholangiopancreatography; FNA, fine-needle aspiration; GI, gastrointestinal; LGI, lower gastrointestinal; PEG, percutaneous endoscopic gastrostomy; UGI, upper gastrointestinal; ±, prophylaxis optional for patients with moderate-risk lesions (insufficient data to make a firm recommendation; physician should choose on case-by-case basis).
Adapted from ASGE Standards of Practice Committee, Banerjee S, Shen B, et al. Antibiotic prophylaxis for GI endoscopy. Gastrointest Endosc. 2008;67(6): 791-798.

Another prospective study evaluated the risk of bacteremia and other infectious complications in patients who underwent EUS FNA of LGI tract lesions. A total of 100 patients underwent a total of 471 FNA procedures to obtain cytologic samples from lymph nodes, the wall of the rectum, or the sigmoid colon. Blood cultures were positive in six patients, with four cultures deemed contaminants, and the remaining two patients had transient bacteremia. Hence it also appears that transrectal EUS FNA of solid lesions in or adjacent to the LGI tract should be considered a low-risk procedure for infectious complications and does not warrant prophylactic antibiotics.[82]

Although the aforementioned studies address the risks of infectious complications following EUS FNA for solid lesions, data support the use of antibiotic prophylaxis for EUS FNA of cystic lesions. In a large retrospective analysis of 603 patients who underwent EUS FNA of cystic lesions of the pancreas, a single infection was reported. Most patients in this study received antibiotic prophylaxis during the procedure and a 3-day course of postprocedure prophylaxis with a fluoroquinolone.[83] The ASGE recommends antibiotic prophylaxis for EUS FNA of pancreatic cystic lesions.[84,85]

Anticoagulants and Antiplatelet Agents

An increasing variety of antithrombotic agents are used in clinical practice, including both anticoagulant and antiplatelet

RISK OF BLEEDING BASED ON ENDOSCOPIC PROCEDURE

Higher Risk	Lower Risk
Polypectomy	Diagnostic endoscopy and
Biliary or pancreatic	colonoscopy (with or
sphincterotomy	without biopsy)
Pneumatic or bougie dilatation	ERCP without
PEG placement	sphincterotomy
Therapeutic balloon-assisted	EUS without FNA
enteroscopy	Enteroscopy and diagnostic
EUS with FNA	balloon-assisted
Endoscopic hemostasis	enteroscopy
Tumor ablation by any technique	Capsule endoscopy
Cystogastrostomy	Enteral stent placement
Treatment of varices	(without dilatation)

ERCP, endoscopic retrograde cholangiopancreatography; FNA, fine-needle aspiration; PEG, percutaneous endoscopic gastrostomy.
Adapted from Anderson MA, Ben-Menachem T, Gan SI, et al. ASGE guideline: management of antithrombotic agents for endoscopic procedures. Gastrointest Endosc. 2009;70(6):1060-1070.

RISK OF THROMBOEMBOLISM BASED ON UNDERLYING MEDICAL CONDITION

High Risk	Low Risk
Atrial fibrillation (with valve disease, active congestive heart failure, left ventricular ejection fraction < 35%, history of thromboembolism, hypertension, diabetes, or age > 75 years)	Uncomplicated or paroxysmal nonvalvular atrial fibrillation
Mechanical valve (mitral)	Mechanical valve (aortic)
Mechanical valve (prior thromboembolic event)	Bioprosthetic valve
Recently placed (less than one year) coronary stent	Deep vein thrombosis
Acute coronary syndrome	
Nonstented percutaneous coronary intervention after myocardial infarction	

Adapted from Anderson MA, Ben-Menachem T, Gan SI, et al. ASGE guideline: management of antithrombotic agents for endoscopic procedures. Gastrointest Endosc. 2009;70(6):1060-1070.

agents. Reviews and expert guidelines regarding the management of these agents before and after invasive surgical and endoscopic procedures have recently been published.[86,87] In this chapter we will review management of these agents in patients undergoing EUS and EUS FNA.

Despite the availability of consensus guidelines, the ideal approach for managing anticoagulation in the perioperative period has not been established and is often controversial.[88–91] Firm conclusions often cannot be made concerning the efficacy and safety of different management strategies based on the current literature, owing to variations in patient populations, procedures, anticoagulation regimens, definitions of events, and duration of follow-up.

Periprocedural management of antithrombotic agents requires an assessment of both the likelihood of procedurally induced bleeding and the patient's underlying risk of thromboembolism. Endoscopic procedures are either high risk or low risk depending on the likelihood of inducing bleeding (Table 4-3).[90] EUS without FNA is regarded as a low-risk procedure. Although patients undergoing EUS FNA are believed to be at low overall risk of FNA-related bleeding, EUS FNA is considered a high-risk procedure because when bleeding results it may be inaccessible or uncontrollable by endoscopic means. Conditions predisposing patients to thromboembolism are classified as high risk or low risk based on the likelihood of developing a thromboembolic event (Table 4-4).

In general, because EUS is a low-risk procedure, antithrombotic therapy does not need to be interrupted in patients undergoing EUS without FNA, so long as anticoagulation is not supratherapeutic. Management of antithrombotic agents in patients undergoing EUS FNA must be individualized. Although EUS FNA is categorized as a higher-risk procedure, there are few empirical data to support this categorization, and discontinuation of antithrombotic therapy may have devastating results, particularly in patients with recently placed coronary stents or deep vein thromboses.

The use of anticoagulants may predispose patients to development of bloody aspirates and may thus impair cytologic analysis. This possibility should be considered when choosing the degree of negative pressure to apply during FNA and the duration of FNA passes.

Warfarin

The incidence of bleeding after EUS FNA in patients on therapeutic doses of warfarin is unknown. However, bleeding risk is increased in patients on warfarin who undergo endoscopic polypectomy or sphincterotomy. Based on these findings, ASGE guidelines recommend discontinuing warfarin prior to EUS FNA.[92] In patients with a low thromboembolic risk (Table 4-4), warfarin may be discontinued three to five doses prior to the endoscopic procedure, aiming for an INR ≤ 1.5 on the day of the procedure. Recommendations vary on the timing of reinitiation of warfarin therapy, but it is often reasonable to resume warfarin on the day of the procedure unless there is a high clinical concern for bleeding. In patients with a higher thromboembolic risk (Table 4-4), bridging therapy with either unfractionated or low molecular weight heparin is often recommended, often beginning 2 days after discontinuation of oral warfarin.

New Oral Anticoagulants

The new oral anticoagulants (NOAs) work by targeting key coagulation factors such as factor Xa and IIa (thrombin). The NOAs approved in the United States are dabigatran (Pradaxa; Boehringer Ingelheim), rivaroxaban (Xarelto; Bayer HealthCare AG and Janssen Research & Development LLC, a Johnson & Johnson Company), and apixaban (Eliquis; Pfizer and Bristol-Myers Squibb). These drugs differ from Warfarin in that their peak onset of action is only 2-4 hours compared with 72-96 hours and their half-life is markedly shorter at 5-17 hours compared to 40 hours. The NOAs unfortunately do not have a reversal agent like warfarin (vitamin K or fresh frozen plasma). Perioperative management of the NOAs is based on the urgency of the procedure, level of bleeding risk, and current renal function.[93–95]

For low-bleeding-risk procedures including EUS without FNA or therapeutic intervention, guidelines recommend that the NOA may be continued, or a morning dose can be held, so that the agent is at trough levels when the procedure is performed.[87] For higher-risk procedures such as EUS FNA, anticoagulation should be interrupted by withholding the drug for at least two to three half-lives. In patients with normal creatinine clearance (CrCl) ($\geq$50 mL/min per 1.73 m^2), dabigatran use should be stopped about 48 hours before the procedure, and rivaroxaban and apixaban use should be stopped 24 to 48 hours before the procedure. In patients with impaired renal function, dabigatran therapy should be stopped 3 to 5 days before the procedure if CrCl is 30-50 mL/min per 1.73 m^2 and at least 4 to 6 days if CrCl is <30 mL/min per 1.73 m^2. Rivaroxaban and apixaban administration should be stopped 2 to 4 days before the procedure in patients with impaired renal function.[87]

Given the rapid clearance of NOAs and rapid onset of action, no bridging therapy with unfractionated heparin or low molecular weight heparin (LMWH) is necessary. When resuming NOAs postprocedure, remember that peak plasma concentrations of these drugs occurs within several hours of the first dose, much different than warfarin. When the post-procedure bleeding risk is low, the NOAs can be reintroduced 4 to 6 hours after the procedure, with or without an initially reduced dose, and then usual maintenance dose the following day. Otherwise, if there is concern about hemostasis, the NOAs should not be reintroduced until the benefit outweighs the risks for the patient.[96]

Heparins

EUS can be performed while patients are anticoagulated with heparin but should be postponed if anticoagulation is supra-therapeutic. Guidelines recommend that both unfractionated heparin (UFH) and LMWH should be discontinued prior to EUS FNA. UFH is often discontinued 4 to 6 hours prior to the planned endoscopic procedure. If the patient is receiving LMWH, a single dose is skipped immediately prior to the endoscopic procedure. These agents are often resumed soon after EUS FNA, for instance, by resuming UFH infusion without a bolus or by resuming LMWH administration at the next scheduled dose. However the timing of anticoagulation resumption must be individualized on the basis of both patient and procedural factors.

Aspirin and Nonsteroidal Anti-inflammatory Drugs

ASGE guidelines recommend that aspirin and nonsteroidal anti-inflammatory drugs may be continued for all endoscopic procedures, including EUS FNA.[92] However, when a higher-risk procedure is planned the clinician may elect to discontinue these drugs for 5 to 7 days before the procedure. The risk of discontinuing aspirin therapy must be carefully weighed prior to stopping aspirin, particularly in patients with a history of cerebral or coronary thrombosis.

Clopidogrel, Ticlopidine

These antiplatelet agents can be continued in patients undergoing EUS. For patients undergoing higher-risk procedures such as EUS FNA, guidelines recommend postponing elective procedures until the thromboembolic risk decreases (for instance, in patients with newly placed coronary stents). When the minimum necessary duration of therapy has elapsed, guidelines recommend withholding clopidogrel and ticlopidine for at least 5 days, and generally 7 to 10 days prior to the procedure. When these drugs are held, consideration should be given to continuing or starting aspirin therapy during the periprocedural therapy to decrease the risk of thromboembolic events.[92]

There are few data available regarding the risks of EUS FNA in patients receiving these agents. However, one recent report describes 12 patients who underwent EBUS-guided FNA while taking clopidogrel with or without aspirin. No bleeding complications were observed. These data suggest that FNA can be safely performed in patients taking clopidogrel, but more data are needed. The authors suggest that FNA should be performed without withdrawing clopidogrel only when the risk of short-term thrombosis is believed to outweigh the risk of bleeding.

Risks and Adverse Effects

EUS shares the risks and adverse effects of other endoscopic procedures, including cardiovascular events, unwanted effects of conscious sedation, and allergic reactions to medications.[97,98] This discussion focuses on adverse effects specifically associated with EUS, EUS FNA, and EUS fine-needle injection procedures. Some of these adverse effects relate primarily to the unique features of echoendoscopes, whereas others are associated with the performance of FNA, TCB, or therapeutic interventions.

Perforation

The incidence of GI perforation during EUS ranged from 0% to 0.4% in prospective series enrolling more than 300 patients. Although available data are limited, perforation is probably more common with UGI EUS than with EGD.[99]

The increased risk is partly accounted for by echoendo-scope design, which combines oblique or side-viewing optics with a relatively long rigid tip that extends well beyond the optical lens. The tip of the endoscope may cause luminal perforation during advancement, particularly in areas of angulation (oropharynx or apex of duodenal bulb), stenosis (esophageal cancer), or a blind lumen (pharyngeal or esophageal diverticula). Some evidence indicates that perforation is more common early in an endosonographer's experience.[100] The risk may also be increased when experienced endosonographers use new equipment with different tip design, length, and deflection characteristics.

Intubation of the esophagus with the echoendoscope remains a partially blind maneuver. A prospective study by Eloubeidi and colleagues[101] reported the frequency of cervical perforations. A total of 4894 patients underwent UGI tract EUS, and only three patients experienced cervical esophageal perforations. Understanding the possible risk factors (age > 65 years, history of swallowing difficulties, known cervical osteophytes, kyphosis of the spine, or hyperextension of the neck) may help to identify high-risk patients.

Approximately 15% to 40% of patients with esophageal cancer have a nontraversable obstructing esophageal tumor.[102–105] Some investigators advocate dilation, given the greater accuracy of EUS for T and N staging for traversable versus nontraversable tumors (81% versus 28% and 86% versus 72%, respectively).[104,105] Other investigators discourage routine dilation given the risk and tendency for advanced disease (85% to 90% likelihood of T3 or T4 disease) in this setting.[105] However, distant lymphadenopathy (meriting M1a tumor staging) is diagnosed in 10% to 40% of patients requiring dilation.[105]

Although initial studies reported perforation rates as high as 24% with esophageal dilation followed by immediate EUS, more recent studies found this practice to be safe. There are several likely explanations for the apparent improvement in safety over time. Radial echoendoscopes introduced in the mid-1990s were of smaller diameter than older devices, so dilation was usually performed to 14 or 15 mm rather than 16 to 18 mm, as in earlier studies. In addition, greater awareness of this potential complication has probably led to less aggressive dilation practices.

For patients with circumferential stenosis, judicious stepwise dilation is undertaken to a maximum of 15 mm. Two large studies reporting on the safety of dilation[105,106] followed the "rule of three" (three stepwise 1-mm increases in dilator diameter above the diameter at which resistance was first encountered) and did not use "unacceptable force" to dilate. Dilation allowed immediate passage of an echoendoscope beyond the tumor in 75% to 85% of cases. Extreme caution is necessary when semicircumferential infiltration is present because the normal (and hence thinner) esophageal wall may be at increased risk of tearing in this setting.

Mini-probes passed through a stenotic malignant esophageal tumor may improve the accuracy of T and N staging, but the limited depth of penetration does not allow a complete examination, particularly with regard to celiac axis nodes.[106,107] Another alternative is the EBUS device. The EBUS scope is approximately 6.9 mm in diameter, can provide staging information, and has the ability to sample celiac nodes and liver lesions through FNA.[108]

Bleeding

The risk of bleeding with EUS is mainly related to the performance of FNA. The incidence of bleeding was 0% to 0.4% in two prospective studies enrolling more than 300 patients, and it was 1.3% in a retrospective study.[109] FNA of pancreatic cystic lesions has been associated with a 6% rate of self-limited bleeding.[110]

A small amount of luminal bleeding is often seen endoscopically at FNA puncture sites, but it is generally without sequelae. Bleeding may also occur in the gut wall, adjacent tissue, or target structure undergoing aspiration. Such bleeding may be detected sonographically as a hypoechoic expansion of soft tissue or an enlargement of a lymph node or mass.[111] Alternatively, echogenic material may be seen filling a previously anechoic cyst or duct lumen or collecting in ascites. As blood clots, it increases in echogenicity and may thus become less apparent. When the bleeding is into a large potential space (e.g., the peritoneal cavity), the extent of blood loss may be difficult to assess because of pooling of blood outside the range of EUS imaging.

EUS-induced extraluminal bleeding is seldom associated with clinically important sequelae such as need for transfusion, angiography, or surgical intervention. Because most endosonographers avoid sonographically visible vessels when selecting a needle path for FNA, bleeding usually occurs from small vessels. Because the bleeding site is often extraintestinal,

methods of endoscopic hemostasis are usually not applicable. In some cases, it is possible to apply transmitted pressure to the bleeding site by deflecting the tip of the echoendoscope against the gut wall[107] or to inject epinephrine. The efficacy of these interventions is unknown.

Infection

Infectious complications have been reported in 0.3% of EUS FNA procedures and may include those associated with the endoscopy itself (aspiration pneumonia) or with FNA (abscess or cholangitis).

Infection may develop secondary to aspiration of cystic lesions in the pancreas, mediastinum, and elsewhere.[112] A 9% rate of infection has been reported after EUS FNA of cysts, the risk of which is markedly decreased by antibiotic administration before and after EUS FNA. The true incidence of cyst infection when antibiotics are given is unknown, but it is likely to be low.[113] Iatrogenic *Candida* infection of a cystic lesion was reported after EUS FNA performed in a patient who received prophylactic antibiotics.[114] Technical issues may also affect the risk of cyst infection. Multiple needle passes into a cyst appear to increase the risk of infection, as does failure to aspirate all the cyst fluid completely.

As reviewed in detail previously, bacteremia after UGI EUS FNA is uncommon. Antibiotic prophylaxis for patients at increased risk of bacterial endocarditis is also discussed earlier.

Pancreatitis

Pancreatitis may occur after EUS FNA of both solid and cystic pancreatic lesions. In a pooled analysis of data from 19 EUS centers in the United States, the incidence of pancreatitis after EUS FNA of solid pancreatic lesions masses was 0.3%.[115,116] The incidence was higher (0.6%) at two centers with prospectively collected data, and it was also 0.6% in another prospective study.[117] Aspiration of cystic lesions has been associated with pancreatitis in 1% to 2% of cases. Pancreatitis occurring after EUS FNA is generally mild, but severe pancreatitis and fatal complications have been reported.

The risk of pancreatitis may be ameliorated by limiting the number of needle passes, minimizing the amount of "normal" pancreatic parenchyma that must be traversed, and avoiding the pancreatic duct during EUS FNA procedures. In one small series, however, 12 patients with dilated pancreatic ducts underwent intentional EUS-guided aspiration of the duct without complications.[118] Cytologic yield on aspirated pancreatic duct fluid was 75%.

Other

The risks associated with EUS-guided cyst ablation therapy include acute pancreatitis, abdominal pain, and possible vascular thrombosis. Venous obliteration and thrombosis in the veins adjacent to the cyst have been reported in two patients who underwent ethanol lavage and paclitaxel injection.[119] Another concerning complication reported after celiac plexus neurolysis is paralysis. Fujii and colleagues[120] describe bilateral lower extremity paralysis after EUS-guided celiac plexus neurolysis from infarct of the anterior spinal artery after injection. The most feared complication after celiac plexus neurolysis is death. Death may occur due to thrombosis or necrosis, with associated perforation of the celiac artery and aorta leading to end organ ischemia.[121,122]

There is a risk of tumor seeding along the needle tract when performing EUS FNA.[123] This risk is of minimal concern for pancreatic head lesions because of inclusion of the needle tract site within the field of resection during pancreaticoduodenectomy.

EUS-guided drainage of peripancreatic fluid collections are associated with complications that include bleeding, visceral perforation, stent migration, and infection. Perforation may be more common when uncinate lesions are drained.[124,125]

Bile peritonitis may result from traversal of the bile duct or gallbladder, especially in the presence of an obstructed biliary system.[126] If biliary puncture occurs, antibiotics should be administered to patients who do not have biliary obstruction. In the presence of biliary obstruction, biliary drainage is also recommended. EUS-guided drainage of obstructed bile ducts and pancreatic ducts is associated with significant risks of leakage and infection.[54,59] If possible, one should avoid the use of a needle-knife when creating the fistula tract to the bile duct as this is reported to be a risk factor for adverse events.[127]

Left adrenal gland hemorrhage has been reported after EUS FNA.[128] Although EUS FNA is a reportedly safe technique, sampling of the left adrenal gland should be limited to cases in which concern for neoplastic involvement exists.

A final adverse effect of EUS is missed or mis-staged lesions. Although this error does no immediate, periprocedural harm to the patient, the long-term consequences have not been fully studied. Careful review of the patient's history and imaging studies, as well as formal training in EUS, may decrease the number of missed lesions encountered in general practice.

REFERENCES

1. Hawes RH. Indications for EUS-directed FNA. *Endoscopy*. 1998;30(suppl 1):A155-A157.
2. Tio TL, Den Hartog Jager FC, Tytgat GN. The role of endoscopic ultrasonography in assessing local respectability of oesophagogastric malignancies. Accuracy, pitfalls, and predictability. *Scand J Gastroenterol Suppl*. 1986;123:78-86.
3. Dittler HJ, Siewert JR. Role of endoscopic ultrasonography in esophageal carcinoma. *Endoscopy*. 1993;25(2):156-161.
4. Grimm H, Binmoller KF, Kamper K, et al. Endosonography for preoperative locoregional staging of esophageal and gastric cancer. *Endoscopy*. 1993;25(3):224-230.
5. Rosch T. Endosonographic staging of esophageal cancer: a review of literature results. *Gastrointest Endosc Clin N Am*. 1995;5(3):537-547.
6. Crabtree TD, Yacoub WN, Puri V, et al. Endoscopic ultrasound for early stage esophageal adenocarcinoma: implications for staging and survival. *Ann Thorac Surg*. 2011;91(5):1509-1515.
7. Zeppa P, Barra E, Napolitano V, et al. Impact of endoscopic ultrasound-guided fine needle aspiration (EUS-FNA) in lymph nodal and mediastinal lesions: a multicenter experience. *Diagn Cytopathol*. 2011;39(10):723-729.
8. Talebian M, von Bartheld MB, Braun J, et al. EUS-FNA in preoperative staging of non–small-cell lung cancer. *Lung Cancer*. 2010;69(1):60-65.
9. Gleeson FC, Rajan E, Levy MJ, et al. EUS-guided FNA of regional lymph nodes in patients with unresectable hilar cholangiocarcinoma. *Gastrointest Endosc*. 2008;67(3):438-443.
10. Dewitt J, Devereaux BM, Lehman GA, et al. Comparison of endoscopic ultrasound and computed tomography for the preoperative evaluation of pancreatic cancer: a systematic review. *Clin Gastroenterol Hepatol*. 2006;4(6):717-725.
11. Chen J, Xu R, Hunt GC, et al. Influence of the number of malignant regional lymph nodes detected by endoscopic ultrasonography on survival stratification in esophageal adenocarcinoma. *Clin Gastroenterol Hepatol*. 2006;4(5):573-579.
12. Bhutani MS, Hawes RH, Hoffman BJ. A comparison of the accuracy of echo features during endoscopic ultrasound (EUS) and EUS-guided fine needle aspiration for diagnosis of malignant lymph node invasion. *Gastrointest Endosc*. 1997;45(6):474-479.
13. Catalano MF, Sivak MV Jr, Rice T, et al. Endosonographic features predictive of lymph node metastasis. *Gastrointest Endosc*. 1994;40(4):442-446.
14. Grimm H, Hamper K, Binmoller KF, et al. Enlarged lymph nodes: malignant or not? *Endoscopy*. 1992;24(suppl 1):320-323.
15. Gleeson FC, Clain JE, Rajan E, et al. EUS-FNA assessment of extramesenteric lymph node status in primary rectal cancer. *Gastrointest Endosc*. 2011;74(4):897-905.
16. Gill KR, Ghabril MS, Jamil LH, et al. Endosonographic features predictive of malignancy in mediastinal lymph nodes in patients with lung cancer. *Gastrointest Endosc*. 2010;72(2):265-271.
17. de Melo SW Jr, Panjala C, Crespo S, et al. Interobserver agreement on the endosonographic features of lymph nodes in aerodigestive malignancies. *Dig Dis Sci*. 2011;56(11):3204-3208.
18. Gleeson FC, Rajan E, Levy MJ, et al. EUS-guided FNA of regional lymph nodes inpatients with unresectable hilar cholangiocarcinoma. *Gastrointest Endosc*. 2008;67(3):438-443.
19. Chen VK, Eloubeidi MA. Endoscopic ultrasound-guided fine needle aspiration is superior to lymph node echofeatures: a prospective evaluation of mediastinal and peri-intestinal lymphadenopathy. *Am J Gastroenterol*. 2004;99(4):628-633.
20. Reddy RP, Levy MJ, Wiersema MJ. Endoscopic ultrasound for luminal malignancies. *Gastrointest Endosc Clin N Am*. 2005;15(3):399-429.
21. DeWitt J, LeBlanc J, McHenry L, et al. Endoscopic ultrasound-guided fine needle aspiration cytology of solid liver lesions: a large single-center experience. *Am J Gastroenterol*. 2003;98(9):1976-1981.
22. TenBerge J, Hoffman BJ, Hawes RH, et al. EUS-guided fine needle aspiration of the liver: indications, yield, and safety based on an international survey of 167 cases. *Gastrointest Endosc*. 2002;55(7):859-862.
23. Hollerbach S, Willert J, Topalidis T, et al. Endoscopic ultrasound-guided fine-needle aspiration biopsy of liver lesions: histological and cytological assessment. *Endoscopy*. 2003;35(9):743-749.
24. Jhala NC, Jhala D, Eloubeidi MA, et al. Endoscopic ultrasound-guided fine-needle aspiration biopsy of the adrenal glands: analysis of 24 patients. *Cancer*. 2004;102(5):308-314.
25. El Hajj II, LeBlanc JK, Sherman S, et al. Endoscopic ultrasound-guided biopsy of pancreatic metastases: a large single center experience. *Pancreas*. 2013;42(3):524-530.
26. Peng HQ, Darwin P, Papadimitriou JC, et al. Liver metastases of pancreatic acinar cell carcinoma with marked nuclear atypia and pleomorphism diagnosed by EUS FNA cytology: a case report with emphasis on FNA cytological findings. *Cytojournal*. 2006;3:29.
27. Crowe DR, Eloubeidi MA, Chhieng DC, et al. Fine-needle aspiration biopsy of hepatic lesions: computerized tomographic-guided versus endoscopic ultrasound-guided FNA. *Cancer*. 2006;108(3):180-185.
28. Stelow EB, Debol SM, Stanley MW, et al. Sampling of the adrenal glands by endoscopic ultrasound-guided fine-needle aspiration. *Diagn Cytopathol*. 2005;33(1):26-30.
29. TenBerge J, Hoffman BJ, Hawes RH, et al. EUS-guided fine needle aspiration of the liver: indications, yield, and safety based on an international survey of 167 cases. *Gastrointest Endosc*. 2002;55(7):859-862.
30. Rice TW. Clinical staging of esophageal carcinoma. CT, EUS, and PET. *Chest Surg Clin N Am*. 2000;10(3):471-485.
31. Choi J, Kim SG, Kim JS, et al. Comparison of endoscopic ultrasonography (EUS), positron emission tomography (PET), and computed tomography (CT) in the preoperative locoregional staging of resectable esophageal cancer. *Surg Endosc*. 2010;24(6):1380-1386.
32. Lowe VJ, Booya F, Fletcher JG, et al. Comparison of positron emission tomography, computed tomography, and endoscopic ultrasound in the initial staging of patients with esophageal cancer. *Mol Imaging Biol*. 2005;7(6):422-430.
33. Stigt JA, Oostdijk AH, Timmer PR, et al. Comparison of EUS-guided fine needle aspiration and integrated PET-CT in restaging after treatment for locally advanced non–small-cell lung cancer. *Lung Cancer*. 2009;66(2):198-204.
34. McDonough PB, Jones DR, Shen KR, et al. Does FDG-PET add information to EUS and CT in the initial management of esophageal cancer? A prospective single center study. *Am J Gastroenterol*. 2008;103(3):570-574.

35. Levy MJ, Gleeson FC, Zhang L. Endoscopic ultrasound fine-needle aspiration detection of extravascular migratory metastasis from a remotely located pancreatic cancer. *Clin Gastroenterol Hepatol.* 2009;7(2):246-248.

36. Singh P, Mukhopadhyay P, Bhatt B, et al. Endoscopic ultrasound versus CT scan for detection of the metastases to the liver: results of a prospective comparative study. *J Clin Gastroenterol.* 2009;43(4):367-373.

37. Levy MJ, Topazian M, Keeney G, et al. Preoperative diagnosis of extrapancreatic neural invasion in pancreatic cancer. *Clin Gastroenterol Hepatol.* 2006;4(12):1479-1482.

38. Micames CG, McCrory DC, Pavey DA, et al. Endoscopic ultrasound-guided fine needle aspiration for non–small-cell lung cancer staging: a systematic review and metaanalysis. *Chest.* 2007;131(2):539-548.

39. Wallace MB, Woodward TA, Raimando M. Endoscopic ultrasound and staging of non–small-cell lung cancer. *Gastrointest Endosc Clin N Am.* 2005;15(1):157-167.

40. Hasan MK, Gill KR, Wallace MB, et al. Lung cancer staging by combined endobronchial ultrasound (EBUS) and endoscopic ultrasound (EUS): the gastroenterologist's perspective. *Dig Liver Dis.* 2010;42(3):156-162.

41. Eloubeidi MA, Seewald S, Tamhane A, et al. EUS-guided FNA of the left adrenal gland in patients with thoracic or GI malignancies. *Gastrointest Endosc.* 2004;59(6):627-633.

42. Yusuf TE, Harewood GC, Clain JE, et al. International survey of knowledge of indications for EUS. *Gastrointest Endosc.* 2006;63(1):107-111.

43. Kipp BR, Pereira TC, Souza PC, et al. Comparison of EUS-guided FNA and Trucut biopsy for diagnosing and staging abdominal and mediastinal neoplasms. *Diagn Cytopathol.* 2009;37(8):549-556.

44. Witt BL, Adler DG, Hilden K, et al. A comparative needle study: EUS-FNA procedures using the HD ProCoreTM and EchoTip® 22-gauge needle types. *Diagn Cytopathol.* 2013[Epub ahead of print].

45. Iwashita T, Nakai Y, Samarasena JB, et al. High single-pass diagnostic yield of a new 25-gauge core biopsy needle for EUS-guided FNA biopsy in solid pancreatic lesions. *Gastrointest Endosc.* 2013;77:909-915.

46. Levy MJ, Reddy RP, Wiersema MJ, et al. EUS-guided Trucut biopsy in establishing autoimmune pancreatitis as the cause of obstructive jaundice. *Gastrointest Endosc.* 2005;61(3):467-472.

47. Levy MJ, Wiersema MJ. EUS-guided Trucut biopsy. *Gastrointest Endosc.* 2005;62(3):417-426.

48. Gress F, Schmitt C, Sherman S, et al. Endoscopic ultrasound-guided celiac plexus block for managing abdominal pain associated with chronic pancreatitis: a prospective single center experience. *Am J Gastroenterol.* 2001;96(2):409-416.

49. Schmulewitz N, Hawes R. EUS-guided celiac plexus neurolysis: technique and indication. *Endoscopy.* 2003;35(8):S49-S53.

50. Seifert H, Dietrich C, Schmitt T, et al. Endoscopic ultrasound-guided one-step transmural drainage of cystic abdominal lesions with a large-channel echo endoscope. *Endoscopy.* 2000;32(3):255-259.

51. Chang KJ, Nguyen PT, Thompson JA, et al. Phase I clinical trial of allogeneic mixed lymphocyte culture (cytoimplant) delivered by endoscopic ultrasound-guided fine-needle injection in patients with advanced pancreatic carcinoma. *Cancer.* 2000;88(6):1325-1335.

52. Ashida R, Chang KJ. Interventional EUS for the treatment of pancreatic cancer. *J Hepatobiliary Pancreat Surg.* 2009;16(5):592-597.

53. Shami VM, Kahaleh M. Endoscopic ultrasound-guided cholangiopancreatography and rendezvous techniques. *Dig Liver Dis.* 2010;42(6):419-424.

54. Fujii LL, Topazian MD, Abu Dayyeh BK, et al. EUS-guided pancreatic duct intervention: outcomes of a single tertiary-care referral center experience. *Gastrointest Endosc.* 2013;in press.

55. Levy MJ, Wong Kee Song LM, Kendrick ML, et al. EUS-guided coil embolization for refractory ectopic variceal bleeding (with videos). *Gastrointest Endosc.* 2008;67(3):572-574.

56. Levy MJ, Wong Kee Song LM, Farnell MB, et al. Endoscopic ultrasound (EUS)-guided angiotherapy of refractory gastrointestinal bleeding. *Am J Gastroenterol.* 2008;103(2):352-359.

57. Levy MJ, Chak A. EUS 2008 Working Group Document: evaluation of EUS-guided vascular therapy. *Gastointest Endosc.* 2009;69(suppl 2):S37-S42.

58. DiMaio CJ, Nagula S, Goodman KA, et al. EUS-guided fiducial placement for image-guided radiation therapy in GI malignancies by using a 22-gauge needle (with videos). *Gastrointest Endosc.* 2010;71(7):1204-1210.

59. Jang JW, Lee SS, Park do H, et al. Feasibility and safety of EUS-guided transgastric/transduodenal gallbladder drainage with single-step placement of a modified covered self-expandable metal stent in patients unsuitable for cholecystectomy. *Gastrointest Endosc.* 2011;74(1):176-181.

60. American Society for Gastrointestinal Endoscopy. Informed consent for gastrointestinal endoscopy. *Gastrointest Endosc.* 1988;34(suppl 3):26S-27S.

61. Plumeri PA. Informed consent for gastrointestinal endoscopy in the '90s and beyond. *Gastrointest Endosc.* 1994;40(3):379.

62. Kopacova M, Bures J. Informed consent for digestive endoscopy. *World J Gastrointest Endosc.* 2012;4(6):227-230.

63. Faigel DO, Eisen GM, Baron TH, et al. Preparation of patients for GI endoscopy. *Gastrointest Endosc.* 2003;57(4):446-450.

64. Kaplan EB, Sheiner LB, Boeckmann AJ, et al. The usefulness of preoperative laboratory screening. *JAMA.* 1985;253(24).

65. Levy MJ, Anderson MA, Baron TH, et al. Position statement on routine laboratory testing before endoscopic procedures. *Gastrointest Endosc.* 2008;68(5):827-832.

66. Smith I, Gaidhane M, Goode A, et al. Safety of endoscopic retrograde cholangiopancreatography in pregnancy: fluoroscopy time and fetal exposure, does it matter? *World J Gastrointest Endosc.* 2013;5(4):148-153.

67. Botoman VA, Surawicz CM. Bacteremia with gastrointestinal endoscopic procedures. *Gastrointest Endosc.* 1986;32(5):342-346.

68. Low DE, Shoenut JP, Kennedy JK, et al. Prospective assessment of risk of bacteremia with colonoscopy and polypectomy. *Dig Dis Sci.* 1987;32(11):1239-1243.

69. Lee TH, Hsueh PR, Yeh WC, et al. Low frequency of bacteremia after endoscopic mucosal resection. *Gastrointest Endosc.* 2000;52(2):223-225.

70. Zuccaro G Jr, Richter JE, Rice TW, et al. Viridans streptococcal bacteremia after esophageal stricture dilation. *Gastrointest Endosc.* 1998;48(6):568-573.

71. Kolars JC, Allen MO, Ansel H, et al. Pancreatic pseudocysts: clinical and endoscopic experience. *Am J Gastroenterol.* 1989;84(3):259-264.

72. Sharma VK, Howden CW. Meta-analysis of randomized controlled trials of antibiotic prophylaxis before percutaneous endoscopic gastrostomy. *Am J Gastroenterol.* 2000;95(11):3133-3136.

73. Dajani AS, Taubert KA, Wilson W, et al. Prevention of bacterial endocarditis: recommendations by the American Heart Association. *Clin Infect Dis.* 1997;25(6):1448-1458.

74. Gould FK, Elliott TS, Foweraker J, et al. Guidelines for the prevention of endocarditis: report of the Working Party of the British Society for Antimicrobial Chemotherapy. *J Antimicrob Chemother.* 2006;57(6):1035-1042.

75. el-Baba M, Tolia V, Lin CH, et al. Absence of bacteremia after gastrointestinal procedures in children. *Gastrointest Endosc.* 1996;44(4):378-381.

76. ASGE Standards of Practice Committee, Banerjee S, Shen B, et al. Antibiotic prophylaxis for GI endoscopy. *Gastrointest Endosc.* 2008;67(6):781-790.

77. Barawi M, Gottlieb K, Cunha B, et al. A prospective evaluation of the incidence of bacteremia associated with EUS-guided fine-needle aspiration. *Gastrointest Endosc.* 2001;53(2):189-192.

78. Lee TH, Hsueh PR, Yeh WC, et al. Low frequency of bacteremia after endoscopic mucosal resection. *Gastrointest Endosc.* 2000;52(2):223-225.

79. Zuccaro G Jr, Richter JE, Rice TW, et al. Viridans streptococcal bacteremia after esophageal stricture dilation. *Gastrointest Endosc.* 1998;48(6):568-573.

80. Levy MJ, Norton ID, Wiersema MJ, et al. Prospective risk assessment of bacteremia and other infectious complications in patients undergoing EUS-guided FNA. *Gastrointest Endosc.* 2003;57(6):672-678.

81. Janssen J, Konig K, Knop-Hammad V, et al. Frequency of bacteremia after linear EUS of the upper GI tract with and without FNA. *Gastrointest Endosc.* 2004;59(3):339-344.

82. Levy MJ, Norton ID, Clain JE, et al. Prospective study of bacteremia and complications with EUS FNA of rectal and perirectal lesions. *Clin Gastroenterol Hepatol.* 2007;5(6):684-689.

83. Lee LS, Saltzman JR, Bounds BC, et al. EUS-guided fine needle aspiration of pancreatic cysts: a retrospective analysis of complications and their predictors. *Clin Gastroenterol Hepatol.* 2005;3(3):231-236.

84. Hirota WK, Petersen K, Baron TH, et al. Guidelines for antibiotic prophylaxis for GI endoscopy. *Gastrointest Endosc.* 2003;58(4):475-482.

85. Hawes RH, Clancy J, Hasan MK. Endoscopic ultrasound-guided fine needle aspiration in cystic pancreatic lesions. *Clin Endosc.* 2012;45(2):128-131.
86. Baron TH, Kamath PS, McBane RD. Management of antithrombotic therapy in patients undergoing invasive procedures. *N Engl J Med.* 2013;368:2113-2124.
87. Desai J, Granger CB, Weitz JI, et al. Novel oral anticoagulants in gastroenterology practice. *Gastrointest Endosc.* 2013;78(2):227-239.
88. Kearon C, Hirsh J. Management of anticoagulation before and after elective surgery. *N Engl J Med.* 1997;336(21):1506-1511.
89. Eisen GM, Baron TH, Dominitz JA, et al. Guideline on the management of anticoagulation and antiplatelet therapy for endoscopic procedures. *Gastointest Endosc.* 2002;55(7):775-779.
90. Douketis JD, Johnson JA, Turpie AG. Low-molecular-weight heparin as bridging anticoagulation during interruption of warfarin: assessment of a standardized periprocedural anticoagulation regimen. *Arch Intern Med.* 2004;164(12):1319-1326.
91. Kwok A, Faigel DO. Management of anticoagulation before and after gastrointestinal endoscopy. *Am J Gastroenterol.* 2009;104(12): 3085-3097.
92. ASGE Standards of Practice Committee, Anderson MA, Ben-Menachem T, et al. Management of antithrombotic agents for endoscopic procedures. *Gastrointest Endosc.* 2009;70(6):1060-1070.
93. Huisman MV, Lip GY, Diener HC, et al. Dabigatran eteilate for stroke prevention in patients with atrial fibrillation: resolving uncertainties in routine practice. *J Thromb Hemost.* 2012;107(5):838-847.
94. Turpie AG, Kreutz R, Llau J, et al. Management consensus guidance for the use of rivaroxaban: an oral, direct factor Xa inhibitor. *Throm Haemost.* 2012;108(5):876-886.
95. Schulman S, Crowther MA. How I treat with anticoagulants in 2012: new and old anticoagulants, and when and how to switch. *Blood.* 2012;119(13):3016-3023.
96. Stather DR, MacEachern P, Chee A, et al. Safety of endobronchial ultrasound-guided transbronchial needle aspiration for patients taking clopidogrel: a report of 12 consecutive cases. *Respiration.* 2012;83(4): 330-334.
97. O'Toole D, Palazzo L, Arotcarena R, et al. Assessment of complications of EUS-guided fine-needle aspiration. *Gastrointest Endosc.* 2001;53(4): 470-474.
98. Wiersema MJ, Vilmann P, Giovanni M, et al. Endosonography-guided fine-needle aspiration biopsy: diagnostic accuracy and complication assessment. *Gastroenterology.* 1997;112(4):1087-1095.
99. Cotton PB, Eisen GM, Aabakken L, et al. A lexicon for endoscopic adverse events: report of an ASGE workshop. *Gastrointest Endosc.* 2010;71(3):446-454.
100. Gonsalves WI, Pruthi RK, Patnaik MM. The new oral anticoagulants in clinical practice. *Mayo Clin Proc.* 2013;88(5):495-511.
101. Eloubeidi MA, Tamhane A, Lopes TL, et al. Cervical esophageal perforations at the time of endoscopic ultrasound: a prospective evaluation of frequency, outcomes, and patient management. *Am J Gastroenterol.* 2009;104(1):53-56.
102. Kallimanis GE, Gupta PK, Al-Kawas FH, et al. Endoscopic ultrasound for staging esophageal cancer, with or without dilation, is clinically safe and important. *Gastrointest Endosc.* 1995;41(6):540-546.
103. Van Dam J, Rice TW, Catalano MF, et al. High-grade malignant stricture is predictive of esophageal tumor stage: risks of endosonographic evaluation. *Cancer.* 1993;71(10):2910-2917.
104. Wallace MB, Hawes RH, Sahai AV, et al. Dilation of malignant esophageal stenosis to allow EUS guided fine-needle aspiration: safety and effect on patient management. *Gastrointest Endosc.* 2000;51(3): 309-313.
105. Pfau PR, Ginsberg GG, Lew RJ, et al. Esophageal dilation for endosonographic evaluation of malignant esophageal strictures is safe and effective. *Am J Gastroenterol.* 2000;95(10):2813-2815.
106. Menzel J, Hoepffner N, Nottberg H, et al. Preoperative staging of esophageal carcinoma miniprobe sonography versus conventional endoscopic ultrasound in a prospective histopathologically verified study. *Endoscopy.* 1999;31(4):291-297.
107. Mennigen R, Tuebergen D, Koehler G, et al. Endoscopic ultrasound and conventional probe and miniprobe in preoperative staging of esophageal cancer. *J Gastrointest Surg.* 2008;12(2):256-262.
108. Liberman M, Hanna N, Duranceau A, et al. Endobronchial ultrasonography added to endoscopic ultrasonography improves staging in esophageal cancer. *Ann Thorac Surg.* 2013;96(1):232-238.
109. Affi A, Vazquez-Sequeiros E, Norton ID, et al. Acute extraluminal hemorrhage associated with EUS-guided fine needle aspiration: frequency and clinical significance. *Gastrointest Endosc.* 2001;53(2):221-225.
110. Varadarajulu S, Eloubeidi MA. Frequency and significance of acute intracystic hemorrhage during EUS-FNA of cystic lesions of the pancreas. *Gastrointest Endosc.* 2004;60(4):631-635.
111. Al-Haddad M, Wallace MB, Woodward TA, et al. The safety of fine-needle aspiration guided by endoscopic ultrasound: a prospective study. *Endoscopy.* 2008;40(3):204-208.
112. Annema JT, Veseli ÇM, Versteegh MI, et al. Mediastinitis caused by EUS-FNA of a bronchogenic cyst. *Endoscopy.* 2003;35(9):791-793.
113. Fabbri C, Luigiano C, Cennama V, et al. Complications of endoscopic ultrasonography. *Minerva Gastroenterol Dietol.* 2011;57(2):159-166.
114. Ryan AG, Zamvar V, Robert SA. Iatrogenic candidal infection of a mediastinal foregut cyst following endoscopic ultrasound-guided fine needle aspiration. *Endoscopy.* 2002;34(10):838-839.
115. Eloubeidi MA, Tamhane A, Varadarajulu S, et al. Frequency of major complications after EUS-guided FNA of solid pancreatic masses: a prospective evaluation. *Gastrointest Endosc.* 2006;63(4):622-629.
116. Eloubeidi MA, Gress FG, Savides TJ, et al. Acute pancreatitis after EUS-guided FNA of solid pancreatic masses: a pooled analysis from EUS centers in the United States. *Gastrointest Endosc.* 2004;60(3): 385-389.
117. Eloubeidi MA, Chen VK, Eltoum IA, et al. Endoscopic ultrasound-guided fine needle aspiration biopsy of patients with suspected pancreatic cancer: diagnostic accuracy and acute and 30-day complications. *Am J Gastroenterol.* 2003;98(12):2663-2668.
118. Lai R, Stanley MW, Bardales R, et al. Endoscopic ultrasound-guided pancreatic duct aspiration: diagnostic yield and safety. *Endoscopy.* 2002;34(9):715-720.
119. Oh HC, Seo DW, Kim SC. Portal vein thrombosis after EUS-guided pancreatic cyst ablation. *Dig Dis Sci.* 2012;57:1965-1967.
120. Fujii L, Clain JE, Morris JM, Levy MJ. Anterior spinal cord infarction with permanent paralysis following endoscopic ultrasound celiac plexus neurolysis. *Endoscopy.* 2012;44:E265-E266.
121. Gimeno-Garcia AZ, Ekwassuef A, Paquin SC, Sahai AV. Fatal complication after endoscopic ultrasound-guided celiac plexus neurolysis. *Endoscopy.* 2012;44:E267.
122. Loeve US, Mortensen MB. Lethal necrosis and perforation of the stomach and the aorta after multiple EUS-guided celiac plexus neurolysis procedures in a patient with chronic pancreatitis. *Gastrointest Endosc.* 2013;77(1):151-152.
123. Shaw JN, Fraker D, Guerry D, et al. Melanoma seeding of an EUS-guided fine needle track. *Gastrointest Endosc.* 2004;59(7): 923-924.
124. Topazian M. Endoscopic ultrasound-guided drainage of pancreatic fluid collections (with video). *Clin Endosc.* 2012;45:337-340.
125. Varadarajulu S, Christein JD, Wilcox CM. Frequency of complications during EUS-guided drainage of pancreatic fluid collections in 148 consecutive patients. *J Gastroenterol Hepatol.* 2011;26:1504-1508.
126. Chen HY, Lee CH, Hsieh CH. Bile peritonitis after EUS-guided fine needle aspiration. *Gastrointest Endosc.* 2002;56(4):594-596.
127. Park do H, Jang JW, Lee SS, et al. EUS-guided biliary drainage with transluminal stenting after failed ERCP: predictors of adverse events and long-term results. *Gastrointest Endosc.* 2011;74(6): 1276-1284.
128. Haseganu LE, Diehl DL. Left adrenal gland hemorrhage as a complication of EUS-FNA. *Gastrointest Endosc.* 2009;69(6):e51-e52.

5

New Techniques in EUS: Real-Time Elastography, Contrast-Enhanced EUS, and Fusion Imaging

Adrian Săftoiu and Peter Vilmann

Key Points

- EUS has improved considerably in the past years through development of real-time EUS elastography, contrast-enhanced EUS, and fusion imaging.
- Real-time EUS elastography provides qualitative and semiquantitative data about tissue stiffness, possibly allowing differentiation of benign and malignant tumors.
- Contrast-enhanced harmonic EUS using specific software (with low mechanical index capabilities) is already established as a procedure useful for the differential diagnosis of focal pancreatic masses.
- Fusion EUS imaging as a combination of EUS and CT/MRI is still under development, with the aim of decreasing the difficult learning curve of EUS but also increasing diagnostic confidence and better orientation of multiple target lesions.

Endoscopic ultrasound (EUS) represents a high-resolution imaging technique used mainly for the diagnosis and staging of digestive cancers situated in the vicinity of the gastrointestinal (GI) tract. The method is increasingly used in tertiary academic medical centers around the world due to a significant clinical impact, especially after the addition of EUS-guided fine-needle aspiration (EUS FNA), which confirms a tissue diagnosis of malignancy. Due to the increased resolution of EUS technology, even as compared to other cross-sectional imaging methods (such as computed tomography [CT] or magnetic resonance [MR] imaging), several other methods were further developed to extend its capabilities, including real-time EUS elastography, contrast-enhanced EUS, and fusion imaging.[1,2]

Real-Time EUS Elastography

Elasticity imaging has been reported useful for the characterization and differentiation of benign and malignant tissues due to the inherent differences in the hardness of tissues. Thus, malignant tumors are usually stiffer as compared with benign masses, whereas the strain information induced by small tissue deformations can be computed and displayed in real time. Initial clinical applications included breast[3–6] and prostate cancer,[6–10] as well as lymph nodes,[11–15] thyroid masses,[16–19] or focal liver lesions.[20] Recently, real-time elastography was extensively used to characterize liver fibrosis in chronic liver diseases, including chronic hepatitis B or C, and

also liver cirrhosis.[21–24] The technique has the distinct advantage that it can be used with a large variety of ultrasound transducers, thus extending the method to virtually all organs. The method has been successfully applied with intraoperative[25,26] or intracavitary[27] transducers, as well as EUS probes.

Technical Details

Real-time sonoelastography represents a technical improvement of gray-scale ultrasound, which allows the estimation of tissue strain, during slight compressions induced by transducer or small heart/vessel movements.[28] The method works in real time in a similar manner as color Doppler, the strain information being visually converted into a hue color scale and displayed as a transparent overlay imposed on the gray-scale ultrasound information.[29,30] The principle of real-time elastography consists of measurement of tissue displacement induced by small compressions, which are inducing strain that is usually smaller in harder tissues as compared to soft tissues (Figure 5-1). A complex algorithm called combined autocorrelation method allows the calculation of axial strain along the direction of ultrasound waves, which also corresponds to the direction of compressions.[28] Consequently, soft tissues are easy to compress because they are displayed in low-hue values approaching green, whereas hard tissues are difficult to strain because they are displayed in high-hue values approaching blue. The information can be further quantified by taking into consideration a hue scale from 0 to

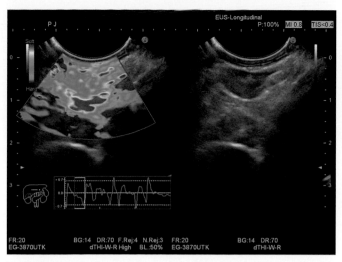

FIGURE 5-1 Benign mediastinal lymph node. EUS elastography showing a relatively homogeneous mixture of green and yellow, indicating a relatively soft structure as compared to the surrounding tissues (*left*).

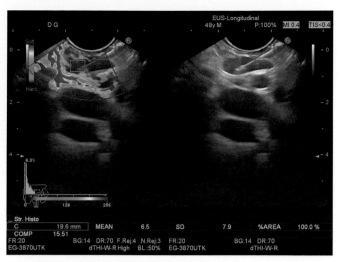

FIGURE 5-3 Malignant mediastinal lymph node. EUS elastography with EUS-guided FNA showing a relatively hard (*blue*) homogeneous lymph node (*left*). A smaller rectangular region of interest is selected at the level of the lymph node and a hue histogram can be displayed, showing low mean elasticity (strain) values.

255, although this method involves relative calculations inside the region of interest. Both the basic principles, as well as the clinical applications for the usage of ultrasound elastography, are carefully reviewed in two comprehensive guidelines and recommendations issued by the European Federation Societies in Ultrasound in Medicine and Biology (EFSUMB).[31,32]

EUS elastography equipment includes a state-of-the-art ultrasound system with real-time sonoelastography capabilities, coupled with conventional endoscopic radial or linear EUS transducers. There is no need for additional devices that induce pressure or vibrations. The usual setting includes a two-panel EUS image, with the conventional gray-scale (B-mode) image on the right panel and the transparent overlay elastography image on the left side (Figure 5-2). The elastography region of interest is trapezoidal in shape and can be freely selected to encompass at least half of the examined targeted lesion, as well as the surrounding tissues. Tissue

elasticity values are represented in a hue color scale, with values from 0 to 255. Consequently, the color information can be semiquantified as average values, whereas all the necessary statistical data (average strain histograms and standard deviation) can be easily calculated by using the latest versions of software (Figures 5-3 to 5-5). The system also includes the possibility of calculation of strain ratio (i.e., an estimation of the modulus ratio between two user-defined areas of interest), thus representing a semiquantitative evaluation of strain differences between the areas.[33] However, it should be taken into consideration that changing the reference area to a deeper position significantly influences strain ratio measurements, which are otherwise independent of the size and other parameters (for example, the elastography dynamic range). It is not

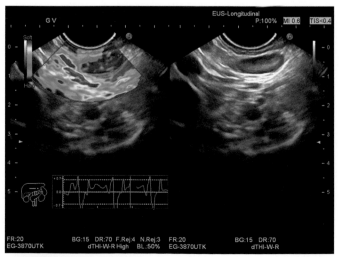

FIGURE 5-2 Malignant mediastinal lymph node. EUS elastography showing a relatively homogeneous mixture of blue, indicating a relatively hard structure as compared to the surrounding tissues (*left*).

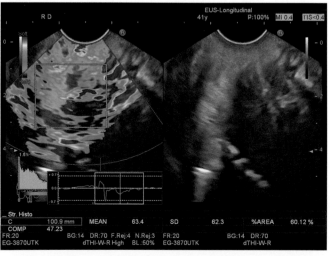

FIGURE 5-4 Chronic pseudotumoral pancreatitis. EUS elastography showing a relatively heterogeneous mixture of blue, green, and red, indicating a relatively intermediate elasticity structure as compared to the surrounding tissues (*left*). Hue histogram analysis can be also performed to obtain semiquantitative data on the elasticity of the focal mass (mean 63.4, SD 62.3).

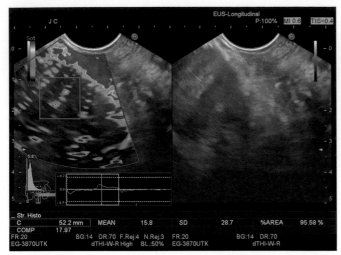

FIGURE 5-5 Pancreatic adenocarcinoma. EUS elastography showing a relatively homogeneous hard *(blue)* mass, indicating a relatively hard elasticity structure as compared to the surrounding tissues *(left)*. Hue histogram analysis can be also performed to obtain semiquantitative data on the elasticity of the focal mass (mean 15.8, SD 28.7).

TABLE 5-1

SENSITIVITY AND SPECIFICITY OF EUS ELASTOGRAPHY FOR THE DIFFERENTIAL DIAGNOSES OF LYMPH NODES

Reference	Number of Lymph Nodes	Sensitivity (%)	Specificity (%)
Giovannini et al[35] (2006)	25	100	50
Săftoiu et al[38] (2006)	42	91.7	94.4
Janssen et al[39] (2007)	66	87.9	86.4
Săftoiu et al[40] (2007)	78	85.4	91.9
Giovannini et al[36] (2009)	101	91.8	82.5
Larsen et al[37] (2012)	56	55	82

yet clear if the usage of strain ratios or strain histograms should be the preferred method, as further studies will be necessary to show the differences between various methodologies.[34]

Clinical Applications

Real-time EUS elastography was initially reported to be useful in a pilot study, which included a low number of patients with focal pancreatic masses ($n = 24$) and lymph nodes ($n = 25$).[35] A high sensitivity of 100% but a low specificity of 67% and 50% for pancreatic masses and lymph nodes, respectively, determined criticism of the study methodology, including qualitative pattern evaluation and establishment of diagnostic criteria in the same group of patients. The study was, however, continued with a multicenter trial that analyzed 222 patients with focal pancreatic masses ($n = 121$) and lymph nodes ($n = 101$), accompanied by interobserver variability data that indicated good values of the kappa coefficient of 0.785 for pancreatic masses and 0.657 for lymph nodes.[36] EUS elastography was proven to have higher sensitivity and specificity values as compared with conventional gray-scale EUS images of 92.3% and 80.0% for the differential diagnosis of focal pancreatic masses and of 91.8% and 82.5% for the differential diagnosis of lymph nodes. Based on the published data, EUS elastography was thus suggested to be superior as compared with conventional B-mode (gray-scale) imaging that might be utilized in patients with pancreatic masses and negative EUS FNA and also to increase the yield of EUS FNA for patients with multiple lymph nodes. Moreover, several prospective studies using qualitative or quantitative criteria were subsequently published and supported the value of real-time EUS elastography in larger patient subgroups and multicenter trial designs (Tables 5-1 and 5-2).

Lymph Nodes

An initial feasibility study that aimed to establish the value of EUS elastography for the differential diagnosis of lymph nodes was based on qualitative pattern analysis of 42 cervical,

mediastinal, or abdominal lymph nodes, taking into consideration five characteristic patterns previously described for breast lesions, which allowed the establishment of a provisional diagnosis of benign (Figure 5-1, Video 5-1) or malignant (Figure 5-2, Video 5-2) lymph nodes.[38] Sensitivity,

TABLE 5-2

SENSITIVITY AND SPECIFICITY OF EUS ELASTOGRAPHY FOR THE DIFFERENTIAL DIAGNOSES OF FOCAL PANCREATIC MASSES

Reference	Number of Patients	Sensitivity (%)	Specificity (%)
Giovannini et al[35] (2006)	24	100	67
Hirche et al[44] (2008)	70	41	53
Săftoiu et al[45] (2008)	43	93.8	63.6
Giovannini et al[36] (2009)	121	92.3	80.0
Iglesias-Garcia et al[46] (2009)	130	100	85.5
Iglesias-Garcia et al[47] (2010)	86	100	92.9
Săftoiu et al[48] (2010)	54	84.8	76.2
Schrader et al[49] (2011)	86	100	100
Săftoiu et al[50] (2011)	258	93.4	66.0
Dawwas et al[51] (2012)	111	100	16.7

Video 5-1. Benign mediastinal lymph node. EUS elastography showing a relatively homogeneous mixture of green and yellow, indicating a relatively soft structure as compared to the surrounding tissues (*left*).

specificity, and accuracy for the qualitative pattern analysis were 91.7%, 94.4%, and 92.86%, respectively, with an area below the receiver operating characteristic curve (AUROC) of 0.949. Quantitative analyses based on RGB color histograms for red, green, and blue channels were further performed, with excellent values calculated for the "elasticity ratio" based on histogram analysis of green versus blue channels. Thus, even higher values were reported for the sensitivity, specificity, and accuracy of the differential diagnosis between benign and malignant lymph nodes of 95.8%, 94.4%, and 95.2%, respectively, with an AUROC of 0.965. Several limitations of the method were acknowledged in the initial papers, including selection bias of the best EUS images, chosen arbitrarily by the examiner from a longer EUS elastography video. Similar results were obtained by another group that analyzed 66 mediastinal lymph nodes based on the same qualitative analysis of color patterns.[39] The accuracy was variable for three examiners, between 81.8% and 87.9% for benign lymph nodes and between 84.6% and 86.4% for malignant lymph nodes, with an excellent interobserver analysis (kappa = 0.84).

Another prospective study was designed to test the accuracy of computer-enhanced dynamic analysis of EUS elastography movies for the differential diagnosis between benign and malignant lymph nodes.[40] A total number of 78 lymph nodes were included, and average hue histograms were calculated for each EUS elastography video in order to better describe the elasticity of each lymph node according to calculations based on the hue scale of the ultrasound system. The receiver operating characteristic (ROC) analysis for the average hue histogram values inside lymph nodes yielded an AUROC of 0.928 for the differential diagnosis, with a sensitivity, specificity, and accuracy of 85.4%, 91.9%, and 88.5%, respectively, based on a cutoff level situated in the middle of

Video 5-2. Malignant mediastinal lymph node. EUS elastography showing a relatively homogeneous mixture of blue, indicating a relatively hard structure as compared to the surrounding tissues (*left*).

the green-blue rainbow scale. The study also reported a high positive predictive value (PPV) of 92.1% and a high negative predictive value (NPV) of 85%, implying that the most probable malignant lymph nodes could be targeted by EUS FNA (Figure 5-3), whereas EUS FNA could be avoided in the lymph nodes that are considered most probably benign.

Another group looked at the intraobserver and interobserver agreement of EUS elastography, including the values of strain ratios, for the differential diagnosis of benign and malignant lymph nodes.[41] Both elastography and elastography strain ratio evaluations of lymph nodes were feasible and had a good interobserver agreement of 0.58 and 0.59 (based on a cutoff of 3.81 for the strain ratio), respectively. Nevertheless the study used only cytology as the gold standard for the 55 out of 62 patients included. The same group further looked at EUS elastography and elastography strain ratios based on histology results after marking of lymph nodes with EUS FNA.[37] The sensitivity of EUS was higher than elastography, while the specificity was lower as compared to elastography and strain ratios.

A recent meta-analysis that included 368 patients with 431 lymph nodes was also published recently, indicating a pooled sensitivity of EUS elastography of 88% with a specificity of 85% for the differential diagnosis of benign and malignant lymph nodes.[43] After subgroup analysis with exclusion of outliers, the sensitivity and specificity were 85% and 91%, respectively, leading the authors to conclude that EUS elastography is a valuable noninvasive method used to differentiate benign and malignant lymph nodes.

Pancreatic Masses

Similar qualitative pattern analysis was used for the visualization and differentiation of pancreatic lesions in a prospective study that included 73 patients: 20 with normal pancreas, 20 with chronic pancreatitis, and 33 with focal pancreatic lesions.[42] Although EUS elastography videos were considered reproducible and could be easily obtained in all the patients included, there was no visible difference between chronic pancreatitis and pancreatic adenocarcinoma. Another study included 70 patients with focal pancreatic masses assessed by qualitative EUS elastography.[44] Again, only 56% of the patients with solid pancreatic lesions had reproducible elastographic tracings, probably because of an incomplete delineation of large lesions (>35 mm in diameter) or due to the large distance from transducer. Due to the inherent problems encountered in the qualitative assessment of EUS elastography videos, it became obvious that the solution might be represented by semiquantitative assessment through quantification of the color (hue) information in the region of interest (focal pancreatic mass).

Thus, semiquantitative analysis based on average hue histograms of the EUS elastography videos showed that the method can be reliably used for the differentiation of normal pancreas, chronic pancreatitis (Figure 5-4, Video 5-3), and pancreatic cancer (Figure 5-5, Video 5-4).[45] A subgroup analysis performed for the patients with focal pancreatic masses (pseudotumoral chronic pancreatitis and pancreatic cancer) yielded an AUROC of 0.847, with good sensitivity, specificity, and accuracy rates of 93.8%, 63.6%, and 86.1%, respectively. The PPV and NPV were 88.2% and 77.8%, respectively. To increase the accuracy, an artificial neural network (ANN) model was further applied and showed a good testing

Video 5-3. Chronic pseudotumoral pancreatitis. EUS elastography showing a relatively heterogeneous mixture of blue, green, and red, indicating a relatively intermediate elasticity structure as compared to the surrounding tissues (*left*). Hue histogram analysis can be also performed to obtain semiquantitative data on the elasticity of the focal mass (mean 63.4, SD 62.3).

performance of 90% on average, with a very good stability of the ANN model and an AUROC of 0.965, indicating also a very good classification performance. EUS elastography thus offers complementary information added to the conventional gray-scale information, whereas the technology has constantly progressed, as hue histogram analysis is nowadays incorporated into the commercial software of the ultrasound systems.

Several other studies using various methodologies also tested the value of real-time EUS elastography in the clinical practice. A large, single-center study involving 130 patients used qualitative pattern analysis with four patterns (homogeneous or heterogeneous, predominantly green or blue patterns) to yield a sensitivity, specificity, and accuracy of 100%, 85.5%, and 94%, respectively.[46] Due to the large subjectivity of the method, the same group published a further study with semiquantitative EUS elastography based on strain ratio, calculated as a quotient between two regions of interest (ROIs): the representative reference area and the focal mass.[47] Based on a total number of 86 consecutive patients with solid focal pancreatic mases, the method was found to be useful with an AUROC of 0.983 and very high sensitivity and specificity of 100% and 92.9%, respectively. Strain ratio measurements were recently used by another group in 109 patients with pancreatic lesions (normal pancreas, chronic pancreatitis, pancreatic cancer, and neuroendocrine tumors).[48] A separate analysis for the red, green, and blue channels achieved a better separation between the groups with normal pancreas and malignant pancreatic lesions, with a high sensitivity and specificity of 100%. Based on quantitative morphometry for pancreatic fibrosis, another group tried to correlate it with pancreatic stiffness but found no relationship.[49] Although

Video 5-4. Pancreatic adenocarcinoma. EUS elastography showing a relatively homogeneous hard (*blue*) mass, indicating a relatively hard elasticity structure as compared to the surrounding tissues (*left*). Hue histogram analysis can also be performed to obtain semiquantitative data on the elasticity of the focal mass (mean 15.8, SD 28.7).

important, this study lacked a group of patients with chronic pancreatitis and thus lacked the most significant and difficult cases of differential diagnosis. A combination of contrast-enhanced power Doppler and real-time EUS elastography also yielded good results for the differentiation of focal pancreatic masses, even though the sensitivity, specificity, and accuracy of elastography had lower values of 84.8%, 76.2%, and 81.5%, respectively, as compared to the combined approach.[50] A recent prospective study included 111 semiquantitative EUS elastography procedures based on strain ratio measurements performed in 104 patients with solid pancreatic masses with the final diagnosis confirmed by pancreatic cytology or histology.[51] The reported areas under the ROC curves for detection of pancreatic malignancy were 0.69 and 0.72 for strain ratio and mass elasticity, respectively, with an overall accuracy of 86.5% and 83.8% (based on cutoffs of 4.65 for SR and 0.27% for mass elasticity), respectively. In concordance with previous studies, the authors suggested that the modest diagnostic role indicates that EUS elastography could supplement EUS FNA and does not replace tissue sampling.

Although EUS elastography brings significant complementary information when added to conventional EUS imaging, the methodology is not yet firmly established, and the choice of either qualitative or semiquantitative methods of evaluation of EUS elastography images or movies is not yet clear.[34] This explains the significant heterogeneity between the published studies (Table 5-2) and also the variability of the results encountered for sensitivity, specificity, and accuracy. Nevertheless, a large European, prospective multicenter trial was performed by the European EUS elastography study group comprising 13 centers and 258 patients.[52] Both a qualitative evaluation by two doctors and also a semiquantitative evaluation by average hue histograms of three separate videos were performed blindly in order to test intraobserver and interobserver variability. For interobserver analysis, qualitative diagnosis of the recorded videos revealed a kappa value of 0.72, whereas for intraobserver analysis the single measure intraclass coefficient ranged between 0.86 and 0.94. Based on a cutoff of 175 for the average hue histograms, the sensitivity, specificity, and accuracy were 94.4%, 66.0%, and 85.4%, respectively, with a corresponding AUROC of 0.894. The PPV was 92.5%, whereas the NPV was 68.9%, implying that EUS elastography could be used in cases with a strong suspicion of pancreatic cancer and negative EUS FNA (which represent up to 25% of focal pancreatic masses). Thus the patients with negative EUS FNA and high-hue histogram values (>185) might be referred to repeat EUS FNA (Figure 5-6) or even directly to surgery, whereas those with negative EUS FNA and relatively lower high-hue histogram values (<170) could be followed-up.

Four meta-analyses have been published concerning the value of EUS elastography for the differential diagnosis of benign and malignant focal pancreatic masses.[53–56] Besides the fact that the meta-analyses are based on the same original studies included, they all found a high pooled sensitivity (85% to 99%) and lower pooled specificity (64% to 76%). Different values of the area under the ROC curve (0.8695 to 0.9624) were dependent on the qualitative or semiquantitative analysis (based on strain ratios or strain histograms), although there was no significant difference between methods. Consequently, all authors concluded that EUS elastography might bring additional information to EUS FNA for the

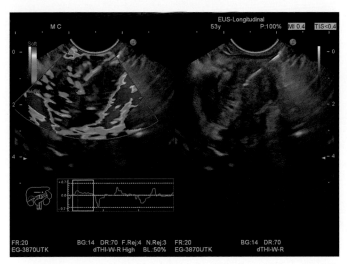

FIGURE 5-6 Pancreatic adenocarcinoma. EUS elastography with EUS-guided FNA, showing the same appearance of a relatively homogeneous hard *(blue)* focal pancreatic mass as compared to the surrounding tissues *(left)*.

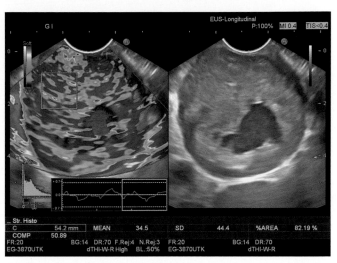

FIGURE 5-8 Malignant GIST (gastrointestinal stromal tumor). EUS elastography showing a relatively heterogeneous hard *(predominantly blue)* mass, indicating a relatively hard elasticity structure as compared to the surrounding tissues *(left)*. Areas of necrosis are not displayed by the elastography software.

differential diagnosis of focal pancreatic masses without being able to exclude EUS FNA for the confirmation of malignancy.

Other Applications

The feasibility of EUS elastography for the characterization of focal liver lesions was reported in only a few papers and case presentations.[57–62] The left liver lobe and part of the right liver lobe can be examined by EUS during staging of other GI tract tumors, with malignant liver masses (especially metastasis) showing a consistent "hard" pattern surrounded by "soft" tissue.

Other indications were proposed for EUS elastography because most of the solid tumors have a "hard" appearance, including esophageal tumors, gastric tumors (Figure 5-7),[63] gastrointestinal stromal tumors (GISTs) (Figure 5-8),[64] or

adrenal tumors. However, the clinical utility of these findings remains to be established in further studies.

Future Techniques

Three-dimensional EUS elastography is a feasible technique, implementing either freehand or automatic reconstruction techniques, through use of the usual transducers or high-quality transducer arrays.[65] The technology is already available in real-time for transabdominal ultrasound (four-dimensional real-time elastography) by using dedicated transducers, thus raising the hope that it will soon be available for EUS also. A significant advantage might be conferred during the follow-up of radiofrequency ablation (RFA) lesions, which are extremely difficult to visualize through conventional ultrasound methods.

Contrast-Enhanced EUS

This technique was initially established using the usual Doppler techniques (color or power Doppler flow imaging) in combination with administration of second-generation microbubble ultrasound contrast agents (UCAs) as Doppler signal enhancers. Due to recent advances in EUS systems, second-generation intravenous UCAs can now be used in association with low mechanical index (MI) techniques in order to improve visualization of tissue perfusion and to differentiate benign from malignant focal lesions, as well as to guide therapeutic procedures.[66,67] Contrast-enhanced EUS (CE EUS) has become an established indication for the discrimination of focal pancreatic masses (especially hypoenhancing pancreatic adenocarcinomas as compared to other isoenhancing or hyperenhancing lesions, including mass-forming chronic pancreatitis or neuroendocrine tumors) and possibly for the discrimination of pseudocysts from pancreatic cystic tumors. Furthermore, dynamic quantification of microvascularization and tissue perfusion can be easily performed based on various software programs embedded in the ultrasound systems or available for off-line use with

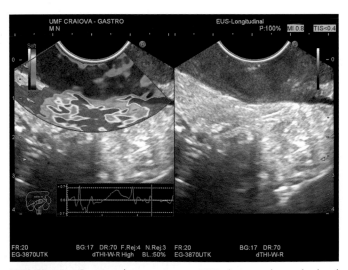

FIGURE 5-7 Gastric adenocarcinoma. EUS elastography at the level of the enlarged and invaded gastric wall showing a relatively homogeneous hard *(blue)* mass, indicating a relatively hard elasticity structure as compared to the surrounding tissues *(left)*.

visualization of time-intensity curves (TIC analysis) and calculation of various quantitative variables.[68]

Technical Details

CE EUS examinations should be performed in association with a careful evaluation of the lesions through conventional gray-scale examinations. There are several techniques used for EUS examinations based on second-generation microbubble UCAs. Initially, these consisted of Doppler signal enhancement during color Doppler and/or power Doppler, although the usage of these high-MI methods was hampered by the presence of both flash (induced by tissue motion) and blooming (induced by signal saturation) artifacts. Recently, the same specific contrast harmonic imaging techniques used in transabdominal US have been developed for usage with both radial and linear EUS transducers.[69] Contrast-specific EUS modes are based on separation of linear ultrasound signals induced by the tissues and utilization of the nonlinear response produced by the microbubbles, thus obtaining a better signal (contrast to tissue) to noise ratio.[70,71]

The most commonly used agent in Europe contains phospholipid-stabilized microbubbles of sulfurhexafluoride (Sono-Vue), which are injected into a large peripheral vein and able to pass through the lung circulation without being destroyed. This agent is classified as a blood pool agent and is restricted in the intravascular compartment until it is eliminated through expired air. Dosage for EUS examinations should be higher than transabdominal US due to the high frequency of EUS transducers, usually 2.4-4.8 mL of Sono-Vue.[71] For the pancreas and other GI tract organs (except the liver, which has a dual blood supply), there is an initial early arterial phase (usually 10 to 30 seconds after contrast injection), followed by a late venous phase usually lasting from approximately 30 to 120 seconds.[72]

Further details of the examination techniques are outside the scope of this chapter and are described in detail elsewhere.[66–72] Thus, the examination uses a low MI (usually below 0.3), defined as a standard measure of the acoustic power, that is, the amplitude of an ultrasound wave at peak negative pressure (PNP) estimated in situ, divided by the square root of the center frequency (Fc) of the ultrasound wave. Examinations are based on nondestructive low-MI nonlinear imaging techniques, whereas the MI can be set up to values between 0.08 and 0.12. Relatively higher values can be used (usually between 0.1 and 0.2), but some microbubbles will be destroyed, although the enhancement will be better delineated. The usual method of low-MI ultrasound examination is called dynamic contrast harmonic imaging (dCHI) and uses a wideband pulse inversion technique, including two pulses with inverted phase and received information with addition of the frequency spectrum of the pulses, thus eliminating the linear information from the tissues and showing the harmonic information produced by the microbubbles.

Clinical Applications

Initial feasibility studies proved the value of CE EUS using a technique that is quite similar to contrast-enhanced transabdominal ultrasound. The first pilot study used a linear EUS prototype and low MI (0.09 to 0.25) in conjuction with a second-generation microbubble contrast agent (Sono-Vue),

allowing the delineation of the arterial and venous phase of the pancreas.[73] The same results were obtained by using a different radial EUS prototype system, showing the real-time continuous images of finely branching vessels of the pancreas, with a slightly higher MI (0.4) and the same second-generation contrast agent (Sono-Vue).[74] This opened up the clinical usage of CE EUS, although some of the contrast agents are still considered off-label indications. Thus, Sono-Vue is registered in the European Union for liver, breast, and vascular applications but pancreatic imaging is not mentioned, although the pancreatic parenchyma is in close contact with the pancreatic vessels and they can be visualized altogether in the same image. Consequently, as mentioned in the current EFSUMB guidelines, an informed consent should be obtained from the patient for the usage of second-generation contrast agents during CE EUS with examinations of pancreas and GI tract; the examination and safety of the patient are within the responsibility of the examining doctor.[68]

Pancreatic Masses

There are several reports in the literature concerning the usage of CE EUS for detection, characterization, staging, and resectability of focal pancreatic masses, using the technique as a one-stop shop for complete analysis of the tumors.[1,2] This is based on the proven hypovascular nature of pancreatic adenocarcinomas in more than 90% of cases, a feature that was reliably and consistently shown by contrast-enhanced CT or angiography. However, none of the cross-sectional techniques (including dynamic contrast-enhanced CT or MR imaging) reaches the high resolution of EUS examinations, which usually allow a confirmation of the final cytologic or histologic diagnosis through EUS-guided fine-needle aspiration.

Initial studies used color Doppler or power Doppler with the addition of the second-generation contrast agent and usage of conventional software with high MI values that usually destroy the microbubbles quickly.[75–81] Also, there are certain artifacts (flash or blooming artifacts), usually induced by movement or saturation of the transducer. An initial feasibility study of power Doppler EUS assessed perfusion by contrast-enhanced power Doppler EUS in 23 patients with inflammatory pseudotumor (Figure 5-9, Video 5-5) and pancreatic carcinoma (Figure 5-10, Video 5-6), with a sensitivity and specificity of 94% and 100%, respectively.[75] These results were further confirmed by other authors using the same qualitative approach (Table 5-3). Another study showed the same hypovascular pattern encountered in most of the pancreatic adenocarcinomas, whereas an isovascular or hypervascular pattern was displayed in all other masses (neuroendocrine tumors, serous microcystic adenomas, and even one teratoma). Considering hypovascularity as a sign of malignancy in pancreatic tumors led to a sensitivity of 92% and a specificity of 100%.[76] The method is useful in small pancreatic carcinomas (less than 2 cm), with a sensitivity of 83.3%, significantly higher than the sensitivity of contrast-enhanced CT, which was only 50%.[77]

Furthermore, the vascularity index (i.e., the percentage of positive Doppler areas reported to the total area of the focal mass) obtained during the late phase of contrast enhancement, after disappearance of the initial blooming effect induced by contrast injection, is useful for the differential diagnosis of pancreatic adenocarcinoma and pseudotumoral chronic pancreatitis.[78,79] These kinds of quantitative techniques

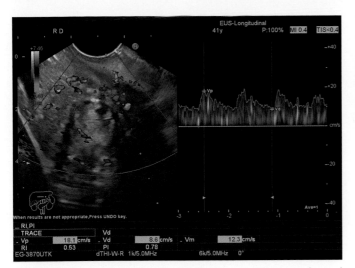

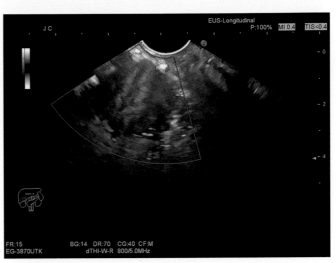

FIGURE 5-9 Pseudotumoral chronic pancreatitis. Contrast-enhanced color Doppler showing multiple Doppler signals inside the hypervascular pancreatic mass (*left*), some with arterial-type signal inside proven by pulsed Doppler (*right*).

FIGURE 5-10 Pancreatic adenocarcinoma. Contrast-enhanced power Doppler showing multiple power Doppler signals (collaterals) surrounding the hypovascular pancreatic mass.

Video 5-5. Pseudotumoral chronic pancreatitis. Contrast-enhanced color Doppler showing multiple Doppler signals inside the hypervascular pancreatic mass (*left*), some with arterial-type signal inside proven by pulsed Doppler (*right*).

Video 5-6. Pancreatic adenocarcinoma. Contrast-enhanced power Doppler showing multiple power Doppler signals (collaterals) surrounding the hypovascular pancreatic mass.

TABLE 5-3

SENSITIVITY AND SPECIFICITY OF CONTRAST-ENHANCED EUS FOR THE DIFFERENTIAL DIAGNOSES OF FOCAL PANCREATIC MASSES

Reference	Number of Patients	Sensitivity (%)	Specificity (%)
High Mechanical Index			
Becker et al[75] (2001)	23	94	100
Hocke et al[78] (2006)	86	91.1	93.3
Dietrich et al[76] (2008)	93	92	100
Sakamoto et al[77] (2008)	156	83.3	100
Săftoiu et al[79] (2010)	54	90.9	71.4
Low Mechanical Index			
Fusaroli et al[82] (2010)	90	96	98
Napoleon et al[83] (2010)	35	89	88
Seicean et al[84] (2010)	30	80	91.7
Romagnuolo et al[85] (2011)	24	100	72.7
Matsubara et al[86] (2011)	91	95.8	92.6
Gheonea et al[87] (2013)	51	93.8	89.5

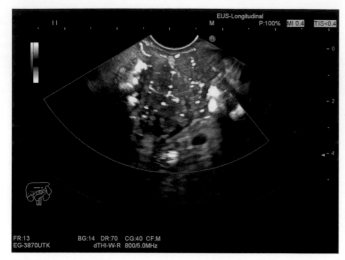

FIGURE 5-11 Malignant neuroendocrine tumor. Contrast-enhanced power Doppler showing multiple power Doppler signals inside the hypervascular pancreatic mass.

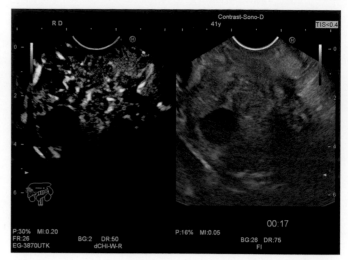

FIGURE 5-12 Pseudotumoral chronic pancreatitis. Low mechanical index contrast-enhanced EUS showing intense uptake of the contrast in the arterial phase, with a small (avascular) pseudocyst at the level of the pancreatic mass (*left*).

seem more appropriate, despite the artifacts induced by contrast enhancement during color and power Doppler EUS. Vascularity index can also be used in combination with the pulsed Doppler sampling of various vessels inside the pancreatic masses, including calculation of resistivity index (RI) and pulsatility index (PI), with values of the RI over 0.7 being indicative of a malignant lesion.

Moreover, most of the intratumoral vessels in pancreatic adenocarcinomas are arterioles, whereas inflammatory chronic pancreatitis masses have both arterioles and venules, both detectable by pulsed Doppler sampling used during CE EUS. Using this approach for differentiation between inflammatory masses and pancreatic carcinoma, the sensitivity was improved, reaching 91.1% with an excellent specificity of 93.3%.[78] Lower values were obtained in a subsequent study that used a cutoff value of 20% for the vascularity index, yielding a sensitivity of 90.9% and a specificity of 71.4%.[79] However, contrast-enhanced power Doppler has been combined in the same study with real-time EUS elastography, yielding a sensitivity of 75.8% and a specificity of 95.2% for the differential diagnosis of focal pancreatic masses. The differential diagnosis is complicated by the fact that around 10% of the patients with pancreatic adenocarcinomas have hypervascular tumors, either due to a neuroendocrine differentiation or to the poor differentiation and advanced stage of the tumor. Neuroendocrine tumors can be characterized as hypervascular lesions (Figure 5-11, Video 5-7), easily visualized by CE EUS, which has a higher sensitivity of 95.1% in comparison with CT or US and is very useful for the assessment of necrotic or hemorrhagic areas inside the tumors.[80] Autoimmune pancreatitis can be differentiated from pancreatic adenocarcinoma, as both focal and diffuse forms show hyperenhancement during CE EUS.[81]

Low MI (harmonic) CE EUS seems to be more advantageous, although the currently published data is still limited (Table 5-3). However, the technique, which is significantly superior to transabdominal US techniques, allows the assessment of microvessel architecture when hampered by the presence of bowel air or obesity, which induce significant artifacts and impede a good visualization of the pancreas.[68] After the initial pilot studies[82,83] and the appearance of commercial EUS systems with low MI (harmonic) CE EUS availability, several articles described the technique and the results in focal pancreatic masses, including pseudotumoral chronic pancreatitis (Figure 5-12, Video 5-8), pancreatic adenocarcinoma (Figure 5-13, Video 5-9), and neuroendocrine tumors (Figure 5-14, Video 5-10). The initial studies varied in methodology (e.g., with variable MI settings from 0.08 to 0.4 as well various qualitative or quantitative methods for signal processing), whereas better multicenter prospective studies are still needed to establish the value of the technique for the characterization, staging, and follow-up of patients with focal pancreatic

Video 5-7. Malignant neuroendocrine tumor. Contrast-enhanced power Doppler showing multiple power Doppler signals inside the hypervascular pancreatic mass.

Video 5-8. Pseudotumoral chronic pancreatitis. Low mechanical index contrast-enhanced EUS showing intense uptake of the contrast in the arterial phase, with a small (avascular) pseudocyst at the level of the pancreatic mass (*left*).

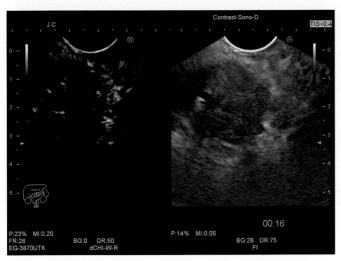

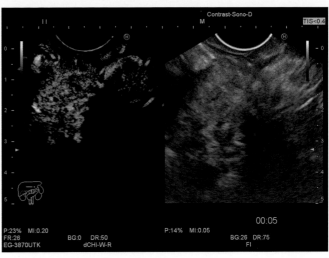

FIGURE 5-13 Pancreatic adenocarcinoma. Low mechanical index contrast-enhanced EUS showing discrete uptake of the contrast in the arterial phase at the level of the hypovascular pancreatic mass, in comparison with the neighboring pancreatic parenchyma (*left*).

FIGURE 5-14 Malignant neuroendocrine tumor. Low mechanical index contrast-enhanced EUS showing intense uptake of the contrast in the arterial phase, at the level of the focal pancreatic mass (*left*).

masses. In the presence of hypoenhancing masses, the sensitivity and specificity reached 96% and 98%, respectively, for the diagnosis of pancreatic adenocarcinoma, while CE EUS allowed the detection of small lesions that could not be visualized during conventional EUS due to the presence of biliary stents or chronic pancreatitis.[82] The sensitivity and specificity had lower values in another study that analyzed qualitatively the pancreatic microcirculation in 35 patients, being 89% and 88%, respectively.[83] Although these values were not improved by quantitative analysis, a more objective way for reporting the results of the CE EUS procedures might be based on histograms and index of contrast uptake, methods that yielded a sensitivity and specificity of 80% and 91.7%, respectively.[84] A small study also tested the feasibility of another second generation perflutren lipid microsphere contrast agent with good sensitivity and specificity of 100% and 72.7%, respectively, although it was based on a limited number of patients.[85] Recently, another group described a dynamic quantitative analysis of CE EUS for the diagnosis of pancreatic diseases, reaching high values of sensitivity and specificity of 95.8% and 92.6% through the use of TIC analysis based on 91 patients with focal pancreatic masses, including 48 patients with pancreatic adenocarcinoma, 14 patients with autoimmune pancreatitis, 13 patients with mass-forming pancreatitis, and 16 patients with pancreatic neuroendocrine tumors.[86]

This was also reported by a recent study published by our group based on quantitative low MI CE EUS used for the differential diagnosis of chronic pseudotumoral pancreatitis and pancreatic cancer, which showed a sensitivity and specificity of 93.75% and 89.47%, respectively, based on TIC analysis.[87]

There has been a significant improvement in the software options needed for semiquantification of perfusion inside focal masses based on TIC analysis with wash-in and wash-out times after bolus injection of contrast performed through curve fitting by computer-enhanced algorithms.[68] Several parameters proportional to the tissue blood flow can be determined (like the peak intensity, area under the curve, time to peak intensity, slope of the wash-in, and mean transit time), which might considerably improve the characterization and follow-up of the patients.[88] Moreover, new software, which is independent of the ultrasound system and user variables, has automatic motion compensation, allowing for a more standardized quantification process through linearization of the DICOM clips during off-line analysis of the CE EUS video clips.[89] This is an area of ongoing research, and future multicenter randomized studies will be necessary to expand the current role of CE EUS in the differential diagnosis of focal pancreatic masses and also for the follow-up of inoperable patients during chemotherapy and radiotherapy.

Video 5-9. Pancreatic adenocarcinoma. Low mechanical index contrast-enhanced EUS showing discrete uptake of the contrast in the arterial phase at the level of the hypovascular pancreatic mass, in comparison with the neighboring pancreatic parenchyma (*left*).

Video 5-10. Malignant neuroendocrine tumor. Low mechanical index contrast-enhanced EUS showing intense uptake of the contrast in the arterial phase, at the level of the focal pancreatic mass (*left*).

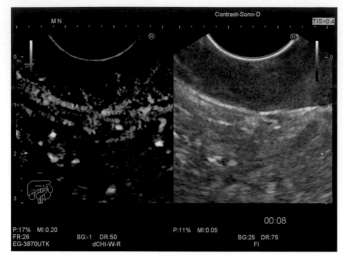

FIGURE 5-15 Gastric adenocarcinoma. Low mechanical index contrast-enhanced EUS showing uptake of the contrast in the arterial phase, at the periphery of the gastric tumor (*left*).

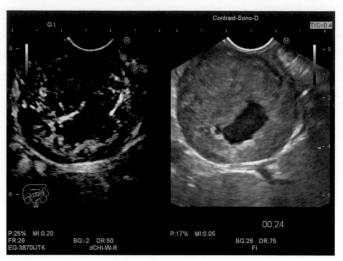

FIGURE 5-16 Gastrointestinal stromal tumor (GIST). Low mechanical index contrast-enhanced EUS showing increased uptake of the contrast in the arterial phase, with a central zone of necrosis (*left*).

Nevertheless, a recent meta-analysis including 12 studies and 1139 patients showed clearly that pooled sensitivity of CE EUS for the differential diagnosis of pancreatic adenocarcinomas was 94% (95% CI, 0.91-0.95), with a specificity of 89% (95% CI, 0.85-0.92).[90] Furthermore, the area under the ROC curve was 0.9732. Both studies based on enhanced color/power Doppler and including harmonic EUS consistently showed that visualization of a hypoenhanced pancreatic lesion was an accurate predictor of pancreatic adenocarcinoma.

Other Applications

Although EUS is certainly useful for staging of GI tract cancer (esophageal, gastric, and colorectal), the usage of CE EUS is not yet established clinically for these patients. Initial studies proved that CE EUS improves the overall accuracy for assessment of depth of invasion of GI tract cancer,[91] as well as a better visualization of the microvasculature and follow-up during treatment (Figure 5-15, Video 5-11). A recent study assessed the correlations between contrast-enhanced power Doppler EUS and the values of angiogenesis markers, showing that postcontrast values of vascularity index were correlated with intratumoral microvascular density assessed by CD34 immunohistochemical analysis as well as with the values of vascular endothelial growth factor (VEGF) assessed by real-time polymerase chain reaction (RT-PCR).[92]

A small study indicated that CE EUS can be used to differentiate GISTs from other benign tumors (lipoma or leiomyoma) based on the hyperenhanced appearance of GISTs.[93] Contrast-enhanced EUS has recently been used for the assessment of tumor vascularity in order to predict the preoperative malignancy risk of GISTs through identification of irregular vessels (Figure 5-16, Video 5-12).[94] The sensitivity, specificity, and accuracy for identification of irregular vessels and thus prediction of malignancy was 100%, 63%, and 83%, respectively, being comparable to EUS-guided FNA, which had similar figures of 63%, 92%, and 81%, respectively. The yield of detection of irregular vessels was better than power Doppler EUS and contrast-enhanced CT.

Microvascularity of intraabdominal lesions can be easily depicted by CE EUS, the method being useful for differentiation of benign and malignant lesions.[95] This has been tested in 43 patients with indeterminate abdominal lesions and reached a high interobserver agreement of 0.953. The sensitivity, specificity, and accuracy for the differential diagnosis of benign and malignant lesions were very high, being equal to 96.3%, 100%, and 97.6%, respectively.

Future Techniques

Three-dimensional EUS has been described previously in order to better assess the relationship between tumors and

Video 5-11. Gastric adenocarcinoma. Low mechanical index contrast-enhanced EUS showing uptake of the contrast in the arterial phase, at the periphery of the gastric tumor (*left*).

Video 5-12. Gastrointestinal stromal tumor (GIST). Low mechanical index contrast-enhanced EUS showing increased uptake of the contrast in the arterial phase, with a central zone of necrosis (*left*).

neighboring structures,[65] whereas the technology allowed freehand reconstructions during contrast-enhanced power Doppler EUS. More recently, low MI contrast-enhanced harmonic three-dimensional EUS was proven to be feasible, showing a good characterization of vascularity and outer borders on tumor lesions.[96] However, automatic acquisition and real-time four-dimensional techniques with quantification software would be necessary to better define the clinical impact of this exciting technique.

Contrast-enhanced transabdominal ultrasound has been proposed for longitudinal monitoring of antiangiogenic treatment effects, especially in association with the use of specific quantification software that allows perfusion assessment.[68] Current recommendations endorse the use of dynamic CE US for the assessment of response to biologic therapy in some hypervascular tumors (e.g., hepatocellular carcinoma, metastatic GIST, or metastatic renal cell carcinoma), provided that appropriate software for contrast signal quantification is available.[97] Contrast-enhanced harmonic EUS would possibly be used due to the increased resolution as well as decreased artifacts, although studies are still ongoing.

By using specific ligands conjugated to the surface of microbubble UCAs, targeted contrast agents can be directed in vivo toward specific endothelial cell surface receptors.[98] One of the most used targeted UCAs is linked with monoclonal antibodies directed toward VEGF receptor 2 (VEGFR2), allowing quantification of VEGFR2 expression inside tumor vessels and monitoring of treatment response.[99] This kind of microbubble carrier can also be used for targeted treatment through incorporation of chemotherapeutic or gene vectors delivered at cellular levels based on the enhanced uptake in the presence of contrast-enhanced ultrasound, a mechanism called sonoporation.[100] However, none of these agents is currently available for clinical use in human patients; all of them are awaiting clinical translation.

Fusion Imaging

Fusion imaging based on ultrasound represents a combination of ultrasound with CT/MR based on electromagnetic positioning tracking of the ultrasound transducer and coregistration with the corresponding CT/MR image obtained based on the three-dimensional cube data set obtained previously.[101] Various applications have been described, including transabdominal ultrasound (TUS),[102] EUS,[103] laparoscopic ultrasound (LUS),[104] and natural orifice transluminal endoscopic surgery (NOTES) procedures,[105] with the aim of improving lesion targeting and increasing the endoscopist's confidence and performance during interventional procedures. The procedure has also been tested in patients, showing an easier image interpretation based on multiple imaging modalities, better lesion targeting during FNA or other interventional procedures, as well as possible shortening of the learning curve.[106] Based on the advance of current imaging systems, other techniques can be easily fused, like elastography and low MI contrast-enhanced EUS with CT, MR, or positron emission tomography (PET)-CT images. A recent review described in detail the current techniques of fusion imaging based on ultrasound and EUS, with several applications in the field of enhanced diagnosis, staging, and follow-up of oncologic patients.[107]

REFERENCES

1. Săftoiu A. State-of-the-art imaging techniques in endoscopic ultrasound. *World J Gastroenterol.* 2011;17:691-696.
2. Gheonea DI, Săftoiu A. Beyond conventional endoscopic ultrasound: elastography, contrast enhancement and hybrid techniques. *Curr Opin Gastroenterol.* 2011;27:423-429.
3. Céspedes I, Ophir J, Ponnekanti H, Maklad N. Elastography: elasticity imaging using ultrasound with application to muscle and breast in vivo. *Ultrason Imaging.* 1993;15:73-88.
4. Hiltawsky KM, Krüger M, Starke C, et al. Freehand ultrasound elastography of breast lesions: clinical results. *Ultrasound Med Biol.* 2001;27(11):1461-1469.
5. Itoh A, Ueno E, Tohno E, et al. Breast disease: clinical application of US elastography for diagnosis. *Radiology.* 2006;239:341-350.
6. Ginat DT, Destounis SV, Barr RG, et al. US elastography of breast and prostate lesions. *Radiographics.* 2009;29:2007-2016.
7. Cochlin DL, Ganatra RH, Griffiths DF. Elastography in the detection of prostatic cancer. *Clin Radiol.* 2002;57:1014-1020.
8. König K, Scheipers U, Pesavento A, et al. Initial experiences with real-time elastography guided biopsies of the prostate. *J Urol.* 2005;174:115-117.
9. Pallwein L, Aigner F, Faschingbauer R, et al. Prostate cancer diagnosis: value of real-time elastography. *Abdom Imaging.* 2008;33:729-735.
10. Kapoor A, Kapoor A, Mahajan G, Sidhu BS. Real-time elastography in the detection of prostate cancer in patients with raised PSA level. *Ultrasound Med Biol.* 2011;37:1374-1381.
11. Alam F, Naito K, Horiguchi J, et al. Accuracy of sonographic elastography in the differential diagnosis of enlarged cervical lymph nodes: comparison with conventional B-mode sonography. *AJR Am J Roentgenol.* 2008;191:604-610.
12. Tan R, Xiao Y, He Q. Ultrasound elastography: its potential role in assessment of cervical lymphadenopathy. *Acad Radiol.* 2010;17:849-855.
13. Bhatia KS, Cho CC, Yuen YH, et al. Real-time qualitative ultrasound elastography of cervical lymph nodes in routine clinical practice: interobserver agreement and correlation with malignancy. *Ultrasound Med Biol.* 2010;36:1990-1997.
14. Choi JJ, Kang BJ, Kim SH, et al. Role of sonographic elastography in the differential diagnosis of axillary lymph nodes in breast cancer. *J Ultrasound Med.* 2011;30:429-436.
15. Taylor K, O'Keeffe S, Britton PD, et al. Ultrasound elastography as an adjunct to conventional ultrasound in the preoperative assessment of axillary lymph nodes in suspected breast cancer: a pilot study. *Clin Radiol.* 2011;66(11):1064-1071.
16. Park SH, Kim SJ, Kim EK, et al. Interobserver agreement in assessing the sonographic and elastographic features of malignant thyroid nodules. *AJR Am J Roentgenol.* 2009;193(5):W416-W423.
17. Bojunga J, Herrmann E, Meyer G, et al. Real-time elastography for the differentiation of benign and malignant thyroid nodules: a meta-analysis. *Thyroid.* 2010;20:1145-1150.
18. Ding J, Cheng HD, Huang J, et al. An improved quantitative measurement for thyroid cancer detection based on elastography. *Eur J Radiol.* 2011;81(4):800-805.
19. Xing P, Wu L, Zhang C, et al. Differentiation of benign from malignant thyroid lesions: calculation of the strain ratio on thyroid sonoelastography. *J Ultrasound Med.* 2011;30:663-669.
20. Kapoor A, Kapoor A, Mahajan G, et al. Real-time elastography in differentiating metastatic from nonmetastatic liver nodules. *Ultrasound Med Biol.* 2011;37:207-213.
21. Gheonea DI, Săftoiu A, Ciurea T, et al. Real-time sono-elastography in the diagnosis of diffuse liver diseases. *World J Gastroenterol.* 2010;16:1720-1726.
22. Wang J, Guo L, Shi X, et al. Real-time elastography with a novel quantitative technology for assessment of liver fibrosis in chronic hepatitis B. *Eur J Radiol.* 2012;81:e31-e36.
23. Koizumi Y, Hirooka M, Kisaka Y, et al. Liver fibrosis in patients with chronic hepatitis C: noninvasive diagnosis by means of real-time tissue elastography—establishment of the method for measurement. *Radiology.* 2011;258:610-617.
24. Hirooka M, Koizumi Y, Hiasa Y, et al. Hepatic elasticity in patients with ascites: evaluation with real-time tissue elastography. *AJR Am J Roentgenol.* 2011;196:W766-W771.
25. Inoue Y, Takahashi M, Arita J, et al. Intra-operative freehand real-time elastography for small focal liver lesions: "visual palpation" for nonpalpable tumors. *Surgery.* 2010;148:1000-1011.

26. Kato K, Sugimoto H, Kanazumi N, et al. Intra-operative application of real-time tissue elastography for the diagnosis of liver tumours. *Liver Int.* 2008;28(9):1264-1271.

27. Waage JE, Havre RF, Odegaard S, et al. Endorectal elastography in the evaluation of rectal tumours. *Colorectal Dis.* 2010;13(10):1130-1137.

28. Frey H. [Realtime elastography. A new ultrasound procedure for the reconstruction of tissue elasticity]. *Radiologe.* 2003;43:850-855.

29. Săftoiu A, Vilmann P. Endoscopic ultrasound elastography—a new imaging technique for the visualization of tissue elasticity distribution. *Journal Gastrointest Liv Dis.* 2006;15:161-165.

30. Dietrich CF, Săftoiu A, Jenssen C. Real time elastography endoscopic ultrasound (RTE-EUS), a comprehensive review. *Eur J Radiol.* 2013; [Epub ahead of print].

31. Bamber J, Cosgrove D, Dietrich CF, et al. EFSUMB guidelines and recommendations on the clinical use of ultrasound elastography. Part 1: basic principles and technology. *Ultraschall Med.* 2013;34:169-184.

32. Cosgrove D, Piscaglia F, Bamber J, et al. EFSUMB guidelines and recommendations on the clinical use of ultrasound elastography. Part 2: clinical applications. *Ultraschall Med.* 2013;34:238-253.

33. Havre RF, Waage JR, Gilja OH, et al. Real-time elastography: strain ratio measurements are influenced by the position of the reference area. *Ultraschall Med.* 2011; [Epub ahead of print].

34. Săftoiu A, Vilmann P. Differential diagnosis of focal pancreatic masses by semiquantitative EUS elastography: between strain ratios and strain histograms. *Gastrointest Endosc.* 2013;78:188-189.

35. Giovannini M, Hookey LC, Bories E, et al. Endoscopic ultrasound elastography: the first step towards virtual biopsy? Preliminary results in 49 patients. *Endoscopy.* 2006;38:344-348.

36. Giovannini M, Thomas B, Erwan B, et al. Endoscopic ultrasound elastography for evaluation of lymph nodes and pancreatic masses: a multicenter study. *World J Gastroenterol.* 2009;15:1587-1593.

37. Larsen MH, Fristrup C, Hansen TP, et al. Endoscopic ultrasound, endoscopic sonoelastography, and strain ratio evaluation of lymph nodes with histology as gold standard. *Endoscopy.* 2012;44:759-766.

38. Săftoiu A, Vilmann P, Hassan H, Gorunescu F. Analysis of endoscopic ultrasound elastography used for characterisation and differentiation of benign and malignant lymph nodes. *Ultraschall Med.* 2006;27: 535-542.

39. Janssen J, Dietrich CF, Will U, Greiner L. Endosonographic elastography in the diagnosis of mediastinal lymph nodes. *Endoscopy.* 2007;39: 952-957.

40. Săftoiu A, Vilmann P, Ciurea T, et al. Dynamic analysis of EUS used for the differentiation of benign and malignant lymph nodes. *Gastrointest Endosc.* 2007;66:291-300.

41. Larsen MH, Fristrup CW, Mortensen MB. Intra- and interobserver agreement of endoscopic sonoelastography in the evaluation of lymph nodes. *Ultraschall Med.* 2011;32(suppl 2):E45-E50.

42. Janssen J, Schlörer E, Greiner L. EUS elastography of the pancreas: feasibility and pattern description of the normal pancreas, chronic pancreatitis, and focal pancreatic lesions. *Gastrointest Endosc.* 2007;65:971-978.

43. Xu W, Shi J, Zeng X, et al. EUS elastography for the differentiation of benign and malignant lymph nodes: a meta-analysis. *Gastrointest Endosc.* 2011;74(5):1001-1009.

44. Hirche TO, Ignee A, Barreiros AP, et al. Indications and limitations of endoscopic ultrasound elastography for evaluation of focal pancreatic lesions. *Endoscopy.* 2008;40:910-917.

45. Săftoiu A, Vilmann P, Gorunescu F, et al. Neural network analysis of dynamic sequences of EUS elastography used for the differential diagnosis of chronic pancreatitis and pancreatic cancer. *Gastrointest Endosc.* 2008;68:1086-1094.

46. Iglesias-Garcia J, Larino-Noia J, Abdulkader I, et al. EUS elastography for the characterization of solid pancreatic masses. *Gastrointest Endosc.* 2009;70:1101-1108.

47. Iglesias-Garcia J, Larino-Noia J, Abdulkader I, et al. Quantitative endoscopic ultrasound elastography: an accurate method for the differentiation of solid pancreatic masses. *Gastroenterology.* 2010;139: 1172-1180.

48. Itokawa F, Itoi T, Sofuni A, et al. EUS elastography combined with the strain ratio of tissue elasticity for diagnosis of solid pancreatic masses. *J Gastroenterol.* 2011;46:843-853.

49. Schrader H, Wiese M, Ellrichmann M, et al. Diagnostic value of quantitative EUS elastography for malignant pancreatic tumors: relationship with pancreatic fibrosis. *Ultraschall Med.* 2011;33(7):E196-E201.

50. Săftoiu A, Iordache SA, Gheonea DI, et al. Combined contrast-enhanced power Doppler and real-time sonoelastography performed during EUS, used in the differential diagnosis of focal pancreatic masses (with videos). *Gastrointest Endosc.* 2010;72:739-747.

51. Dawwas MF, Taha H, Leeds JS, et al. Diagnostic accuracy of quantitative EUS elastography for discriminating malignant from benign solid pancreatic masses: a prospective, single-center study. *Gastrointest Endosc.* 2012;76:953-961.

52. Săftoiu A, Vilmann P, Gorunescu F, et al. Accuracy of endoscopic ultrasound elastography used for differential diagnosis of focal pancreatic masses: a multicenter study. *Endoscopy.* 2011;43:596-603.

53. Pei Q, Zou X, Zhang X, et al. Diagnostic value of EUS elastography in differentiation of benign and malignant solid pancreatic masses: a meta-analysis. *Pancreatology.* 2012;12:402-408.

54. Xu W, Shi J, Li X, et al. Endoscopic ultrasound elastography for differentiation of benign and malignant pancreatic masses: a systemic review and meta-analysis. *Eur J Gastroenterol Hepatol.* 2013;25: 218-224.

55. Hu DM, Gong TT, Zhu Q. Endoscopic ultrasound elastography for differential diagnosis of pancreatic masses: a meta-analysis. *Dig Dis Sci.* 2013;58:1125-1131.

56. Ying L, Lin X, Xie ZL, et al. Clinical utility of endoscopic ultrasound elastography for identification of malignant pancreatic masses: a meta-analysis. *J Gastroenterol Hepatol.* 2013;28:1434-43.

57. Rustemovic N, Hrstic I, Opacic M, et al. EUS elastography in the diagnosis of focal liver lesions. *Gastrointest Endosc.* 2007;66:823-824.

58. Iglesias García J, Lariño Noia J, Souto R, et al. Endoscopic ultrasound (EUS) elastography of the liver. *Rev Esp Enferm Dig.* 2009;101: 717-719.

59. Gheorghe L, Gheorghe C, Cotruta B, Carabela A. CT aspects of gastrointestinal stromal tumors: adding EUS and EUS elastography to the diagnostic tools. *J Gastrointestin Liver Dis.* 2007;16:346-347.

60. Kato K, Sugimoto H, Kanazumi N, et al. Intra-operative application of real-time tissue elastography for the diagnosis of liver tumours. *Liver Int.* 2008;28:1264-1271.

61. Gheorghe L, Iacob S, Iacob R, et al. Real time elastography—a noninvasive diagnostic method of small hepatocellular carcinoma in cirrhosis. *J Gastrointestin Liver Dis.* 2009;18:439-446.

62. Kapoor A, Kapoor A, Mahajan G, et al. Real-time elastography in differentiating metastatic from nonmetastatic liver nodules. *Ultrasound Med Biol.* 2011;37:207-213.

63. Carrara S, Doglioni C, Arcidiacono PG, Testoni PA. Gastric metastasis from ovarian carcinoma diagnosed by EUS-FNA biopsy and elastography. *Gastrointest Endosc.* 2011;74:223-225.

64. Gheorghe L, Gheorghe C, Cotruta B, Carabela A. CT aspects of gastrointestinal stromal tumors: adding EUS and EUS elastography to the diagnostic tools. *J Gastrointestin Liver Dis.* 2007;16:346-347.

65. Saftoiu A, Gheonea DI. Tridimensional (3D) endoscopic ultrasound—a pictorial review. *J Gastrointestin Liver Dis.* 2009;18:501-505.

66. Reddy NK, Ioncică AM, Săftoiu A, et al. Contrast-enhanced endoscopic ultrasonography. *World J Gastroenterol.* 2011;17:42-48.

67. Săftoiu A, Dietrich CF, Vilmann P. Contrast-enhanced harmonic endoscopic ultrasound. *Endoscopy.* 2012;44:612-617.

68. Piscaglia F, Nolsoe C, Dietrich CF, et al. The EFSUMB guidelines and recommendations on the clinical practice of contrast-enhanced ultrasound (CEUS): update 2011 on non-hepatic applications. *Ultraschall Med.* 2012;33:33-59.

69. Greis C, Dietrich CF. Ultrasound contrast agents and contrast enhanced sonography. In: Dietrich CF, ed. *Endoscopic Ultrasound, an Introductory Manual and Atlas.* 2nd ed. Thieme Verlag; 2011.

70. Dietrich CF. Contrast-enhanced low mechanical index endoscopic ultrasound (CELMI-EUS). *Endoscopy.* 2009;41(suppl 2):E43-E44.

71. Sanchez MVA, Varadarajulu S, Napoleon B. EUS contrast agents: what is available, how do they work, and are they effective? *Gastrointest Endosc.* 2009;69:S71-S77.

72. Claudon M, Cosgrove D, Albrecht T, et al. Guidelines and good clinical practice recommendations for contrast enhanced ultrasound (CEUS)—update 2008. *Ultraschall Med.* 2008;29:28-44.

73. Dietrich CF, Ignee A, Frey H. Contrast-enhanced endoscopic ultrasound with low mechanical index: a new technique. *Z Gastroenterol.* 2005;43:1219-1223.

74. Kitano M, Takagi T, Sakamoto H, et al. Dynamic imaging of pancreatic tumors by contrast-enhanced harmonic EUS with long-lasting contrast. *Gastrointest Endosc.* 2009;67:141-150.

75. Becker D, Strobel D, Bernatik T, Hahn EG. Echo-enhanced color- and power-Doppler EUS for the discrimination between focal pancreatitis and pancreatic carcinoma. *Gastrointest Endosc.* 2001;53: 784-789.

76. Dietrich CF, Ignee A, Braden B, et al. Improved differentiation of pancreatic tumors using contrast-enhanced endoscopic ultrasound. *Clin Gastroenterol Hepatol.* 2008;6:590-597, e1.

77. Sakamoto H, Kitano M, Suetomi Y, et al. Utility of contrast-enhanced endoscopic ultrasonography for diagnosis of small pancreatic carcinomas. *Ultrasound Med Biol.* 2008;34:525-532.

78. Hocke M, Schulze E, Gottschalk P, et al. Contrast-enhanced endoscopic ultrasound in discrimination between focal pancreatitis and pancreatic cancer. *World J Gastroenterol.* 2006;12:246-250.

79. Săftoiu A, Iordache SA, Gheonea DI, et al. Combined contrast-enhanced power Doppler and real-time sonoelastography performed during EUS, used in the differential diagnosis of focal pancreatic masses (with videos). *Gastrointest Endosc.* 2010;72:739-747.

80. Ishikawa T, Itoh A, Kawashima H, et al. Usefulness of EUS combined with contrast-enhancement in the differential diagnosis of malignant versus benign and preoperative localization of pancreatic endocrine tumors. *Gastrointest Endosc.* 2010;71:951-959.

81. Hocke M, Ignee A, Dietrich CF. Contrast-enhanced endoscopic ultrasound in the diagnosis of autoimmune pancreatitis. *Endoscopy.* 2011;43(2):163-165.

82. Fusaroli P, Spada A, Mancino MG, Caletti G. Contrast harmonic echoendoscopic ultrasound improves accuracy in diagnosis of solid pancreatic masses. *Clin Gastroenterol Hepatol.* 2010;8:629-634.

83. Napoleon B, Alvarez-Sanchez MV, Gincoul R, et al. Contrast-enhanced harmonic endoscopic ultrasound in solid lesions of the pancreas: results of a pilot study. *Endoscopy.* 2010;42:564-570.

84. Seicean A, Badea R, Stan-Iuga R, et al. Quantitative contrast-enhanced harmonic endoscopic ultrasonography for the discrimination of solid pancreatic masses. *Ultraschall Med.* 2010;31:571-576.

85. Romagnuolo J, Hoffman B, Vela S, et al. Accuracy of contrast-enhanced harmonic EUS with a second-generation perflutren lipid microsphere contrast agent (with video). *Gastrointest Endosc.* 2011;73:52-63.

86. Matsubara H, Itoh A, Kawashima H, et al. Dynamic quantitative evaluation of contrast-enhanced endoscopic ultrasonography in the diagnosis of pancreatic diseases. *Pancreas.* 2011;40:1073-1079.

87. Gheonea DI, Streba CT, Ciurea T, Săftoiu A. Quantitative low mechanical index contrast-enhanced endoscopic ultrasound for the differential diagnosis of chronic pseudotumoral pancreatitis and pancreatic cancer. *BMC Gastroenterol.* 2013;13:2.

88. Gauthier TP, Averkiou MA, Leen EL. Perfusion quantification using dynamic contrast-enhanced ultrasound: the impact of dynamic range and gain on time-intensity curves. *Ultrasonics.* 2011;51:102-106.

89. Peronneau P, Lassau N, Leguerney I, et al. Contrast ultrasonography: necessity of linear data processing for the quantification of tumor vascularization. *Ultraschall Med.* 2010;31:370-378.

90. Gong TT, Hu DM, Zhu Q. Contrast-enhanced EUS for differential diagnosis of pancreatic mass lesions: a meta-analysis. *Gastrointest Endosc.* 2012;76:301-309.

91. Nomura N, Goto H, Niwa Y, et al. Usefulness of contrast-enhanced EUS in the diagnosis of upper GI tract diseases. *Gastrointest Endosc.* 1999;50:555-560.

92. Iordache S, Filip MM, Georgescu CV, et al. Contrast-enhanced power Doppler endosonography and pathological assessment of vascularization in advanced gastric carcinomas—a feasibility study. *Med Ultrason.* 2012;14:101-107.

93. Kannengiesser K, Mahlke R, Petersen F, et al. Contrast-enhanced harmonic endoscopic ultrasound is able to discriminate benign submucosal lesions from gastrointestinal stromal tumors. *Scand J Gastroenterol.* 2012;47:1515-1520.

94. Sakamoto H, Kitano M, Matsui S, et al. Estimation of malignant potential of GI stromal tumors by contrast-enhanced harmonic EUS (with videos). *Gastrointest Endosc.* 2011;73:227-237.

95. Xia Y, Kitano M, Kudo M, et al. Characterization of intra-abdominal lesions of undetermined origin by contrast-enhanced harmonic EUS (with videos). *Gastrointest Endosc.* 2010;72:637-642.

96. Hocke M, Dietrich CF. New technology—combined use of 3D contrast enhanced endoscopic ultrasound techniques. *Ultraschall Med.* 2011;32:317-318.

97. Casali PG, Blay JY, Experts ECECPo. Gastrointestinal stromal tumours: ESMO clinical practice guidelines for diagnosis, treatment and follow-up. *Ann Oncol.* 2010;(suppl 5):v98-v102.

98. Kruskal JB. Can contrast-enhanced US with targeted microbubbles monitor the response to antiangiogenic therapies? *Radiology.* 2008;246:339-340.

99. Willmann JK, Paulmurugan R, Chen K, et al. US imaging of tumor angiogenesis with microbubbles targeted to vascular endothelial growth factor receptor type 2 in mice. *Radiology.* 2008;246:508-518.

100. Postema M, Gilja OH. Ultrasound-directed drug delivery. *Curr Pharm Biotechnol.* 2007;8:355-361.

101. Estépar RS, Stylopoulos N, Ellis R, et al. Towards scarless surgery: an endoscopic ultrasound navigation system for transgastric access procedures. *Comput Aided Surg.* 2007;12:311-324.

102. Ewertsen C, Henriksen BM, Torp-Pedersen S, Bachmann Nielsen M. Characterization by biopsy or CEUS of liver lesions guided by image fusion between ultrasonography and CT, PET/CT or MRI. *Ultraschall Med.* 2011;32:191-197.

103. Vosburgh KG, Stylopoulos N, Estepar RS, et al. EUS with CT improves efficiency and structure identification over conventional EUS. *Gastrointest Endosc.* 2007;65:866-870.

104. Estépar RS, Westin CF, Vosburgh KG. Towards real time 2D to 3D registration for ultrasound-guided endoscopic and laparoscopic procedures. *Int J Comput Assist Radiol Surg.* 2009;4:549-560.

105. Fernández-Esparrach G, Estépar SR, Guarner-Argente C, et al. The role of a computed tomography-based image registered navigation system for natural orifice transluminal endoscopic surgery: a comparative study in a porcine model. *Endoscopy.* 2010;42:1096-1103.

106. Obstein KL, Estépar RS, Jayender J, et al. Image Registered Gastroscopic Ultrasound (IRGUS) in human subjects: a pilot study to assess feasibility. *Endoscopy.* 2011;43:394-399.

107. Ewertsen C, Săftoiu A, Gruionu LG, et al. Real-time image fusion involving diagnostic ultrasound. *AJR Am J Roentgenol.* 2013;200(3):W249-W255.

SECTION II

Mediastinum

How to Perform EUS in the Esophagus and Mediastinum

Robert H. Hawes • Shyam Varadarajulu • Paul Fockens

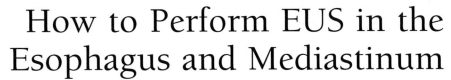

Esophagus

Obtaining high-quality images of the esophageal wall is one of the more difficult tasks that an endosonographer will encounter. One has to deal with the "catch 22" that pits adequate coupling of the ultrasound signal to the esophageal wall against wall compression. This situation can lead to inaccurate assessment of invasion depth in patients with early esophageal cancer or to missing lesions completely in the case of varices. Numerous techniques can be employed to overcome these conflicting goals.

In the case of a relatively advanced mass in the esophagus, minimal or no balloon inflation is sufficient to couple the ultrasound signal to the esophageal wall without causing compression that adversely affects staging accuracy. In this circumstance, the electronic radial instrument has an advantage over the mechanical radial device because of the absence of ringdown artifact and the superior near-field resolution of electronic array technology. Periesophageal structures (e.g., lymph nodes) are not affected by the amount of balloon inflation.

When compression of the esophageal wall needs to be avoided, several different techniques can be employed. The simplest is to instill water into the gut lumen by pressing the air/water button to its first position. This maneuver sprays water across the endoscopic image lens. Remarkably, this does a very good job of filling the lumen with water while reducing the risk of aspiration. This technique can be employed with the standard radial echoendoscope or when using a high-frequency catheter probe in conjunction with a single- or dual-channel forward-viewing endoscope. The images generated are often fleeting because of peristalsis and variability in water filling. As a result, the cine function on the console becomes important in that it allows one to freeze the image and then scroll through the stored images to save the best one. High-resolution esophageal images can be obtained only when the esophagus is in its relaxed state, and this occurs only periodically. Agents normally used to paralyze the stomach, duodenum, and colon have little to no effect on esophageal contractions.

A second method that can be used with a radial scanning echoendoscope is to instill water through the biopsy channel. If this technique is employed, it is recommended that water be slowly siphoned into the esophagus rather than actively pumped or vigorously instilled by syringe. There is a very real risk of aspiration if high volumes are instilled over a short time, especially when topical pharyngeal anesthesia has also been applied.

Until the advent of the electronic radial echoendoscope, the device of choice for high-quality images of the esophageal wall was a high-frequency ultrasound probe. However, the newer electronic radial echoendoscopes have excellent near-field resolution and provide superb images without the need for significant balloon inflation. Nonetheless, if one wishes to stage early (T1m,sm) esophageal cancer (to determine the presence or absence of penetration through the muscularis mucosa), high-frequency catheter probes (20 to 30 MHz) would still be considered the instruments of choice.

When catheter probes are used for esophageal imaging, several techniques can be employed. One method is to use a bare catheter and instill water through the air/water channel. A second method is to use an ultrasound catheter with an attachable balloon. This technique still risks compression of the esophageal wall layers with inflation of the balloon. However, because the focal length of the catheter is very short, only a small amount of balloon inflation is necessary, thereby minimizing this risk.

Another technique that has been described is to affix a transparent, low-compliance condom onto the end of a double-channel endoscope (Figure 6-1). The condom is taped onto the end of the endoscope such that approximately 2 to 3 cm of the condom protrude beyond the tip of the endoscope. This redundant portion of the condom is folded across the imaging lens as the endoscope is passed into the esophagus. During the intubation process, it is extremely important to avoid instilling air (a common habit) because this will inflate the condom and could compromise the patient's airway. After entering the esophagus, the instrument is passed into the stomach lumen, and air is "bled" from the condom tip (instill water-aspirate; reinstill; reaspirate and repeat until all the air is gone). Once the condom has been bled, the endoscope is withdrawn to the level of the lesion, and the condom is filled with water. Because of the low compliance of the condom, it tends to elongate rather than compress the wall layers. The ultrasound catheter is then advanced into the lumen of the condom, and imaging proceeds (Video 6-1). With this technique, the coupling of the ultrasound waves to the esophageal wall is virtually perfect. With the transparent condom, the lesion can be viewed endoscopically in real time, thus assuring that the catheter probe is positioned correctly. Because the water is completely contained within the condom, there is no risk of aspiration.

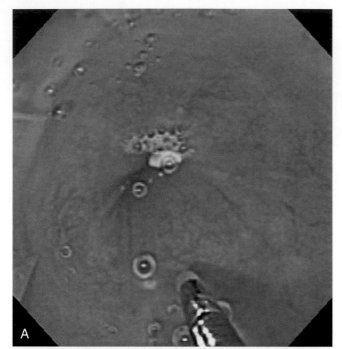

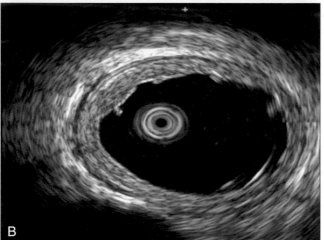

FIGURE 6-1 Endoscopic view of the esophageal lumen. **A,** View with a water-filled condom. **B,** The esophageal wall layers as visualized with a high-frequency catheter probe using the condom technique.

Video 6-1 (with narration). Examination of the esophagus using a high-frequency catheter probe passed via a dual-channel gastroscope using the condom technique.

esophageal wall associated with blurring and triangulation of the deep border of the esophageal wall (Figure 6-2). If one recognizes tangential imaging, the corrective action is usually to use all four directional dials (*do not torque the scope shaft*) to move the transducer in the direction where tangential imaging is seen. When the deep edge of the muscularis propria layer becomes smooth and the layer is seen sharply, tangential imaging has been corrected.

Mediastinum
Radial Echoendoscope

Examination of the mediastinum with a radial echoendoscope is relatively straightforward. The learning curve should be short (compared with endoscopic ultrasonography [EUS] of the pancreas) because the EUS images correlate with a thoracic computed tomography (CT) scan. It is recommended that a systemic approach be applied to all EUS examinations and that images be presented with a standard orientation. This approach holds true for mediastinal imaging. To begin the mediastinal study, the echoendoscope tip is placed in the distal esophagus near the gastroesophageal junction. The aorta is a round, anechoic structure that is a constant anatomic finding throughout the examination until withdrawal proximal to the aortic arch. It is recommended that the endoscopic ultrasound image be presented on the monitor in an orientation that exactly matches a CT slice. To accomplish

Whichever technique is employed, the risk of aspiration should be minimized while good coupling of the ultrasound waves to the esophageal wall is achieved without inducing compression. These techniques are employed for patients with early esophageal cancer, with Barrett's esophagus with or without nodules, and with small submucosal lesions.

The other major problem with esophageal EUS is tangential imaging. The esophagus is often perceived as a straight tube, but in most cases it has some tortuosity. The imaging section of an echoendoscope, as well as a catheter probe, is straight and rigid. Imaging a tortuous tube with a straight instrument creates tangential imaging. The endosonographer must be trained to recognize tangential imaging and must be aware of the maneuvers that will correct it. The consequence of unrecognized tangential imaging is overstaging malignant lesions or missing the layer of origin of a submucosal lesion. Tangential imaging is characterized by focal thickening of the

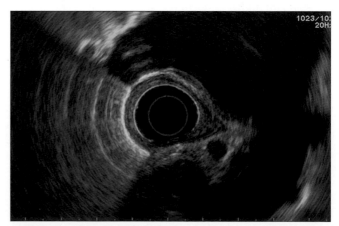

FIGURE 6-2 Muscularis layer of the esophageal wall. The muscularis layer of the esophageal wall appears blurred and focally thickened secondary to tangential imaging.

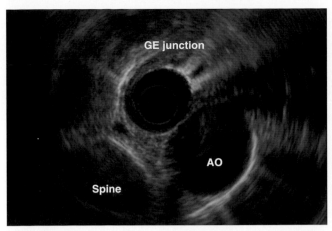

FIGURE 6-3 EUS image when the radial echoendoscope is positioned at the gastroesophageal (GE) junction. The aorta (AO) is located at the 5-o'clock position, and the spine is at 7 o'clock.

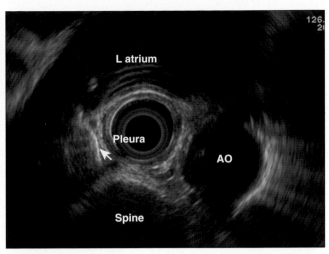

FIGURE 6-4 View of the left atrium. On gradual withdrawal of the radial echoendoscope from the gastroesophageal junction, the left atrium (L atrium) appears as a pulsating structure in the upper half of the EUS screen. AO, aorta; arrow, pleura.

this, the aorta should be rotated (using the rotation function on the instrument panel, *not* by torquing the scope shaft) to the 5-o'clock position. This will present the spine at 7 o'clock (Figure 6-3), and the heart and respiratory tree will emerge in the 12-o'clock position.

With the transducer placed in the distal esophagus and the aorta located in the 5-o'clock position, the examination begins (Video 6-2). The balloon should be inflated sufficiently to displace any intraluminal air, and the transducer itself should be placed roughly in the center of the balloon (again using right/left and up/down dials and *not* by torquing the scope shaft). With this starting position, the echoendoscope is then slowly withdrawn.

The anatomy around the distal esophagus is not complex, and as the examination begins, the aorta, spine, and portions of the left and right lung are the only anatomic structures that can be identified. The lungs are seen only as a very bright white line. The area of the mediastinum surrounding the distal esophagus corresponds to area 8 of the American Thoracic Society (ATS) areas.[1]

As the instrument is slowly withdrawn, usually approximately 35 cm from the incisors, an anechoic structure begins to emerge at roughly the 12-o'clock position (it could emerge anywhere from 10 to 2 o'clock). This structure is the left atrium (Figure 6-4). As the echoendoscope is withdrawn further, the left atrium gradually disappears. The subcarinal space is located from 10 to 12 o'clock and extends from where the left atrium disappears to where the left and right main stem bronchi come together to form the trachea (Figure 6-5).

Video 6-2 (with narration). Examination of the mediastinum using a radial echoendoscope.

The subcarinal space may be 3 to 4 cm in length and is designated area 7 by the ATS. The subcarina should be examined by withdrawing the echoendoscope in 1-cm increments while observing the 10- to 2-o'clock area for lymph nodes. Lymph nodes are typically well-circumscribed, relatively echo-poor structures that may be triangular, elongated, or round and located adjacent to the esophagus (see Figure 6-5C). The inner echo architecture can vary from being almost anechoic to having a very bright central echo. On withdrawal of the endoscope, after the disappearance of the left atrium, eventually the right or left main stem bronchus emerges. Obviously, the left main stem bronchus is present on the same side of the screen as the aorta. Air-filled structures on EUS show up as very bright "ribs" on the monitor (see Figure 6-5B).

On further withdrawal of the endoscope, three distinctive findings are seen over the span of 2 to 3 cm: the trachea, the elongated azygous vein, and the aortic arch (Figure 6-6). First, the left and right main stem bronchi come together to form the trachea, which is represented as a typical air-filled structure (echogenic ribs) at the 12-o'clock position. The second anatomic landmark is the azygous vein, up to now seen as a round, anechoic structure near the spine, or occasionally between the spine and the aorta, that elongates and moves anteriorly to join the superior vena cava. The third anatomic landmark is the elongation of the aorta, representing the aortic arch.

The area at 3 o'clock, just distal to the arch of the aorta, is the aortopulmonary window (area 4L/5) (Figure 6-7). After the aortic arch, further withdrawal of the endoscope demonstrates the great vessels coming off the aortic arch. Other than the trachea and the spine, however, this area is devoid of any significant anatomic landmarks. Nonetheless, this area is extremely important to image in order to look for periesophageal and paratracheal lymph nodes (area 2). Any confirmed metastatic lymph node found above the aortic arch in association with upper gastrointestinal cancer essentially represents unresectable disease.

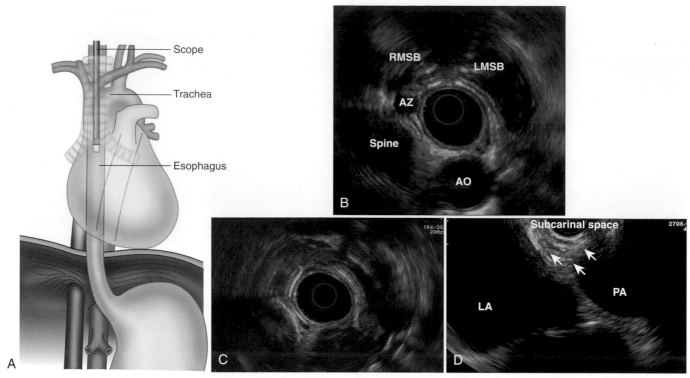

FIGURE 6-5 Subcarinal region. **A,** The position of the scope when visualizing the subcarinal region. At this site, on radial imaging, (**B**) the right (RMSB) and the left main stem bronchi (LMSB) come together to form the trachea, and (**C**) the characteristic draping lymph nodes are seen in this station. **D,** On linear imaging, two structures characterize the subcarinal space *(arrows)*: the one on the left is the left atrium (LA), and the one on the right is the pulmonary artery (PA). AO, aorta; AZ, azygous vein.

Linear Array Echoendoscope

Examination of the mediastinum with the linear array echo-endoscope is more time consuming and tedious when compared with examination with the radial instrument. Because of the narrow field of view, it is critical to adopt a systematic approach to the examination. When examining the area around the distal esophagus (area 8), the starting point is the aorta, which appears as a linear, anechoic structure that essentially fills the field of view. From here, it is necessary to rotate the echoendoscope purposefully 180 degrees in a clockwise fashion, return to the neutral position (aorta), and then rotate 180 degrees in a counterclockwise direction. This needs to be done initially and then repeated after withdrawing 1 to 2 cm. Effective rotating (torquing) of the linear echoendoscope is a fundamental skill required to perform linear EUS competently. A simple method to determine whether the torquing technique is correct is to watch the distance numbers on the scope shaft. If they rotate around the axis of the scope 1 to 1 during torquing, the maneuver is being performed correctly (Video 6-3).

The two most important areas in the mediastinum in which to look for lymph nodes are the subcarinal space (area 7) and the aortopulmonary window (area 4L/5). One should take a systematic approach to locate and image both areas with the linear echoendoscope. There are two ways to locate the subcarinal space. The first is to begin the examination in

FIGURE 6-6 Trachea, azygous vein, and aortic arch (AO). On upward withdrawal of the radial echoendoscope 2 to 3 cm from the subcarina, the trachea, azygous vein, and the aortic arch are seen.

Video 6-3 (with narration). Examination of the mediastinum using a curvilinear array echoendoscope.

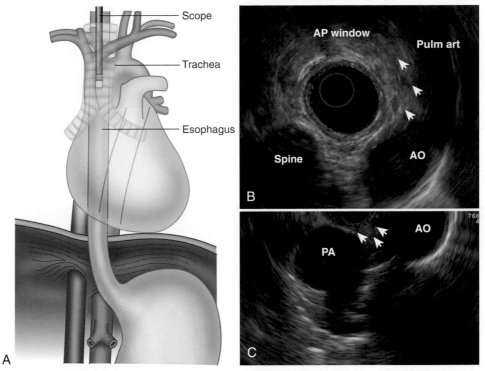

FIGURE 6-7 Aortopulmonary window. **A,** The position of the echoendoscope for visualizing the aortopulmonary (AP) window. **B,** On radial imaging, at 3 o'clock, the pulmonary artery is seen superior to the arch of the aorta (AO). **C,** On linear imaging, the anechoic structure on the left of the screen is the pulmonary artery (PA), and the anechoic structure on the right is the aorta (AO), with arrows pointing to the left paratracheal space.

the distal esophagus (at 35 to 40 cm on the scope shaft). The instrument should be rotated in a clockwise or counterclockwise direction until the aorta is found. Once the aorta has been located, the instrument should be torqued 180 degrees (clockwise or counterclockwise, whichever is more comfortable) and then slowly withdrawn. The aorta is positioned posteriorly, and this maneuver orients the image anteriorly.

As the instrument is withdrawn, usually approximately 35 cm from the incisors, a large anechoic structure is seen, and this represents the left atrium. The instrument should then be subtly torqued either clockwise or counterclockwise until the left atrium is centered. The instrument is then further withdrawn until the left atrium is situated on the left side of the ultrasound image. When this has been achieved, a slight tip deflection upward will bring a round, anechoic structure into view on the right side of the screen; this represents the pulmonary artery. The area between the left atrium and the pulmonary artery represents the subcarinal space (see Figure 6-5D). Full interrogation of the subcarinal space then requires careful clockwise and counterclockwise torquing.

The second way to find the subcarinal space is to locate the aorta in the middle of the esophagus. With the aorta occupying the screen, the echoendoscope is slowly withdrawn until the aorta disappears; this represents the aortic arch. At this point, 180 degrees of clockwise torque are applied. This maneuver orients the image anteriorly, and one encounters the typical echogenic ribs, which represent the trachea. Once the trachea has been located, the scope is advanced 1 to 2 cm. When the trachea disappears, this represents the bifurcation into the left and right main stem bronchi. Thus, one is now viewing the subcarinal space. Just as with the first maneuver,

the left atrium is seen on the left side of the screen, and the pulmonary artery is on the right.

The other important anatomic station in the mediastinum is the aortopulmonary window (area 4L/5). This is essentially the area underneath the arch of the aorta. This area can be found most easily by locating the aorta in the middle of the esophagus and then withdrawing the instrument until the aorta disappears. From this position, one advances the scope by 1 to 2 cm, at a level underneath the aortic arch. The scope is rotated 60 degrees in a clockwise direction and comes slightly "up" on the up/down dial. With the linear echoendoscope, the aortopulmonary window is seen as the space between the aorta (round, anechoic structure on the right side of the screen) and the pulmonary artery (round, anechoic structure on the left side of the screen; see Figure 6-7C).

Above the area of the aortic arch, the left and right paratracheal area can be examined by torquing the scope clockwise and counterclockwise off the trachea every 2 cm (area 2). This is a critical area to examine in patients with distal esophageal cancer because malignant lymph nodes in this area represent metastatic disease.

Another alternative technique to examine the mediastinum using the linear array echoendoscope is to identify the aorta at the gastroesophageal junction. The echoendoscope is then torqued 360 degrees in a clockwise or counterclockwise direction to identify the aorta once more and then withdrawn 3 cm into the esophagus. This 360-degree torquing maneuver is continued proximally at 3-cm intervals until the upper esophageal sphincter is reached. This technique enables access to all the posterior mediastinal stations for lymph node sampling (Video 6-4).

Video 6-4 (with narration). The 360-degree torquing technique for evaluation of the posterior mediastinum using a curvilinear array echoendoscope.

Video 6-5 (with narration). Evaluation of the left adrenal gland using a linear array echoendoscope.

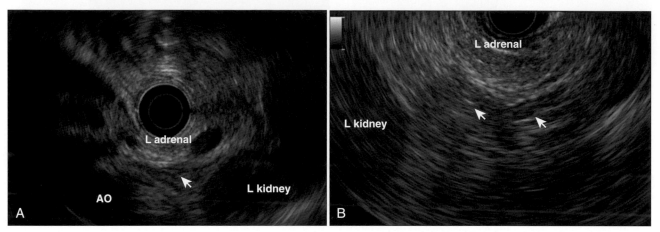

FIGURE 6-8 Left adrenal gland. The left adrenal gland *(arrows)* with the typical "seagull" appearance as seen using (**A**) radial and (**B**) linear echoendoscopes. AO, aorta; L, left.

How to Examine the Adrenal Glands

The left adrenal gland is an important landmark in lung cancer staging. This gland can be identified in more than 95% of EUS examinations by using either of the two techniques described here. It is easier to locate the adrenal gland with the linear scope as compared with the radial instrument. However, the technique for locating the adrenal gland is the same. The most straightforward approach involves locating the aorta at the gastroesophageal junction and then advancing the scope to the point where the celiac artery takes off. The scope is advanced along the celiac artery, and then slight clockwise torque is applied to the echoendoscope. The left adrenal gland is seen as a structure with a central "body" and two "wings" (Video 6-5). It is often described as resembling a seagull in flight. An echogenic line frequently runs in the middle of the wings (Figure 6-8).

In the second technique, the echoendoscope is advanced into the proximal stomach, and the abdominal aorta is identified just below the gastroesophageal junction. The splenic vein is then identified by advancing the transducer forward with a clockwise rotation. The splenic hilum is found by following the splenic vein laterally. The left kidney is then imaged by advancing the scope from the splenic hilum. The left kidney is seen in cross section with a central echo-rich area representing the renal pelvis and caliceal system and a surrounding homogeneous echo-poor area representing the cortex. The left adrenal gland is found just below the splenic vein between the left kidney and the abdominal aorta.

The right adrenal gland generally cannot be well visualized by EUS because it is located farther away from the stomach and is superior to the duodenal sweep. In 20% of cases, it can be seen with the transducer deep into the duodenal lumen beyond the ampulla and with morphologic characteristics similar to those of the left adrenal gland. Even when detected by EUS, the right adrenal gland usually is located deep or adjacent to the inferior vena cava, thereby making EUS-guided fine-needle aspiration difficult but not impossible.

Summary

Evaluation of the mediastinum by EUS is relatively straightforward. Images obtained by the radial scanning instrument correlate very precisely with images of a CT scan. Linear images are more difficult to interpret, and successful examination of the mediastinum using a linear array echoendoscope requires a systematic approach.

REFERENCE

1. Mountain CF, Dresler CM. Regional lymph node classification for lung cancer staging. *Chest.* 1997;111:1718-1723.

EUS and EBUS in Non–Small-Cell Lung Cancer

Jouke T. Annema

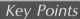

Key Points

- EUS and EBUS are the techniques of choice in case mediastinal nodal sampling is indicated for the diagnosis and staging of lung cancer.
- Complete endosonographic nodal staging improves staging versus either of the methods alone.
- Incorporation of endosonography in the staging algorithm for non–small-cell lung cancer improves locoregional staging, reduces both the number of mediastinoscopies and unnecessary thoracotomies, and is additionally cost effective.
- EUS fine-needle aspiration can diagnose intrapulmonary tumors adjacent to the esophagus directly and assess mediastinal tumor invasion (T4).

Transesophageal endoscopic ultrasonography (EUS)-guided fine-needle aspiration (FNA) and endobronchial ultrasound (EBUS)-guided transbronchial needle aspiration (TBNA) are novel techniques for the diagnosis and staging of lung cancer. Worldwide, more than 1 million patients are diagnosed with lung cancer annually, and one third of these patients present with mediastinal metastases. Accurate diagnosis and staging are important for both prognostic and therapeutic reasons. Patients with non–small-cell lung cancer (NSCLC) and mediastinal lymph node metastases or mediastinal tumor invasion (stage III) are preferably treated with chemoradiation therapy, whereas patients without locally advanced disease are treated primarily by surgical resection of the lung tumor.[1] Starting mediastinal nodal tissue sampling by endosonography has been proven to be superior to initial surgical staging,[2] and therefore 2013 guidelines recommend that for mediastinal staging endosonography is the technique of choice.[3,4] In this chapter, the role of EUS FNA and EBUS TBNA for the diagnosis and staging of lung cancer is evaluated. The indications for both methods are addressed (Table 7-1), as well as the concept of complete (esophageal and endobronchial) echoendoscopic staging of the mediastinum. The impact of EUS and EBUS on patient management is also discussed, in particular the role of these imaging techniques in preventing surgical staging procedures as well as the position of endosonography in staging algorithms for NSCLC.

EUS Fine-Needle Aspiration for the Diagnosis and Staging of Lung Cancer

General Procedure

Evaluation of the mediastinum by EUS should be performed in a standardized fashion (see Chapter 6) to examine all mediastinal lymph node stations that can be detected from the esophagus (EUS FNA Examination Checklist). The EUS assessment tool (EUSAT) can be helpful for a structural

---

EUS FNA Examination Checklist[a]

Aorta and celiac axis
Left adrenal gland
Left liver lobe (optional)
Peri-esophageal space below carina (station 8L/R)
Subcarinal space (station 7)
Aortopulmonary window/pulmonary trunk (station 4L/5)
Paratracheal space (stations 2R and 2L)
Intrapulmonary tumor visible?
Mediastinal tumor invasion (T4)

[a]See also reference 4 and Chapter 6.

INDICATIONS FOR ENDOSONOGRAPHY FOR THE DIAGNOSIS AND STAGING OF LUNG CANCER

Mediastinal Lymph Nodes	EUS FNA	EBUS TBNA
Paratracheal to the left	++	++
Paratracheal to the right	–	++
Aortopulmonary window	+	–
Subcarinal	++	++
Lower mediastinum	++	–
Hilar	–	++
Mediastinal restaging	+	+
FDG PET uptake in lymph node within reach	++	++
Lung tumor located adjacent to the esophagus	++	–
Lung tumor located adjacent to the trachea or main bronchi	–	++
Suspected left adrenal metastasis	++	–

++, strong evidence; +, moderate evidence; -, no evidence; FDG, fluorodeoxyglucose; FNA, fine-needle aspiration; PET, positron emission tomography; TBNA, transbronchial needle aspiration.

assessment.[5] Lymph nodes should be described in relation to the anatomic (vascular) landmarks and given a number according to the tumor, node, metastasis (TNM) classification.[6,7] After an initial orientation, enlarged (short axis >10 mm) or sonographically suspicious nodes should be sampled for biopsy, starting with contralateral (N3) nodes before ipsilateral (N2) lymph nodes are analyzed.

Biopsy of Intrapulmonary Tumors

Intrapulmonary tumors that are located adjacent to or near the esophagus can be visualized by EUS.[8,9] Once the primary tumor has been identified, real-time EUS-guided biopsy of the intrapulmonary lesion is possible (Figure 7-1). Left upper lobe tumors located adjacent to the aorta are often detected by EUS (Figure 7-2). In a retrospective study of 18 patients with intrapulmonary tumors abutting the esophagus, EUS identified intrapulmonary tumors and obtained a tissue diagnosis in all patients.[9] In a prospective study of 32 patients with suspected lung cancer and a primary tumor located adjacent to the esophagus, intrapulmonary masses were detected in all patients, and the diagnosis of lung cancer was established in 97% of patients.[8]

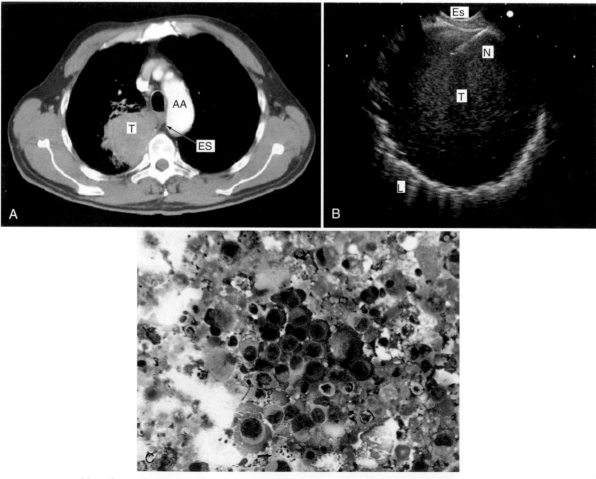

FIGURE 7-1 A 53-year-old smoker with suspected lung cancer in whom bronchoscopy did not establish a diagnosis. **A,** Computed tomography of the chest demonstrating an intrapulmonary tumor (T) in the right upper lobe located adjacent to the esophagus (ES). AA, aortic arch. **B,** Corresponding EUS fine-needle aspiration image. Notice the needle (N) located in the tumor (T). Es, esophagus; L, compromised lung tissue. **C,** Cytology of fine-needle aspirate demonstrating a squamous cell carcinoma.

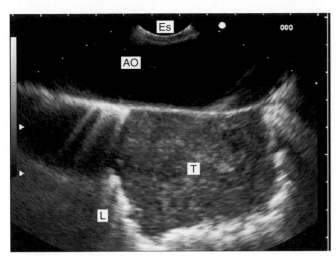

FIGURE 7-2 Left upper lobe tumor (T) located adjacent to the aorta (AO). There are no signs of tumor invasion in the aorta (T4). Es, esophagus; L, compromised lung tissue.

Mediastinal Tumor Invasion (T4)

Once the primary tumor has been identified in a subset of patients, one can assess the presence or absence (see Figure 7-2) of mediastinal tumor invasion (T4), defined as invasion in the mediastinum, centrally located large vessels, or vertebrae. Patients with T4 lung tumors (stage IIIB) are generally not considered eligible for surgical resection. Currently, mediastinal tumor invasion is frequently assessed during surgery because computed tomography (CT) has limited sensitivity and specificity (<75%) for mediastinal invasion,[10] and positron emission tomography (PET) has no value in detecting T4 tumors because of its limited anatomic resolution.[11] In a retrospective study that evaluated T4 staging in 308 patients, EUS had sensitivity, specificity, and positive and negative predictive values of 88%, 98%, 70%, and 99%, respectively.[12] Most cases of tumor invasion were assessed based on EUS images alone. Tumor invasion in large vessels (Figure 7-3B) or the heart is easier to assess than invasion in the mediastinum (see Figure 7-3A), as a result of the increased ultrasound contrasts between tumor and blood as well as the possibility of using a Doppler signal (see Figure 7-3C). In a few patients in the foregoing study, surgical verification of EUS T4 findings occurred, and, therefore the definitive value of EUS in T4 staging requires further investigation.

In conclusion, intrapulmonary tumors can be visualized and sampled for biopsy safely by EUS FNA provided the tumors are located adjacent to the esophagus. In addition to establishing a tissue diagnosis, EUS can detect mediastinal tumor invasion, especially of vascular structures.

Mediastinal Nodal Staging by EUS

Diagnostic Reach

Regional lymph nodes in NSCLC are classified using the TNM classification.[7] Only lymph nodes that lie adjacent to the esophagus or centrally located vessels can be visualized by EUS. These lymph nodes are located in the following regions: low paratracheal on the left (station 4L; Figure 7-4), aortopulmonary window (station 5; Figure 7-5), para-aortal (station

6; Figure 7-6), subcarinal (station 7; Figures 7-7 and 7-8), lower paraesophageal (station 8), and pulmonary ligamentum (station 9; Figures 7-9 and 7-10). Lymph nodes located in the aortopulmonary window can be detected by EUS but only sampled in selected cases because of the interposition of the pulmonary artery. Para-aortal nodes are located on the other

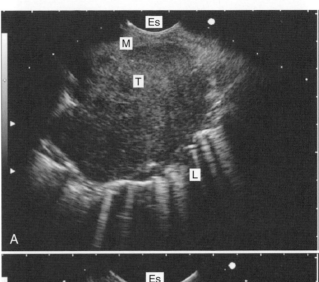

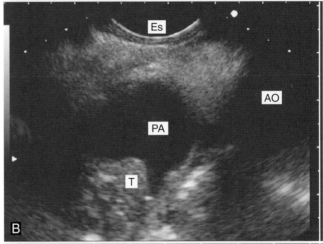

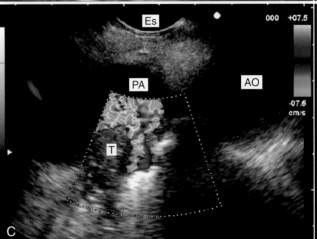

FIGURE 7-3 Large cell carcinoma. **A,** Centrally located large cell carcinoma (T) invading the mediastinum (M). Es, esophagus; L, compromised lung tissue. **B** and **C,** Centrally located left-sided tumor (T) invading the pulmonary artery (PA), with (**C**) and without (**B**) color Doppler. AO, aorta.

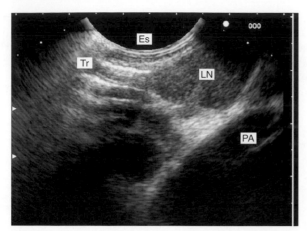

FIGURE 7-4 Lower paratracheal lymph node (LN) on the left (station 4L) located between the esophagus (Es), trachea (Tr), and pulmonary artery (PA).

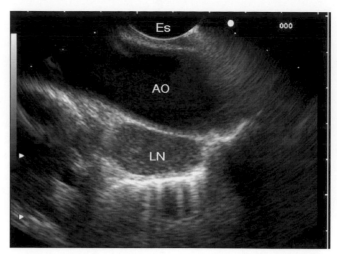

FIGURE 7-6 Lymph node (LN) located adjacent to the aortic arch (AO) (station 6). Es, esophagus.

side of the aorta and can be well visualized by EUS (see Figure 7-6). In carefully selected cases, these lymph nodes can be aspirated either transaortally [13] or by a long approach (7-8 cm) from the proximal esophagus to obtain a tissue diagnosis.[14] Otherwise this region can only be reached by surgical methods such as mediastinotomy or video-assisted thoracoscopy (VATS). EUS has limitations in its diagnostic reach because air in the trachea and main bronchi inhibits visualization of the upper paratracheal lymph node (station 2) and the lower paratracheal station on the right (4R). EUS FNA can be used for the assessment of mediastinal nodes in patients with known (Figure 7-11) or suspected lung cancer or in patients with mediastinal masses suspected of being lung cancer (Figure 7-12). In addition to lymph node sampling, EUS FNA can be used for biopsy of the left adrenal gland and intrapulmonary tumors, provided these structures lie adjacent to the esophagus (Figure 7-13).

EUS versus EUS Fine-Needle Aspiration

Specific ultrasonographic features of mediastinal lymph nodes (size [short axis >10 mm], round shape, homogeneous hypoechoic pattern, sharp distinctive borders) are associated with malignant involvement,[15,16] for which EUS has a sensitivity, specificity, and positive and negative predictive values of 78%, 71%, 75%, and 79%, respectively.[17] Elastography is a newer technical application that depicts the mechanical properties of tissue during endosonography. An accuracy of 85% for differentiating benign from malignant mediastinal nodes has been reported.[18] The value of elastography is investigational, and this technique may be helpful in selecting target lymph nodes for biopsy. EUS in combination with FNA is more accurate than is EUS imaging alone.[15,17,19,20] Therefore FNA is always required before a lymph node can be designated as malignant (Video 7-1). For this reason, curved linear, not radial, ultrasound probes are required for mediastinal staging of NSCLC. Of the different needle sizes (19, 22, and 25 G) available for nodal staging, the 22 G is regarded as the standard size.

The recommended number of biopsies per lymph node depends on the presence or absence of on-site cytologic examination. If on-site cytologic examination is not available, a minimum of three needle passes is recommended to obtain

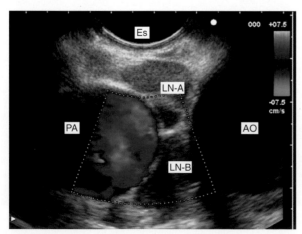

FIGURE 7-5 Left paratracheal lymph node (station 4L, LN-A) located between the aorta (AO), pulmonary artery (PA), and esophagus (ES) and the aortopulmonary node (station 5, LN-B).

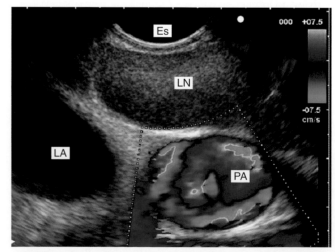

FIGURE 7-7 Subcarinal lymph node (LN) located between the esophagus (Es), pulmonary artery (PA), with color Doppler signal, and left atrium (LA).

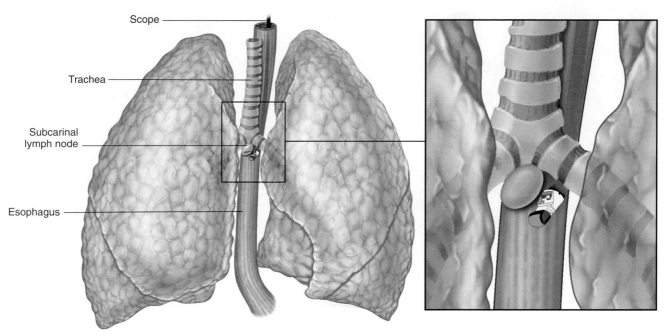

Scope

Trachea

Subcarinal
lymph node

Esophagus

FIGURE 7-8   Diagram showing transesophageal ultrasound-guided fine-needle aspiration of a subcarinal lymph node.

an optimal yield.[21,22] No benefit in diagnostic yield has been correlated with the position of the needle in the lymph node (central versus peripheral) or the application of suction.[22] In addition to conventional cytologic evaluation, cell blocks can be made of EUS fine-needle aspirates on which immunohistochemistry and molecular analysis can be performed. EUS FNA of mediastinal lymph nodes is safe, and complications such as a mediastinitis are rare.[23]

Accuracy of Mediastinal Staging

Mediastinal nodal staging in patients with known or suspected lung cancer has been investigated in multiple studies.[22,24–41] In a meta-analysis of 18 studies of EUS FNA for the mediastinal staging of lung cancer, sensitivity was 83% (95% confidence interval [CI], 78% to 87%) and specificity was 97% (95% CI, 96% to 98%).[42] In those patients with enlarged lymph nodes, sensitivity was 90% (95% CI, 84% to 94%). Another meta-analysis, which partly discussed the

same studies, of 1003 patients in whom the overall prevalence of mediastinal disease was 61%, EUS had a sensitivity of 84% and a false-negative rate of 19%.[43] Although positive predictive values were reported in most studies, tumor-positive findings were verified by surgical-pathologic staging in only one study.[25] Although false-positive EUS FNA findings have seldom been reported, they are possible when the primary tumor is located immediately adjacent to a lymph node, a situation in which the EUS images can be misinterpreted.[25] Most studies are performed in selected patients with enlarged (>1 cm) mediastinal lymph nodes at CT, and therefore the results apply only to patients in that category. Few studies have focused specifically on small (short axis ≤10 mm) nodes; sensitivity has varied between 35% and 93%.[33,37,39] The pooled sensitivity in a meta-analysis for this subgroup was 58% (95% CI, 39% to 75%).[42] Investigators have also reported that EUS FNA of mediastinal lymph nodes can be performed with a convex linear EBUS probe (Figure 7-14).[44,45]

Mediastinal restaging after induction chemotherapy is an increasingly common indication for EUS FNA. Accurate restaging is important to identify those patients who are successfully downstaged because they benefit most from subsequent surgical resection.[46,47] In two studies the sensitivity of EUS FNA for mediastinal restaging was inferior (44% and 75%), with a low negative predictive value of 58% in

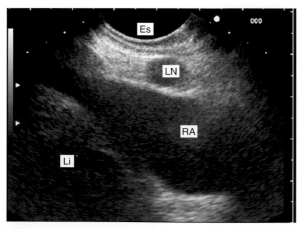

FIGURE 7-9   Lymph node (LN) located in the pulmonary ligamentum (station 9). Es, esophagus; Li, liver; RA, right atrium.

Video 7-1. Demonstrating EUS-guided FNA of the subcarinal lymph node in a patient with non–small-cell lung cancer.

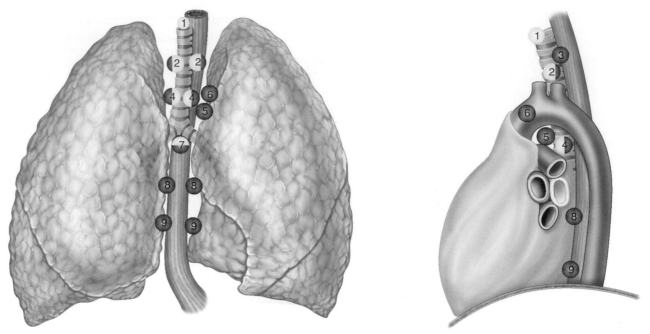

FIGURE 7-10   Mediastinal staging techniques and their diagnostic reach. *Yellow ball,* within reach of EBUS and mediastinoscopy; *red ball,* within reach of EUS; *black ball,* within reach of mediastinotomy or video-assisted thoracoscopy.

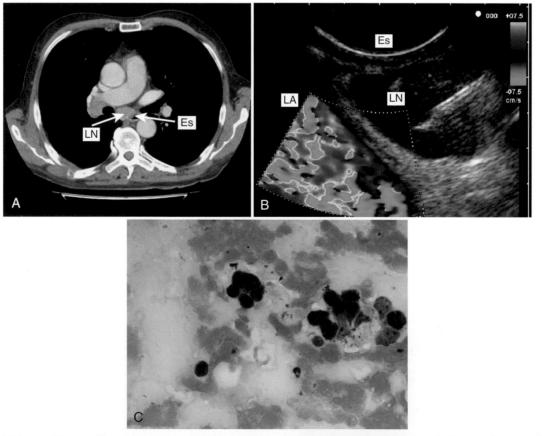

FIGURE 7-11   A 54-year-old man with proven non–small-cell lung cancer who was fit for surgical resection. **A**, Computed tomography of the chest demonstrating a centrally located non–small-cell lung carcinoma of the right lung and an enlarged subcarinal lymph node (LN). Es, esophagus. **B**, Real-time EUS-guided aspiration of the subcarinal lymph node (LN) located between the esophagus (Es) and the left atrium (LA). **C**, Cytologic appearance of a lymph node metastasis.

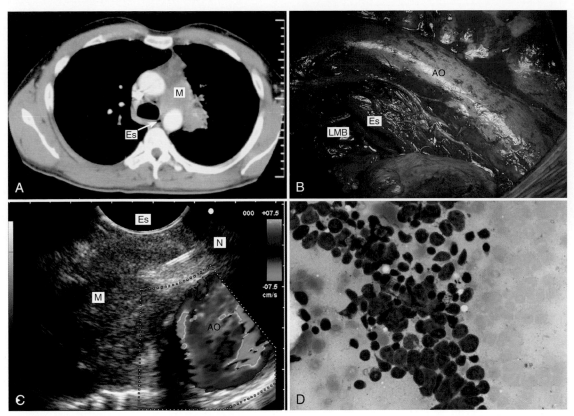

FIGURE 7-12 A 66-year-old man, a heavy smoker with suspected lung cancer, in whom bronchoscopy was nondiagnostic. **A,** Computed tomography of the chest demonstrating a mass (M) in the aortopulmonary window. Es, esophagus. **B,** In another patient just after left-sided pneumonectomy, the close relationship between the esophagus (ES) and the aortopulmonary window. AO, aorta; LMB, left main bronchus. **C,** Corresponding EUS image with fine-needle aspiration of the mass (M) located between the esophagus (Es) and the aorta (AO) (with color Doppler). N, needle. **D,** Cytologic appearance of small cell carcinoma.

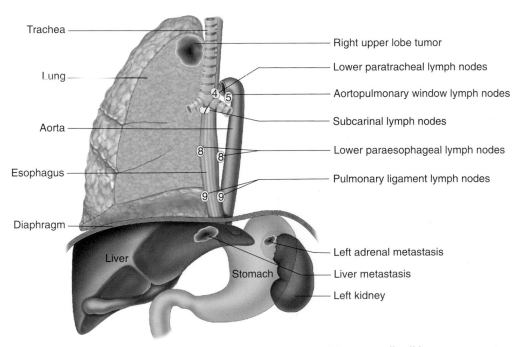

FIGURE 7-13 EUS fine-needle aspiration (FNA) in non–small-cell lung cancer. EUS FNA in non–small-cell lung cancer can sample intrapulmonary tumors for biopsy and detect mediastinal tumor invasion (T4), assess mediastinal lymph nodes, and identify distant metastases located in the left liver lobe and left adrenal gland.

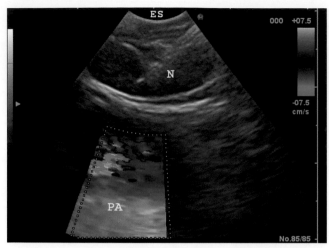

FIGURE 7-14 EUS fine-needle aspiration of a subcarinal lymph node (station 7) with an EBUS scope. Notice the smaller ultrasound range in comparison with an investigation with a conventional EUS scope (see Figure 7-7). ES, esophagus; N, needle; PA, pulmonary artery.

comparison to conventional staging, mostly as a result of the sampling error of small residual tumor metastases.[48,49] In a study of 28 patients with locally advanced NSCLC, EUS had both an accuracy and negative predictive value of 92% for mediastinal restaging and was superior to fluorodeoxyglucose (FDG) PET.[50] Therefore EUS can be used to confirm but not to exclude persistent mediastinal nodal metastases.

Assessment of Distant Metastases

Approximately 40% of patients with lung cancer present with distant metastases, mostly in liver, brain, bone, and adrenal glands. Of these common locations of distant lung cancer metastases, lesions located in the left liver lobe and adrenal gland can be identified (Figure 7-15) and sampled for biopsy by EUS (Video 7-2). In a study of highly selected patients (both with and without lung cancer) with enlarged left adrenal glands, EUS assessed malignant left adrenal involvement in 42% of patients.[51] In 40 patients with (suspected) lung cancer and an enlarged left adrenal gland, EUS FNA altered TNM

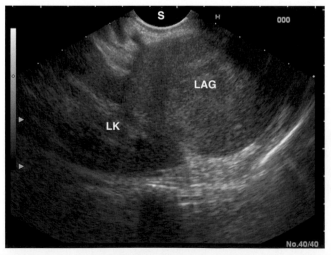

FIGURE 7-15 Transgastric EUS image of the left kidney (LK) and metastatic-involved left adrenal gland (LAG). S, stomach.

Video 7-2. Demonstrating EUS-guided FNA of the left adrenal gland in a patient with metastatic non–small-cell lung cancer.

staging in 70% of patients after analysis of the left adrenal gland.[52] In a study in 85 patients with lung cancer, the sensitivity of left adrenal gland analysis was at least 86%.[53] Whether the left adrenal gland should be examined routinely during EUS procedures in patients with lung cancer is the subject of debate.[54] Recently, in a study in 150 consecutive patients with lung cancer the right adrenal gland was visualized in 87% of patients—the left adrenal gland in all.[55] Patients with disseminated lung cancer often present with liver metastases. The standard procedure for the detection of liver metastases is transabdominal ultrasonography. Investigators have reported that liver metastases can be assessed by EUS FNA using a transgastric approach.[56–58] Whether EUS FNA has additional benefits compared with transabdominal ultrasound-guided liver biopsy is unknown.

EBUS Transbronchial Needle Aspiration for the Diagnosis and Staging of Lung Cancer

EBUS enables visualization of intrapulmonary lesions, mediastinal and hilar lymph nodes, and mediastinal masses located adjacent to the main airways (EBUS TBNA Examination Checklist). Similar to EUS in gastroenterology, EBUS development started with radial probes. With radial EBUS, lesions can be detected but not sampled under real-time ultrasound control. Radial EBUS is mainly used for the detection of peripheral lung lesions that can be subsequently sampled using fluoroscopy or guide sheets. Linear EBUS, commercially available since 2004, enables real-time controlled sampling of mediastinal or hilar nodes and centrally located lung tumors, similar to EUS FNA. In this chapter, only linear EBUS applications for the diagnosis and staging of lung cancer are discussed. Current guidelines state that EBUS TBNA is the technique of choice for mediastinal nodal staging.[3,4]

EBUS TBNA Examination Checklist*
Upper left paratracheal region (station 2L)
Lower left paratracheal region (station 4L)
Upper right paratracheal region (station 2R)
Lower right paratracheal region (station 4R)
Subcarinal area (station 7)
Left hilar region (station 10L)
Left intrapulmonary region (station 11L)
Right hilar region (station 10R)
Right intrapulmonary region (station 11R)
Intrapulmonary tumor visible?

*See also reference 4.

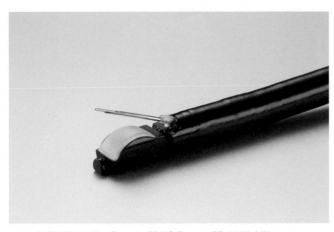

FIGURE 7-16   Convex EBUS Pentax EB 1970 UK scope.

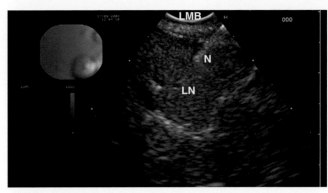

FIGURE 7-18   Real-time EBUS transbronchial needle aspiration of a subcarinal lymph node (station 7). Notice that when contact between the ultrasound transducer and the airway mucosa is made, the optical image disappears *(left upper corner)*. LMB, position of the endoscope in the left main bronchus; LN, lymph node; N, needle.

EBUS Procedure

Linear EBUS scopes (Olympus XBF UC 160 F, Fujinon EB-530 US, Pentax EB 1970 UK; Figure 7-16) are modified bronchoscopes with an electronic linear ultrasound transducer (scanning range, 5 to 12 MHz) integrated in the distal end of the scope. A light source is also available and is positioned at a 10- to 30-degree angle. EBUS investigations are commonly performed with the patient under conscious sedation using low-dose midazolam or propofol sedation. The examination takes approximately 15 to 20 minutes. Before endoscopy, the pharynx is sprayed with lidocaine, and often codeine is administered to suppress the cough reflex. Patients are investigated lying in a supine position, and the scope is introduced orally into the trachea. During an EBUS investigation, both white optical light and transbronchial ultrasound images are available. With the endobronchial view, the position of the EBUS scope in the tracheobronchial tree is evident (Figure 7-17). When the ultrasound transducer is directed toward the airway mucosa, lymph nodes adjacent to the airway wall can be visualized (Figure 7-18). Optionally, a water-filled balloon can be attached to the ultrasound head to increase contact. During visualization of the lymph nodes, the endoscopic view is often limited because of the close proximity of the optical source to the airway wall (see Figure 7-18). After positioning a sheet (see Figure 7-16) that protects the working channel

of the scope from the needle, lymph nodes can be aspirated in a real-time controlled fashion (see Figure 7-18). Three needle passes are advised for an optimal yield.[59] Regarding needle size, 22-G needles are standard; 21- and 25-G needles are also available with forceps biopsy devices under investigation. EBUS-related complications are very rare; a case of pneumothorax[60] and infections[61] have been reported.

Diagnosing Intrapulmonary Tumors by EBUS

Conventional bronchoscopy fails to detect the primary lung tumor in approximately 30% of patients.[62] Intrapulmonary tumors that are located immediately adjacent to the trachea or the main bronchi can be visualized (Figure 7-19) and sampled by EBUS TBNA. In two studies in patients with a centrally located lung tumor without abnormalities noted on conventional bronchoscopy, the diagnosis was made by EBUS in 77%[63] and 94%[64] of patients, respectively. Biopsy of intrapulmonary tumors after a nondiagnostic conventional bronchoscopy is an important indication for EBUS because it is often difficult to procure tissue safely in centrally located lung

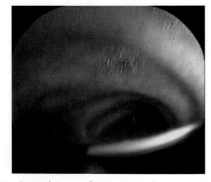

FIGURE 7-17   Optical image during EBUS demonstrating the position of the endoscope in the distal trachea. The main carina and ostia of the left and right main bronchi can be seen. Notice the white line at the bottom end of the image representing the ultrasound head of the scope.

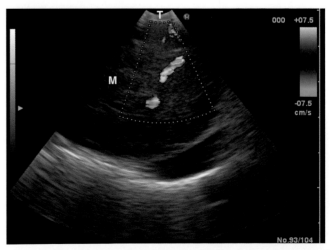

FIGURE 7-19   Adenocarcinoma (M) of the right upper lobe detected by EBUS from the trachea (T). Note the vessel running through the intrapulmonary tumor.

Video 7-3. Demonstrating EBUS TBNA in a patient with mediastinal adenopathy and non–small-cell lung cancer.

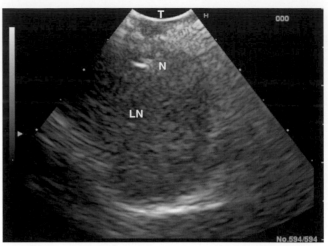

FIGURE 7-21 EBUS transbronchial needle aspiration image of a paratracheal node (LN) on the right (station 4R). N, needle; T, position of the scope in the trachea.

lesions. In these patients, a CT-guided lung biopsy is often unattractive, given the close proximity of the tumor to centrally located vessels that pose an increased risk of pneumothorax and hemoptysis. For the primary diagnosis of lung cancer, and especially for distinguishing among the different subtypes of adenocarcinoma, it remains to be seen how EBUS samples relate to histologic findings for accurate tumor subclassification. No data are available on the value of linear EBUS for mediastinal tumor invasion.

Nodal Staging by EBUS

Mediastinal nodal sampling is the major indication for EBUS TBNA (Video 7-3). Mediastinal lymph nodes that can be reached are located adjacent to the trachea (above the level of the aortic arch, stations 2L and 2R; below the aortic arch, stations 4L [Figure 7-20] and 4R [Figure 7-21]) or main bronchi (station 7, which can be reached from both the left and right main bronchi). Lymph nodes in the aortopulmonary window (station 5) can sometimes be detected but not safely sampled because of the intervening pulmonary artery. In addition to mediastinal nodes, EBUS can also be used to sample intrapulmonary lymph nodes (Figure 7-22) or nodes located in the hilum of the lung (station 10). With the experimental elastography technique, the stiffness of a node can be assessed (Figure 7-23). Whether elastography influences the biopsy procedure or diagnostic yield needs to be investigated. It is of critical importance that the lymph nodes identified by EBUS are given the appropriate number according to the revised

seventh edition of the TNM classification[7] in order to prevent understaging or overstaging.[6]

In 2009, three meta-analyses were published, partly discussing the same studies, on EBUS for mediastinal staging.[65-67] In 11 studies of 1299 patients, EBUS had a pooled sensitivity of 93% (95% CI, 91% to 94%) and a pooled specificity of 100% (95% CI, 0.99% to 1.0%). Selected patients with either enlarged or PET-positive lymph nodes had a higher sensitivity, 0.94% (95% CI, 0.93% to 0.96%), in comparison with those patients unselected by CT or PET, in whom sensitivity was 0.76% (95% CI, 0.65% to 0.85%).[65] In this meta-analysis, no correlation was found between the prevalence of nodal metastases and sensitivity in the various studies. As in EUS, most studies were performed in selected patients with enlarged nodes.[59,68-74] In patients whose PET scans were suspected of showing nodal metastases, EBUS had sensitivities between 90% and 95% and negative predictive values between 60% and 97%.[60,75,76]

In a study in 100 patients with NSCLC without nodal enlargement at CT, sensitivity and negative predictive value

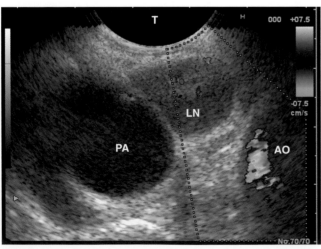

FIGURE 7-20 EBUS image of a left paratracheal lymph node (LN) (station 4L) detected by EBUS from the trachea (T). AO, aorta; PA, pulmonary artery.

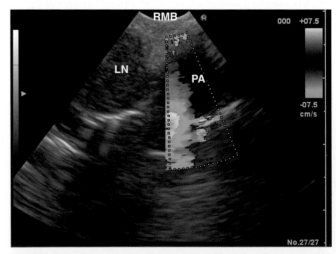

FIGURE 7-22 EBUS image of intrapulmonary node (LN) on the right detected from the right upper lobe carina (station 11R). The Doppler signal demonstrates a branch from the pulmonary artery (PA). RMB, position of the scope in the right main bronchus.

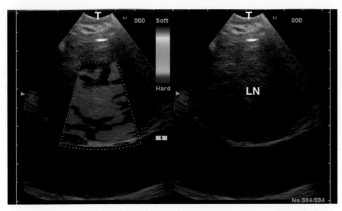

FIGURE 7-23 Enlarged right-sided lower paratracheal node. EBUS image (*on the right*) of an enlarged right-sided lower paratracheal node (station 4R). The blue color at elastography (*on the left*) shows the increased stiffness of the nodal tissue.

were 92% and 96%, respectively.[77] In another series of 100 patients with NSCLC with small (mean diameter, 7.9 mm) and PET-negative nodes, EBUS detected mediastinal malignancy in 9% of patients and had a sensitivity and a negative predictive value of 89% and 99%, respectively.[78] EBUS is also the technique of choice for sampling lymph nodes located in the hilum of the lung. In 213 patients with either enlarged or FDG PET-active hilar nodes, EBUS had a sensitivity of 91%.[79] EBUS can also be used for mediastinal restaging after induction chemotherapy. Herth and colleagues[80] found a sensitivity of 76% and a negative predictive value of only 20%. The low negative predictive value was mainly the result of sampling errors. In another mediastinal restaging study in 61 patients, EBUS had sensitivity and a negative predictive value of 67% and 78%, respectively.[81] In one study, it has been show that analysis of 22 G TBNA samples revealed an adequate tissue for cytological analysis in 97% of samples, and the specimens were adequate for EGFR testing in 88% of cases.[82]

Impact of Endosonography on Patient Management

The impact of endosonography on patient management depends on the prevalence of mediastinal metastases in the target population, the location of the primary tumor, and the extent and location of mediastinal disease.[41] Important in this discussion is the detection of nodal metastases versus excluding them.

Preventing Mediastinoscopies

In a prospective study of 84 patients with mediastinal masses suspected of being malignant, EUS prevented thoracotomy or thoracoscopy in 48% and mediastinoscopy in 68% of patients by demonstrating lymph node metastases.[32] In a similar study population of 59 patients, all scheduled for mediastinoscopy, EUS FNA proved mediastinal metastases in 39% of patients, and mediastinoscopy was eventually performed in only 22%.[34] In a prospective study of 242 patients with (suspected) NSCLC and enlarged mediastinal lymph nodes (all candidates for mediastinoscopy or mediastinotomy), EUS FNA demonstrated lymph node metastases, tumor invasion, or an alternative diagnosis in 70% of patients, and surgical interventions were thus prevented.[24] Routine use of EUS FNA in 152 patients with NSCLC (unselected by CT) reduced the need for surgical staging in nearly half the patients.[36]

In a randomized trial in patients with resectable NSCLC, EUS significantly reduced the need for surgical staging.[38] In other studies, EBUS omitted the need for surgical staging in half of patients with enlarged nodes at CT.[70,73] In patients with suspected nodal metastases based on PET, surgical staging was avoided in up to 71% of patients based on EBUS findings.[76] In a lung cancer staging strategy including PET, the diminished need for surgical staging based on EUS outcomes resulted in a cost reduction of 40%.[31]

Reducing Unnecessary Thoracotomies

In a prospective study of 108 patients with NSCLC, staging by EUS added to mediastinoscopy identified significantly more patients with either tumor invasion or lymph node metastasis (36%) compared with staging by mediastinoscopy alone (20%). Had EUS results been taken into account, one in six thoracotomies could have been prevented.[25] Additionally, in a randomized study of 104 patients, routine staging by EUS FNA resulted in a 16% decrease in the number of futile thoracotomies compared with staging of selected patients by EUS.[83] In the ASTER randomized trial, it was shown that unnecessary thoracotomies could be reduced by more than half by starting mediastinal tissue staging with endosonography in comparison to immediate surgical staging.[2]

Endosonography versus Other Mediastinal Staging Methods

How do EUS FNA and EBUS TBNA compare with other mediastinal staging techniques? It is important to distinguish between imaging techniques that provide information about lymph node size (CT scan of the chest) or metabolic activity (PET) and those staging techniques by which tissue is obtained ("blind" TBNA, mediastinoscopy, mediastinotomy, or VATS).

In mediastinal staging, EUS FNA is more sensitive (88% versus 57%) and specific (91% versus 82%) than CT scan of the chest.[17,19] EUS FNA and PET have similar sensitivities (88% versus 84%) and specificities (91% versus 89%) in identifying mediastinal lymph node metastases.[17,19]

In a direct comparison study that had identification of inoperable patients as the outcome, EUS FNA and PET had comparable sensitivities (63% versus 68%) and negative predictive values (68% versus 64%), but EUS was more specific (100% versus 72%).[84] Obviously, tissue verification of PET-positive lymph nodes should occur, given the limited positive predictive value of FDG PET.[85] Analysis of PET-positive mediastinal nodes by either EUS[31,86] or EBUS[60,75,76] is a minimally invasive mediastinal staging strategy for NSCLC that has sensitivities of approximately 90%.

All available biopsy techniques have a different diagnostic reach, and, unfortunately, none can sample all mediastinal N2 to N3 lymph node stations. For the various sampling techniques, sensitivity and specificity are regularly based on the specific area that can be reached by the technique under investigation, and not on the mediastinum as a whole.

Mediastinoscopy provides access to the upper and lower para-tracheal regions (stations 2 and 4) and the ventral part of the subcarinal station (region 7) and has a sensitivity of 78%.[43] EUS is complementary to mediastinoscopy because it provides access to both the ventral and the dorsal parts of station 7, the aortopulmonary window, the lower paraesophageal lymph nodes (station 8), and the nodes located in the pulmonary ligamentum (station 9; see Figure 7-9). VATS has been shown to be more accurate than EUS FNA for lymph nodes located in stations 5 and 6.[87]

A limitation of EUS is its inability to detect upper paratracheal lesions as well as those located paratracheally on the right (see Figure 7-10) because of the interposition of air in the trachea by which the ultrasound waves are reflected. As a result of their complementary diagnostic reach, the combination of EUS FNA and mediastinoscopy detects significantly more patients with lymph node metastases than either EUS FNA or mediastinoscopy alone.[2] EBUS TBNA has a diagnostic reach similar to that of mediastinoscopy (the paratracheal areas [stations 2L, 4L, 2R, 4R] and the subcarinal space [station 7]), but it can additionally reach the hilar regions (station 10). In a comparison between EBUS and mediastinoscopy, a slight advantage for EBUS was found.[88] When EUS and EBUS are combined, virtually all mediastinal nodal stations can be investigated.[89–92] The combined esophageal (EUS) and endobronchial staging results in improved outcomes versus either technique alone.[93]

Complete Echoendoscopic Staging

In combination, EUS FNA and EBUS TBNA can reach virtually all mediastinal nodal stations. EBUS has access to the paratracheal zones (stations 2R, 4R, 2L, 4L), and EUS reaches the lower mediastinum (stations 8 and 9; see Figure 7-9). The subcarinal area (station 7) and the left paratracheal station 4L can be reached by both methods. Herth and colleagues[94] found that a combined EUS and EBUS approach had an added value for the subcarinal station. Vilmann and colleagues[91] proposed the concept of complete mediastinal staging of lung cancer by investigating patients with both EUS FNA and EBUS TBNA.

Initially, two small series demonstrated the combined value of EUS FNA and EBUS TBNA for mediastinal staging.[91,95] In 138 patients with (suspected) lung cancer who were investigated by this combined approach, Wallace and colleagues[92] found a sensitivity for lymph nodes of 93% and a negative predictive value of 97%. In 120 patients with NSCLC without nodal enlargement at CT, complete echoendoscopic staging of the mediastinum resulted in a sensitivity of 68% and a negative predictive value of 91%.[90] Complete echoendoscopic staging of the mediastinum with a single EBUS scope was reported in two studies evaluating 150 patients each.[44,45] In a recent meta-analysis, it was shown that combined EBUS and EUS evaluation is more sensitive than EBUS TBNA or EUS FNA alone.[96]

Position of EUS and EBUS in Lung Cancer Staging Algorithms

Where should endosonography (EUS or EBUS or both) be positioned in staging algorithms for the diagnosis and staging of lung cancer? The strength of endosonography is the minimally invasive confirmation of mediastinal lymph node metastases or mediastinal tumor invasion. Endosonography is complementary to PET, which has, under defined circumstances, a high negative predictive value in excluding advanced disease.[85] In a randomized design investigating nodal staging, the ASTER trial found that endosonography (followed by mediastinoscopy in case no nodal metastases were found) had a sensitivity of 94% versus 79% by immediate surgical staging.[2] The endosonographic approach also resulted in significant reduction of unnecessary thoracotomies and was cost effective.[97]

Implementation of endosonography in local lung cancer staging protocols obviously depends on the availability and expertise of EUS and EBUS and its practitioners, the presence of imaging modalities such as integrated CT-PET, and surgical expertise. Current guidelines recommend the use of EUS or EBUS as the tissue sampling technique of choice to confirm mediastinal metastases. Importantly, in cases of suspected mediastinal metastases on imaging (CT/PET or endosonography) but in the absence of malignancy at tissue sampling, subsequent surgical staging (mediastinoscopy) should be performed to rule out false-negative endosonography cases.[3,4]

Increasingly, EUS and EBUS are being advocated to be used early in diagnostic and staging algorithms for NSCLC, especially in those patients with a high pretest probability of mediastinal disease.

In hospitals that have access to both endosonography and integrated PET-CT scanning, the following strategy is proposed for patients with (suspected) lung cancer who are candidates for surgical resection: PET-CT followed by bronchoscopy, including conventional "blind" TBNA (Figure 7-24). In patients with centrally located tumors or enlarged (>1 cm) or PET-positive mediastinal lymph nodes, further staging is required by EUS or EBUS (first) and mediastinoscopy (when EUS or EBUS does not provide proof of mediastinal metastasis or tumor invasion). In peripherally located lung lesions, performance of a conventional bronchoscopy is under discussion, because it rarely adds to any new information following an EBUS investigation.

In patients with a peripherally located tumor without enlarged or PET-positive mediastinal lymph nodes, thoracotomy can be performed directly because the probability of mediastinal metastases is very low.[85]

In centers without access to PET, the recommendation is for staging of patients by EUS or EBUS, followed by mediastinoscopy in the absence of mediastinal metastases at endosonography (Figure 7-25). Combined staging with EUS and mediastinoscopy significantly improves staging compared with EUS or mediastinoscopy alone.[25] The concept of complete echoendoscopic staging of NSCLC is very promising and is currently under investigation.[90–92,95]

Future Perspectives

A large body of evidence indicates that both EUS FNA and EBUS TBNA are accurate endoscopic methods for the diagnosis and staging of NSCLC. By demonstrating mediastinal lymph node metastases or tumor invasion, endosonography provides a minimally invasive alternative for surgical staging and therefore qualifies as the diagnostic technique of choice

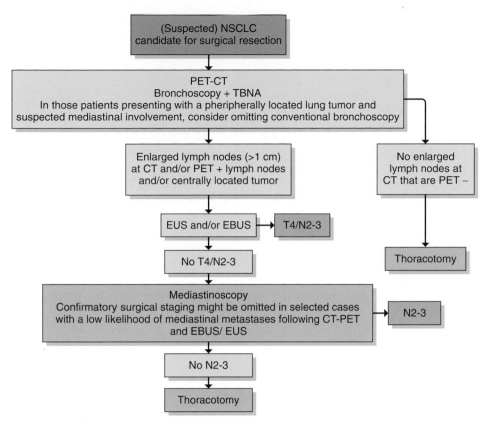

FIGURE 7-24 Proposed role of EUS fine-needle aspiration (FNA) and EBUS transbronchial needle aspiration (TBNA) in the mediastinal staging of non–small-cell lung cancer (NSCLC) (with availability of positron emission tomography [PET]). CT, computed tomography.

in many patients. The 2013 guidelines clearly position endosonography—and not surgical mediastinoscopy—as the test of choice for lung cancer staging.[3,4] As combined EBUS and EUS yields improved sensitivity over either method alone,[93] much is expected of the single endosonographic approach in which, following EBUS, an esophageal examination is performed using the EBUS scope.

Although the safety record of endosonography is impressive, monitoring for complications during these interventional techniques is recommended. Additionally, data on patient preferences for the various mediastinal tissue sampling methods (EBUS versus EUS) are indicated. Further development of echoendoscopes (improved imaging) and needles (larger EBUS needles) is ongoing.

Targeted therapy, addressing specific treatments for different subtypes of NSCLC, will be more important in the years to come. Investigators will need to determine the extent to which the fine-needle aspirates and cell blocks obtained by EUS and EBUS can obtain the same molecular information (EGFR/K-ras receptor status)[45,98,99] as lymph node biopsies at surgical staging.

Regarding the high incidence of lung cancer, vast numbers of patients will qualify for mediastinal staging by endosonography. The dissemination of EUS and EBUS from specialized academic institutions to large regional hospitals is needed to facilitate general availability of these techniques. Investments in equipment, needles, training, and cytopathologic expertise are requirements for a successful endosonography service. To achieve this goal, key professionals in lung cancer care, including chest physicians and surgeons who perform lung surgery, should be aware of the indications of

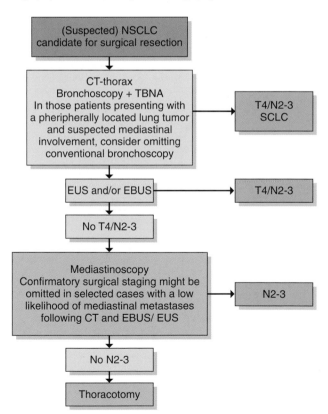

FIGURE 7-25 Proposed role of EUS fine-needle aspiration (FNA) and EBUS transbronchial needle aspiration (TBNA) in the mediastinal staging of non–small-cell lung cancer (NSCLC) (without the availability of positron emission tomography). CT, computed tomography; SCLC, small cell lung cancer; TBNA, transbronchial needle aspiration.

endosonography and the alternative it provides to surgical staging. Furthermore, specialists need to be trained to perform EUS and EBUS procedures. The fact that gastroenterologists are not generally familiar with lung cancer staging, and chest physicians are not used to performing EUS, may be a barrier. With a dedicated training and EUS implementation strategy, however, chest physicians have obtained results similar to those achieved by experts.[26] Training data regarding EBUS TBNA are needed; one study reported a plateau in diagnostic performance after 50 investigations.[100] Virtual reality simulators[5,101] and assessment tools[102] might play an important role for endosonography training. The challenge will be to implement both EUS and EBUS in a short time span to guarantee general accessibility of these important diagnostic and staging methods for patients with NSCLC.

REFERENCES

1. Spira A, Ettinger DS. Multidisciplinary management of lung cancer. *N Engl J Med.* 2004;350:379-392.
2. Annema JT, van Meerbeeck JP, Rintoul RC, et al. Mediastinoscopy vs endosonography for mediastinal nodal staging of lung cancer: a randomized trial. *JAMA.* 2010;304:2245-2252.
3. Vansteenkiste J, De Ruysscher D, Eberhardt WEE, et al. Early and locally advanced non–small-cell lung cancer (NSCLC): ESMO Clinical Practice Guidelines for diagnosis, treatment and follow-up. *Ann Oncol.* 2013;24:vi89-vi98.
4. Silvestri GA, Gonzalez AV, Jantz MA, et al. Methods for staging non–small-cell lung cancer: diagnosis and management of lung cancer, 3rd ed: American College of Chest Physicians evidence-based clinical practice guidelines. *Chest.* 2013;143:e211S-e250S.
5. Konge L, Vilmann P, Clementsen P, et al. Reliable and valid assessment of competence in endoscopic ultrasonography and fine-needle aspiration for mediastinal staging of non–small-cell lung cancer. *Endoscopy.* 2012;44:928-933.
6. Tournoy KG, Annema JT, Krasnik M, et al. Endoscopic and endobronchial ultrasonography according to the proposed lymph node map definition in the seventh edition of the tumor, node, metastasis classification for lung cancer. *J Thorac Oncol.* 2009;4:1576-1584.
7. Rusch VW, Asamura H, Watanabe H, et al. The IASLC lung cancer staging project: a proposal for a new international lymph node map in the forthcoming seventh edition of the TNM classification for lung cancer. *J Thorac Oncol.* 2009;4:568-577.
8. Annema JT, Veselic M, Rabe KF. EUS-guided FNA of centrally located lung tumours following a non-diagnostic bronchoscopy. *Lung Cancer.* 2005;48:357-361, discussion 63-64.
9. Varadarajulu S, Hoffman BJ, Hawes RH, Eloubeidi MA. EUS-guided FNA of lung masses adjacent to or abutting the esophagus after unrevealing CT-guided biopsy or bronchoscopy. *Gastrointest Endosc.* 2004;60:293-297.
10. Venuta F, Rendina EA, Ciriaco P, et al. Computed tomography for preoperative assessment of T3 and T4 bronchogenic carcinoma. *Eur J Cardiothorac Surg.* 1992;6:238-241.
11. Pieterman RM, van Putten JW, Meuzelaar JJ, et al. Preoperative staging of non–small-cell lung cancer with positron-emission tomography. *N Engl J Med.* 2000;343:254-261.
12. Varadarajulu S, Schmulewitz N, Wildi SM, et al. Accuracy of EUS in staging of T4 lung cancer. *Gastrointest Endosc.* 2004;59:345-348.
13. von Bartheld MB, Rabe KF, Annema JT. Transaortic EUS-guided FNA in the diagnosis of lung tumors and lymph nodes. *Gastrointest Endosc.* 2009;69:345-349.
14. Liberman M, Duranceau A, Grunenwald E, et al. New technique performed by using EUS access for biopsy of para-aortic (station 6) mediastinal lymph nodes without traversing the aorta (with video). *Gastrointest Endosc.* 2011;73:1048-1051.
15. Bhutani MS, Hawes RH, Hoffman BJ. A comparison of the accuracy of echo features during endoscopic ultrasound (EUS) and EUS-guided fine-needle aspiration for diagnosis of malignant lymph node invasion. *Gastrointest Endosc.* 1997;45:474-479.
16. Catalano MF, Sivak MV Jr, Rice T, et al. Endosonographic features predictive of lymph node metastasis. *Gastrointest Endosc.* 1994;40:442-446.
17. Toloza EM, Harpole L, Detterbeck F, McCrory DC. Invasive staging of non–small-cell lung cancer: a review of the current evidence. *Chest.* 2003;123:S157-S166.
18. Janssen J, Dietrich CF, Will U, Greiner L. Endosonographic elastography in the diagnosis of mediastinal lymph nodes. *Endoscopy.* 2007;39:952-957.
19. Toloza EM, Harpole L, McCrory DC. Noninvasive staging of non–small-cell lung cancer: a review of the current evidence. *Chest.* 2003;123:S137-S146.
20. Wiersema MJ, Vazquez-Sequeiros E, Wiersema LM. Evaluation of mediastinal lymphadenopathy with endoscopic US-guided fine-needle aspiration biopsy. *Radiology.* 2001;219:252-257.
21. LeBlanc JK, Ciaccia D, Al-Assi MT, et al. Optimal number of EUS-guided fine needle passes needed to obtain a correct diagnosis. *Gastrointest Endosc.* 2004;59:475-481.
22. Wallace MB, Silvestri GA, Sahai AV, et al. Endoscopic ultrasound-guided fine needle aspiration for staging patients with carcinoma of the lung. *Ann Thorac Surg.* 2001;72:1861-1867.
23. Aerts JG, Kloover J, Los J, et al. EUS-FNA of enlarged necrotic lymph nodes may cause infectious mediastinitis. *J Thorac Oncol.* 2008;3:1191-1193.
24. Annema JT, Versteegh MI, Veselic M, et al. Endoscopic ultrasound-guided fine-needle aspiration in the diagnosis and staging of lung cancer and its impact on surgical staging. *J Clin Oncol.* 2005;23:8357-8361.
25. Annema JT, Versteegh MI, Veselic M, et al. Endoscopic ultrasound added to mediastinoscopy for preoperative staging of patients with lung cancer. *JAMA.* 2005;294:931-936.
26. Annema JT, Bohoslavsky R, Burgers S, et al. Implementation of endoscopic ultrasound for lung cancer staging. *Gastrointest Endosc.* 2010;71:64-70, e1.
27. Eloubeidi MA, Tamhane A, Chen VK, Cerfolio RJ. Endoscopic ultrasound-guided fine-needle aspiration in patients with non–small-cell lung cancer and prior negative mediastinoscopy. *Ann Thorac Surg.* 2005;80:1231-1239.
28. Fritscher-Ravens A, Sriram PV, Bobrowski C, et al. Mediastinal lymphadenopathy in patients with or without previous malignancy: EUS-FNA-based differential cytodiagnosis in 153 patients. *Am J Gastroenterol.* 2000;95:2278-2284.
29. Fritscher-Ravens A. Endoscopic ultrasound evaluation in the diagnosis and staging of lung cancer. *Lung Cancer.* 2003;41:259-267.
30. Gress FG, Hawes RH, Savides TJ, et al. Endoscopic ultrasound-guided fine-needle aspiration biopsy using linear array and radial scanning endosonography. *Gastrointest Endosc.* 1997;45:243-250.
31. Kramer H, van Putten JW, Post WJ, et al. Oesophageal endoscopic ultrasound with fine needle aspiration improves and simplifies the staging of lung cancer. *Thorax.* 2004;59:596-601.
32. Larsen SS, Krasnik M, Vilmann P, et al. Endoscopic ultrasound guided biopsy of mediastinal lesions has a major impact on patient management. *Thorax.* 2002;57:98-103.
33. LeBlanc JK, Devereaux BM, Imperiale TF, et al. Endoscopic ultrasound in non–small-cell lung cancer and negative mediastinum on computed tomography. *Am J Respir Crit Care Med.* 2005;171:177-182.
34. Savides TJ, Perricone A. Impact of EUS-guided FNA of enlarged mediastinal lymph nodes on subsequent thoracic surgery rates. *Gastrointest Endosc.* 2004;60:340-346.
35. Silvestri GA, Hoffman BJ, Bhutani MS, et al. Endoscopic ultrasound with fine-needle aspiration in the diagnosis and staging of lung cancer. *Ann Thorac Surg.* 1996;61:1441-1445, discussion 5-6.
36. Talebian M, von Bartheld MB, Braun J, et al. EUS-FNA in the preoperative staging of non–small-cell lung cancer. *Lung Cancer.* 2010;69:60-65.
37. Tournoy KG, Ryck FD, Vanwalleghem L, et al. The yield of endoscopic ultrasound in lung cancer staging: does lymph node size matter? *J Thorac Oncol.* 2008;3:245-249.
38. Tournoy KG, De Ryck F, Vanwalleghem LR, et al. Endoscopic ultrasound reduces surgical mediastinal staging in lung cancer: a randomized trial. *Am J Respir Crit Care Med.* 2008;177:531-535.
39. Wallace MB, Ravenel J, Block MI, et al. Endoscopic ultrasound in lung cancer patients with a normal mediastinum on computed tomography. *Ann Thorac Surg.* 2004;77:1763-1768.
40. Williams DB, Sahai AV, Aabakken L, et al. Endoscopic ultrasound guided fine needle aspiration biopsy: a large single centre experience. *Gut.* 1999;44:720-726.
41. Witte B, Neumeister W, Huertgen M. Does endoesophageal ultrasound-guided fine-needle aspiration replace mediastinoscopy in mediastinal

staging of thoracic malignancies? *Eur J Cardiothorac Surg.* 2008;33:1124-1128.

42. Micames CG, McCrory DC, Pavey DA, et al. Endoscopic ultrasound-guided fine-needle aspiration for non–small-cell lung cancer staging: a systematic review and metaanalysis. *Chest.* 2007;131:539-548.

43. Detterbeck FC, DeCamp MM Jr, Kohman LJ, Silvestri GA, American College of Chest Physicians. Lung cancer. Invasive staging: the guidelines. *Chest.* 2003;123:167S-175S.

44. Herth FJ, Krasnik M, Kahn N, et al. Combined endoscopic-endobronchial ultrasound-guided fine-needle aspiration of mediastinal lymph nodes through a single bronchoscope in 150 patients with suspected lung cancer. *Chest.* 2010;138:790-794.

45. Hwangbo B, Lee GK, Lee HS, et al. Transbronchial and transesophageal fine-needle aspiration using an ultrasound bronchoscope in mediastinal staging of potentially operable lung cancer. *Chest.* 2010;138:795-802.

46. Bueno R, Richards WG, Swanson SJ, et al. Nodal stage after induction therapy for stage IIIA lung cancer determines patient survival. *Ann Thorac Surg.* 2000;70:1826-1831.

47. Voltolini L, Luzzi L, Ghiribelli C, et al. Results of induction chemotherapy followed by surgical resection in patients with stage IIIA (N2) non–small-cell lung cancer: the importance of the nodal downstaging after chemotherapy. *Eur J Cardiothorac Surg.* 2001;20:1106-1112.

48. Annema JT, Veselic M, Versteegh MI, et al. Mediastinal restaging: EUS-FNA offers a new perspective. *Lung Cancer.* 2003;42:311-318.

49. von Bartheld MB, Versteegh MI, Braun J, et al. Transesophageal ultrasound-guided fine-needle aspiration for the mediastinal restaging of non–small-cell lung cancer. *J Thorac Oncol.* 2011;6:1510-1515.

50. Stigt JA, Oostdijk AH, Timmer PR, et al. Comparison of EUS-guided fine needle aspiration and integrated PET-CT in restaging after treatment for locally advanced non–small-cell lung cancer. *Lung Cancer.* 2009;66:198-204.

51. Eloubeidi MA, Seewald S, Tamhane A, et al. EUS-guided FNA of the left adrenal gland in patients with thoracic or GI malignancies. *Gastrointest Endosc.* 2004;59:627-633.

52. Bodtger U, Vilmann P, Clementsen P, et al. Clinical impact of endoscopic ultrasound-fine needle aspiration of left adrenal masses in established or suspected lung cancer. *J Thorac Oncol.* 2009;4:1485-1489.

53. Schuurbiers OC, Tournoy KG, Schoppers HJ, et al. EUS-FNA for the detection of left adrenal metastasis in patients with lung cancer. *Lung Cancer.* 2011;73:310-315.

54. Ringbaek TJ, Krasnik M, Clementsen P, et al. Transesophageal endoscopic ultrasound/fine-needle aspiration diagnosis of a malignant adrenal gland in a patient with non–small-cell lung cancer and a negative CT scan. *Lung Cancer.* 2005;48:247-249.

55. Uemura S, Yasuda I, Kato T, et al. Preoperative routine evaluation of bilateral adrenal glands by endoscopic ultrasound and fine-needle aspiration in patients with potentially resectable lung cancer. *Endoscopy.* 2013;45:195-201.

56. Prasad P, Schmulewitz N, Patel A, et al. Detection of occult liver metastases during EUS for staging of malignancies. *Gastrointest Endosc.* 2004;59:49-53.

57. Hollerbach S, Willert J, Topalidis T, et al. Endoscopic ultrasound-guided fine-needle aspiration biopsy of liver lesions: histological and cytological assessment. *Endoscopy.* 2003;35:743-749.

58. Nguyen P, Feng JC, Chang KJ. Endoscopic ultrasound (EUS) and EUS-guided fine-needle aspiration (FNA) of liver lesions. *Gastrointest Endosc.* 1999;50:357-361.

59. Lee HS, Lee GK, Lee HS, et al. Real-time endobronchial ultrasound-guided transbronchial needle aspiration in mediastinal staging of non–small-cell lung cancer: how many aspirations per target lymph node station? *Chest.* 2008;134:368-374.

60. Bauwens O, Dusart M, Pierard P, et al. Endobronchial ultrasound and value of PET for prediction of pathological results of mediastinal hot spots in lung cancer patients. *Lung Cancer.* 2008;61:356-361.

61. Haas AR. Infectious complications from full extension endobronchial ultrasound transbronchial needle aspiration. *Eur Respir J.* 2009;33:935-938.

62. Mazzone P, Jain P, Arroliga AC, Matthay RA. Bronchoscopy and needle biopsy techniques for diagnosis and staging of lung cancer. *Clin Chest Med.* 2002;23:137-158, ix.

63. Tournoy KG, Rintoul RC, van Meerbeeck JP, et al. EBUS-TBNA for the diagnosis of central parenchymal lung lesions not visible at routine bronchoscopy. *Lung Cancer.* 2009;63:45-49.

64. Nakajima T, Yasufuku K, Fujiwara T, et al. Endobronchial ultrasound-guided transbronchial needle aspiration for the diagnosis of intrapulmonary lesions. *J Thorac Oncol.* 2008;3:985-988.

65. Gu P, Zhao YZ, Jiang LY, et al. Endobronchial ultrasound-guided transbronchial needle aspiration for staging of lung cancer: a systematic review and meta-analysis. *Eur J Cancer.* 2009;45:1389-1396.

66. Adams K, Shah PL, Edmonds L, Lim E. Test performance of endobronchial ultrasound and transbronchial needle aspiration biopsy for mediastinal staging in patients with lung cancer: systematic review and meta-analysis. *Thorax.* 2009;64:757-762.

67. Varela-Lema L, Fernandez-Villar A, Ruano-Ravina A. Effectiveness and safety of endobronchial ultrasound-transbronchial needle aspiration: a systematic review. *Eur Respir J.* 2009;33:1156-1164.

68. Gilbert S, Wilson DO, Christie NA, et al. Endobronchial ultrasound as a diagnostic tool in patients with mediastinal lymphadenopathy. *Ann Thorac Surg.* 2009;88:896-900, discussion 1-2.

69. Herth FJ, Eberhardt R, Vilmann P, et al. Real-time endobronchial ultrasound guided transbronchial needle aspiration for sampling mediastinal lymph nodes. *Thorax.* 2006;61:795-798.

70. Steinfort DP, Hew MJ, Irving LB. Bronchoscopic evaluation of the mediastinum using endobronchial ultrasound: a description of the first 216 cases carried out at an Australian tertiary hospital. *Intern Med J.* 2011;41:815-824.

71. Szlubowski A, Kuzdzal J, Kolodziej M, et al. Endobronchial ultrasound-guided needle aspiration in the non–small-cell lung cancer staging. *Eur J Cardiothorac Surg.* 2009;35:332-335, discussion 5-6.

72. Yasufuku K, Chiyo M, Sekine Y, et al. Real-time endobronchial ultrasound-guided transbronchial needle aspiration of mediastinal and hilar lymph nodes. *Chest.* 2004;126:122-128.

73. Yasufuku K, Chiyo M, Koh E, et al. Endobronchial ultrasound guided transbronchial needle aspiration for staging of lung cancer. *Lung Cancer.* 2005;50:347-354.

74. Omark Petersen H, Eckardt J, Hakami A, et al. The value of mediastinal staging with endobronchial ultrasound-guided transbronchial needle aspiration in patients with lung cancer. *Eur J Cardiothorac Surg.* 2009;36:465-468.

75. Hwangbo B, Kim SK, Lee HS, et al. Application of endobronchial ultrasound-guided transbronchial needle aspiration following integrated PET/CT in mediastinal staging of potentially operable non–small-cell lung cancer. *Chest.* 2009;135:1280-1287.

76. Rintoul RC, Tournoy KG, El Daly H, et al. EBUS-TBNA for the clarification of PET positive intra-thoracic lymph nodes-an international multi-centre experience. *J Thorac Oncol.* 2009;4:44-48.

77. Nakajima T, Yasufuku K, Iyoda A, et al. The evaluation of lymph node metastasis by endobronchial ultrasound-guided transbronchial needle aspiration: crucial for selection of surgical candidates with metastatic lung tumors. *J Thorac Cardiovasc Surg.* 2007;134:1485-1490.

78. Herth FJ, Eberhardt R, Krasnik M, Ernst A. Endobronchial ultrasound-guided transbronchial needle aspiration of lymph nodes in the radiologically and positron emission tomography-normal mediastinum in patients with lung cancer. *Chest.* 2008;133:887-891.

79. Ernst A, Eberhardt R, Krasnik M, Herth FJ. Efficacy of endobronchial ultrasound-guided transbronchial needle aspiration of hilar lymph nodes for diagnosing and staging cancer. *J Thorac Oncol.* 2009;4:947-950.

80. Herth FJ, Annema JT, Eberhardt R, et al. Endobronchial ultrasound with transbronchial needle aspiration for restaging the mediastinum in lung cancer. *J Clin Oncol.* 2008;26:3346-3350.

81. Szlubowski A, Herth FJ, Soja J, et al. Endobronchial ultrasound-guided needle aspiration in non–small-cell lung cancer restaging verified by the transcervical bilateral extended mediastinal lymphadenectomy—a prospective study. *Eur J Cardiothorac Surg.* 2010;37:1180-1184.

82. Esterbrook G, Anathhanam S, Plant PK. Adequacy of endobronchial ultrasound transbronchial needle aspiration samples in the subtyping of non–small-cell lung cancer. *Lung Cancer.* 2013;80:30-34.

83. Larsen SS, Vilmann P, Krasnik M, et al. Endoscopic ultrasound guided biopsy performed routinely in lung cancer staging spares futile thoracotomies: preliminary results from a randomised clinical trial. *Lung Cancer.* 2005;49:377-385.

84. Fritscher-Ravens A, Davidson BL, Hauber HP, et al. Endoscopic ultrasound, positron emission tomography, and computerized tomography for lung cancer. *Am J Respir Crit Care Med.* 2003;168:1293-1297.

85. De Wever W, Stroobants S, Coolen J, Verschakelen JA. Integrated PET/CT in the staging of non–small-cell lung cancer: technical aspects and clinical integration. *Eur Respir J.* 2009;33:201-212.

86. Annema JT, Hoekstra OS, Smit EF, et al. Towards a minimally invasive staging strategy in NSCLC: analysis of PET positive mediastinal lesions by EUS-FNA. *Lung Cancer.* 2004;44:53-60.
87. Cerfolio RJ, Bryant AS, Eloubeidi MA. Accessing the aortopulmonary window (#5) and the paraaortic (#6) lymph nodes in patients with non–small-cell lung cancer. *Ann Thorac Surg.* 2007;84:940-945.
88. Ernst A, Anantham D, Eberhardt R, et al. Diagnosis of mediastinal adenopathy-real-time endobronchial ultrasound guided needle aspiration versus mediastinoscopy. *J Thorac Oncol.* 2008;3:577-582.
89. Rintoul RC, Skwarski KM, Murchison JT, et al. Endobronchial and endoscopic ultrasound-guided real-time fine-needle aspiration for mediastinal staging. *Eur Respir J.* 2005;25:416-421.
90. Szlubowski A, Zielinski M, Soja J, et al. A combined approach of endobronchial and endoscopic ultrasound-guided needle aspiration in the radiologically normal mediastinum in non–small-cell lung cancer staging—a prospective trial. *Eur J Cardiothorac Surg.* 2010;37: 1175-1179.
91. Vilmann P, Krasnik M, Larsen SS, et al. Transesophageal endoscopic ultrasound-guided fine-needle aspiration (EUS-FNA) and endobronchial ultrasound-guided transbronchial needle aspiration (EBUS-TBNA) biopsy: a combined approach in the evaluation of mediastinal lesions. *Endoscopy.* 2005;37:833-839.
92. Wallace MB, Pascual JM, Raimondo M, et al. Minimally invasive endoscopic staging of suspected lung cancer. *JAMA.* 2008;299:540-546.
93. Zhang R, Mietchen C, Kruger M, et al. Endobronchial ultrasound guided fine needle aspiration versus transcervical mediastinoscopy in nodal staging of non–small-cell lung cancer: a prospective comparison study. *J Cardiothorac Surg.* 2012;7:51.
94. Herth FJ, Rabe KF, Gasparini S, Annema JT. Transbronchial and transoesophageal (ultrasound-guided) needle aspirations for the analysis of mediastinal lesions. *Eur Respir J.* 2006;28:1264-1275.
95. Rintoul RC, Skwarski KM, Murchison JT, et al. Endoscopic and endobronchial ultrasound real-time fine-needle aspiration for staging of the mediastinum in lung cancer. *Chest.* 2004;126:2020-2022.
96. Zhang R, Ying K, Shi L, et al. Combined endobronchial and endoscopic ultrasound-guided fine needle aspiration for mediastinal lymph node staging of lung cancer: a meta-analysis. *Eur J Cancer.* 2013;49: 1860-1867.
97. Sharples LD, Jackson C, Wheaton E, et al. Clinical effectiveness and cost-effectiveness of endobronchial and endoscopic ultrasound relative to surgical staging in potentially resectable lung cancer: results from the ASTER randomised controlled trial. *Health Technol Assess.* 2012;16:1-75, iii-iv.
98. Garcia-Olive I, Monso E, Andreo F, et al. Endobronchial ultrasound-guided transbronchial needle aspiration for identifying EGFR mutations. *Eur Respir J.* 2010;35:391-395.
99. Nakajima T, Yasufuku K, Suzuki M, et al. Assessment of epidermal growth factor receptor mutation by endobronchial ultrasound-guided transbronchial needle aspiration. *Chest.* 2007;132:597-602.
100. Steinfort DP, Liew D, Conron M, et al. Cost-benefit of minimally invasive staging of non–small-cell lung cancer: a decision tree sensitivity analysis. *J Thorac Oncol.* 2010;5:1564-1570.
101. Konge L, Annema J. Assessment of endobronchial ultrasound-guided transbronchial needle aspiration performance. *Am J Respir Crit Care Med.* 2013;188:254.
102. Davoudi M, Colt HG, Osann KE, et al. Endobronchial ultrasound skills and tasks assessment tool: assessing the validity evidence for a test of endobronchial ultrasound-guided transbronchial needle aspiration operator skill. *Am J Respir Crit Care Med.* 2012;186:773-779.

EUS in Esophageal Cancer

Mohamad A. Eloubeidi

8

Key Points

- Treatment and outcomes in patients with esophageal cancer are stage dependent.
- One important role for endoscopic ultrasound is the initial triage of patients to receive neoadjuvant therapy or to undergo immediate surgical resection or, in very early stages, endoscopic mucosal resection with or without ablation by photodynamic therapy or radiofrequency ablation.
- EUS is superior to conventional and spiral CT scan for T and N staging.
- EUS is superior to computed tomography and positron emission tomography in celiac and peritumoral lymph node detection.
- Dilation risk should be explained in detail to the patient. Less accurate staging might be a trade off for safety in patients with very stenotic tumors, and those who are high risk for surgery. Alternatives such as high-frequency catheter probes, blind probe or thin caliber echoendoscope might be used instead. Imaging of the tumor with the radial echoendoscope might provide enough, albeit less accurate, information to proceed with radiation and chemotherapy in very stenotic tumors.
- According to the revised American Joint Committee on Cancer, the number of lymph nodes is important and more relevant than their location. In addition, the definition of T4 has been revised according to which organ is invaded.
- Application of EUS after administration of neoadjuvant therapy in esophageal cancer may provide a general idea of response but cannot accurately differentiate residual tumor from radiation effect.

Treatment and outcomes of patients with esophageal cancer are stage dependent. Since its introduction in the early 1980s, endoscopic ultrasound (EUS) played a central and growing role in the staging of patients with esophageal cancer. The purpose of this chapter is to review data pertaining to the accuracy of EUS in staging patients with esophageal cancer and to compare its operating characteristics to other staging modalities such as positron emission tomography (PET) scan and computed tomography (CT) scan. Data on the role of EUS in early and superficial esophageal cancer arising in Barrett's esophagus are reviewed, particularly in the light of development of new ablative methods such as radiofrequency ablation. In addition, techniques of dilation of stricture to facilitate EUS and the use of alternative strategies are explored. The stepwise staging including celiac axis area and liver evaluation are described. Data on restaging after chemotherapy and radiation therapy are reviewed. Finally, the vital role of EUS fine-needle aspiration (FNA) in sampling lymph node to complete the staging of patients with esophageal cancer is explored.

Importance of Staging

Esophageal cancer (ECA) is a leading health problem worldwide. In 2013, about 17,990 cases were diagnosed in the United States of which 15,210 will die of the disease.[1] Survival has slightly improved in patients with esophageal adenocarcinoma in the United States, but overall 5-year survival remains dismal.[2] Treatment and outcomes of patients with esophageal cancer are stage dependent.[2-5] (Figure 8-1 and Figure 8-2). EUS plays a vital role in the management and treatment planning of patients with ECA by providing accurate T and N staging that are vital to triage patients for therapy.[6] Perhaps the most important role for EUS is to initially triage patients to receive neoadjuvant therapy or undergo immediate surgical resection. Patients with any nodal involvement would typically receive preoperative therapy, while patients with either T1 or T2 tumors (without nodal involvement) would go directly for surgical resection (Figure 8-2). The second important role for EUS is restaging after patients receive chemotherapy and radiation therapy. While EUS is less accurate in determining the true stage in these patients, it helps choose the group of patients who are less likely to benefit from surgical resection or the group who could potentially benefit from additional chemotherapy prior to surgical resection, such as those with recalcitrant lymph nodes or persistent T4 disease. The recent American Joint Commission on Staging for Esophageal Cancer classification is shown in Table 8-1.

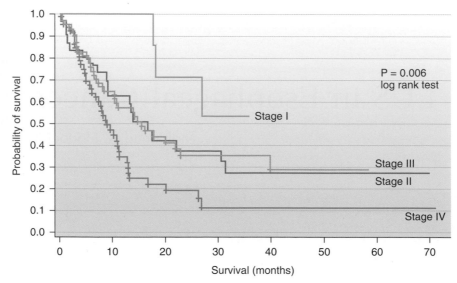

FIGURE 8-1 Survival of patients as staged by EUS using the America Joint Committee on Cancer System.

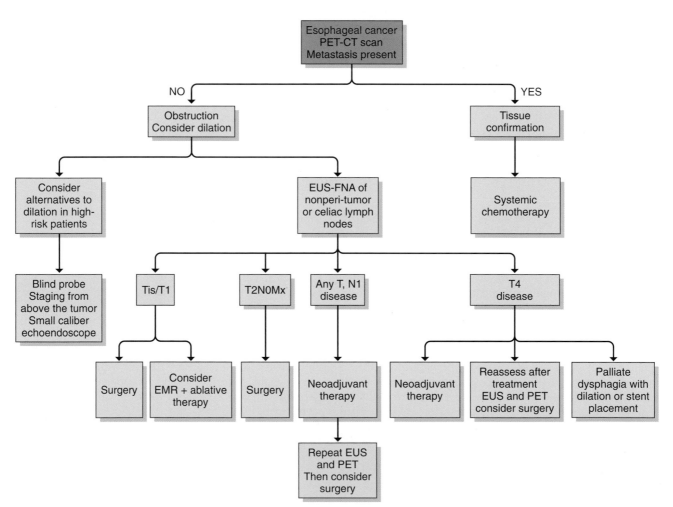

FIGURE 8-2 EUS-based algorithm for the management of esophageal cancer. CT, computed tomography, EMR, endoscopic mucosal resection; EUS, endoscopic ultrasound; FNA, fine-needle aspiration; PET, positron emission tomography.

TABLE 8-1

THE AMERICAN JOINT COMMISSION ON CANCER TNM CLASSIFICATION

Anatomic Stage/Prognostic Groups

Stage	T	N	M	Grade	Tumor Location[a]
Squamous Cell Carcinoma[b]					
0	Tis (HGD)	N0	M0	1, X	Any
IA	T1	N0	M0	1, X	Any
IB	T1	N0	M0	2–3	Any
	T2–3	N0	M0	1, X	Lower, X
IIA	T2–3	N0	M0	1, X	Upper, middle
	T2–3	N0	M0	2–3	Lower, X
IIB	T2–3	N0	M0	2–3	Upper, middle
	T1–2	N1	M0	Any	Any
IIIA	T1–2	N2	M0	Any	Any
	T3	N1	M0	Any	Any
	T4a	N0	M0	Any	Any
IIIB	T3	N2	M0	Any	Any
IIIC	T4a	N1–2	M0	Any	Any
	T4b	Any	M0	Any	Any
	Any	N3	M0	Any	Any
IV	Any	Any	M1	Any	Any

Stage	T	N	M	Grade
Adenocarcinoma				
0	Tis (HGD)	N0	M0	1, X
IA	T1	N0	M0	1–2, X
IB	T1	N0	M0	3
	T2	N0	M0	1–2, X
IIA	T2	N0	M0	3
IIB	T3	N0	M0	Any
	T1–2	N1	M0	Any
IIIA	T1–2	N2	M0	Any
	T3	N1	M0	Any
	T4a	N0	M0	Any
IIIB	T3	N2	M0	Any
IIIC	T4a	N1–2	M0	Any
	T4b	Any	M0	Any
	Any	N3	M0	Any
IV	Any	Any	M1	Any

Definitions of TNM

Primary Tumor (T)[c]

Tx	Tumor cannot be assessed
T0	No evidence of primary tumor
Tis	High-grade dysplasia[d]
T1	Tumor invades lamina propria, muscularis mucosa, or submucosa
T1a	Tumor invades lamina propria or muscularis mucosa
T1b	Tumor invades submucosa
T2	Tumor invades muscularis propria
T3	Tumor invades adventitia
T4	Tumor invades adjacent structures
T4a	Resectable tumor invading pleura, pericardium, or diaphragm
T4b	Unresectable tumor invading other adjacent structures, such as aorta, vertebral body, trachea

Regional Lymph Nodes (N)[e]

Nx	Regional lymph nodes cannot be assessed
N0	No regional lymph node metastasis
N1	Metastases in 1-2 regional lymph nodes
N2	Metastases in 3-6 regional lymph nodes
N3	Metastases in seven or more regional lymph nodes

Distant Metastasis (M)

M0	No distant metastasis
M1	Distant metastasis

HGD, high-grade dysplasia.

[a]Location of the primary cancer site is defined by the position of the upper (proximal) edge of the tumor in the esophagus.

[b]Or mixed histology, including a squamous component or NOS.

[c](1) At least maximal dimension of the tumor must be recorded and (2) multiple tumors require T(m) suffix.

[d]High-grade dysplasia includes all noninvasive neoplastic epithelia that was formerly called carcinoma in situ, a diagnosis that is no longer used for columnar mucosae anywhere in the gastrointestinal tract.

[e]Number must be recorded for total number of regional nodes sampled and total number of reported nodes with metastasis.

(From Edge S, Byrd DR, Compton CC, Fritz AG, Greene FL, Trotti A, eds. AJCC Cancer Staging Manual. 7th ed. New York, NY: Springer; 2010:103-109.)

TABLE 8-2

COMPARISON OF ACCURACY OF COMPUTERIZED TOMOGRAPHY AND ENDOSCOPIC ULTRASOUND IN THE LOCOREGIONAL STAGING OF ESOPHAGEAL CANCER

Technique	Number of Studies	Sensitivity % (Range)	Specificity % (Range)
CT T stage	5	40-80	14-97
CT N stage	7	40-73	25-67
EUS T stage	13	71-100	67-100
EUS N stage	20	60-97	40-100

Data adapted from: Kelly S, Harris KM, Berry E, Hutton J, Roderick P, Cullingworth J et al. A systematic review of the staging performance of endoscopic ultrasound in gastroesophageal carcinoma. Gut. 2001 Oct;49(4):534-9.

TABLE 8-3

COMPARISON OF OPERATING CHARACTERISTICS OF CT, EUS, AND EUS FNA IN THE PREOPERATIVE LYMPH NODE STAGING OF ESOPHAGEAL CANCER PATIENTS

Technique	Sensitivity % (95% CI)	Specificity % (95% CI)	Accuracy % (95% CI)
CT	29 (17-44)	89 (72-98)	51 (40-63)
EUS	71 (56-83)	79 (59-92)	74 (62-83)
EUS FNA	83 (70-93)	93 (77-99)	87 (77-94)

Modified from: Vazquez-Sequeiros E, Wiersema MJ, Clain JE, Norton ID, Levy MJ, Romero Y et al. Impact of lymph node staging on therapy of esophageal carcinoma. Gastroenterology. 2002;125:1626-35.

EUS, CT Scan and PET SCAN

Numerous studies to date have shown that EUS is superior to CT scan in the individual detection of tumor stage (T stage) in patients with esophageal cancer[7,8] (Table 8-2). This superiority stems from the fact that EUS can determine and examine esophageal wall layers with histological correlates.[9] In addition, EUS is superior to CT in the detection of peritumoral and celiac adenopathy[7,10] (Tables 8-2 to 8-4) When compared to PET, which relies on metabolic imaging, EUS can better delineate the wall layers, and hence has better operating characteristics compared to PET for T staging. In addition, EUS is superior in detecting peri-tumoral and celiac lymph nodes (CLNs) compared to PET.[15] In a systematic review of the literature, fluorodeoxyglucose (FDG) PET showed moderate sensitivity and specificity for the detection of locoregional metastasis and reasonable sensitivity and specificity in detection of distant lymphatic and hematogenous metastases.[16] False-positive results were found in 13 out of 86 patients or 15% in one study.[17] Proper interpretation of FDG PET in staging esophageal cancer is impeded by false-positive results; hence, positive FDG PET findings still have to be confirmed by additional investigations.[17] EUS FNA can be used in this setting to confirm positive findings by PET scan.[18] While EUS is superior to PET and CT for locoregional recurrence, CT and PET are better for the detection of liver and lung metastasis.[10,16] Therefore, it is logical to perform EUS in those patients with CT and PET scans that did not reveal distant metastasis, and EUS thus helps triage patient to surgery alone versus neoadjuvant therapy followed by surgery. Often, many investigations are needed in the same patient to complete staging. A recent study has shown that the combination of CT/PET/EUS reduced the number of unnecessary surgeries.[19] The number of unnecessary surgeries decreased from 44% when CT alone was used to 21% when the three modalities were incorporated in the preoperative staging protocol. Moreover, the presence of celiac axis metastasis during surgical exploration was significantly reduced in patients who underwent EUS (13%) or PET (7%) compared to CT (32%).[19] Finally, while not statistically significant, patients who underwent the trimodality staging had better survival compared to those who underwent staging with CT alone (48 versus 28 months).[19] The integration of PET-CT promises better resolution and hence better staging of patients with esophageal cancer.

Equipment
Echoendoscopes

The full detailed description of equipment is discussed elsewhere in this book. EUS equipment consists of radial (mechanical or electronic) and curvilinear array (CLA, electronic) echoendoscopes with their respective processors. The radial (electronic or mechanical) echoendoscope is the most popular instrument used in the United States for the staging of esophageal cancer, whereas the CLA echoendoscope is the most popular in Europe. The image created by the radial echoendoscope is in a 360° transverse plane perpendicular to the long axis of the echoendoscope. The electronic radial instrument provides a 360° ultrasound field of view (a portion of the image is obscured by the fiberoptic bundle in forward viewing instruments) via an electronic multielement transducer. Image orientation is similar to that of radial mechanical instruments; however, it is augmented by the addition of pulsed, color and power Doppler.

TABLE 8-4

OPERATING CHARACTERISTICS OF EUS FNA IN CELIAC LYMPH NODES

Study (Year)	Number of Patients	Sensitivity % (n)	Specificity % (n)	Accuracy % (n)
Giovanini[11] 1995	26	100 (21/21)	—	80 (21/26)
Reed[12] 1997	17	100 (15/15)	—	86 (15/17)
Williams[13] 1999	27	96 (25/26)	100 (1/1)	96 (26/27)
Eloubeidi[14] 2001	51	98 (45/46)	100 (5/5)	98 (50/51)

Curvilinear array instruments scan along the long axis of the endoscope thereby permitting real-time visualization of a needle passed through the biopsy channel. The field of view of CLA echoendoscopes is narrower than with the radial echoendoscopes, which appears to lengthen the learning curve for CLA endosonography and make luminal tumor staging more tedious.

High-Frequency Catheter Probes (HFCP)

High-frequency transducers (12-30 MHz) can be incorporated into small catheters (2-3 mm in diameter). Currently, the best images are produced when the transducer is mechanically rotated 360° as is done with radial endosonography. The most commonly used catheters in the United States are produced by Olympus (UM-2R, 20 MHz; UM-3R, 30 MHz). These catheters produce very high resolution images of the gut wall and are important adjuncts to endoscopic mucosal resection for early malignancies of the esophagus, stomach, and rectum. With the advent of the EUM-30S, a free standing ultrasound unit, catheter probes are more accessible to use in general endoscopy units.

Blind Probes

Passing standard echoendoscopes past a tight stricture can be quite problematic. Perforation of the esophagus has been reported and can result from aggressive dilation or applying too much force when passing a malignant stricture. Characteristics that make use of the echoendoscope in esophageal strictures more difficult include the large diameter of the echoendoscope shaft, oblique optics, and a long rigid distal tip. The outer diameter of both a radial and a CLA echoendoscope is approximately 13 mm; typically, the diameter of the lumen should be dilated to 45 FR or greater to predictably allow the passage of the echoendoscope.[20] Earlier studies reported an unacceptably high perforation rate in patients with esophageal cancer when dilation was performed in conjunction with endosonography.[21] Several studies since have confirmed that esophageal dilation prior to EUS is safe as long as the rules of sequential dilation are followed.[20,22,23] The use of a small diameter nonoptic probe that can be inserted over a guidewire provides an alternative to esophageal dilation.[24,25] The ultrasonic esophagoprobe (Olympus MH-908) has an Eden-Peustow shaped metal tip and is passed over a guide wire in a "monorail" fashion. The probe has an outer diameter of 7.9 mm and can usually be passed through an esophageal cancer without dilation.

Technique
Patient Preparation

Endoscopic evaluation is an important step in the evaluation of patients with dysphagia and esophageal strictures. By the time a patient is referred for endosonography for the staging of esophageal cancer, the diagnosis is usually established. Review of the patient's prior barium swallow examination, recent endoscopy reports from referring colleagues, and assessment of the patient's degree of dysphagia will allow optimal planning for performing the EUS. If the patient has difficulty swallowing soft (pureed) foods, one can predict that dilation will be required to pass the echoendoscope. This information should be communicated to the staff so that dilation equipment and appropriate endoscopes can be prepared. An upper endoscopy is a must prior to endosonography, even in patients without significant dysphagia, to assess the degree of stenosis and distance of the stricture from incisors, and to look for tortuosity within the stricture that might impact on the safety of EUS. Adequate landmarks, the extent of coexisting Barrett's esophagus, and the location of the lower and upper esophageal sphincter should also be noted to help the surgeon plan his or her surgery.

Radial Endosonography

Initial passage of the echoendoscope should be done carefully, gently, and slowly. Once in the esophagus, the instrument is usually advanced past the tumor "by feel" rather by direct visualization of the stenosed lumen. Once the echoendoscope is in position, ultrasound is switched on and imaging begins. In patients with esophageal cancer (see later discussion), imaging actually begins in the duodenum and antrum of the stomach to examine the liver for possible metastasis. The area surrounding the fundus and cardia of the stomach are scanned to look for perigastric and celiac axis lymphadenopathy. Once in the esophagus, attention is turned to the primary tumor with particular attention to the wall layers. At frequencies raging from 5 to 10 MHz, the esophageal wall is imaged as a five-layer structure (*first hyperechoic layer*: superficial mucosa; *second hypoechoic layer*: deep mucosa; *third hyperechoic layer*: submucosa; *fourth hypoechoic layer*: muscularis propria; and *fifth hyperechoic layer*: adventitia). Based on these special characteristics, EUS allows the endosonographer to assess the degree of tumor infiltration into the wall layers and subsequently determine the tumor stage (T stage). It is important to avoid tangential imaging since it might lead to overstaging of the tumor. Imaging with 12 MHz (GF-UM 130) or 20 MHz (GF-UM Q 130) allows superior resolution of the esophageal wall layers. After adequate interrogation of the tumor, several passes are performed at 5 or 7.5 MHz to evaluate the surrounding mediastinum looking for lymph nodes. Other data suggests that staging patients with more advanced esophageal cancer can be performed equally well with the curvilinear echoendoscope alone.[26] Using the CLA echoendoscope permits lymph node sampling without switching to a second echoendoscope. The author uses the CLA echoendoscope first if prior imaging suggests enlarged lymph nodes and liver lesions, and T staging becomes less important. However, using the radial echoendoscope for staging the primary tumor is more complete and less cumbersome than the CLA echoendoscope.

High-Frequency Catheter Probes

High-frequency catheter probes provide high resolution imaging of the gastrointestinal wall layers. They have proven to be indispensable in the staging of superficial esophageal cancer, and selection of patients for endoscopic mucosal resection (EMR). High-frequency miniprobes (20 MHz) provide a more detailed visualization, allowing one to delineate nine layers in the esophageal wall (first and second layer: superficial mucosa [hyperechoic and hypoechoic, respectively], third layer: lamina propria [hyperechoic], fourth layer: muscularis mucosa [hypoechoic], fifth layer: submucosa [hyperechoic], sixth, seventh, and eighth layer: [hypoechoic, hyperechoic, and hypoechoic, respectively], inner circular muscle and outer longitudinal muscle of the muscularis propria with intermuscular connective tissue, and ninth layer: adventitia [hyperechoic]). Visualization of the muscularis mucosa is important when evaluating superficial lesions and nonsurgical alternatives are being considered (endoscopic mucosal resection or ablative therapy such as radiofrequency ablation or photodynamic therapy).

Imaging of small superficial esophageal lesions with a radial echoendoscope is quite difficult because achieving proper positioning is cumbersome, and balloon inflation compresses the lesion causing inaccuracies in staging. High-quality esophageal wall imaging depends on maintaining a water-filled lumen (despite esophageal peristalsis), positioning the transducer perpendicular to the lesion, and being able to adjust the distance between the probe and the lesion. There are few methods that are currently used to achieve safe imaging of the esophageal wall with the high-frequency catheter probes: free floating catheter technique, the condom technique, or the most recently introduced balloon sheath.[27,28] The free technique does not rely on a sheath or a condom to retain water in the esophagus. Whereas achieving a column of water in the distal esophagus is possible for the expert endosonographer, this technique is limited by its short duration due to peristalsis that washes the water down to the stomach. Occasionally, suctioning some of the air out from a hernia sac can bring the column of water back up in the esophagus. If the lesion cannot be demonstrated in a short period of time, it is necessary to refill the distal esophagus is repeatedly. The most dreaded complication from this procedure is aspiration. Therefore, if attempted, the head of the bed should be elevated to at least 45 degrees to minimize the risk of aspiration. In this author's experience, patients with Barrett's esophagus tend to tolerate this technique well. In addition, it is impossible to use this technique to image superficial lesions in the mid- or upper esophagus. Because of the impracticality of these techniques, alternative methods were sought to image early esophageal lesions: the condom and the balloon sheath techniques.[27,28]

Fixing a condom to the end of a two-channel endoscope optimizes imaging by providing a contained column of water within the esophagus (that is not affected by peristalsis) and permits perpendicular imaging while being able to adjust the position of the catheter relative to the lesion.[28] Additionally, condoms are soft and very compliant and thus do not compress esophageal wall layers. Adequate preparation in the success of this technique is important. A standard, nonlubricated, translucent latex condom is attached to a two-channel therapeutic endoscope. One inch of condom extends beyond the endoscope tip. The condom is fixed to the endoscope shaft at three locations with a rubber band, and then 2 cm wide strips of waterproof transparent dressing are wrapped full circle around the condom. Because the condom is transparent, intubation can be performed under direct visualization, but one *must* avoid air insufflation during intubation. The endoscope is passed into the stomach and the condom is filled with water; then residual air and water are aspirated. The collapsed condom is then withdrawn into the esophagus and water is gently instilled. The lesion should be visible through the condom. Once in position, the ultrasound catheter is passed down the second channel and positioned against

Video 8-1. Examination of the esophagus using a high-frequency probe with the condom technique.

the lesion using visual contact. Withdrawing the scope is relatively easy, but if advancement is necessary, it is best to aspirate some water first. The limitation of this technique is the formation of air pockets between the condom and the esophageal wall, resulting in image artifacts. (Video 8-1)

Another recently developed method is the balloon sheath technique.[27,28] The HFCP is fitted with a sheath that has an acoustic coupling balloon at the distal end. The balloon can be filled with water and expanded by means of an adapter at the proximal end outside the endoscope. With this device, standard endoscopy can performed, and then the HFCP with balloon sheath can be advanced through the accessory channel of the endoscope and placed in the area of interest. With the balloon filled with water and enhanced acoustic coupling, high resolution images can be obtained.

Esophageal Dilation and Alternatives

Up to one third of patients with esophageal cancer present with marked luminal stenosis that does not allow the passage of the 13-mm tipped echoendoscope.[20] EUS examination from a position proximal to the tumor has been shown to result in inaccurate T staging and inadequate evaluation of the celiac axis. An earlier study using older model echoendoscopes and dilation practices that did not adhere to the "rule of threes" reported an unacceptably high rate of esophageal perforation (24%) when dilation was employed before EUS.[21] Several studies have recently reported that dilation is safe and increases the yield of detection of CLN involvement.[20,23] Dilation to 45 Fr or 15 mm is usually needed to allow the passage of the echoendoscope. Repeated dilation over a 2-day period should be employed if necessary.

In patients with inadequate dilation or in situations where dilation is not preferred or impractical, a narrow caliber, tapered-tipped, wire-guided echoendoscope was shown to traverse high-grade malignant esophageal strictures with ease.[24,25] In addition, this probe has been shown to improve staging in this situation by evaluating both the primary tumor and the celiac axis. This esophagoprobe markedly reduced the occurrence of incomplete esophageal cancer staging and improved the detection of celiac nodal disease in one study. However, the celiac axis could not be identified in 10% of the patients with esophagoprobe due to either an extremely stenotic tumor or retained gastric air. Obviously, this instrument lacks the image orientation to permit EUS-guided FNA. In case of T4 cancers (invasion into adjacent organ), FNA might not be required. Finally, in patients with esophageal stenosis that could not be overcome with dilation or tumors with

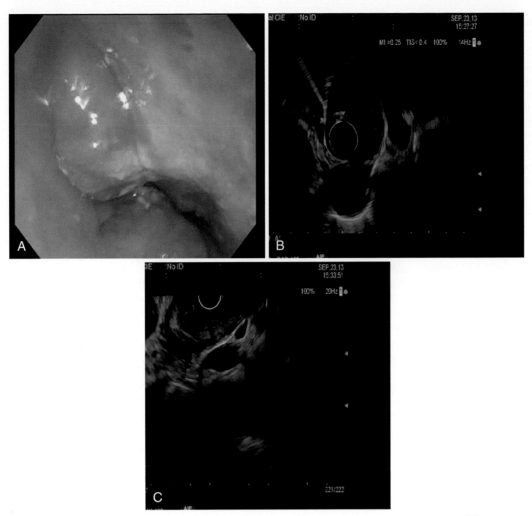

FIGURE 8-3 **A**, On gastroscopy a tight stricture is seen at the distal esophagus due to adenocarcinoma. (**B**, On radial imaging the tumor invades the muscularis layer consistent with T3 disease (T3N0). (**C**) On "wedging" the linear echoendoscope transducer at the tumor site, additional disease burden such as nodal involvement could be recognized in the same patient (T3N1).

significant angulations, obtaining information from above the tumor (T3) can be sufficient to initiate chemotherapy and radiation therapy. In such situations, repeat EUS after neoadjuvant therapy might be appropriate to evaluate the presence of residual disease. Alternatively, a small caliber echoendoscope used for EBUS could be useful in documenting nodal disease in patients with significant stenosis, or where the risk of perforation is either high or detrimental (personal observations). Moreover, the inability to cross a malignant stricture at the time of EUS carries important implications for staging that cannot be assessed without EUS staging. Hence it is believed that all esophageal cancer patients should undergo EUS staging since most surgeons now rely on this technology as a road map prior to providing preoperative neoadjuvant therapy. When evaluating a very tight stricture using the radial echoendoscope, adequate/accurate visualization may not be possible due to air artifacts or tangential imaging. Although not well studied, "wedging" the transducer of the linear array echoendoscope within the tumor can provide a more adequate/accurate staging information (Figures 8-3A-C and Video 8-2).

Finding and Evaluating the Celiac Axis

Celiac lymph node (CLN) metastasis carries a grave implication in patients with esophageal cancer.[4,29,30] Patients with esophageal cancer and CLN metastasis have worse survival than patients without CLN involvement.[2] It is therefore crucial, when possible, to both identify and inspect the celiac

Video 8-2. Examination of esophageal cancer by "wedging" the transducer of a curvilinear echoendoscope.

axis in all patients with esophageal cancer. To identify and evaluate the celiac axis with the radial instrument, the echoendoscope is usually placed at the gastroesophageal junction and the aorta (anechoic and posterior) is located. Once identified, the aorta is placed at the 6-o'clock position on the screen and as the echoendoscope is advanced forward, the aorta will move away from the echoendoscope towards the 5-o'clock position. With further advancement, the celiac axis emerges as a branching point from the descending aorta at the 7-o'clock position. Pushing further by 1-2 cm will usually demonstrate the bifurcation of the celiac axis into the splenic artery and the common hepatic artery ("whale's tail sign") and is typically seen at about 45 cm from the incisors. Sometimes it is not possible to locate the celiac axis by advancing the echoendoscope from the gastroesophageal junction (most commonly due to a hiatal hernia). In this case, beginning the examination in the gastric antrum and withdrawing slowly (while keeping the liver in the "11-o'clock" position) will enable identification of the splenic-portal confluence, and then with an additional 2-3 cm withdrawal, the celiac axis can be seen.[31]

To identify the celiac axis with the CLA echoendoscope, the aorta is found at approximately 35 cm from the incisors (distal esophagus) as a long tubular structure. The endoscope is slowly advanced while maintaining the aorta in view. The first branching artery from the descending aorta is the celiac axis trunk (the superior mesenteric artery follows a few centimeters more distally). When in doubt, Doppler allows for proper identification and verification of the celiac axis trunk. Careful interrogation is performed to assess for lymphadenopathy.

Lymph node characteristics are helpful in differentiating benign from malignant lymph nodes. Malignant lymph nodes tend to be greater than 1 cm, round, sharply demarcated, and hypoechoic.[32] Successively more criteria enhances the likelihood the lymph node is malignant.[31] In patients with esophageal cancer, the identification of celiac lymph nodes is virtually synonymous with malignant involvement. Regardless of echo features and size, 90% of all detected CLNs were proven to be malignant in one study.[14] Moreover, 100% of all those lymph nodes greater than 1 cm were malignant. The clinical impact that malignant celiac lymph nodes have on therapy leads us to perform EUS FNA, providing a means of documenting nodal involvement prior to neoadjuvant therapy.[14,34]

Once lymph nodes are identified and deemed suitable for biopsy, EUS FNA is performed with a CLA echoendoscope.[14,31] The instrument is placed in the stomach lumen opposite the identified celiac lymph node. The FNA needle-sheath system is inserted through the biopsy channel of the echoendoscope and screwed into the Luer lock or the channel hub of the echoendoscope and EUS FNA is performed. Some have suggested suction during FNA of lymph nodes increases the bloodiness of the specimen but does not necessarily increase yield.[35] When this occurs, additional passes without suction are warranted. After 30 to 60 seconds, the needle is retracted. The aspirate is placed on a glass slide, processed with a Diff-Quick stain (American Scientific Products, McGraw Park, IL), and preferably reviewed immediately by an on-site cytologist or pathologist to ensure an adequate specimen. The availability of on-site interpretation is variable from center to center. Malignant diagnosis is usually obtained in the first two passes in the majority of malignant lymph nodes. Typically, four passes are performed in lymph nodes with benign EUS

features to insure that adequate sampling has been performed. The operating characteristics of EUS FNA for assessing celiac lymph nodes are shown in Table 8-4.

Evaluation of the Liver

EUS can detect occult liver metastases in patients in whom noninvasive hepatic imaging studies are normal, although the frequency at which such lesions are detected is low. In addition, EUS FNA can be performed to document liver metastasis.[36,37] The echoendoscope is usually placed in the antrum of the stomach to evaluate the parenchyma of the left lobe of the liver. Restricted by anatomic relations, not all segments of the liver can be viewed with endosonography. The latex balloon is inflated with water to allow better acoustic coupling and therefore better imaging. Installation of water in the stomach is not necessary. Imaging begins by pulling the endoscope slowly from the antrum. Metastasis usually appear as discrete relatively hypoechoic areas in the liver. Once identified, EUS FNA can be performed (Video 8-3) yielding important diagnostic and prognostic information for patient management.[36,37]

Staging of Malignant Strictures

Accurate preoperative staging of esophageal cancer allows appropriate selection of therapy and prognostication (Figure 8-2). After dilation of the tumor (if necessary), staging is performed according to the revised TNM classification[38] (Table 8-1). Inspection of the liver and the celiac axis and the gastrohepatic ligament areas is performed to assess the presence of liver metastasis and lymph nodes, respectively. Attention is then turned to the primary tumor and the mediastinum to identify depth of tumor invasion and the presence of peritumoral and mediastinal adenopathy. The TNM system is based on the determination of depth of tumor invasion (T stage), the presence or absence of regional lymph node metastasis (N stage), and the presence or absence of distant metastasis (M stage). A global stage can be obtained by combining these components. There is an emerging body of data to suggest that EUS staging, similar to surgical staging, predicts long-term survival in patient with esophageal cancer[4,39] (Figure 8-1).

T Stage

T stage is determined by the depth of tumor invasion and esophageal wall layers involvement. The earliest stage (Tis) is present when the cancer is limited to the epithelium and the

Video 8-3. EUS-guided FNA of a mass in the left lobe of the liver that was proven to be a metastatic adenocarcinoma.

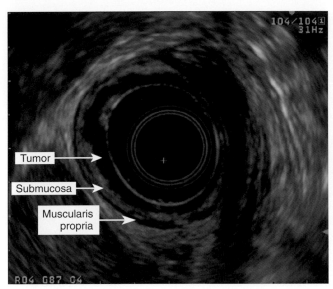

FIGURE 8-4 EUS staging showed a tumor that invaded into but not through the submucosa consistent with a T1 tumor. Findings were confirmed at surgery. (Olympus electronic radial array scanning at 12 MHz.)

Video 8-4. At radial examination, an esophageal tumor mass invading the muscularis propria is seen but has not progressed all the way through the muscle layer consistent with T2 disease. An elongated peritumoral node is seen with a central scar that appears benign.

lamina propria is intact. This stage is detected by biopsy and cannot be imaged by EUS. T1 tumors are those where cancerous cells invade the lamina propria and the submucosa. (Figures 8-4, Figure 8-5A,B) With the advent of HFCPs, T1 tumors are further classified into T1a (confined to mucosa) or T1b (tumor invaded submucosa). This classification becomes important in countries where esophageal cancer is detected at early stages. These two tumors differ in their propensity to have early spread to lymph nodes through a dense network of esophageal lymphatics. This classification helps to identify appropriate therapy commensurate with stage of disease. For example, endoscopic mucosal resection is appropriate treatment because rarely is there involvement with local LN. T1b disease has a 15% to 30% rate of lymph node metastasis and therefore surgery or EMR is the most appropriate

treatment if lymph nodes are not detected. A recent retrospective study evaluated the value of EUS in nodular and nodular high-grade dysplasia or intra-mucosal carcinoma.[40] The authors suggested that EUS does not alter the plan in these patients with high-grade dysplasia. In patients with nodular intramucosal carcinoma (IMC), EMR might be preferable. Another study suggested that EUS leads to over staging in patients with early neoplasia in Barrett's esophagus.[41] It is believed that EUS with the electronic radial array (ERA) echo-endoscope or HFCP should be performed prior to EMR in order to rule out lymph node metastasis and assess for T1a or T1b disease. When the tumor invades the muscularis propria, the tumor is classified as T2 tumor (Video 8-4). When the tumor progresses further to invade the adventitia, the tumor is classified as T3 tumor (Figure 8-6A,B). Involvement of mediastinal structures is now classified as resectable (T4a) involving the diaphragm, the pleura, and pericardium or unresectable (T4b) such as tumors invading the aorta (Figure 8-7), azygous vein (Video 8-5), trachea, or vertebrae. The accuracy of EUS and CT for various T stages is shown in Table 8-2. A systematic review of the literature that included 13 studies that met inclusion criteria found that EUS has a sensitivity range of 71.4% to 100% and a specificity range of 66.7% to 100% for T staging. The true positive rate was 89% (95% CI 0.88-0.93). In articles that compared EUS directly

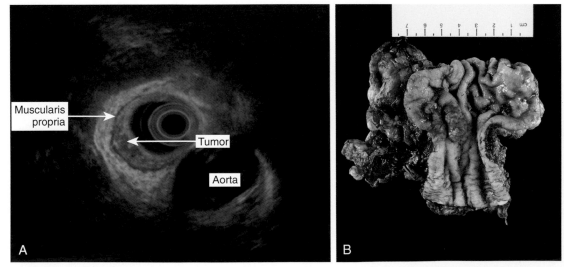

FIGURE 8-5 A, EUS revealed a tumor limited to the submucosa (muscularis propria is intact) with no lymph nodes observed (T1N0). Surgery was recommended after EUS. B, Surgical resection confirmed no involvement of lymph nodes and disease that invaded the submucosa consistent with T1 tumor.

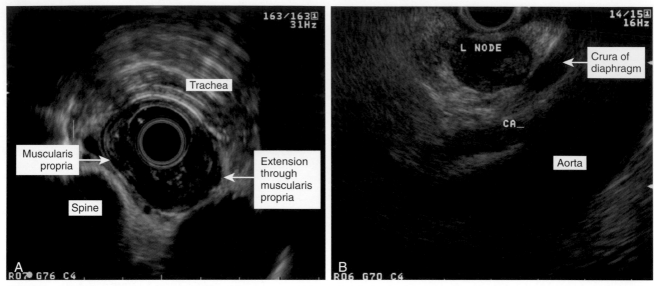

FIGURE 8-6   A, EUS reveals a circumferential hypoechoic mass that invaded the muscularis propria to the adventitia consistent with T3 disease. **B,** Inspection of the celiac axis area revealed an enlarged hypoechoic lymph node with sharp boarders. Transgastric EUS-guided FNA confirmed the presence of malignant involvement. Adjuvant therapy was recommended after EUS. (Olympus UC-30P, frequency 5 MHz.)

with incremental computed tomography, EUS was shown to perform better.[42]

It is noteworthy that T stage accuracy is dependent in part on the learning curve of the endosonographer. An earlier study showed that at least 100 examinations are required to provide accurate T staging in patients with esophageal cancer.[43] Appropriate hands-on and mentored training is mandatory to achieve safe, accurate and reproducible results.

N Stage

Due to rich esophageal lymphatics, esophageal cancer has the propensity to spread early to local lymph nodes. It is clear that those patients with N1 (nodal involvement) disease as classified by EUS have poorer survival compared to N0 (no lymph node involvement) (Figures 8-8 and 8-9).[4,44] Furthermore, per the revised American Joint Committee on Cancer

(AJCC) classification, the number of involved lymph nodes determines N stage (Figure 8-9). For example, N1 reflects the presence of two lymph nodes, N2 the presence of three to six lymph nodes, and N3 reflects the presence of more than seven lymph nodes. The advantage of EUS is that these lymph nodes can be accurately detected preoperatively. Lymph nodes characteristics are helpful in distinguishing benign from malignant lymph nodes. Malignant lymph nodes tend to be greater than 1 cm, round, sharply demarcated, and hypoechoic.[32] The higher the number of criteria a lymph node acquires, the more likely it is to be malignant.[33] The location of the lymph node can help determine if it contains cancer cells. For example, unlike the mediastinum, patients without upper abdominal pathology generally do not have CLN detectable by EUS. In patients with esophageal cancer, the identification of CLNs is synonymous with malignant involvement.[14] Regardless of echo features and size, 90% of all detected CLNs were proven to be malignant in one study. Moreover, 100% of all those lymph nodes greater than 1 cm were malignant.[14]

A systematic review of the literature that included 13 studies that met inclusion criteria found that EUS has a sensitivity range of 59.5% to 100% and a specificity range of 40% to 100% for T staging. The true positive rate was 79% (95% CI 0.75-0.83).[42]

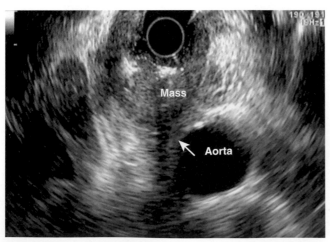

FIGURE 8-7   EUS reveals adherence to the descending aorta consistent with vascular invasion. (Olympus Electronic radial array scanning at 7.5 MHz.)

Video 8-5. At radial examination, an esophageal tumor mass is seen invading the muscularis layer and also the azygos vein. Also, several peritumoral nodes are noted. The lesion was staged to be T4bN1.

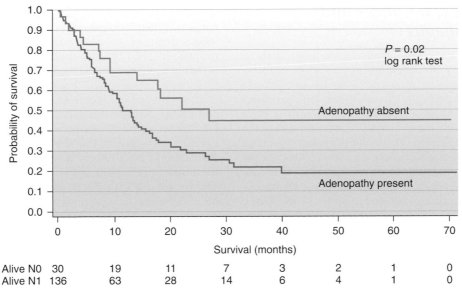

| Alive N0 | 30 | 19 | 11 | 7 | 3 | 2 | 1 | 0 |
| Alive N1 | 136 | 63 | 28 | 14 | 6 | 4 | 1 | 0 |

FIGURE 8-8 Survival of patients with esophageal cancer according to celiac adenopathy status in the group who underwent surgery. Patients who had celiac lymph nodes at the time of surgery had shorter survival.

To eliminate or reduce uncertainty, EUS FNA provides a means of documenting nodal involvement prior to neoadjuvant therapy.[14,34,45] A major limitation to EUS FNA is the fact that an intervening tumor does not allow sampling of these lymph nodes without the risk of contamination. The revised AJCC TNM classification does not take into account the location of the primary tumor for classification of lymph nodes as local disease (N1) or metastatic disease (M1).[38] With the new classification based on numbers of lymph nodes, the location in the abdomen formerly known as celiac carries less importance, and patients' tumors should be considered resectable pending treatment effects on the eradication of these lymph nodes. With this new classification, it is imperative to improve the identification of malignant lymph nodes by non-invasive means, particularly for lymph nodes in the peritumoral area. One study suggested that malignant lymph nodes can be better identified by a combination of elastography and image analysis than by EUS lymph nodes characteristics alone.[46]

M Stage

Involvement of distant sites from the primary tumor via hematogenous seeding of distant organs (liver, lung, bones) is considered metastatic disease.[38] EUS provides excellent imaging of the medial two thirds of the liver but cannot exclude with certainty metastatic disease to all areas of the liver. According to the new TNM classification, metastasis to celiac lymph nodes is not considered as M1a or M1b disease anymore.[38] In contradistinction, the number of lymph nodes, rather than their location, is what further determines the AJCC group staging (Video 8-6).

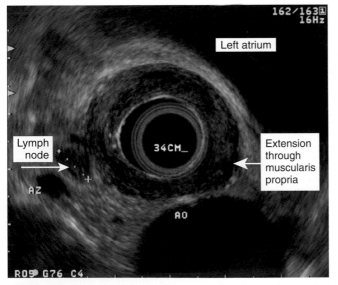

FIGURE 8-9 EUS appearance of a tumor that invaded muscularis propria to adventitia. One peritumoral lymph nodes is seen consistent with malignant involvement (T3N1). These lymph nodes are not amenable to EUS FNA (Olympus electronic radial array, scanning at 12 MHz.)

Video 8-6. At radial EUS, an esophageal tumor mass invading the muscularis propria is seen with more than three peritumoral nodes. The tumor was staged T3N2.

EUS in Superficial Cancer and Barrett's Esophagus

With the advent of EMR and ablative procedures such as photodynamic therapy or radiofrequency ablation, accurate assessment of depth of tumor invasion is a mandate prior to their application. Since depth of tumor invasion correlates with lymph node metastasis, it is crucial to identify T stage prior to EMR. One study has shown that cancer limited to the epithelium and lamina propria (m1 and m2), have 5% chance of metastasis to lymph nodes. In contrast, cancer invading the muscularis mucosa or the submucosa has 12% to 27% chance of metastasis to lymph nodes. Invasion of the deep submucosa reaching the proper muscle could lead to 36% to 46% chance of lymph node metastasis.[47] The accuracy of HFCP in distinguishing between mucosal cancer and cancer invading the submucosa is 81% to 100%.[48] The accuracy of EUS in patients with Barrett's esophagus and high-grade dysplasia or intramucosal carcinoma has been reported. The sensitivity, specificity, and negative predictive values of preoperative EUS for submucosa invasion were 100%, 94%, and 100%, and for lymph node involvement were 100%, 81%, and 100%, respectively.[49] A nodule or stricture noted by endoscopy was associated with an increased likelihood of submucosa invasion.[49] Of note, this study used the regular echoendoscope and not the HFCP. With the exception of patients with BE, early esophageal cancer is rarely seen in the United States and, therefore, HFCP is less frequently used than in Japan.

EUS-Guided Fine-Needle Aspiration Biopsy of Celiac and Peri-Intestinal Lymph Nodes

Prior to the advent of EUS FNA, endosonographers relied on lymph nodes echofeatures to identify malignancy in lymph nodes. Features included size greater than 1 cm, sharp borders, round shape, and hypoechoic echo texture. Recent work suggests that EUS FNA improves the accuracy of lymph node staging and is superior to EUS echofeatures.[33] EUS alone was only 33.3% accurate in differentiating between malignant and benign lymphadenopathy, whereas EUS FNA had a significantly higher accuracy of 99.4%.[33] This study also found that LN echofeatures are particularly unreliable in the mediastinum. In patients with esophageal cancer, EUS FNA was found superior to helical CT and EUS for the preoperative staging of lymph nodes.[34] Due to a small number, EUS was equivalent to CT for the detection of celiac lymph nodes. EUS has previously been shown to be superior to both CT and PET for the detection of celiac lymph nodes.[10] The operating characteristics of EUS FNA compared to CT and EUS and the accuracy of EUS FNA in sampling celiac lymph nodes are shown in Tables 8-3 and 8-4, respectively.

Controversies in EUS Staging

The role of EUS in the staging of esophageal cancer has been challenged by a study from the Cleveland Clinic. Zuccaro and colleagues assert that in previous studies, advanced staged patients were overrepresented.[50] They reviewed their cohort who went directly to surgery following EUS (without neoadjuvant therapy) between 1987 and 2001. The T stage was misclassified in 45% of patients and N stage in 25% of patients. When T classification was dichotomized into tumors whose depth of invasion was not beyond the muscularis propria (pTis-pT2) and those beyond (pT3-pT4), errors occurred in 42 patients (16%).[50]

It has been suggested that the 14-year time period of the study might make it less reflective of contemporary methods and results. Shimpi and colleagues designed a study with an equivalent standard, surgery immediately following EUS (without neoadjuvant therapy), but limited the duration to their cohort from 1999 to 2004.[51] This group also emphasized the importance of dilating stricture to optimize evaluation. They reported a T stage accuracy of 76% and N stage accuracy of 89%, more consistent with what has been previously reported in the literature. However, they did observe that EUS may perform less well in assigning T1 and T2 stage compared to T3 and T4, but that the high-frequency probe could improve the yield for T1. It was noted that FNA in the Zuccaro and colleagues study was not routinely performed and that a critical strength of EUS compared to other staging modalities is the ability to confirm lymph node involvement with tissue sampling.[50]

Role and limitation of EUS Following Neoadjuvant Therapy

Due to its ability to image the gastrointestinal tract wall layers with accuracy and histologic correlates,[9] EUS is currently the best staging modality for locoregional disease in esophageal cancer. However, several studies have shown that standard EUS criteria are not accurate after neoadjuvant chemoradiation because its performance is poor in differentiating tumor from necrosis or inflammatory reaction.[52,53] A recent study evaluated the utility of EUS after neoadjuvant therapy.[54] The authors studied 97 consecutive esophageal cancer patients treated with preoperative chemoradiotherapy and a potentially curative surgical procedure. All patients had EUS examination prior to chemoradiation, and 53 had a repeat EUS examination after chemoradiation but prior to surgery. Surgical resection specimens were analyzed for absence or presence of residual tumor and its location. Patients with residual tumor in the esophagus and patients without residual tumor had similar cumulative survival. Patients with residual cancer in lymph nodes showed a trend towards shorter cumulative survival compared to patients without residual tumor in lymph nodes. The actuarial survival in patients with involved lymph nodes group was lower than patients with no lymph node group at 1-, 2-, and 3-years posttreatment. Patients with significant residual lymphadenopathy detected by EUS after therapy had significantly worse postoperative survival compared to patients with no residual lymphadenopathy.[54] In eight patients, the authors reliably obtained cytology and were able to identify residual malignancy by EUS FNA after chemoradiotherapy. The authors concluded that EUS and EUS-guided FNA can be helpful in identifying residual tumor in the lymph nodes after preoperative chemoradiotherapy to select patients who benefit maximally from surgery.

Another study[55] evaluated the accuracy of EUS in restaging 83 patients with esophageal adenocarcinoma after induction therapy. T classification was assessed correctly by EUS in 22 patients (29%). The proportion of individual T classifications by EUS that were correct were 0% for T0 tumors, 19% for T1 tumors, 27% for T2 tumors, 52% for T3 tumors, and 0% for T4 tumors when comparing results from the EUS restaging examination with the findings at surgical pathology. Nineteen of 83 patients (25%) were assigned the correct group stage by restaging EUS, 42 patients (55%) were over staged, and 15 patients (20%) were under staged. The overall accuracy of the restaging EUS examination for predicting the N classification of the tumor was (49%). The sensitivity of EUS for N classification was 48% for N0 disease and 52% for N1 disease. Interestingly, EUS FNA was not routinely performed in this study to assess for residual disease. A more recent study that evaluated 73 patients with esophageal cancer that underwent EUS staging after chemotherapy and radiation revealed a very poor correlation between EUS staging and pathology; hence the group abandoned using EUS for restaging esophageal cancer.[56]

The current practice is to sample lymph nodes after chemoradiotherapy; patients with residual disease especially in the celiac axis undergo more treatment prior to consideration of surgical resection. Since neoadjuvant therapy was used initially to shrink and reduce the bulk of the tumor, perhaps it is more important to ask the question whether residual tumor is resectable so that the patient will undergo surgical resection. In addition, and more importantly, EUS FNA has the ability to sample lymph node after chemotherapy and therefore can identify persistent disease necessitating further chemotherapy (Figure 8-10). Experience with esophageal cancer staged as N0 by EUS either with or without neoadjuvant therapy was recently published. From January 2002 to June 2009, 207 patients underwent Ivor Lewis esophagogastrectomy. Of 95 patients who did not undergo neoadjuvant therapy 82 were staged as N0. Seventy-seven (94%) were confirmed as N0 on final pathology (sensitivity 94%, accuracy 95%). Neoadjuvant chemoradiotherapy was administered to the remaining 112 patients and 107 had a restaging EUS FNA. Ninety of these patients were staged by EUS as N0. Seventy patients (78%) were N0 on final pathology (sensitivity 82%, accuracy 68%). There was no EUS FNA-related procedural morbidity or mortality. It was concluded that EUS FNA is very accurate and sensitive when it clinically stages patients with

esophageal cancer as N0. In addition, it is even accurate and sensitive when restaging patients as N0 after neo-adjuvant chemoradiotherapy.

Another useful measure of tumor response is reduction in cross-sectional area. Reduction in maximal cross-sectional area of tumor (MAX) offers promise as a useful measure for assessing response to preoperative therapy.[52]

In one study, responders (patients who had > 50% reduction in the MAX) as assessed by EUS were more likely to survive compared to nonresponders.[52] Moreover, it is apparent that responders with adenocarcinoma were more likely to survive compared to nonresponders. However, this finding did not hold true for patients with squamous cell carcinoma of the esophagus. It is noteworthy that five of six patients in the R0 group were among the responders. None of the other clinical, endoscopic, or endosonographic variables studied predicted survival. This study was limited by a small sample size. The lack of effect of known important variables on survival (e.g., T stage, N stage, the presence of celiac adenopathy, or overall AJCC stage, is probably due to a type two error, i.e., the study was underpowered to detect such a difference). The development of three-dimensional EUS that has the ability to measure the total volume of the tumor, rather than the cross-sectional area, might prove to be a superior modality in the assessment of response to multimodality therapy in patients with esophageal cancer.

Impact of EUS on Survival in Patients with Esophageal Cancer

Because EUS provides accurate preoperative staging, initial data obtained at the time of EUS is predictive of survival. It has previously been shown that EUS (AJCC) stage, the presence of adenopathy, and the presence of celiac adenopathy are all predictive factors of survival.[4] More recently, a study showed that distinct survival advantages was seen in patients with fewer malignant-appearing regional lymph nodes seen by EUS.[57] The median survivals were 66 months, 14.5 months, and 6.5 months for 0, 1-2, and >2 malignant-appearing lymph nodes, respectively. Survival was also influenced by the presence of celiac lymph nodes and tumor length, both of which were associated with increased number of malignant nodes.[57] The authors concluded that the number of malignant-appearing periesophageal lymph nodes detected by EUS is associated with improved survival stratification in patients with esophageal adenocarcinoma and should be considered in the pre-surgical staging of esophageal cancer.[57] These findings were supportive of previous work from the Surveillance, Epidemiology, and End Results database suggesting that tumor length and the number of lymph nodes should be routinely reported as part of the staging system because these findings independently predicted survival in patients with esophageal cancer.[3]

Summary

EUS is currently the only available modality that images the esophageal wall layers with histologic correlates. EUS is superior to CT and PET scan in the detection of peritumoral and celiac lymph nodes. EUS FNA allows for documentation of locoregional and distant lymph node status prior to

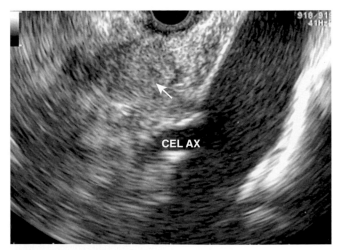

FIGURE 8-10 EUS performed after chemotherapy and radiation identified a soft tissue density in the celiac axis area. EUS-guided FNA confirmed the presence of squamous cell carcinoma.

neoadjuvant therapy. EUS can select patients for surgical resection after neoadjuvant therapy. Future efforts should focus on implementing EUS as part of research protocols evaluating therapies for esophageal cancer.

Examination Checklist

Liver
Celiac axis
Primary tumor
Periesophageal area above the aortic arch for lymph nodes
Note relationship of tumor to carina
For distal esophageal tumors, look for invasion into the diaphragm
Full report that incorporates TNM staging should supplied. The length of the tumor, and number of lymph nodes and their respective location should be listed. Finally, the extent of Barrett's esophagus, location of GE junction and the upper esophageal sphincter should be included to alert the surgeon to import landmarks prior to the operation.

REFERENCE

1. Siegel R, Naishadham D, Jemal A. Cancer statistics. *CA Cancer J Clin.* 2013;63(1):11-30.
2. Eloubeidi MA, Mason AC, Desmond RA, El Serag HB. Temporal trends (1973-1997) in survival of patients with esophageal adenocarcinoma in the United States: a glimmer of hope? *Am J Gastroenterol.* 2003;98(7):1627-1633.
3. Eloubeidi MA, Desmond R, Arguedas MR, et al. Prognostic factors for the survival of patients with esophageal carcinoma in the U.S.: the importance of tumor length and lymph node status. *Cancer.* 2001;95:1434-1443.
4. Eloubeidi MA, Wallace MB, Hoffman BJ, et al. Predictors of survival for esophageal cancer patients with and without celiac axis lymphadenopathy: impact of staging endosonography. *Ann Thorac Surg.* 2001;72:212-219.
5. Fockens P, Kisman K, Merkus MP, et al. The prognosis of esophageal carcinoma staged irresectable (T4) by endosonography. *J Am Coll Surg.* 1998;186:17-23.
6. Buxbaum JL, Eloubeidi MA. Endoscopic evaluation and treatment of esophageal cancer. *Minerva Gastroenterol Dietol.* 2009;55(4):455-469.
7. Rosch T. Endosonographic staging of esophageal cancer: a review of literature results. *Gastrointest Endosc Clin N Am.* 1995;5:537-547.
8. Romagnuolo J, Scott J, Hawes RH, et al. Helical CT versus EUS with fine needle aspiration for celiac nodal assessment in patients with esophageal cancer. *Gastrointest Endosc.* 2002;55:648-654.
9. Kimmey MB, Martin RW, Haggitt RC, et al. Histologic correlates of gastrointestinal ultrasound images. *Gastroenterology.* 1989;96:433-441.
10. Akdamar M, Eloubeidi MA. A prospective comparison of computerized tomography (CT), 18 fluoro-deoxyglucose positron emission tomography (FDG-PET) and endoscopic ultrasonography (EUS) in the preoperative evaluation of potentially operable esophageal cancer (ECA) patients. *Am J Gastroenterol.* 2005;98:s5.
11. Giovannini M, Seitz JF, Monges G, et al. Fine-needle aspiration cytology guided by endoscopic ultrasonography: results in 141 patients. *Endoscopy.* 1995;27:171-177.
12. Reed CE, Mishra G, Sahai AV, et al. Esophageal cancer staging: improved accuracy by endoscopic ultrasound of celiac lymph nodes. *Ann Thorac Surg.* 1999;67:319-321.
13. Williams DB, Sahai AV, Aabakken L, et al. Endoscopic ultrasound guided fine needle aspiration biopsy: a large single centre experience. *Gut.* 1999;44:720-726.
14. Eloubeidi MA, Wallace MB, Reed CE, et al. The utility of EUS and EUS-guided fine needle aspiration in detecting celiac lymph node metastasis in patients with esophageal cancer: a single-center experience. *Gastrointest Endosc.* 2001;54:714-719.
15. Pfau PR, Perlman SB, Stanko P, et al. The role and clinical value of EUS in a multimodality esophageal carcinoma staging program with CT

and positron emission tomography. *Gastrointest Endosc.* 2007;65(3):377-384.
16. van Westreenen HL, Westerterp M, Bossuyt PM, et al. Systematic review of the staging performance of 18F-fluorodeoxyglucose positron emission tomography in esophageal cancer. [Review] [59 refs]. *J Clin Oncol.* 2004;22(18):3805-3812.
17. van Westreenen HL, Heeren PA, Jager PL, et al. Pitfalls of positive findings in staging esophageal cancer with F-18-fluorodeoxyglucose positron emission tomography. *Ann Surg Oncol.* 2003;10(9):1100-1105.
18. Eloubeidi MA, Cerfolio RJ, Chen VK, et al. Endoscopic ultrasound-guided fine needle aspiration of mediastinal lymph node in patients with suspected lung cancer after positron emission tomography and computed tomography scans. *Ann Thorac Surg.* 2005;79(1):263-268.
19. van Westreenen HL. Heeren PA, van Dullemen HN, et al. Positron emission tomography with F-18-fluorodeoxyglucose in a combined staging strategy of esophageal cancer prevents unnecessary surgical explorations. *J Gastrointest Surg.* 2005;9:54-61.
20. Wallace MB, Hawes RH, Sahai AV, et al. Dilation of malignant esophageal stenosis to allow EUS guided fine-needle aspiration: safety and effect on patient management. *Gastrointest Endosc.* 2000;51:309-313.
21. Van Dam J, Rice TW, Catalano MF, et al. High-grade malignant stricture is predictive of esophageal tumor stage. Risks of endosonographic evaluation. *Cancer.* 1993;71:2910-2917.
22. Kallimanis GE, Gupta PK, al-Kawas FH, et al. Endoscopic ultrasound for staging esophageal cancer, with or without dilation, is clinically important and safe. *Gastrointest Endosc.* 1995;41:540-546.
23. Pfau PR, Ginsberg GG, Lew RJ, et al. Esophageal dilation for endosonographic evaluation of malignant esophageal strictures is safe and effective. *Am J Gastroenterol.* 2000;95:2813-2815.
24. Binmoeller KF, Seifert H, Seitz U, et al. Ultrasonic esophagoprobe for TNM staging of highly stenosing esophageal carcinoma. *Gastrointest Endosc.* 1995;41:547-552.
25. Mallery S, Van DJ. Increased rate of complete EUS staging of patients with esophageal cancer using the nonoptical, wire-guided echoendoscope. *Gastrointest Endosc.* 1999;50:53-57.
26. Siemsen M, Svendsen LB, Knigge U, et al. A prospective randomized comparison of curved array and radial echoendoscopy in patients with esophageal cancer. *Gastrointest Endosc.* 2003;58(5):671-676.
27. Vazquez-Sequeiros E, Wiersema MJ. High-frequency US catheter-based staging of early esophageal tumors. *Gastrointest Endosc.* 2002;55(1):95-99.
28. Wallace MB, Hoffman BJ, Sahai AS, et al. Imaging of esophageal tumors with a water-filled condom and a catheter US probe. *Gastrointest Endosc.* 2000;51:597-600.
29. Christie NA, Rice TW, DeCamp MM, et al. M1a/M1b esophageal carcinoma: clinical relevance. *J Thorac Cardiovasc Surg.* 1999;118:900-907.
30. Hiele M, De LP, Schurmans P, et al. Relation between endoscopic ultrasound findings and outcome of patients with tumors of the esophagus or esophagogastric junction. *Gastrointest Endosc.* 1997;45:381-386.
31. Eloubeidi MA, Vilmann P, Wiersema MJ. Endoscopic ultrasound-guided fine-needle aspiration of celiac lymph nodes. *Endoscopy.* 2004;36(10):901-908.
32. Catalano MF, Sivak MVJ, Rice T, et al. Endosonographic features predictive of lymph node metastasis. *Gastrointest Endosc.* 1994;40:442-446.
33. Chen VK, Eloubeidi MA. Endoscopic ultrasound-guided fine needle aspiration is superior to lymph node echofeatures: a prospective evaluation of mediastinal and peri-intestinal lymphadenopathy. *Am J Gastroenterol.* 2004;99(4):628-633.
34. Vazquez-Sequeiros E, Wiersema MJ, Clain JE, et al. Impact of lymph node staging on therapy of esophageal carcinoma. *Gastroenterology.* 2002;125:1626-1635.
35. Wallace MB, Kennedy T, Durkalski V, et al. Randomized controlled trial of EUS-guided fine needle aspiration techniques for the detection of malignant lymphadenopathy. *Gastrointest Endosc.* 2001;54:441-447.
36. Prasad P, Schmulewitz N, Patel A, et al. Detection of occult liver metastases during EUS for staging of malignancies. *Gastrointest Endosc.* 2004;59(1):49-53.
37. tenBerge J, Hoffman BJ, Hawes RH, et al. EUS-guided fine needle aspiration of the liver: indications, yield, and safety based on an international survey of 167 cases. *Gastrointest Endosc.* 2002;55(7):859-862.
38. AJCC. Esophageal and esophagogastric junction. In: Edge SB, Byrd DR, Compton CC, et al, eds. *AJCC Cancer Staging Manual.* 7th ed. New York, NY: Springer; 2010:103-115.

39. Harewood GC, Kumar KS. Assessment of clinical impact of endoscopic ultrasound on esophageal cancer. *J Gastroenterol Hepatol*. 2004;19(4): 433-439.

40. Bulsiewicz WJ, Dellon ES, Rogers AJ, et al. The impact of endoscopic ultrasound findings on clinical decision making in Barrett's esophagus with high-grade dysplasia or early esophageal adenocarcinoma. *Dis Esophagus*. 2012;1442-2050.

41. Fernández-Sordo JO, Konda VJ, Chennat J, et al. Is Eendoscopic ultrasound (EUS) necessary in the pre-therapeutic assessment of Barrett's esophagus with early neoplasia? *J Gastrointest Oncol*. 2012;3(4): 314-321.

42. Kelly S, Harris KM, Berry E, et al. A systematic review of the staging performance of endoscopic ultrasound in gastro-oesophageal carcinoma. *Gut*. 2001;49(4):534-539.

43. Fockens P, van den Brande JH, van Dullemen MH, et al. Endosonographic T-staging of esophageal carcinoma: a learning curve. *Gastrointest Endosc*. 1996;44:58-62.

44. Pfau PR, Ginsberg GG, Lew RJ, et al. Endoscopic ultrasound predictors of long term survival in esophageal carcinoma. *Gastrointest Endosc*. 2000;51:AB136.

45. Penman ID, Williams DB, Sahai AV, et al. Ability of EUS with fine-needle aspiration to document nodal staging and response to neoadjuvant chemoradiotherapy in locally advanced esophageal cancer: a case report. *Gastrointest Endosc*. 1999;49:783-786.

46. Knabe M, Gunter E, Ell C, Pech O. Can EUS elastography improve lymph node staging in esophageal cancer? *Surg Endo*. 2013;17(4):1196-1202.

47. Kodama M, Kakegawa T. Treatment of superficial cancer of the esophagus: a summary of responses to a questionnaire on superficial cancer of the esophagus in Japan. *Surgery*. 1998;123(4):432-439.

48. Murata Y, Napoleon B, Odegaard S. High-frequency endoscopic ultrasonography in the evaluation of superficial esophageal cancer. *Endoscopy*. 2003;35(5):429-435, discussion 436.

49. Scotiniotis IA, Kochman ML, Lewis JD, et al. Accuracy of EUS in the evaluation of Barrett's esophagus and high-grade dysplasia or intramucosal carcinoma. *Gastrointest Endosc*. 2001;54(6):689-696.

50. Zuccaro G Jr, Rice TW, Vargo JJ, et al. Endoscopic ultrasound errors in esophageal cancer. *Am J Gastroenterol*. 2005;100(3):601-606.

51. Shimpi RA, George J, Jowell P, Gress FG. Staging of esophageal cancer by EUS: staging accuracy revisited. *Gastrointest Endosc*. 2007;66(3): 475-482.

52. Chak A, Canto MI, Cooper GS, et al. Endosonographic assessment of multimodality therapy predicts survival of esophageal carcinoma patients. *Cancer*. 2000;88:1788-1795.

53. Isenberg G, Chak A, Canto MI, et al. Endoscopic ultrasound in restaging of esophageal cancer after neoadjuvant chemoradiation. *Gastrointest Endosc*. 1998;48:158-163.

54. Agarwal B, Swisher S, Ajani J, et al. Endoscopic ultrasound after preoperative chemoradiation can help identify patients who benefit maximally after surgical esophageal resection. *Am J Gastroenterol*. 2004;99(7): 1258-1266.

55. Kalha I, Kaw M, Fukami N, et al. The accuracy of endoscopic ultrasound for restaging esophageal carcinoma after chemoradiation therapy. *Cancer*. 2004;101(5):940-947.

56. Griffin JM, Reed CE, Delinger CE. Utility of restaging endoscopic ultrasound after neoadjuvant therapy for esophageal cancer. *Ann Thorac Surg*. 2012;93(6):1855-1859.

57. Chen J, Xu R, Hunt GC, et al. Influence of the number of malignant regional lymph nodes detected by endoscopic ultrasonography on survival stratification in esophageal adenocarcinoma. *Clin Gastroenterol Hepatol*. 2006;4(5):573-579.

9

EUS in the Evaluation of Posterior Mediastinal Lesions

Thomas J. Savides

Key Points

- Criteria exist to differentiate benign from malignant mediastinal lymph nodes, but used alone these criteria are not sufficiently accurate. EUS-guided fine-needle aspiration is required to make sound clinical decisions.
- The overall accuracy for the diagnosis of posterior mediastinal malignancies with transesophageal EUS FNA is greater than 90%.
- The diagnosis of lymphoma in the posterior mediastinum is made by cytology and flow cytometry studies on EUS FNA specimens.
- EUS FNA can be valuable in helping to establish a diagnosis of granulomatous disease involving the mediastinum (sarcoidosis, histoplasmosis, tuberculosis).
- Most mediastinal cysts are benign, and because the risk of infection is high, EUS FNA should not be performed. If a high suspicion of malignancy exists, the cyst should undergo one puncture and be fully drained, and antibiotics should be administered.

Transesophageal endoscopic ultrasonography (EUS) with fine-needle aspiration (FNA) offers a unique ability for the evaluation and biopsy of posterior mediastinal lesions.[1] Usually these lesions are first detected with computed tomography (CT), but occasionally lesions are detected during passage of the echoendoscope through the esophagus on the way to image gastrointestinal or pancreatic disease. Transesophageal EUS is well suited to image the posterior mediastinum, but it cannot visualize the middle or anterior mediastinum. This chapter focuses on EUS diagnosis of posterior mediastinal masses, lymph nodes, and cysts. The role of EUS FNA in lung cancer staging is discussed in Chapter 7.

EUS Evaluation of Enlarged Posterior Mediastinal Lymph Nodes

EUS Appearance of Benign Posterior Mediastinal Lymph Nodes

Mediastinal lymph nodes are commonly encountered during EUS for nonthoracic indications. The most common EUS feature of these benign lymph nodes is a triangular or crescent shape, with possibly an echogenic center (Figure 9-1). The echogenic center represents the hilum of the lymph node. Intranodal blood vessels also suggest benign lymph nodes.[2,3]

The prevalence of posterior mediastinal adenopathy varies with geographic region of the world, depending on the risk of endemic pulmonary infections. The prevalence of benign posterior mediastinal adenopathy in a study from Indianapolis that evaluated patients undergoing EUS for nonthoracic indications was 86%, with an average of 3.6 periesophageal lymph nodes per patient.[4] These lymph nodes had mean short-axis and long-axis diameters of 5 and 10 mm, respectively. The high prevalence of lymph nodes in this study may be explained by the high rate of respiratory histoplasmosis in the state of Indiana. In contrast, a prospective study from England and Sweden revealed that only 62% of patients had posterior mediastinal lymph nodes, with a mean of 1.4 lymph nodes per patient. Nearly all of these lymph nodes had a short-axis diameter of 5 mm or less.[5]

EUS Appearance of Malignant Posterior Mediastinal Lymph Nodes

EUS findings associated with malignant lymph nodes include round shape, short-axis diameter greater than 5 mm, hypoechoic echotexture, and well-demarcated borders (Figure 9-2).[4,6] If all four features are present in a lymph node, the chance of malignancy is 80% to 100%.[6,7] However, all four features are seen in only 25% of malignant lymph nodes.[6] For this reason, tissue sampling is important to obtain diagnostic cytopathologic material of enlarged mediastinal lymph nodes.

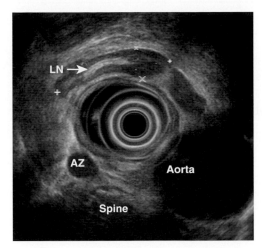

FIGURE 9-1 Benign mediastinal lymph node. Note the triangular appearance with a central hyperechoic stripe. AZ, azygos vein; LN, lymph node.

Elastography has been reported in the evaluation of mediastinal lymph nodes and masses.[8] However, the sensitivity and specificity (in the range of 80% to 90%) of this technique are lower than those of transesophageal or transbronchial EUS-guided FNA (>90% range). Therefore elastography needs further assessment and improvement before widespread use of this method can be recommended.

Transesophageal EUS Fine-Needle Aspiration of Mediastinal Lymph Nodes

The first report of EUS-assisted FNA of mediastinal lymph nodes was in 1992 at Indiana University Medical Center.[9] A diagnostic radial EUS endoscope was used to mark the site on the esophageal wall adjacent to a mass lesion, followed by FNA using a sclerotherapy needle through a standard forward-viewing endoscope.[9] The first use of a dedicated linear array echoendoscope to perform transesophageal EUS FNA of posterior mediastinal lymph nodes was reported in

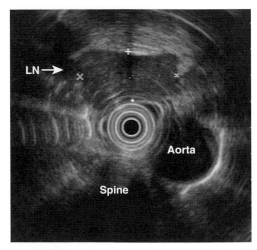

FIGURE 9-2 Malignant-appearing lymph node (LN). Note the round shape, well-demarcated border, hypoechoic echo pattern, and size larger than 5 mm.

TABLE 9-1

POSTERIOR MEDIASTINAL LESIONS THAT CAN BE DIAGNOSED WITH EUS FINE-NEEDLE ASPIRATION

Malignant	Benign
Lung cancer	Reactive
Primary or metastatic	Granulomatous disease
Non–small-cell (NSCLC)	Histoplasmosis
Small-cell	Sarcoid
Mesothelioma	Tuberculosis
Lymphoma	Duplication cyst
Metastatic from nonlung primary	Leiomyoma
Gastrointestinal stromal tumor	Mediastinitis/
(GIST)	abscess
Spindle cell neoplasm	Pleural effusion

1993.[10] Table 9-1 shows the types of pathologic lesions that can be diagnosed with transesophageal EUS FNA cytology.

Technique for EUS Fine-Needle Aspiration of Posterior Mediastinal Lesions

Transesophageal EUS FNA is generally performed as an outpatient procedure. Patients are asked to stop taking antiplatelet medications, nonsteroidal anti-inflammatory drugs, and warfarin before the procedure. Patients usually receive intravenous moderate sedation using meperidine and midazolam. EUS can be performed first using a radial echoendoscope to identify lesions, followed by a linear array echoendoscope to perform the FNA, or directly with the linear array scope to find and biopsy a lesion based on prior CT findings. The echoendoscope is passed through the patient's mouth and into the stomach, and then ultrasound imaging is performed as the scope is withdrawn. The liver, celiac axis, left adrenal gland, and posterior mediastinum are evaluated for lesions.

The location of each lesion is documented in terms of the distance in centimeters of the transducer tip from the incisors and the anatomic site (e.g., subcarinal, left paraesophageal, right paratracheal, posterior aortopulmonic window). For each lesion, the short-axis and long-axis dimensions are measured, and the degree of demarcation is described (well demarcated or poorly demarcated). The shape is described in terms of round, oval, triangular, or draping. The echogenicity is described in terms of hypoechoic, hyperechoic, heterogeneous, or anechoic.

Transesophageal EUS FNA is performed using a linear array echoendoscope and a 22- or 25-G aspiration needle. If there is more than one possible lesion to sample for biopsy, the lesion that is most likely to be malignant (i.e., rounder, larger, more demarcated) is chosen as the target.[11] If any question exists about whether the structure to undergo biopsy is vascular, color Doppler imaging can be used to assess for blood flow. Needle passage through an adjacent blood vessel can usually be avoided by displacing the esophagus with the scope tip to create a different needle path. However, in some reported cases, transaortic EUS FNA puncture with 22- and 25-G needles was successfully and safely used for biopsy of mediastinal lesions where the aorta was between the lesion and the esophagus.[12,13]

Once the lesion has been brought into view, the needle is passed through the esophageal wall and into the lymph node under constant ultrasound visualization. The internal stylet is then removed, intermittent suction is applied, and the needle is moved back and forth within the lesion to sample the edges as well as the center of the lesion. The needle is then pulled out of the scope, the stylet is slowly reintroduced into the needle, and the aspirated material is slowly expressed onto a microscope slide and into medium for cell block or flow cytometry.

In the United States, it is common for a cytotechnologist in the procedure room to prepare the slides using Quik-Dip stain (Mercedes Medical, Sarasota, FL). The cytopathologist then provides immediate cytologic evaluation of the slides under the microscope to determine whether there is adequate material on the slide for a preliminary diagnosis. The availability of immediate cytologic evaluation may increase the diagnostic yield.[14,15] If immediate cytologic evaluation raises the possibility of lymphoma, additional passes may be obtained for flow cytometry. If immediate cytologic evaluation suggests infection, additional passes may be made for microbiologic studies. A final diagnosis is provided only after the cytopathologist has evaluated all processed specimen slides and cell block material. In general, fewer EUS FNA passes are needed to obtain diagnostic material for posterior mediastinal lesions (on average approximately two to five passes for diagnostic material) in contrast to pancreatic masses, which usually require five to seven EUS FNA passes.[16–19]

EUS-guided core biopsy can also be performed in mediastinal lesions. The advantages of this technique are the acquisition of a core of tissue for pathologic evaluation, the potentially shorter procedure duration, and perhaps reduced cost when immediate cytologic evaluation is not used. However, the potential disadvantages are that the method can be technically difficult, core needles are more expensive than standard FNA needles, and patients have a potentially increased safety risk. The 19-G Tru-Cut FNA has been reported to increase the diagnostic yield in suspected lymphoma.[20] However, more recent studies suggest that the routine use of "rescue" endoscopic ultrasound-guided Tru-Cut biopsy following nondiagnostic EUS FNA using on-site cytology did not improve the diagnostic yield.[21]

Endobronchial Ultrasound

Endobronchial ultrasound (EBUS)-guided FNA has become increasingly widely available, especially as performed by interventional pulmonologists and thoracic surgeons.[22,23] EBUS provides unique access to lymph nodes and masses adjacent to the trachea, as well as the subcarinal and perihilar areas. The combination of transesophageal and transbronchial EUS provides nearly complete mediastinal evaluation.[24–26]

Accuracy of EUS Fine-Needle Aspiration for Diagnosing Posterior Mediastinal Lesions

The overall accuracy rate for diagnosing posterior mediastinal malignancy with transesophageal EUS FNA is approximately 93%.[11] A meta-analysis of 76 studies (n = 9310 patients) found a pooled sensitivity of 88% and specificity of 96%.[27] Table 9-2 shows a summary of the accuracy rates for EUS FNA for diagnosing malignancy in posterior mediastinal lesions. Several studies showed that the diagnostic accuracy of malignant posterior mediastinal lymph nodes increases with the use of EUS FNA cytology over simple EUS appearance alone.[27,28,41,42]

Risks of EUS Fine-Needle Aspiration of Posterior Mediastinal Lesions

EUS FNA of posterior mediastinal lesions is extremely safe, with few complications reported in the thousands of patients described in retrospective and prospective trials. A pooled review of prospective studies revealed a 0.43% risk of

---

TABLE 9-2

SUMMARY OF STUDIES EVALUATING THE OPERATING CHARACTERISTICS OF EUS FINE-NEEDLE ASPIRATION FOR DIAGNOSING MALIGNANT POSTERIOR MEDIASTINAL LESIONS

Authors (year)	n	Sensitivity (%)	Specificity (%)	Accuracy (%)	PPV (%)	NPV (%)
Giovannini et al[28] (1995)	24	81	100	83	—	—
Silvestri et al[29] (1996)	27	89	100	—	—	—
Gress et al[30] (1997)	52	95	81	96	—	—
Hunerbein et al[31] (1998)	23	89	83	87	—	—
Serna et al[32] (1998)	21	86	100	—	—	—
Wiersema et al[33] (2001)	82	96	100	98	94	100
Fritscher-Ravens et al[34] (2000)	153	92	100	95	—	—
Wallace et al[35] (2001)	121	87	100	—	—	—
Devereaux et al[36] (2002)	49	—	—	94	—	—
Larsen et al[37] (2002)	79	92	100	94	100	80
Hernandez et al[38] (2004)	59	—	—	84	—	—
Savides and Perricone[39] (2004)	59	96%	100	98	100	97
Eloubedi et al[40] (2005)	104	93%	100	97	100	97
Overall	91	97	100	97	99	94

NPV, negative predictive value; PPV, positive predictive value.

complications with mediastinal EUS FNA, mostly pain, bleeding, and perforation.[43] However, several cases of mediastinitis have also been reported after transesophageal EUS FNA.[44–55] Although most of these cases have involved mediastinal cysts, some patients with solid lesions (nodes or masses) have also developed post-EUS FNA mediastinitis.

There has been a single case of esophageal wall seeding with tumor after EUS FNA of a posterior mediastinal malignant node from a primary gastric cancer.[56] This occurred in the setting of several passes using a large 19-G needle, which may have contributed to the seeding. A case of esophagomediastinal fistula formation after EUS FNA of a posterior mediastinal lymph node resulting from tuberculosis has also been reported.[57]

EUS Fine-Needle Aspiration Compared with Other Modalities for Evaluation and Biopsy of Posterior Mediastinal Lymph Nodes or Masses

The noninvasive imaging modalities commonly used to evaluate enlarged mediastinal lymph nodes are CT scan and positron emission tomography (PET) scan. These modalities have mostly been compared with EUS FNA in the setting of suspected lung cancer. Both EUS alone and EUS FNA have been shown to be more accurate than CT alone (using short-axis lymph node diameter >10 mm) for diagnosing malignant posterior mediastinal lymph nodes.[80,58]

PET scanning detects increased uptake of the glucose analog ^{18}F-2-deoxy-D-glucose. Increased uptake can occur both in malignancy and in inflammatory conditions. A meta-analysis comparing CT with PET scan for evaluation of mediastinal adenopathy in patients with lung cancer revealed that when the CT scan showed enlarged lymph nodes, the sensitivity of PET was 100%, but the specificity was only 78%, in contrast to no CT findings of lymph node enlargement (sensitivity of 82% and specificity of 93%).[59] The low specificity of PET scan implies that 22% of patients with PET-positive enlarged mediastinal lymph nodes actually do not have malignancy (false-positive PET scan). Therefore these PET-positive lymph nodes should undergo tissue biopsy if it is critical to be certain about the diagnosis of malignancy in the nodes.[59]

Several studies confirmed the poor specificity of PET compared with transesophageal EUS FNA.[42,58–60] One large study found that the EUS FNA positive predictive value of malignancy was 100% compared with 40% for PET.[42] One report noted an EUS FNA diagnosis of malignancy in an enlarged posterior mediastinal lymph node that had a false-negative PET scan result.[61] The combination of PET and EUS FNA can help improve the specificity and overall accuracy as compared with PET alone.[62,63]

The other modalities for obtaining tissue samples from posterior mediastinal lesions are percutaneous CT-guided transthoracic FNA, bronchoscopy with transbronchial biopsy, EBUS with transbronchial FNA, and mediastinoscopy with biopsy. Percutaneous transthoracic FNA is generally not used for biopsy of posterior mediastinal lesions because of the risk of pneumothorax or puncture of a major vessel. The diagnostic yield of transbronchial FNA without EBUS is lower than that of EUS FNA, whereas EBUS has a similar diagnostic yield in the biopsying of adenopathy locations visualized by both transesophageal EUS and EBUS.[25] Mediastinoscopy is associated with greater difficulty (and potentially increased risk) in accessing the lymph nodes in stations that are the most easily visualized and biopsied with transesophageal EUS FNA (subcarina, posterior aortopulmonic window, and periesophageal stations). Therefore the less invasive EUS FNA and EBUS FNA are increasingly replacing mediastinoscopy at most referral centers.

Differential Diagnosis of Enlarged Posterior Mediastinal Lymph Nodes

Enlarged mediastinal lymph nodes are usually defined by CT findings of lymph nodes 10 mm diameter or larger. In the setting of a peripheral lung mass and mediastinal lymph nodes, the main concern is primary lung cancer with metastatic disease. The finding of numerous posterior mediastinal and hilar lymph nodes raises the question of whether the diagnosis is benign (sarcoid, histoplasmosis, tuberculosis, reactive) or malignant (especially lymphoma). Often the clinical history suggests the origin.

Malignant Posterior Mediastinal Lymph Nodes

The rate of diagnosis of malignancy with EUS FNA of posterior mediastinal nodes in patients without a known diagnosis of cancer varies depending on prior bronchoscopic evaluation and local referral patterns; however, it is approximately 50%, and most cancers are of pulmonary origin.[36,41,64] Table 9-2 shows the reported operating characteristics of EUS FNA for diagnosing malignancy in posterior mediastinal adenopathy. The overall sensitivity, specificity, and accuracy are greater than 90%.

Metastatic Disease from Thoracic Tumors

Lung Cancer

Most thoracic tumors originate as primary lung cancer. This disease is generally divided into small-cell and non–small-cell lung cancer (NSCLC) pathologic types, and 80% of lung cancer is NSCLC. EUS FNA cytology can diagnose and stage metastatic lung cancer to mediastinal lymph nodes from both small-cell carcinoma and NSCLC.[11,28] Further discussion of EUS FNA for lung cancer staging is discussed in detail in Chapter 7.

Mesothelioma

Mesothelioma is a much rarer pleura-based tumor of the thoracic cavity associated with asbestos exposure. EUS FNA can diagnose mesothelioma metastases in posterior mediastinal lymph nodes.[65–67] The combination of transbronchial EBUS FNA and transesophageal EUS FNA may increase the sensitivity of diagnosed metastatic mesothelioma, especially because mesothelioma can also metastasize or directly extend below the diaphragm into the abdominal cavity, where EUS FNA can detect metastases.[68]

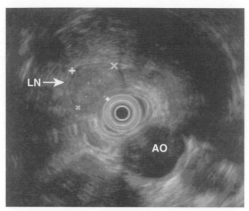

FIGURE 9-3 EUS of renal cell carcinoma metastatic to the mediastinum. AO, aorta; LN, lymph node.

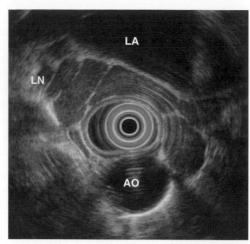

FIGURE 9-4 EUS image of presumed sarcoid lymph node (LN). Note that several lymph nodes are adjacent to each other. AO, aorta; LA, left atrium.

Metastatic Disease from Extrathoracic Malignancy

Various tumors result in metastases to the posterior mediastinum, and they appear as either a lymph node or a mass (Figure 9-3). Metastatic lymph nodes from breast, colon, renal, testicular, laryngeal, pancreas, and esophageal cancers have been diagnosed by transthoracic EUS FNA.[38,69–71]

Lymphoma

EUS FNA can diagnose lymphoma in posterior mediastinal lymph nodes by obtaining material that can be evaluated with cytology, flow cytometry, and immunohistochemistry. In one study, the sensitivity of lymphoma diagnosis increased from 44% to 86% with the addition of flow cytometry and immunocytochemistry.[72] Sometimes it can be difficult to obtain large quantities of adequate material during transesophageal EUS FNA to diagnose lymphoma, and therefore more needle passes may be needed than for NSCLC. Tru-Cut needle biopsies may provide additional material for architectural evaluation of low-grade lymphomas.[20,73]

Benign Posterior Mediastinal Lymph Nodes

Reactive Lymph Nodes

Reactive lymph nodes are usually the result of previous pulmonary infections. Cytologically, they appear as a mixture of lymphoid elements, with reactive and hyperplastic features.

Granulomatous Lymph Nodes

EUS FNA cytology is able to demonstrate granulomatous disease in lymph nodes. The cytologic appearance is that of histiocytes in a swirling pattern. The differential diagnosis usually includes sarcoid, histoplasmosis, tuberculosis, and coccidiomycosis. The presence or absence of caseating granulomas does not necessarily help with the diagnosis because caseation can be seen in all of the foregoing disorders. Sending EUS FNA cytology material for fungal stains and culture, acid-fast bacillus stain, and mycobacterial culture can help to determine whether the cause is infectious. Lymphoma is also rarely associated with granulomas.

Sarcoid

Sarcoid is a multisystemic granulomatous disease of unknown origin. It typically involves mediastinal lymph nodes. The final diagnosis is made by using clinical criteria and by excluding other causes of granulomatous disease. No pathognomic laboratory or pathologic finding exists for this disease. Elevated serum angiotensin-converting enzyme levels may suggest this diagnosis. The diagnosis of noncaseating granulomas in a mediastinal lymph node supports the diagnosis of sarcoid.

The usual endosonographic appearance of posterior mediastinal sarcoid is the presence of numerous enlarged lymph nodes (Figure 9-4). EUS FNA can obtain granulomatous material to support the diagnosis of sarcoid with a high degree of accuracy (Table 9-3).[74–78] One retrospective study found the sensitivity and specificity of EUS FNA for diagnosing granulomas in suspected sarcoid to be 89% and 96%, respectively.[79] Another study found that EUS FNA demonstrated noncaseating granulomas in 41 of 50 patients (82%) with a final clinical diagnosis of sarcoidosis.[76] A study of patients with bilateral hilar lymphadenopathy, in whom EUS FNA was performed with a 19-G needle and whose material was sent for both cytologic and histopathologic examination, found

TABLE 9-3

DIAGNOSTIC ACCURACY OF EUS FINE-NEEDLE ASPIRATION FOR SARCOIDOSIS

Authors (year)	n	Sensitivity (%)	Specificity (%)
Fritscher-Ravens et al[75] (2000)	19	100	94
Wildi et al[79] (2004)	28	89	96
Annema et al[76] (2005)	50	82	—
Overall		90	95

that 94% of the histopathology specimens had noncaseating granulomas, compared with 79% of the cytology specimens (P = 0.04).[52] Recent studies suggest that sarcoid lymph nodes aspirated via the transesophageal route may be at increased risk for mediastinitis (albeit rare) compared to EBUS FNA.[54,55] EBUS FNA has been shown to be superior to blind transbronchial FNA in the diagnosis of sarcoid.[80,81]

Histoplasmosis

Histoplasmosis is caused by infection with *Histoplasma capsulatum*. Within the United States, infection is most common in the midwestern states located in the Ohio and Mississippi River valleys. The diagnosis is typically made by histopathology, serologic testing, or antigen testing.[82] Histoplasmosis usually is suspected either because of pulmonary symptoms or because of incidentally found mediastinal adenopathy on CT scan.

EUS FNA can diagnose granulomas in patients with suspected histoplasmosis.[83,84] Histoplasmosis should be suspected in patients with enlarged posterior mediastinal lymph nodes and granulomas on EUS FNA, particularly if these patients have spent time in areas endemic for *Histoplasma* infection.

Histoplasmosis can also cause dysphagia resulting from compression of the esophagus by enlarged, fibrosing lymph nodes (Figure 9-5). The EUS appearance of mediastinal histoplasmosis that causes dysphagia includes the finding of a large mass of matted together, calcified lymph nodes that are adherent to a focally thickened esophageal wall.[84]

Tuberculosis

Mycobacterium tuberculosis can cause enlarged mediastinal lymph nodes, as well as a lymph node tuberculoma mass (Figure 9-6). EUS findings suggestive of tuberculosis in mediastinal lymph nodes include patchy anechoic/hypoechoic areas or hyperechoic foci.[85] EUS FNA can obtain material for *M. tuberculosis* culture.[36,75,85–88] Patients with granulomas identified on EUS FNA should have material submitted for mycobacterial culture. The addition of polymerase chain reaction testing for *M. tuberculosis* in samples obtained by EUS FNA

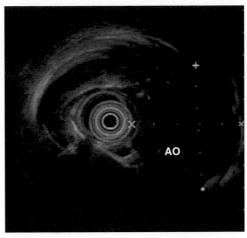

FIGURE 9-6 Posterior mediastinal tuberculoma. AO, aorta.

may help increase the diagnostic yield compared with cytologic study and culture in patients suspected to have tuberculosis.

Other Infections

EUS FNA has also been reported to diagnosis infection with *Coccidioides immitis*, *Mycobacterium kansasii*, and *Nocardia*.[89,90]

Eosinophilic Esophagitis

Eosinophilic esophagitis is an increasingly recognized condition of diffuse esophageal strictures resulting from eosinophilic inflammation that may lead to dysphagia in adults. EUS often reveals thickening of the esophageal wall. One report noted patients with enlarged periesophageal lymph nodes who underwent EUS FNA after steroid treatment of eosinophilic esophagitis.[91] Results of the procedure revealed eosinophilic infiltrate of the lymph node, a finding suggesting that enlarged eosinophilic mediastinal lymph nodes may occur in the setting of eosinophilic esophagitis.[91]

Impact of EUS Fine-Needle Aspiration of Mediastinal Lymph Nodes on Subsequent Thoracic Surgery Rates

One study found that among 59 patients with mediastinal adenopathy who were referred for surgical mediastinoscopy but instead underwent EUS FNA first, only 22% of them eventually needed thoracic surgery.[41] Based on initial CT scan findings, 42% of the patients who had a lung mass and mediastinal lymph nodes underwent surgery, compared with only 6% of patients with only mediastinal lymph nodes without an associated lung mass. The reason for this difference was that patients with lung masses and negative lymph nodes underwent surgical resection of the primary cancer, whereas those with only mediastinal adenopathy did not undergo surgery because either they had benign disease (i.e., sarcoid or reactive lymph nodes) or unresectable disease (i.e., lymphoma).

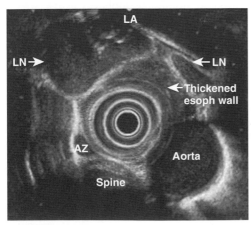

FIGURE 9-5 Lymph nodes (LN) in histoplasmosis. Note the matted together lymph nodes and calcification. AZ, azygos vein; esoph, esophageal; LA, left atrium.

Only 4% of patients with a positive EUS FNA result underwent subsequent surgery. These results are similar to those of other studies in which 38% to 41% of patients who underwent EUS FNA subsequently underwent thoracic surgery.[39,92]

Mediastinal Masses

The distinction between a posterior mediastinal mass and a lymph node can be difficult because some lymph nodes are very large, whereas some masses are extremely small. Additionally, numerous lymph nodes matted together can form a "lymph node mass" (Figure 9-7). Usually, a mass is larger than an enlarged lymph node (i.e., several centimeters in diameter), but no standardized terminology exists. Generally, when the term *mass* is used, there is only a single lesion, or one lesion that is significantly larger than adjacent lymph nodes. For the purpose of this section, only discrete, nonlymph node masses are discussed.

The differential diagnosis of a posterior mediastinal mass includes primary lung cancer extending into the posterior mediastinum, metastatic cancer (either primary lung cancer or nonthoracic cancer), neurogenic tumor, cyst, and infection. Transesophageal EUS FNA can easily sample large posterior mediastinal masses for biopsy.

Malignant Posterior Mediastinal Masses

Just as with mediastinal lymph nodes, approximately 50% of mediastinal masses that undergo EUS FNA are malignant.[38,69,93,94] Primary lung cancer masses that abut the esophagus can easily and safely undergo biopsy with transesophageal EUS FNA.[95,96] Mediastinal metastases from primary cancer of the lung, breast, colon, kidney, testicle, cervix, larynx, and esophagus have been diagnosed with transesophageal EUS FNA (see Figure 9-3).[38,69,95] EUS FNA has also been reported to diagnose cases of primary mediastinal plasmacytoma and mediastinal granular cell tumor.[97,98]

Neurogenic Tumors

Primary neoplasms of the posterior mediastinum are rare. Neurogenic tumors account for approximately 75% of

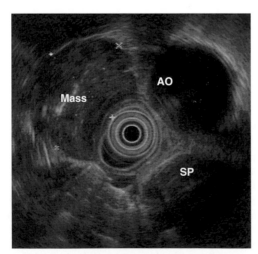

FIGURE 9-7 Mass of matted together lymph nodes. "Lymph node mass." *AO,* aorta; *SP,* spine.

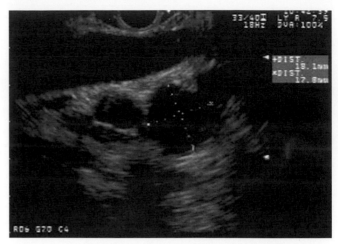

FIGURE 9-8 Posterior mediastinal schwannoma. Note the tumor located between the descending thoracic aorta and the spine.

these primary posterior mediastinal neoplasms.[99] Neurogenic tumors may arise from peripheral nerves (schwannoma, neurilemoma, neurofibroma, nerve-sheath tumors), sympathetic ganglia (ganglioneuroma, ganglioneuroblastoma, neuroblastoma), or parasympathetic ganglia (paraganglionoma).[59] These are usually benign tumors, but approximately 10% to 20% may be malignant.[100] EUS FNA cytologic examination can diagnose mediastinal schwannoma (Figure 9-8).[101,102]

Leiomyoma and Gastrointestinal Stromal Tumors

Gastrointestinal spindle cell tumors can arise from the muscularis propria of the esophagus and extend predominantly into the posterior mediastinum, rather than into the esophageal lumen. These tumors can have a CT and endoscopic appearance that more closely resembles that of a posterior mediastinal mass than an esophageal wall mass.[103–105] Esophageal spindle cell neoplasms are usually c-kit–negative leiomyomas, although occasionally they can be c-kit–positive gastrointestinal stromal tumors (GISTs).[103,104] These tumors have an EUS appearance of a hypoechoic mass with some internal signal and occasional acoustic enhancement, which sometimes makes them difficult to distinguish from cysts.[104] Because GISTs are highly metabolically active, they can often be diagnosed and followed with PET scans.[106] Although leiomyomas generally are PET-negative tumors, there have been reports of PET-positive esophageal or posterior mediastinal leiomyomas.[105] EUS FNA can be used to diagnose both posterior mediastinal leiomyomas and GISTs and can be considered when the distinction between a cyst and a GIST is uncertain.

Mesothelioma

Mesothelioma is a rare malignant tumor associated with asbestos exposure. This tumor is usually recognized as pleural thickening on CT, but sometimes the initial appearance is that of a mediastinal mass. The presence of metastatic lymphadenopathy is considered in the decision regarding surgical resection. EUS FNA has been used to diagnosis mesothelioma in both mediastinal masses and lymph nodes.[107,108]

Benign Posterior Mediastinal Masses

Benign causes of mediastinal "masses" that can be diagnosed with EUS FNA include histoplasmosis, sarcoidosis, leiomyoma, duplication cysts, and teratomas.[36] Tuberculosis can also appear as a tuberculoma mass (see Figure 9-6). A case of lymphangiohemangioma, a rare malformation of the lymphatic system, has been reported as a posterior mediastinal mass detected with EUS.[109]

Mediastinal Cysts

Congenital foregut cysts are the most common benign mediastinal cysts, and they account for 10% to 15% of mediastinal masses.[110-113] These cysts probably arise as a result of aberrant development of the primitive foregut. These foregut cysts may be categorized on the basis of the embryonic origin into bronchogenic or neuroenteric (esophageal duplication cysts and neuroenteric cysts). Esophageal duplication cysts are adherent to the esophagus, whereas those away from the esophageal wall are suggestive of bronchogenic cysts. The pathologic evaluation of duplication cysts reveals them to be typically lined by columnar epithelium.

Most patients with posterior mediastinal cysts are asymptomatic, and the cysts are discovered incidentally during other imaging studies. When symptoms occur, they can include chest pain, cough, dyspnea, and dysphagia. CT scan findings include well-defined, homogeneous lesions ranging in size from 2 to 10 cm. These cysts are nonenhancing with intravenous contrast. They can sometimes be mistaken for a mass based on CT findings. Surgical resection may be indicated in symptomatic patients. Because the risk of malignancy is so rare, incidentally found lesions can usually be followed clinically.

The EUS appearance of a mediastinal cyst is usually a round or tubular anechoic structure with acoustic enhancement (Figure 9-9).[114-117] Because it is usually difficult to determine whether the cyst is bronchogenic or esophageal in origin, the term *duplication cyst* is often used to describe the lesion. Some cysts appear to be mass lesions because of a more hypoechoic (rather than anechoic) echotexture and minimal acoustic enhancement. Sometimes these can be confused with esophageal leiomyomas or GISTs because of the heterogeneous hypoechoic appearance, and for this reason sometimes undergo EUS FNA. These mass-like cysts usually consist of thick, gelatinous cyst material.[46,48,117]

Mediastinal cysts can easily be aspirated with EUS FNA, but this is usually performed only when the EUS appearance is not compatible with a cyst and the lesion appears to be a possible mass.[44,48,114,117,118] Cytologic examination may reveal benign amorphous debris, degenerated cells, macrophages, needle-like crystals, mucinous material, or detached ciliary tufts.[109]

The risk of aspirating cystic mediastinal lesions was demonstrated by several reports of patients who developed mediastinitis after undergoing EUS FNA, including at least one patient who underwent Tru-Cut needle biopsy.[45,46,48,119] These patients required treatment with antibiotics, surgery, or endoscopic cyst drainage. None of the patients with reported bacterial mediastinitis after EUS FNA had received preprocedure or intraprocedure antibiotics. This situation raises the possibility that mediastinitis after EUS FNA of cysts may be prevented or minimized by the use of preprocedure or intraprocedure antibiotics. One series in which 22 patients underwent EUS FNA of posterior mediastinal cysts with 22-G needles and received intravenous ciprofloxacin followed by 5 days of oral ciprofloxacin reported no cases of mediastinitis.[120] This finding suggests that periprocedure antibiotics may prevent infection or mediastinitis when FNA of a cyst is performed.[120]

Despite the use of preprocedure antibiotics, in one reported case, EUS FNA of a duplication cyst resulted in *Candida albicans* infection of the cyst.[44] A 5-cm paratracheal cyst was aspirated, and gelatinous material was obtained. The patient subsequently underwent surgical resection, and culture grew *C. albicans*, which was not present on the original EUS FNA. This organism was believed to have been introduced at the time of EUS FNA. The patient, who had been administered prophylactic antibiotics, did not develop mediastinitis. However, this finding again emphasizes the possible infectious risks in mediastinal cysts even with prophylactic antibiotics.

Because of these reports of mediastinitis after aspirating posterior mediastinal duplication cysts, and given the benign nature of these cysts, any obvious posterior mediastinal duplication cyst should not be aspirated with EUS FNA. If there is a question that the lesion may be a cyst versus a malignant tumor, then the safest next diagnostic test may be thoracic magnetic resonance imaging or CT or PET scan to confirm the presence of a cyst and to exclude malignancy.[48] If EUS FNA is performed, a smaller gauge (i.e., 25-G) needle ideally should be used to minimize introduction of infection into the cyst. If the lesion turns out to be a cyst (i.e., mucinous fluid), then the cyst should be completely drained if possible, and prophylactic antibiotics should be administered. A typical approach is to administer intravenous antibiotics during the procedure and oral antibiotics for the next 3 to 5 days afterward to minimize any risk of mediastinitis.[120] EUS-guided 19-G Tru-Cut needle biopsies should be avoided in suspected posterior mediastinal cysts because of the even higher risk of mediastinitis reported with the use of these larger needles.

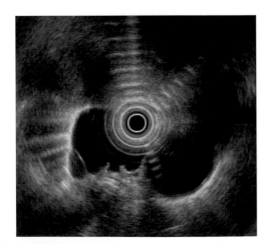

FIGURE 9-9 Mediastinal duplication cyst. Note the acoustic enhancement of the ultrasound signal.

Mediastinal Abscess and Mediastinitis

Acute mediastinitis and abscess occur most commonly after thoracic surgery or esophageal perforation. Patients generally have symptoms of sepsis. CT scan may show mediastinal fluid collections. Fritscher-Ravens and colleagues reported a series of 18 critically ill patients with clinical mediastinitis (mostly after thoracic surgery) who underwent EUS FNA.[88] The EUS appearance of the abscesses were 2-4 cm, inhomogeneous, well-demarcated hypoechoic areas. Some lesions had hyperechoic 2- to 3-mm spots with shadowing that were thought to represent air. EUS FNA revealed purulent material and bacterial organisms on microbiology culture. No apparent complications resulted from performing EUS FNA in the mediastinal abscesses. EUS FNA has also been reported to diagnose candidal mediastinitis.[121] There has been a case report of a mediastinal abscess drained by EUS FNA aspiration, followed by placement of a transesophageal pigtail stent.[122]

Pleural Effusions

EUS FNA can also sample pleural effusions that abut the esophagus. This is important in the staging of non–small-cell lung cancer as it upstages the patient to stage IV disease if positive for malignancy.[123]

Summary

EUS is a very safe and effective means of visualizing and characterizing posterior mediastinal lesions. EUS FNA allows the ability to biopsy posterior mediastinal lesions accurately and safely to determine malignancy. Because of the high rate of reported infectious complications after EUS FNA of mediastinal cysts, biopsy should be avoided if a cyst is suspected.

REFERENCES

1. Jue TL, Sharaf RN, Appalaneni V, et al. Role of EUS for the evaluation of mediastinal adenopathy. *Gastrointest Endosc.* 2011;74(2):239-245.
2. Sawhney MS, Debold SM, Kratzke RA, et al. Central intranodal blood vessel: a new EUS sign described in mediastinal lymph nodes. *Gastrointest Endosc.* 2007;65(4):602-608.
3. Hall JD, Kahaleh M, White GE, et al. Presence of lymph node vasculature: a new EUS criterion for benign nodes? *Dig Dis Sci.* 2009;54(1):118-121.
4. Wiersema MJ, Hassig WM, Hawes RH, Wonn MJ. Mediastinal lymph node detection with endosonography. *Gastrointest Endosc.* 1993;39(6):788-793.
5. Kalaitzakis E, Sadik R, Doig L, Meenan J. Defining the lymph node burden in a Northern European population without malignancy: the potential effect of geography in determining a need for FNA? *Dis Esophagus.* 2009;22(5):409-417.
6. Catalano MF, Sivak MV Jr, Rice T, et al. Endosonographic features predictive of lymph node metastasis. *Gastrointest Endosc.* 1994;40(4):442-446.
7. Bhutani MS, Hawes RH, Hoffman BJ. A comparison of the accuracy of echo features during endoscopic ultrasound (EUS) and EUS-guided fine-needle aspiration for diagnosis of malignant lymph node invasion. *Gastrointest Endosc.* 1997;45(6):474-479.
8. Janssen J, Dietrich CF, Will U, Greiner L. Endosonographic elastography in the diagnosis of mediastinal lymph nodes. *Endoscopy.* 2007;39(11):952-957.
9. Wiersema MJ, Hawes RH, Tao LC, et al. Endoscopic ultrasonography as an adjunct to fine needle aspiration cytology of the upper and lower gastrointestinal tract. *Gastrointest Endosc.* 1992;38(1):35-39.
10. Wiersema MJ, Kochman ML, Chak A, et al. Real-time endoscopic ultrasound-guided fine-needle aspiration of a mediastinal lymph node. *Gastrointest Endosc.* 1993;39(3):429-431.
11. Wallace MB, Fritscher-Ravens A, Savides TJ. Endoscopic ultrasound for the staging of non–small-cell lung cancer. *Endoscopy.* 2003;35(7):606-610.
12. Wallace MB, Woodward TA, Raimondo M, et al. Transaortic fine-needle aspiration of centrally located lung cancer under endoscopic ultrasound guidance: the final frontier. *Ann Thorac Surg.* 2007;84(3):1019-1021.
13. von Bartheld MB, Rabe KF, Annema JT. Transaortic EUS-guided FNA in the diagnosis of lung tumors and lymph nodes. *Gastrointest Endosc.* 2009;69(2):345-349.
14. Klapman JB, Logrono R, Dye CE, Waxman I. Clinical impact of on-site cytopathology interpretation on endoscopic ultrasound-guided fine needle aspiration. *Am J Gastroenterol.* 2003;98(6):1289-1294.
15. Tournoy KG, Praet MM, Van MG, Van Meerbeeck JP. Esophageal endoscopic ultrasound with fine-needle aspiration with an on-site cytopathologist: high accuracy for the diagnosis of mediastinal lymphadenopathy. *Chest.* 2005;128(4):3004-3009.
16. Emery SC, Savides TJ, Behling CA. Utility of immediate evaluation of endoscopic ultrasound-guided transesophageal fine needle aspiration of mediastinal lymph nodes. *Acta Cytol.* 2004;48(5):630-634.
17. LeBlanc JK, Ciaccia D, Al-Assi MT, et al. Optimal number of EUS-guided fine needle passes needed to obtain a correct diagnosis. *Gastrointest Endosc.* 2004;59(4):475-481.
18. Wallace MB, Kennedy T, Durkalski V, et al. Randomized controlled trial of EUS-guided fine needle aspiration techniques for the detection of malignant lymphadenopathy. *Gastrointest Endosc.* 2001;54(4):441-447.
19. Erickson RA, Sayage-Rabie L, Beissner RS. Factors predicting the number of EUS-guided fine-needle passes for diagnosis of pancreatic malignancies. *Gastrointest Endosc.* 2000;51(2):184-190.
20. Levy MJ, Wiersema MJ. EUS-guided Trucut biopsy. *Gastrointest Endosc.* 2005;62(3):417-426.
21. Cho CM, Al-Haddad M, Leblanc JK, et al. Rescue endoscopic ultrasound (EUS)-guided Trucut biopsy following suboptimal EUS-guided fine needle aspiration for mediastinal lesions. *Gut Liver.* 2013;7(2):150-156.
22. Herth FJ, Eberhardt R, Vilmann P, et al. Real-time endobronchial ultrasound guided transbronchial needle aspiration for sampling mediastinal lymph nodes. *Thorax.* 2006;61(9):795-798.
23. Gilbert S, Wilson DO, Christie NA, et al. Endobronchial ultrasound as a diagnostic tool in patients with mediastinal lymphadenopathy. *Ann Thorac Surg.* 2009;88(3):896-900, discussion 901-902.
24. Khoo KL, Ho KY, Nilsson B, Lim TK. EUS-guided FNA immediately after unrevealing transbronchial needle aspiration in the evaluation of mediastinal lymphadenopathy: a prospective study. *Gastrointest Endosc.* 2006;63(2):215-220.
25. Wallace MB, Pascual JM, Raimondo M, et al. Minimally invasive endoscopic staging of suspected lung cancer. *JAMA.* 2008;299(5):540-546.
26. Zhang R, Ying K, Shi L, et al. Combined endobronchial and endoscopic ultrasound-guided fine needle aspiration for mediastinal lymph node staging of lung cancer: a meta-analysis. *Eur J Cancer.* 2013;49(8):1860-1867.
27. Puli SR, Batapati Krishna Reddy J, Bechtold ML, et al. Endoscopic ultrasound: its accuracy in evaluating mediastinal lymphadenopathy? A meta-analysis and systematic review. *World J Gastroenterol.* 2008;14(19):3028-3037.
28. Giovannini M, Seitz JF, Monges G, et al. Fine-needle aspiration cytology guided by endoscopic ultrasonography: results in 141 patients. *Endoscopy.* 1995;27(2):171-177.
29. Silvestri GA, Hoffman BJ, Bhutani MS, et al. Endoscopic ultrasound with fine-needle aspiration in the diagnosis and staging of lung cancer. *Ann Thorac Surg.* 1996;61(5):1441-1445, discussion 1445-1446.
30. Gress FG, Savides TJ, Sandler A, et al. Endoscopic ultrasonography, fine-needle aspiration biopsy guided by endoscopic ultrasonography, and computed tomography in the preoperative staging of non–small-cell lung cancer: a comparison study. *Ann Intern Med.* 1997;127(8 Pt 1):604-612.
31. Hunerbein M, Ghadimi BM, Haensch W, Schlag PM. Transesophageal biopsy of mediastinal and pulmonary tumors by means of endoscopic ultrasound guidance. *J Thorac Cardiovasc Surg.* 1998;116(4):554-559.
32. Serna DL, Aryan HE, Chang KJ, et al. An early comparison between endoscopic ultrasound-guided fine-needle aspiration and

mediastinoscopy for diagnosis of mediastinal malignancy. *Am Surg.* 1998;64(10):1014-1018.

33. Wiersema MJ, Vazquez-Sequeiros E, Wiersema LM. Evaluation of mediastinal lymphadenopathy with endoscopic US-guided fine-needle aspiration biopsy. *Radiology.* 2001;219(1):252-257.

34. Fritscher-Ravens A, Sriram PV, Bobrowski C, et al. Mediastinal lymphadenopathy in patients with or without previous malignancy: EUS-FNA-based differential cytodiagnosis in 153 patients. *Am J Gastroenterol.* 2000;95(9):2278-2284.

35. Wallace MB, Silvestri GA, Sahai AV, et al. Endoscopic ultrasound-guided fine needle aspiration for staging patients with carcinoma of the lung. *Ann Thorac Surg.* 2001;72(6):1861-1867.

36. Devereaux BM, LeBlanc JK, Yousif E, et al. Clinical utility of EUS-guided fine-needle aspiration of mediastinal masses in the absence of known pulmonary malignancy. *Gastrointest Endosc.* 2002;56(3):397-401.

37. Larsen SS, Krasnik M, Vilmann P, et al. Endoscopic ultrasound guided biopsy of mediastinal lesions has a major impact on patient management. *Thorax.* 2002;57(2):98-103.

38. Hernandez LV, Mishra G, George S, Bhutani MS. A descriptive analysis of EUS-FNA for mediastinal lymphadenopathy: an emphasis on clinical impact and false negative results. *Am J Gastroenterol.* 2004;99(2):249-254.

39. Savides TJ, Perricone A. Impact of EUS-guided FNA of enlarged mediastinal lymph nodes on subsequent thoracic surgery rates. *Gastrointest Endosc.* 2004;60(3):340-346.

40. Eloubeidi MA, Cerfolio RJ, Chen VK, et al. Endoscopic ultrasound-guided fine needle aspiration of mediastinal lymph node in patients with suspected lung cancer after positron emission tomography and computed tomography scans. *Ann Thorac Surg.* 2005;79(1):263-268.

41. Vazquez-Sequeiros E, Wiersema MJ, Clain J, et al. Impact of lymph node staging on therapy of esophageal carcinoma. *Gastroenterology.* 2003;125(6):1626-1635.

42. Chen VK, Eloubeidi MA. Endoscopic ultrasound-guided fine needle aspiration is superior to lymph node echofeatures: a prospective evaluation of mediastinal and peri-intestinal lymphadenopathy. *Am J Gastroenterol.* 2004;99(4):628-633.

43. Wang KX, Ben QW, Jin ZD, et al. Assessment of morbidity and mortality associated with EUS-guided FNA: a systematic review. *Gastrointest Endosc.* 2011;73(2):283-290.

44. Ryan AG, Zamvar V, Roberts SA. Iatrogenic candidal infection of a mediastinal foregut cyst following endoscopic ultrasound-guided fine-needle aspiration. *Endoscopy.* 2002;34(10):838-839.

45. Annema JT, Veselic M, Versteegh MI, Rabe KF. Mediastinitis caused by EUS-FNA of a bronchogenic cyst. *Endoscopy.* 2003;35(9):791-793.

46. Wildi SM, Hoda RS, Fickling W, et al. Diagnosis of benign cysts of the mediastinum: the role and risks of EUS and FNA. *Gastrointest Endosc.* 2003;58(3):362-368.

47. Varadarajulu S, Fraig M, Schmulewitz N, et al. Comparison of EUS-guided 19-gauge Trucut needle biopsy with EUS-guided fine-needle aspiration. *Endoscopy.* 2004;36(5):397-401.

48. Westerterp M, van den Berg JG, van Lanschot JJ, Fockens P. Intramural bronchogenic cysts mimicking solid tumors. *Endoscopy.* 2004;36(12):1119-1122.

49. Pai KR, Page RD. Mediastinitis after EUS-guided FNA biopsy of a posterior mediastinal metastatic teratoma. *Gastrointest Endosc.* 2005;62(6):980-981.

50. Savides TJ, Margolis D, Richman KM, Singh V. *Gemella morbillorum* mediastinitis and osteomyelitis following transesophageal endoscopic ultrasound-guided fine-needle aspiration of a posterior mediastinal lymph node. *Endoscopy.* 2007;39(suppl 1):E123-E124.

51. Aerts JG, Kloover J, Los J, et al. EUS-FNA of enlarged necrotic lymph nodes may cause infectious mediastinitis. *J Thorac Oncol.* 2008;3(10):1191-1193.

52. Iwashita T, Yasuda I, Doi S, et al. The yield of endoscopic ultrasound-guided fine needle aspiration for histological diagnosis in patients suspected of stage I sarcoidosis. *Endoscopy.* 2008;40(5):400-405.

53. Diehl DL, Cheruvattath R, Facktor MA, Go BD. Infection after endoscopic ultrasound-guided aspiration of mediastinal cysts. *Interact Cardiovasc Thorac Surg.* 2010;10(2):338-340.

54. von Bartheld M, van der Heijden E, Annema J. Mediastinal abscess formation after EUS-guided FNA: are patients with sarcoidosis at increased risk? *Gastrointest Endosc.* 2012;75(5):1104-1107.

55. Allen BD, Penman I. Mediastinal abscess formation after EUS-guided FNA in patients with sarcoidosis. *Gastrointest Endosc.* 2012;76(5):1078-1079, author reply 1079.

56. Doi S, Yasuda I, Iwashita T, et al. Needle tract implantation on the esophageal wall after EUS-guided FNA of metastatic mediastinal lymphadenopathy. *Gastrointest Endosc.* 2008;67(6):988-990.

57. von Bartheld MB, van Kralingen KW, Veenendaal RA, et al. Mediastinal-esophageal fistulae after EUS-FNA of tuberculosis of the mediastinum. *Gastrointest Endosc.* 2010;71(1):210-212.

58. Fritscher-Ravens A, Bohuslavizki KH, Brandt L, et al. Mediastinal lymph node involvement in potentially resectable lung cancer: comparison of CT, positron emission tomography, and endoscopic ultrasonography with and without fine-needle aspiration. *Chest.* 2003;123(2):442-451.

59. Gould MK, Kuschner WG, Rydzak CE, et al. Test performance of positron emission tomography and computed tomography for mediastinal staging in patients with non–small-cell lung cancer: a meta-analysis. *Ann Intern Med.* 2003;139(11):879-892.

60. Fritscher-Ravens A, Davidson BL, Hauber HP, et al. Endoscopic ultrasound, positron emission tomography, and computerized tomography for lung cancer. *Am J Respir Crit Care Med.* 2003;168(11):1293-1297.

61. Rosenberg JM, Perricone A, Savides TJ. Endoscopic ultrasound/fine-needle aspiration diagnosis of a malignant subcarinal lymph node in a patient with lung cancer and a negative positron emission tomography scan. *Chest.* 2002;122(3):1091-1093.

62. Kalade AV, Eddie Lau WF, Conron M, et al. Endoscopic ultrasound-guided fine-needle aspiration when combined with positron emission tomography improves specificity and overall diagnostic accuracy in unexplained mediastinal lymphadenopathy and staging of non–small-cell lung cancer. *Intern Med J.* 2008;38(11):837-844.

63. Bataille L, Lonneux M, Weynand B, et al. EUS-FNA and FDG-PET are complementary procedures in the diagnosis of enlarged mediastinal lymph nodes. *Acta Gastroenterol Belg.* 2008;71(2):219-229.

64. Catalano MF, Nayar R, Gress F, et al. EUS-guided fine needle aspiration in mediastinal lymphadenopathy of unknown etiology. *Gastrointest Endosc.* 2002;55(7):863-869.

65. Kahi CJ, Dewitt JM, Lykens M, et al. Diagnosis of a malignant mesothelioma by EUS-guided FNA of a mediastinal lymph node. *Gastrointest Endosc.* 2004;60(5):859-861.

66. Bean SM, Eloubeidi MA, Cerfolio R, et al. Endoscopic ultrasound-guided fine needle aspiration is useful for nodal staging in patients with pleural mesothelioma. *Diagn Cytopathol.* 2008;36(1):32-37.

67. Tournoy KG, Burgers SA, Annema JT, et al. Transesophageal endoscopic ultrasound with fine needle aspiration in the preoperative staging of malignant pleural mesothelioma. *Clin Cancer Res.* 2008;14(19):6259-6263.

68. Rice DC, Steliga MA, Stewart J, et al. Endoscopic ultrasound-guided fine needle aspiration for staging of malignant pleural mesothelioma. *Ann Thorac Surg.* 2009;88(3):862-868, discussion 868-869.

69. Dewitt J, Ghorai S, Kahi C, et al. EUS-FNA of recurrent postoperative extraluminal and metastatic malignancy. *Gastrointest Endosc.* 2003;58(4):542-548.

70. Kramer H, Koeter GH, Sleijfer DT, et al. Endoscopic ultrasound-guided fine-needle aspiration in patients with mediastinal abnormalities and previous extrathoracic malignancy. *Eur J Cancer.* 2004;40(4):559-562.

71. Hahn M, Faigel DO. Frequency of mediastinal lymph node metastases in patients undergoing EUS evaluation of pancreaticobiliary masses. *Gastrointest Endosc.* 2001;54(3):331-335.

72. Ribeiro A, Vazquez-Sequeiros E, Wiersema LM, et al. EUS-guided fine-needle aspiration combined with flow cytometry and immunocytochemistry in the diagnosis of lymphoma. *Gastrointest Endosc.* 2001;53(4):485-491.

73. Levy MJ, Jondal ML, Clain J, Wiersema MJ. Preliminary experience with an EUS-guided trucut biopsy needle compared with EUS-guided FNA. *Gastrointest Endosc.* 2003;57(1):101-106.

74. Mishra G, Sahai AV, Penman ID, et al. Endoscopic ultrasonography with fine-needle aspiration: an accurate and simple diagnostic modality for sarcoidosis. *Endoscopy.* 1999;31(5):377-382.

75. Fritscher-Ravens A, Sriram PV, Topalidis T, et al. Diagnosing sarcoidosis using endosonography-guided fine-needle aspiration. *Chest.* 2000;118(4):928-935.

76. Annema JT, Veselic M, Rabe KF. Endoscopic ultrasound-guided fine-needle aspiration for the diagnosis of sarcoidosis. *Eur Respir J.* 2005;25(3):405-409.

77. Michael H, Ho S, Pollack B, et al. Diagnosis of intra-abdominal and mediastinal sarcoidosis with EUS-guided FNA. *Gastrointest Endosc.* 2008;67(1):28-34.

78. Cooke JR, Behling CA, Perricone A, Savides TJ. Using trans-esophageal endoscopic ultrasound-guided fine needle aspiration to diagnose sarcoidosis in patients with mediastinal lymphadenopahy. *Clin Pulm Med.* 2008;15(1):13-17.

79. Wildi SM, Judson MA, Fraig M, et al. Is endosonography guided fine needle aspiration (EUS-FNA) for sarcoidosis as good as we think? *Thorax.* 2004;59(9):794-799.

80. Tremblay A, Stather DR, Maceachern P, et al. A randomized controlled trial of standard versus endobronchial ultrasonography-guided transbronchial needle aspiration in patients with suspected sarcoidosis. *Chest.* 2009;136(2):340-346.

81. Tournoy KG, Bolly A, Aerts JG, et al. The value of endoscopic ultrasound after bronchoscopy to diagnose thoracic sarcoidosis. *Eur Respir J.* 2010;35(6):1329-1335.

82. Wheat LJ, Kohler RB, Tewari RP. Diagnosis of disseminated histoplasmosis by detection of *Histoplasma capsulatum* antigen in serum and urine specimens. *N Engl J Med.* 1986;314(2):83-88.

83. Wiersema MJ, Chak A, Wiersema LM. Mediastinal histoplasmosis: evaluation with endosonography and endoscopic fine-needle aspiration biopsy. *Gastrointest Endosc.* 1994;40(1):78-81.

84. Savides TJ, Gress FG, Wheat LJ, et al. Dysphagia due to mediastinal granulomas: diagnosis with endoscopic ultrasonography. *Gastroenterology.* 1995;109(2):366-373.

85. Rana SS, Bhasin DK, Srinivasan R, Singh K. Endoscopic ultrasound (EUS) features of mediastinal tubercular lymphadenopathy. *Hepatogastroenterology.* 2011;58(107-108):819-823.

86. Hainaut P, Monthe A, Lesage V, Weynand B. Tuberculous mediastinal lymphadenopathy. *Acta Clin Belg.* 1998;53(2):114-116.

87. Kramer H, Nieuwenhuis JA, Groen HJ, Wempe JB. Pulmonary tuberculosis diagnosed by esophageal endoscopic ultrasound with fine-needle aspiration. *Int J Tuberc Lung Dis.* 2004;8(2):272-273.

88. Fritscher-Ravens A, Schirrow L, Pothmann W, et al. Critical care transesophageal endosonography and guided fine-needle aspiration for diagnosis and management of posterior mediastinitis. *Crit Care Med.* 2003;31(1):126-132.

89. Chaya CT, Schnadig V, Gupta P, et al. Endoscopic ultrasound-guided fine-needle aspiration for diagnosis of an infectious mediastinal mass and/or lymphadenopathy. *Endoscopy.* 2006;38(suppl 2):E99-E101.

90. Naidu VG, Tammineni AK, Biscopink RJ, et al. *Coccidioides immitis* and *Mycobacterium tuberculosis* diagnosed by endoscopic ultrasound. *J S C Med Assoc.* 2009;105(1):4-7.

91. Bhutani MS, Moparty B, Chaya CT, et al. Endoscopic ultrasound-guided fine-needle aspiration of enlarged mediastinal lymph nodes in eosinophilic esophagitis. *Endoscopy.* 2007;39(suppl 1):E82-E83.

92. Srinivasan R, Bhutani MS, Thosani N, et al. Clinical impact of EUS-FNA of mediastinal lymph nodes in patients with known or suspected lung cancer or mediastinal lymph nodes of unknown etiology. *J Gastrointestin Liver Dis.* 2012;21(2):145-152.

93. Catalano MF, Rosenblatt ML, Chak A, et al. Endoscopic ultrasound-guided fine needle aspiration in the diagnosis of mediastinal masses of unknown origin. *Am J Gastroenterol.* 2002;97(10):2559-2565.

94. Panelli F, Erickson RA, Prasad VM. Evaluation of mediastinal masses by endoscopic ultrasound and endoscopic ultrasound-guided fine needle aspiration. *Am J Gastroenterol.* 2001;96(2):401-408.

95. Varadarajulu S, Hoffman BJ, Hawes RH, Eloubeidi MA. EUS-guided FNA of lung masses adjacent to or abutting the esophagus after unrevealing CT-guided biopsy or bronchoscopy. *Gastrointest Endosc.* 2004;60(2):293-297.

96. Vazquez-Sequeiros E, Levy MJ, Van Domselaar M, et al. Diagnostic yield and safety of endoscopic ultrasound guided fine needle aspiration of central mediastinal lung masses. *Diagn Ther Endosc.* 2013;2013:150492.

97. Mallo R, Gottlieb K, Waggoner D, Wittenkeller J. Mediastinal plasmacytoma detected by echocardiography and biopsied with EUS-FNA. *Echocardiography.* 2008;25(9):997-998.

98. Bean SM, Eloubeidi MA, Eltoum IA, et al. Preoperative diagnosis of a mediastinal granular cell tumor by EUS-FNA: a case report and review of the literature. *Cytojournal.* 2005;2(1):8.

99. Macchiarini P, Ostertag H. Uncommon primary mediastinal tumours. *Lancet Oncol.* 2004;5(2):107-118.

100. Reed JC, Hallet KK, Feigin DS. Neural tumors of the thorax: subject review from the AFIP. *Radiology.* 1978;126(1):9-17.

101. McGrath KM, Ballo MS, Jowell PS. Schwannoma of the mediastinum diagnosed by EUS-guided fine needle aspiration. *Gastrointest Endosc.* 2001;53(3):362-365.

102. Pakseresht K, Reddymasu SC, Oropeza-Vail MM, et al. Mediastinal schwannoma diagnosed by endoscopic ultrasonography-guided fine needle aspiration cytology. *Case Rep Gastroenterol.* 2011;5(2):411-415.

103. Lee JR, Anstadt MP, Khwaja S, Green LK. Gastrointestinal stromal tumor of the posterior mediastinum. *Eur J Cardiothorac Surg.* 2002;22(6):1014-1016.

104. Portale G, Zaninotto G, Costantini M, et al. Esophageal GIST: case report of surgical enucleation and update on current diagnostic and therapeutic options. *Int J Surg Pathol.* 2007;15(4):393-396.

105. Miyoshi K, Naito M, Ueno T, et al. Abnormal fluorine-18-fluorodeoxyglucose uptake in benign esophageal leiomyoma. *Gen Thorac Cardiovasc Surg.* 2009;57(11):629-632.

106. Van den Abbeele AD. The lessons of GIST—PET and PET/CT: a new paradigm for imaging. *Oncologist.* 2008;13(suppl 2):8-13.

107. Bakdounes K, Jhala N, Jhala D. Diagnostic usefulness and challenges in the diagnosis of mesothelioma by endoscopic ultrasound guided fine needle aspiration. *Diagn Cytopathol.* 2008;36(7):503-507.

108. Balderramo DC, Pellise M, Colomo L, et al. Diagnosis of pleural malignant mesothelioma by EUS-guided FNA (with video). *Gastrointest Endosc.* 2008;68(6):1191-1192, dicussion 1192-1193.

109. Tang SJ, Sreenarasimhaiah J, Tang L, et al. Endoscopic injection sclerotherapy with doxycycline for mediastinal and esophageal lymphangiohemangioma. *Gastrointest Endosc.* 2007;66(6):1196-1200.

110. Ribet ME, Copin MC, Gosselin B. Bronchogenic cysts of the mediastinum. *J Thorac Cardiovasc Surg.* 1995;109(5):1003-1010.

111. Strollo DC, Rosado-de-Christenson ML, Jett JR. Primary mediastinal tumors: part II. Tumors of the middle and posterior mediastinum. *Chest.* 1997;112(5):1344-1357.

112. Snyder ME, Luck SR, Hernandez R, et al. Diagnostic dilemmas of mediastinal cysts. *J Pediatr Surg.* 1985;20(6):810-815.

113. Sirivella S, Ford WB, Zikria EA, et al. Foregut cysts of the mediastinum. Results in 20 consecutive surgically treated cases. *J Thorac Cardiovasc Surg.* 1985;90(5):776-782.

114. Van Dam J, Rice TW, Sivak MV Jr. Endoscopic ultrasonography and endoscopically guided needle aspiration for the diagnosis of upper gastrointestinal tract foregut cysts. *Am J Gastroenterol.* 1992;87(6):762-765.

115. Geller A, Wang KK, DiMagno EP. Diagnosis of foregut duplication cysts by endoscopic ultrasonography. *Gastroenterology.* 1995;109(3):838-842.

116. Bhutani MS, Hoffman BJ, Reed C. Endosonographic diagnosis of an esophageal duplication cyst. *Endoscopy.* 1996;28(4):396-397.

117. Faigel DO, Burke A, Ginsberg GG, et al. The role of endoscopic ultrasound in the evaluation and management of foregut duplications. *Gastrointest Endosc.* 1997;45(1):99-103.

118. Eloubeidi MA, Cohn M, Cerfolio RJ, et al. Endoscopic ultrasound-guided fine-needle aspiration in the diagnosis of foregut duplication cysts: the value of demonstrating detached ciliary tufts in cyst fluid. *Cancer.* 2004;102(4):253-258.

119. Wiersema MJ, Vilmann P, Giovannini M, et al. Endosonography-guided fine-needle aspiration biopsy: diagnostic accuracy and complication assessment. *Gastroenterology.* 1997;112(4):1087-1095.

120. Fazel A, Moezardalan K, Varadarajulu S, et al. The utility and the safety of EUS-guided FNA in the evaluation of duplication cysts. *Gastrointest Endosc.* 2005;62(4):575-580.

121. Prasad VM, Erickson R, Contreras ED, Panelli F. Spontaneous candida mediastinitis diagnosed by endoscopic ultrasound-guided, fine-needle aspiration. *Am J Gastroenterol.* 2000;95(4):1072-1075.

122. Kahaleh M, Yoshida C, Kane L, Yeaton P. EUS drainage of a mediastinal abscess. *Gastrointest Endosc.* 2004;60(1):158-160.

123. Lococo F, Cesario A, Attili F, et al. Transoesophageal endoscopic ultrasound-guided fine-needle aspiration of pleural effusion for the staging of non–small-cell lung cancer. *Interact Cardiovasc Thorac Surg.* 2013.

SECTION III

Stomach

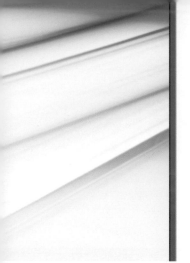

10

How to Perform EUS in the Stomach

Robert H. Hawes • Shyam Varadarajulu • Paul Fockens

The two basic techniques for examining the stomach are the balloon inflation procedure and the water-filled stomach method. Both methods can be employed with either the linear or the radial echoendoscope, but examination with the radial scope is easier and more efficient because of the larger viewing field. The balloon inflation method is preferred for rapid screening of submucosal lesions and for examination of perigastric structures (Figure 10-1). The water-filled method is best for examining the gastric wall layers and for careful and accurate evaluation of specific lesions (Figure 10-2). With the balloon inflation technique, the tip of the echoendoscope is advanced to the immediate prepyloric antrum. The balloon is fully inflated, and continuous suction is applied to remove air from the gastric lumen. When the gastric wall is completely collapsed around the balloon, the balloon is centered as well as possible, and slow withdrawal is performed (Video 10-1).

When one is learning EUS, it is critical that images are displayed in a standard orientation. In the case of gastric imaging, the liver is easily recognized and should be electronically rotated until it is positioned in the 9- to 12-o'clock space. This orientation will cause the pancreas to emerge at the 6-o'clock position on withdrawal, and the spleen and left kidney will appear between 12 and 4 o'clock. The examiner's eyes should then be fixed on both the gastric wall and the perigastric structures. If a lesion or abnormality is recognized, specific maneuvers can be applied to obtain detailed imaging.

With the water-filled method, the stomach is collapsed (removing all air), and 200 to 400 mL of fluid is instilled into the gastric lumen (see Figure 10-2; Video 10-2). High-quality imaging of the gastric wall requires attention to detail on two

Video 10-1. Video demonstrating the balloon-inflation method for examination of the stomach using a radial echoendoscope.

points: (1) the transducer must be positioned at a perpendicular angle to the gastric wall or a specific lesion (Video 10-3) and (2) the tip of the echoendoscope must be positioned within the focal zone of the transducer (see Chapter 1). This second point is absolutely critical when using the mechanical radial echoendoscope but is less important with electronic radial instruments. To obtain superfine images with the water-filled method, one should consider using an agent to paralyze peristalsis and instill water into the gastric lumen in a way that minimizes the production of microbubbles (slow infusion versus a water jet technique).

The difficulty or impossibility of obtaining perpendicular images in some areas presents a significant challenge in gastric endoscopic ultrasonography (EUS). An example is the gastric antrum. It may be impossible to adjust the tip deflection in a way that positions the transducer perpendicular to the antral wall while at the same time not pressing the transducer against

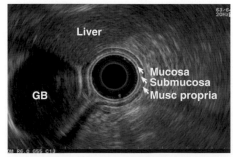

FIGURE 10-1 Balloon inflation method. Gastric wall layers as imaged using a radial echoendoscope. GB, gallbladder.

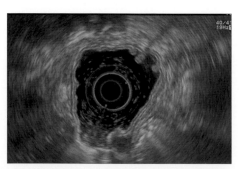

FIGURE 10-2 Water-filled method. With the radial echoendoscope positioned in the gastric lumen and the stomach filled with water, the individual layers of the gastric wall can be well visualized.

Video 10-2. Video demonstrating the water-filled method for examination of the stomach using a radial echoendoscope.

Video 10-4. EUS examination performed using a 20-MHz high-frequency mini-probe (water-filled method) revealing a T1 gastric cancer confined to the mucosal region.

the wall. The consequence of an inability to achieve optimal orientation between the transducer and the surface of the stomach is tangential imaging. If the ultrasound waves pass tangentially across the gastric wall, the layers will appear abnormally thick. This appearance can lead to overstaging of early gastric cancer or inaccurate determination of the layer of origin in submucosal masses. With large bulky tumors, in which one is trying to differentiate stage T3 from stage T4, this is less of an issue than with very superficial lesions in which one is trying to determine whether endoscopic mucosal resection (EMR) is appropriate. In the antrum, it is sometimes easier to use a dual-channel endoscope and a high-frequency catheter probe to achieve good positioning (Video 10-4; Figure 10-3). However, if the lesion is large, the depth of penetration of the catheter probe will be insufficient for accurate staging.

Summary

Two techniques are described for gastric imaging using standard echoendoscopes. Attention to proper technique is critical to accurate imaging. Evaluation of large lesions (>2 cm), global imaging of the stomach, and assessment of the perigastric space are best accomplished with standard echoendoscopes. Imaging of small lesions in which it is advantageous to obtain simultaneous endoscopic and ultrasound images is best accomplished with catheter probes in conjunction with dual-channel endoscopes.

Video 10-3. Radial EUS, performed after instillation of water, reveals a T1 gastric cancer confined to the mucosal layer.

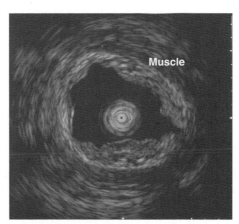

FIGURE 10-3 Imaging in the gastric antrum. Gastric wall layers as visualized using a high-frequency catheter probe with the water-filled technique.

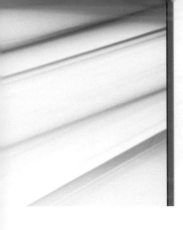

11

Subepithelial Lesions

Eun Young (Ann) Kim

Key Points

- EUS can accurately differentiate a mural lesion from extrinsic compression against the gut wall.
- Determination of the cause of an intramural lesion is based on its layer of origin and internal echo characteristics.
- The finding of an intact submucosal layer running deep into a mural lesion indicates that the lesion can be removed safely by endoscopic mucosal resection.
- Carcinoid tumors can usually be diagnosed with standard mucosal biopsies because these tumors emanate from the deep mucosal layer.
- Gastrointestinal stromal tumors can be differentiated from leiomyomas by immunohistochemical staining for CD117 (c-kit proto-oncogene protein product).

The term *submucosal lesion* is used by endoscopists to describe any bulge covered with normal mucosa, usually found incidentally during gastrointestinal (GI) endoscopy or barium contrast radiography. This lesion could be either an intramural mass or an impression caused by extramural structures. Recently, the term "subepithelial lesion" has been more frequently used than "submucosal lesion" because intramural lesions may arise from any layer of GI wall underneath the epithelium. In the past, the prevalence of suspected gastric submucosal lesions at routine endoscopy was reported to be as low as 0.36%.[1] More recently, however, the detection rate notably increased, especially with regard to small lesions, and the advances in technology and close attention paid to these lesions may be responsible for this augmentation.

To characterize the cause of protrusion, some noninvasive imaging methods, such as transabdominal ultrasonography, computed tomography (CT), and magnetic resonance imaging (MRI), have been used, but they are often insufficient. With endoscopic ultrasonography (EUS), however, the clinician can visualize the structure of gut wall layers clearly. Thus, EUS can not only differentiate subepithelial lesions from extramural structures but also identify the layers of origin and endosonographic characteristics of intraluminal lesions.[2-7] EUS is now accepted as the modality of choice for visualization of subepithelial lesions with high precision.

The differential diagnosis of subepithelial lesions includes a wide variety of benign and malignant subepithelial neoplasms, as well as non-neoplastic lesions (Video 11-1). To evaluate subepithelial lesions, the transition zone (the area where the tumor arises from normal gut wall layers) should be examined carefully to determine the layer of origin. Next, the size and echo pattern of the tumor, such as the smoothness of the border, internal features, echogenicity, and vascularity, should be observed. In addition, the relationship with other adjacent organs and the presence of adenopathy nearby provide valuable information. From the information gathered, an educated guess on the subepithelial tumor for the differential diagnosis can be made with reasonable accuracy (Table 11-1).[7] The reported accuracy of EUS in predicting the pathologic diagnosis of subepithelial lesions showed a wide range from 45.5% to 82.9% (Table 11-2).[8-13] If tissue was obtained from EUS-guided fine-needle aspiration (EUS FNA), the diagnostic accuracy increased markedly, ranging from 63% to 98%.[14,15] Detailed description comes later in this chapter.

Diagnostic information on the subepithelial lesions, including the origin of the wall layer provided by EUS, also helps in deciding whether a lesion should be removed or followed in situ.[16,17] Lesions confined to the mucosal or submucosal layers can be safely removed endoscopically. Surgical resection, if needed, is generally recommended for lesions located in muscularis propria, although advances in endoscopic techniques such as endoscopic submucosal dissection (ESD) have made it possible for these lesions to be removed by experienced clinicians with minimal risk to the patient.[18,19]

Comparison of Accuracy between EUS and Other Imaging Modalities

Differentiation of subepithelial lesions is one of the main indications for EUS. Compared with endoscopy, barium contrast radiography, ultrasonography, CT, and MRI, EUS has a higher accuracy in detecting and assessing the size and location of subepithelial lesions.[20] When viewed endoscopically, the surface of subepithelial lesions is usually smooth and has

TABLE 11-1

EUS CHARACTERISTICS OF VARIOUS SUBEPITHELIAL LESIONS

Cause	EUS Layers[a]	EUS Appearance
Gastrointestinal stromal tumor	Fourth (rarely second)	Hypoechoic (irregular borders, echogenic foci with mixed echogenicity; anechoic areas suggest malignancy)
Leiomyoma	Fourth, second	Hypoechoic
Aberrant pancreas	Second, third, and/or fourth	Hypoechoic or mixed echogenicity (anechoic ductal structure may be present)
Lipoma	Third	Hyperechoic
Carcinoid	Second and/or third	Mildly hypoechoic, homogeneous
Granular cell tumor	Second or third	Homogeneous hypoechoic mass with smooth borders
Cyst	Third	Anechoic, round or oval (three- or five-layer walls suggest duplication cyst)
Varices	Third	Anechoic, tubular, serpiginous
Inflammatory fibroid polyp	Second and/or third	Hypoechoic, homogeneous or mixed echogenicity, indistinct margin
Glomus tumor	Third or fourth	Hypoechoic, smooth margin, internal heterogeneous echo mixed with high echoic spots
Lymphoma	Second, third, and/or fourth	Hypoechoic
Metastatic deposits	Any or all	Hypoechoic, heterogeneous

[a]First layer, interface of luminal fluid and mucosa; second layer, deep mucosa; third layer, submucosa; fourth layer, muscularis propria; fifth layer, serosa or adventitia.

a color similar to that of the surrounding mucosa, without ulceration or erosion. Sometimes these lesions show a slight color change and certain morphologic characteristics, but it is often impossible to differentiate them by endoscopy alone. Ultrasonography provides diagnostic information only for very large subepithelial lesions. In a study of patients with endosonographically diagnosed gastric subepithelial lesions, 82.5% of tumors were visualized and measured by ultrasonography after the stomach was filled with water.[21] Like CT and MRI, ultrasonography can also provide useful information on perigastric structures. CT may be used to evaluate a subepithelial lesion especially when it is malignant and metastasis is suspected. However, a study pointed out that large submucosal tumors previously identified by EUS were visualized in only two thirds of cases from preoperative CT.[20] Reported mean sizes of possibly malignant subepithelial lesions detected and not detected by CT were 27.4 mm and 11 mm, respectively.[22] Currently high-quality images are available through multidetector computed tomography (MDCT). The diagnostic accuracy of MDCT is expected to be improved to even higher levels because MDCT can offer images from multiplanar and three-dimensional reconstructions. Overall accuracy of MDCT in detection and classification of subepithelial lesions from a recent study was 85.3% and 78.8%, respectively.[23]

In addition to detection, only EUS can establish the precise location of the lesion within the GI wall layer and provide information on the sonographic characteristics of the subepithelial tumor. The narrow differential diagnosis of subepithelial lesions afforded by the use of EUS improves decision making. Based on EUS, the clinician can decide between observation with re-examination in patients with suspected benign lesions or resection when the lesion is likely to be malignant.

In the differentiation between subepithelial lesions and extraluminal compression, EUS also demonstrates higher accuracy than endoscopy, ultrasonography, and CT. In a multicenter study, endoscopy was able to differentiate subepithelial lesions from extraluminal compressions with sensitivity and specificity of 87% and 29%, respectively.[24] In another study, ultrasonography and CT established the diagnosis in only 16% of cases, compared with 100% for EUS.[25] Another comparison of ultrasonography, CT, and EUS reported an accuracy of 22%, 28%, and 100%, respectively, in differentiating subepithelial tumors from extraluminal compression.[26]

Video 11-1. Video demonstrating the sonographic features of various subepithelial lesions.

TABLE 11-2

DIAGNOSTIC ACCURACY OF EUS FOR GASTROINTESTINAL SUBEPITHELIAL LESIONS

Authors (year)	Number of Patients	Accuracy (%)
Reddymasu et al[8] (2012)	37	49
Karaca et al[9] (2010)	22	45.5
Ji et al[10] (2008)	76	82.9
Kwon et al[11] (2005)	58	79.3
Kojima et al[12] (1999)	54	74
Matsui et al[13] (1998)	15	60

Extramural Lesions

Examination Checklist

Check the integrity of the five wall layers between the lesion and the gut lumen.

Because EUS is able to visualize the gut wall layers in detail, it can readily differentiate the intramural and extramural nature of subepithelial mass-like lesions. When EUS demonstrates the integrity of all gut wall layers between the gut lumen and the lesion, it is safe to say that the lesion is an impression caused by an extramural structure.

Although the extramural structures that compress the gut wall are on occasion pathologic masses, such findings are more likely to represent adjacent normal structures[24–27] (Table 11-3). A study revealed that when EUS evaluation was done for patients with suspected extraluminal compression or subepithelial lesions during endoscopy, 66.4% of them were proven to be extraluminal compression. It is worth noting that only 11% were due to pathologic lesions, and others were related to adjacent normal organs or vessels.[28]

A normal spleen usually makes an impression in the gastric fundus and upper body (Figure 11-1), and the gallbladder compresses the gastric antrum. Transient gastric impression is often caused by bowel loops. Other causes of gastric impression include vessels in the splenic hilum, the pancreatic tail, and the left lobe of the liver. Abnormal structures such as pancreatic pseudocysts, splenic artery aneurysm, aortic aneurysm, cystic tumor of the pancreas or liver, colonic tumors, and lymphoma may also produce endoscopically visible impressions on the gastric wall. Adjacent structures, such as the aortic arch and vertebrae, can also press on the esophagus. Other potential causes of esophageal impression are vascular anomalies, such as a right descending aortic arch, anomalous branches of the aortic arch, aneurysm, and left atrial dilation. Enlarged mediastinal lymph nodes or mediastinal tumors, lung cancer, and lymphomas are also known to compress the esophagus.

When using EUS, the suspected area of gastric impression should be observed by the two-step method. First, at a low frequency of 7.5 MHz, the examiner should survey the gross relationship between the extramural structure and the gut wall. Then, at a higher frequency of 12 MHz, the outer hyperechoic serosal layer should be observed carefully to determine whether it is intact or disrupted. This method allows reliable differentiation between gastric wall impression and gastric

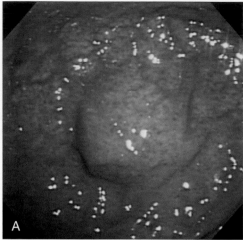

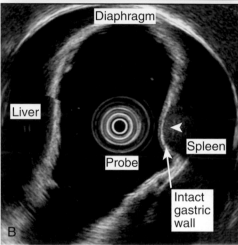

FIGURE 11-1 Extraluminal compression. **A**, Endoscopic image of gastric wall compression by normal spleen. An ill-defined, elevated area is seen at the gastric fundus. **B**, Endosonographic view of spleen *(arrow)* compressing the gastric wall.

wall infiltration caused by an extragastric tumor. For examination of small lesions, a high-frequency catheter ultrasound probe is technically easier to use than is a conventional echoendoscope. In the esophagus, the endosonographer may encounter difficulties in this evaluation owing to interference from the air-filled bronchial system.

Evaluation of Subepithelial Lesions

Examination Checklist

Carefully examine the transition zone between the normal gut wall and the lesion to determine the layer of origin.
Measure the size of the lesion and observe the echo pattern (e.g., echogenicity, internal features, vascularity, and smoothness of the border).
Check the presence of adjacent lymphadenopathy.
Small lesions measuring less than 1 to 2 cm may be better imaged using high-frequency catheter ultrasound probes.
For better imaging of the wall layers and evaluation of subepithelial lesions, it may be necessary to instill water or jelly into the luminal tract to obtain better acoustic coupling. Aspiration precautions should be taken under these circumstances.

TABLE 11-3

CAUSES OF EXTRALUMINAL COMPRESSION MIMICKING SUBEPITHELIAL LESION

Normal Organ	Pathologic Condition
Liver	Pancreatic cystic tumor
Spleen	Pancreatic pseudocyst
Blood vessel	Hepatic cyst
Gallbladder	Vascular anomaly including aneurysm
Pancreas	Lymphoma
Bowel loop	Colonic tumor
Vertebra	Mediastinal tumor or lymphadenopathy
Kidney	Lung cancer

Gastrointestinal Stromal Tumor

Diagnostic Checklist

Origin in second or fourth gastric wall layer.
Generally a well-circumscribed, hypoechoic, relatively homogeneous mass.
If malignant, noticeable characteristics include large size, features of heterogeneous echo texture with hyperechoic foci and/or anechoic necrotic zones, irregular extraluminal border, and adjacent malignant-looking lymphadenopathy.

Gastrointestinal stromal tumors (GISTs) are some of the most common mesenchymal tumors in the GI tract, and they are also the most commonly identified intramural subepithelial mass in the upper GI tract. Previously, these tumors were classified as GI smooth muscle tumors, such as leiomyomas and leiomyosarcomas, owing to histologic findings of circular palisades of spindle cells with prominent nuclei and apparent origin in the muscularis propria layer of the gut wall. However, with the development of newer molecular markers and an improved understanding of the biologic behavior of these tumors, GISTs are now classified as a distinct but heterogeneous group of mesenchymal tumors with varying differentiation. Interstitial cells of Cajal, also known as pacemaker cells of the GI tract, are now believed to be the precursor of GISTs that typically express c-kit proto-oncogene, a transmembrane tyrosine kinase receptor. With immunohistochemical staining techniques, most GISTs stain positive for CD117, epitope of kit protein, and, sometimes, CD34 but negative for desmin. Leiomyomas express smooth muscle actin and desmin, and schwannomas produce S-100 protein and neuron-specific enolase.[29]

According to the more recent classification, approximately 80% of GI mesenchymal tumors are GISTs, and approximately 10% to 30% of GISTs are malignant.[30] Leiomyomas are the most common mesenchymal tumors in the esophagus, but they rarely occur in the stomach and small bowel. In contrast, GISTs are rare in the esophagus and are more common in the stomach (60% to 70%) and small bowel (20% to 25%).[31]

The most common symptoms associated with GISTs are vague abdominal discomfort and pain, but most lesions are small (<2 cm) and asymptomatic. Larger lesions (>2 cm) may be ulcerated on top of the mass, and patients may present with bleeding or anemia. Occasionally, GISTs cause intestinal obstruction.

In defining the prognosis of patients with GIST, it has been recommended that a "grading as to the risk of aggressive behavior" be used instead of the term *benign*. This means that no GIST can be definitively labeled as benign, and all are considered to have some malignant potential. Pathologists classify GISTs as "very low risk," "low risk," "intermediate risk," and "high risk" according to the size of the mass and the mitotic count of the resected specimen.[32]

Endosonographically, a GIST is typically a well-circumscribed, hypoechoic, relatively homogeneous mass that can arise from either the second hypoechoic layer (muscularis mucosa) or more frequently the fourth hypoechoic layer (muscularis propria) (Figure 11-2). In contrast, leiomyomas (Figure 11-3) arise from muscularis mucosa more frequently than do GISTs. The images of GISTs, leiomyomas, and schwannomas are seen as relatively homogeneous hypoechoic masses under EUS and cannot be differentiated unless special immunohistochemical tissue staining is performed. One study suggested that GISTs have a marginal hypoechoic halo and relatively higher echogenicity compared with the adjacent muscular layer.[33] Another study added inhomogeneity and hyperechoic spots to the foregoing features, and the presence of at least two of these four features predicted GISTs with 89.1% sensitivity and 85.7% specificity.[34]

Several studies have attempted to predict the potential malignancy of GISTs based on the EUS characteristics of the lesion, but none of them obtained completely satisfying results. In addition to size and mucosal ulcer, other EUS characteristics were considered as possible predictive factors, but size was the only consistently definitive predictive factor.[34-37] EUS features mentioned by the authors were distorted shape, lobulation, irregular border, increased echogenicity in comparison with the surrounding muscle echo, inhomogeneity, hyperechoic posts, anechoic area, marginal halo, and extraluminal growth pattern. In one study, internal

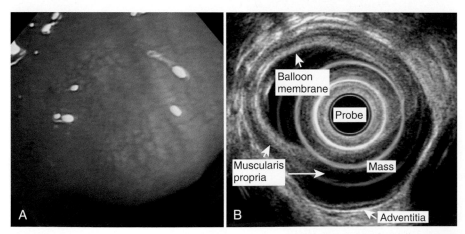

FIGURE 11-2 Esophageal benign gastrointestinal stromal tumor (GIST). **A,** Endoscopic finding of histologically proven esophageal benign GIST. **B,** Radial scanning EUS image showing a homogeneous, hypoechoic mass arising from the fourth sonographic layer, corresponding to the muscularis propria.

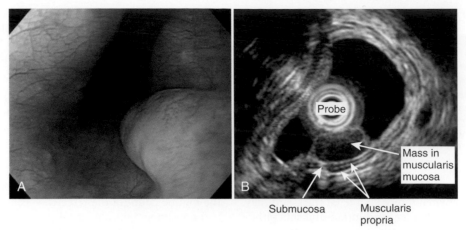

FIGURE 11-3 Esophageal leiomyoma. **A,** Endoscopic image shows an elongated submucosal lesion visible in the mid esophagus. **B,** Endosonographic view using a 20-MHz catheter probe. The lesion is homogeneous, hypoechoic, and associated with muscularis mucosa.

hypoechoic feature was suggested as a predictive marker of tumor progression.[36] When malignant changes occur, GISTs commonly show heterogeneous echo texture with hyperechoic deposits or anechoic necrotic zones inside large tumors (Figure 11-4). In one report, EUS findings of tumor size greater than 4 cm, an irregular extraluminal border, echogenic foci, and anechoic spaces were strong indicators of malignancy.[38] Sensitivity ranged between 80% and 100% in detecting malignancy when at least two of four features were present.[38] Another study found a correlation with malignancy when irregular extraluminal margins, cystic spaces, and lymph nodes were seen. The presence of two of these three features had a positive predictive value of 100% for malignant or borderline-malignant tumors.[39] Nonetheless, a lack of defined risk factors could not exclude a malignant potential. A multicenter study reported that malignancy or indeterminate GIST status correlated with the presence of ulceration, tumor size larger than 3 cm, irregular margins, and gastric location but not with hyperechoic or hypoechoic internal foci.[40]

Recently, contrast-enhanced harmonic EUS (CEH EUS) has been introduced. CEH EUS can demonstrate perfusion characteristics of subepithelial lesions, and it is helpful for establishing a differential diagnosis. The image of GIST is hyperenhanced after infusion of ultrasound contrast; in consequence, CEH EUS signal intensity of GIST is higher than other benign lesions.[41] In addition, another study reported that prediction of malignant GIST was possible with CEH EUS by identifying intratumoral irregular vessels with 83% accuracy.[42]

EUS-guided fine-needle aspiration (EUS FNA) and EUS-guided Tru-Cut biopsy (EUS TCB) can be performed for immunohistochemical examination to achieve better diagnostic accuracy of GIST (Table 11-4).[43–51] A major drawback of EUS FNA is its inability to differentiate with absolute certainty benign from malignant GISTs. However, staining for ki-67 (MIB-1), a marker of cell proliferation, may enable the discrimination of benign from malignant GIST with EUS FNA.[50,51] The role of EUS FNA is further described later in this chapter.

Because small (<1 cm), asymptomatic mesenchymal tumors are rarely malignant, a policy of close follow-up with EUS may be justified, although an optimal surveillance strategy has not yet been established. Excision is advised when

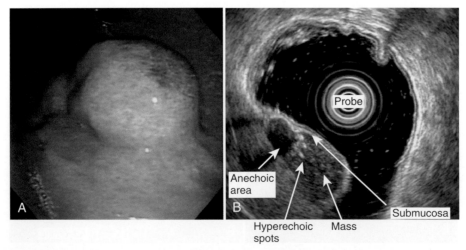

FIGURE 11-4 Malignant gastrointestinal stromal tumor (GIST) of the stomach. **A,** Endoscopy shows a submucosal mass in the body of the stomach. **B,** Radial scanning EUS image of histologically proven malignant GIST showing hyperechoic spots and an anechoic area. The mass is contiguous with the fourth sonographic layer.

TABLE 11-4

DIAGNOSTIC ACCURACY OF EUS-GUIDED FINE-NEEDLE ASPIRATION FOR GASTROINTESTINAL STROMAL TUMORS

Authors (year)	Number of Patients	Accuracy (%)	Diagnostic Method
DeWitt et al[43] (2011)	38	76	EUS FNA[a]
		79	EUS TCB[a]
Watson et al[44] (2011)	65	80	EUS FNA[b]
Fernandez et al[45] (2010)	40	70	EUS FNA[a]
		60	EUS TCB[a]
Sepe et al[46] (2009)	37	78	EUS FNA[b]
Chatzipantelis et al[47] (2008)	17	100	EUS FNA[b]
Akahoshi et al[48] (2007)	29	97	EUS FNA[b]
Mochizuki et al[49] (2006)	18	83	EUS FNA[b]
Okubo et al[50] (2004)	14	79	EUS FNA[c]
Ando et al[51] (2002)	23	91	EUS FNA[d]

EUS, endoscopic ultrasonography; FNA, fine-needle aspiration; GIST, gastrointestinal stromal tumor; TCB, fine-needle biopsy using a Tru-Cut needle.
[a]For diagnosis of gastrointestinal mesenchymal tumors.
[b]For diagnosis of GISTs.
[c]For differentiating between low-grade and high-grade malignancy of GISTs.
[d]For differentiating between benign and malignant GISTs.

growth of the lesion, a change in the echo pattern, or necrosis is noted during yearly follow-up with EUS. Surgical treatment is indicated for lesions greater than 3 cm in diameter with features suggestive of malignancy. For lesions between 1 and 3 cm, EUS FNA can be recommended, or ESD can be chosen as a definite diagnostic and therapeutic tool with some risk of bleeding and perforation (2% to 3% in specialized centers). When the lesion is confirmed to be a GIST, the risk of malignant transformation needs to be discussed with the patient; more careful follow-up or early resection should be considered.

Aberrant Pancreas

Diagnostic Checklist

Origin in the second, third, and/or fourth layers.
Hypoechoic or mixed echogenicity with internal anechoic ductal structure.

The term *aberrant pancreas* is used to describe ectopic pancreatic tissue lying outside its normal location with no anatomic or vascular connection to the pancreas proper. These lesions are also termed *ectopic pancreas, pancreatic rest,* and *heterotopic pancreas.* They are typically discovered incidentally during endoscopy, surgery, or autopsy. Aberrant pancreas is encountered in approximately 1 of every 500 operations performed in the upper abdomen, and the incidence in autopsy series has been estimated to be between 0.6% and 13.7%.[52] Aberrant pancreas is usually located in the stomach wall (frequently along the greater curvature of the antrum), duodenum, small intestine, or anywhere in the GI tract. Patients with aberrant pancreas are usually asymptomatic, but rare complications such as pancreatitis, cyst formation, ulceration, bleeding, gastric outlet obstruction, obstructive jaundice, and malignancy can occur.[53]

On endoscopy, an aberrant pancreas appears as a submucosal nodule, usually small, with a characteristic central umbilication that corresponds to a draining duct. The characteristic EUS features of aberrant pancreas are heterogeneous lesions, mainly hypoechoic or intermediate echogenic masses accompanied by scattered small hyperechoic areas, with indistinct margins within the gut wall (Figure 11-5). Generally, an anechoic area and fourth layer thickening accompany the lesions. Anechoic cystic or tubular structures within the lesion correlate with ductal structures. They commonly arise from the third and fourth layers.[54] However, lesions may develop in any location from the deep mucosal to the serosal layer.

The management of aberrant pancreas remains controversial. It should be guided by symptoms and the possibility of

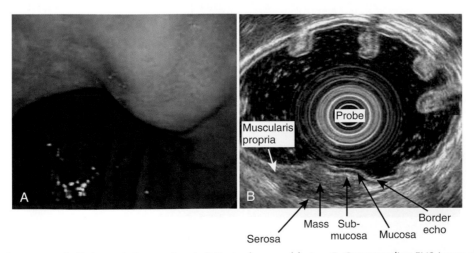

FIGURE 11-5 Aberrant pancreas. **A,** Endoscopic image of an indistinct submucosal lesion. **B,** Corresponding EUS image showing an ill-defined, slightly hypoechoic, inhomogeneous mass involving the third and fourth gastric layers.

malignancy. Asymptomatic lesions do not necessarily require resection and can be followed expectantly. If needed, endoscopic removal is useful for both accurate diagnosis and treatment, although surgical resection is preferred to endoscopic resection when the muscularis propria is involved.

Lipoma

> ### Diagnostic Checklist
>
> Origin in the third layer.
> Hyperechoic, homogeneous lesion with regular margins.

Lipomas are benign tumors composed of mature lipocytes. They are found incidentally in any part of the GI tract and more frequently in the lower tract. Lipomas are rarely symptomatic, but they may result in hemorrhage, abdominal pain, and intestinal obstruction.[55]

Endoscopically, most lipomas are solitary, with a smooth bulge and a yellow hue. They are soft and indented when pressed with biopsy forceps (pillow or cushion sign). On endosonography, lipomas characteristically appear as intensely hyperechoic, homogeneous lesions with clean regular margins arising from the third layer of the GI tract, which corresponds to the submucosa (Figure 11-6).[56,57] The endoscopic and endosonographic characteristics make it possible to diagnose lipoma in most cases. Once lipoma has been confirmed, follow-up EUS is not recommended. The incidentally found lipoma does not require treatment, but local excision is advised for symptomatic lipomas associated with bleeding or obstruction. Resection is also recommended when it is impossible to distinguish between a lipoma and a malignant neoplasm, such as a liposarcoma, even though this lesion is rare in the GI tract.[58]

Carcinoid Tumor

> ### Diagnostic Checklist
>
> Origin in the second layer.
> Homogeneous, well-demarcated, and mildly hypoechoic or
>   isoechoic lesion.

Carcinoid tumors are slow-growing neuroendocrine tumors with malignant potential. They may arise at various sites, most commonly the GI tract and lung. GI carcinoid tumors are generally discovered incidentally during endoscopy, surgery, or autopsy from the appendix, rectum, stomach, and small intestine. Rectal carcinoids are common and represent approximately 20% of all GI carcinoid lesions. Carcinoid tumors are usually asymptomatic, but rare complications include hemorrhage, abdominal pain, intestinal obstruction, and the endocrine carcinoid syndrome that results from secretion of functionally active substances.

Endoscopically, carcinoid tumors are small, round, sessile, or polypoid lesions with a smooth surface and a yellow hue. They usually have normal overlying mucosa and seldom ulcerate. Gastric and ileal carcinoids are commonly multiple, whereas those arising elsewhere are typically solitary. The endosonographic appearance of carcinoids is usually that of a homogeneous, well-demarcated, and mildly hypoechoic or isoechoic mass (Figure 11-7). These lesions arise from the second layer of the GI tract and may invade beyond the third submucosal layer.[59] Deep mucosal biopsy is normally diagnostic. EUS accurately defines the size and extent of masses and can guide management. When the lesion is smaller than 2 cm, does not invade further than the third layer, and no adenopathy is noted, endoscopic resection is possible.[12,60,61]

Granular Cell Tumor

> ### Diagnostic Checklist
>
> Origin in the second or third layer.
> Hypoechoic, homogeneous lesion with smooth margins.

Granular cell tumors (GCTs) are rare lesions of neural derivation, as supported by immunophenotypic and ultrastructural evidence. Granularity of tumor cells results from the accumulation of secondary lysosomes in the cytoplasm. Visceral involvement is encountered as mucosal or submucosal nodules anywhere in the GI tract, larynx, bronchi, gallbladder, and biliary tract. Approximately 2.7% to 8.1% of GCTs involve the digestive tract, and these tumors are multiple in approximately 5% to 12% of patients. GCTs are usually found incidentally during endoscopy or colonoscopy

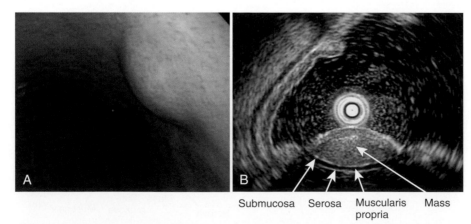

Submucosa   Serosa   Muscularis   Mass
                       propria

FIGURE 11-6   Gastric lipoma. **A,** Endoscopic view of a slightly elevated lesion covered with normal mucosa. **B,** Endosonography reveals a homogeneous, hyperechoic mass with smooth borders within the third gastric wall layer.

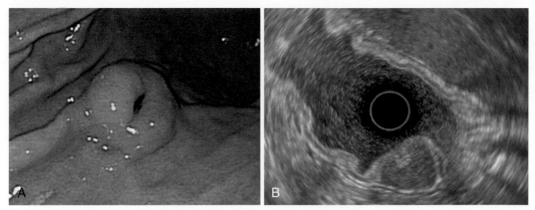

FIGURE 11-7 Gastric carcinoid tumor. **A,** Endoscopic image of a round, umbilicated, submucosal lesion in the gastric body. **B,** Endosonographic view of a homogeneous, hypoechoic, umbilicated mass within the second sonographic layer.

and are located mostly in the esophagus; other locations include the stomach (10%) and rarely the colon or rectum.[62] GCTs are generally considered benign, but in 2% to 3% of cases they are malignant.[63]

The endoscopic appearance of GCTs is that of small, isolated nodules or polyps resembling molar teeth, with normal overlying mucosa having a yellow hue. Most GCTs are small (<4 cm), but larger size is associated with malignant potential. At EUS, GCTs appear as hypoechoic, homogeneous lesions with smooth margins originating from the second or third layer of the GI tract (Figure 11-8).[64] One study using EUS examined 15 patients with 21 GCTs and found that tumor size was less than 2 cm in 95% of cases. In all patients, echo patterns were hypoechoic and solid. The tumors arose in the inner layers in 95% of cases (second layer, 15; third layer, 5).[65] The EUS pattern of leiomyoma originating from the muscularis mucosal layer can be similar to GCT. A study attempted to differentiate GCT from leiomyoma by using EUS characteristics. The authors suggested two differential EUS features: (1) although both lesions were hypoechoic, GCTs demonstrated slightly higher echogenicity compared to the surrounding normal muscle layer; and (2) the margins of GCT were less well-defined than leiomyoma.[66]

For asymptomatic GCTs that are not excised, surveillance EUS every 1 to 2 years is recommended to monitor changes in size. Local endoscopic snare excision can be performed for small tumors limited to the mucosa.

Cysts Including Duplication Cyst

Diagnostic Checklist

Origin in the third layer.
Anechoic, round, or oval lesion showing posterior acoustic enhancement (if the lesion has three- or five-layered walls, this suggests a duplication cyst).
Antibiotics are indicated for EUS FNA of a bronchogenic cyst.

Endosonographically, cysts in the GI tract appear as anechoic structures. But some may be seen as hypoechoic lesions containing echogenic foci.

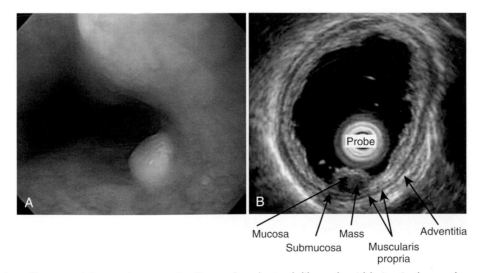

FIGURE 11-8 Granular cell tumor of the esophagus. **A,** Small, round, molar tooth-like, polypoid lesion in the esophagus. **B,** Endosonographic image acquired with a 20-MHz mini-probe shows the nine-layered structure of the esophageal wall. A homogeneous, hypoechoic lesion with smooth margins is noted within the fourth layer.

Cystic submucosal tumors may be classified into three EUS types:[67] simple cystic, multicystic, and solid cystic tumors. The simple cystic type is more frequent in occurrence and, rarely, Brunner's gland hamartomas or heterotopic gastric mucosa can resemble a simple cyst. The multicystic type is common in lymphangiomas, gastric cystic malformations, hemangiomas, and Brunner's gland hamartomas. The solid cystic type includes duplication cysts, heterotopic gastric mucosa, aberrant pancreas, myogenic tumors with advanced cystic degeneration, and gastric tuberculomas.

Gastric cyst is a rare clinical entity and is usually asymptomatic. It may result from a resolved inflammatory process. Endosonographically, the cysts appear in the submucosal layer of the gastric wall as sharply demarcated, anechoic, rounded, or ovoid structures with dorsal acoustic accentuation (Figure 11-9). The inflammatory cyst always shows a single hyperechoic wall layer.

In adults, foregut cysts usually are asymptomatic and are discovered incidentally during radiographic or endoscopic examination. Foregut cysts are categorized on the basis of their anomalous embryonic origin into bronchogenic and neuroenteric cysts. Bronchogenic cysts represent 50% to 60% of all mediastinal cysts,[68] and they can be diagnosed easily with EUS as anechoic mass without wall layers (Figure 11-10). But some lesions may be seen as a hypoechoic or solid mass. In these cases, EUS FNA would cause serious complications, including cyst infection and mediastinitis.[68] Therefore antibiotic prophylaxis is needed and close attention should be paid to avoid accidental instrumentation.

Duplication cysts may involve the entire GI tract, with the ileum being the most common site. The stomach is the least common site for GI duplication cysts. When examined endoscopically, duplication cysts may have a slightly transparent appearance. EUS or EUS FNA (with antibiotic prophylaxis) is useful and safe for the diagnosis of duplication cyst; some of these cysts are misdiagnosed as solid masses on CT or MRI.[69] Duplication cysts on endosonography appear as anechoic, homogeneous lesions with regular margins arising from the third layer or extrinsic to the GI wall. The walls of duplication cysts may be seen as three- or five-layer structures because of the presence of the submucosa and muscle layer.[70,71]

Duplication cysts are believed to have a low malignant potential, but case reports have described malignant transformation. Complications are rare and may include dysphagia, abdominal pain, bleeding, and pancreatitis when the cyst is located near the ampulla of Vater.

Varices

Diagnostic Checklist

Origin in the third layer.
Anechoic, tubular, serpiginous lesion.

Patients with portal hypertension may have varices. Gastric varices can be misdiagnosed endoscopically as submucosal tumors or thickened gastric folds. When varices are found incidentally during endoscopy in a patient with no relevant information, it is highly inappropriate and potentially hazardous to take a biopsy sample from such a lesion without EUS examination. On EUS, fundic varices appear as small, round to oval, and anechoic structures within the submucosa. They can be differentiated from submucosal cysts, which usually occur as solitary lesions, by their shape and easy compressibility using the ultrasound balloon. When gastric varices grow larger, they appear as anechoic, serpentine, tubular structures with smooth margins, accompanied by perigastric collateral vessels (Figure 11-11). In severe portal hypertension, cross sections of multiple fundic varices may show a "Swiss cheese" pattern.[72] Demonstration of flow with Doppler examination is a definite clue for diagnosis.

In portal hypertensive gastropathy, EUS findings are often normal, and endosonographic intramural vessel changes are usually not observed. However, dilation of the azygos vein and thoracic duct and thickening of the gastric mucosa and submucosa have also been reported.[73] In comparative studies, EUS was inferior to endoscopy for detecting and grading esophageal varices, but it permitted detection of fundic varices earlier and more often than endoscopy in patients with portal hypertension.[74] EUS was used in the treatment of varices by making it possible to inject a sclerosing agent into perforating

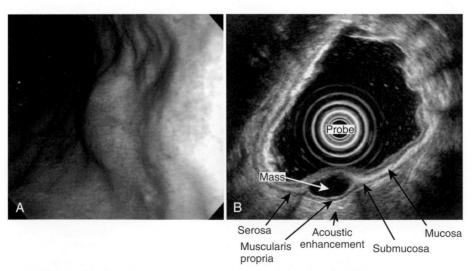

FIGURE 11-9 Gastric cyst. **A,** Endoscopic view of a smooth bulge in the body of the stomach. **B,** EUS revealed a sharply demarcated, anechoic, ovoid structure within the third gastric wall layer.

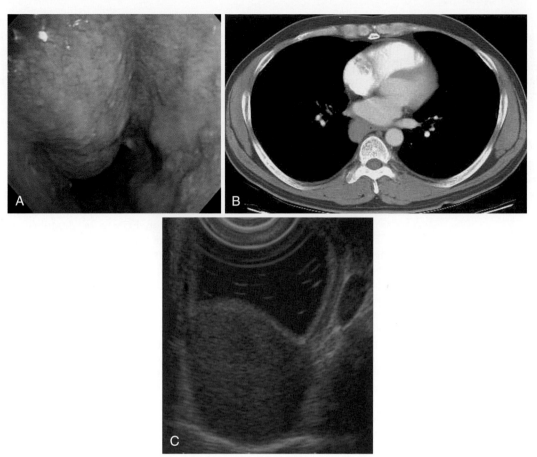

FIGURE 11-10 Bronchogenic cyst. **A**, Endoscopic view of a bulging mass lesion at the mid esophagus. **B**, The mass looks like a solid mass lesion on computed tomography. **C**, EUS demonstrated a round, homogeneous, hypoechoic lesion in the mediastinum.

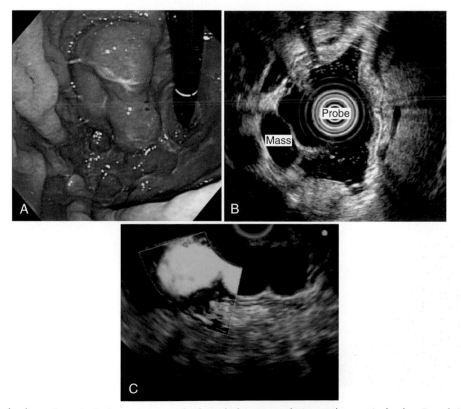

FIGURE 11-11 Gastric fundic varices. **A**, Endoscopic view of a large bulging mass lesion at the gastric fundus. **B** and **C**, EUS confirmed large, anechoic, tubular, submucosal vessels with multiple extramural collateral vascular structures.

veins.[75] Also, there is a report about transesophageal EUS-guided treatment of gastric fundic varices. This procedure was safe and successful in 96% of cases.[76] Because the procedure can be performed in a better scope position with easy accessory manipulation avoiding the thin gastric mucosa overlying the fundic varices, more frequent application of this technique is expected.

Inflammatory Fibroid Polyps

Diagnostic Checklist

Origin in the second and/or third layer.
Hypoechoic, relatively homogeneous lesion with indistinct
   margins.

Inflammatory fibroid polyp is a rare benign polypoid lesion that is usually found in the stomach, occasionally in the small bowel, and rarely in the esophagus or large bowel.[77] The lesion is located in the second or third sonographic layer of the gastric wall, with an intact fourth layer. The usual echoendoscopic features of inflammatory fibroid polyp are indistinct margin and a hypoechoic and homogeneous echo pattern (Figure 11-12). These findings correlate well with the histologic findings of proliferated, nonencapsulated fibrous tissue with vascular elements and eosinophilic infiltration, located in the deep mucosal and submucosal layers. Sometimes the internal echo pattern is heterogeneous or hyperechoic. In that case, the inner hyperechoic area and bright echoes correspond to the presence of small blood vessels.[78]

The EUS patterns of leiomyomas originating from the muscularis mucosa and carcinoid tumors may be similar to that of an inflammatory fibroid polyp. However, those tumors have a distinct margin.

Glomus Tumor

Glomus body is a contractile neuromyoarterial receptor that acts as a thermoregulator. Glomus tumor originates from modified smooth muscle cells of the glomus body. Glomus tumor of the gastrointestinal tract is a rare disease, but most of them are found in the stomach. The majority of gastric glomus tumors are benign and found incidentally as a subepithelial lesion. However, some malignant gastric glomus tumors and cases of bleeding have been reported.

The glomus tumor of the stomach manifests as a circumscribed and hypoechoic mass in the third or fourth layer (Figure 11-13). Usually it appears as an internal heterogeneous echo mixed with hyperechogenic spots.[79-81] Also, a marginal halo is frequently observed. Contrast-enhanced CT reveals a homogeneous hyperdense enhancement on early and delayed phase.

Rare Lesions

Many uncommon lesions have been reported in the endosonographic literature. The number of lesions is too small for their appearance on EUS to be described as characteristic. Some examples are provided here.

Glandular cysts appear as small, nodular to polypoid lesions in the body of the stomach. They create a uniform, relatively hyperechoic, internal echo pattern in the upper mucosa, but they do not disrupt the normal layer pattern of the gastric wall.[72] Lymphoma may occasionally manifest as a submucosal mass. This mass typically appears as a homogeneous, hypoechoic lesion that is contiguous with the second and third gastric wall layers, but it can also invade down to deeper layers. Distant metastases may also appear as submucosal masses in the GI tract. On EUS, they are seen as hypoechoic, heterogeneous masses and may involve any or all of the sonographic layers.

Linitis plastica can sometimes be difficult to diagnose at endoscopy, and biopsy may be unrevealing. The mucosal and submucosal layers appear very thickened at EUS in these patients, who have poor distensibility of the GI lumen even with air insufflation. EUS FNA is diagnostic in most cases. Extrinsic malignant tumors that directly infiltrate the gut wall and manifest as submucosal lesions can be visualized easily by EUS.

Tissue Sampling for Histologic Assessment of Subepithelial Lesions

During endoscopic examination of submucosal lesions, biopsy of the mucosa overlying the lesion is recommended to confirm

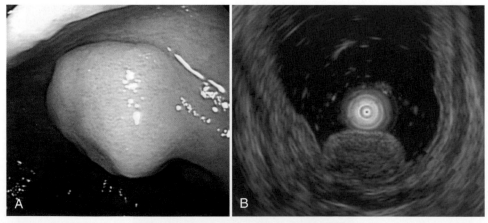

FIGURE 11-12 Inflammatory fibroid polyp. **A,** Endoscopic image of a small, round, polypoid lesion at the gastric antrum. **B,** Gastric EUS demonstrates a homogeneous hypoechoic lesion with indistinct margins located deep in the mucosal layer.

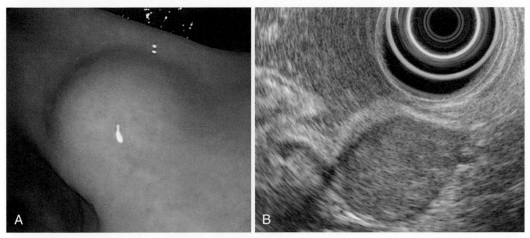

FIGURE 11-13 Glomus tumor. **A**, Endoscopic image of a protruded lesion covered with normal mucosa at the gastric antrum. **B**, Gastric EUS demonstrates a relatively hypoechoic lesion with marginal halo connected with the fourth layer of the gastric wall. *(Courtesy of Gwang Ha Kim, Pusan National University School of Medicine, Busan, South Korea.)*

the presence of intact epithelium. Nevertheless, when the lesion appears cystic or vascular, biopsy should not be attempted before EUS.

Some subepithelial masses arising from the lamina propria or muscularis mucosa may be diagnosed using standard endoscopic forceps biopsy. In particular, when the subepithelial mass is ulcerated, careful biopsy provides an accurate diagnosis. However, for most subepithelial lesions, the results of endoscopic biopsy are inconclusive.[82] Trials with a bite-on-bite technique[83] or an unroofing and partial snaring technique[84] for subepithelial lesions suggest better diagnostic yield than with standard forceps biopsy. However, one thing that should be kept in mind is that manipulation of the mucosal layer overlying the subepithelial lesion may hinder subsequent endoscopic resection procedures such as endoscopic submucosal tunnel dissection for these lesions.

EUS FNA enables the procurement of tissue from subepithelial masses for cytologic examination.[85,86] However, the sensitivity, specificity, and accuracy of cytologic evaluation of intramural lesions are lower than those of lymph nodes or organs adjacent to the GI tract. In one study, the sensitivity of EUS FNA for mediastinal masses, mediastinal lymph nodes, celiac lymph nodes, pancreatic tumors, and submucosal tumors was 88%, 81%, 80%, 75%, and 60%, respectively.[87] No significant difference in diagnostic accuracy was noted according to the size of the FNA needle, but the 25-G needle easily punctured small mobile subepithelial lesions[86] and the 19-G needle showed excellent differentiation between GIST and leiomyoma by enabling tissue procurement for immunohistochemical studies.[88] To overcome some of the limitations of EUS FNA, EUS TCB was introduced. In EUS TCB, use of a needle with a guillotine tip yielded adequate tissue with no major complications in early reports (Figure 11-14).[89] In some later prospective studies, however, the diagnostic yield of EUS TCB in patients with gastric subepithelial lesions was not better than that of EUS FNA, and tissue core obtained with EUS TCB was not sufficient to examine for mitotic index in GIST.[14,90] However, it is clear that EUS TCB can be complementary to EUS FNA, yielding significant additional information, though it cannot be used technically via the transduodenal route.[91] Complications of EUS FNA and EUS TCB include infection, bleeding, and perforation, but they are very rare.

Newly developed ProCore needle (Cook Endoscopy, Winston-Salem, NC, USA) or Side-Port needle (Olympus, Tokyo, Japan) appears promising. Core biopsy along with aspiration material is possible with these types of FNA needles (Figure 11-15), and many endosonographers are eager to learn about their adaptability and efficiency.[82,92] In addition, there is a suggestion that the new forward-array echoendoscope may be helpful to puncture difficult lesions including right colonic subepithelial lesions.[93,94] Further development of new accessories and echoendoscopes will yield better EUS FNA results in the future. The average reported accuracy of EUS FNA in the diagnosis of subepithelial lesions is approximately 80% (Table 11-5).[13–15,47,89,95–101] EUS FNA with histologic and immunohistochemical analysis has a high reported accuracy in the differential diagnosis of mesenchymal tumors of the GI tract.[43–51] However, any form of needle biopsy carries the possibility of sampling error, and a negative finding does not exclude malignancy in GISTs. Because inoperable GIST can now be treated with imatinib, tyrosine kinase inhibitors that specifically block the kit receptor, EUS-guided tissue diagnosis is useful for patients with GIST who have metastasis.

Management of Subepithelial Lesions

Management of subepithelial lesions can be guided by EUS findings (Figure 11-16). Extraluminal compression by adjacent organs and benign submucosal lesions such as lipoma or simple cyst do not need further treatment or follow-up. Pancreatic rest and inflammatory fibroid polyp can be followed in situ. Suspicious superficial lesions, such as carcinoid tumor, can be diagnosed with endoscopic biopsy. Biopsy should be avoided in lesions that are suspected varices. For deeply located hypoechoic lesions, EUS FNA or EUS TCB can be performed for tissue diagnosis. If resection is planned, ESD can be used as a therapeutic tool for small mass lesions arising from the submucosal or inner circular muscularis propria layer instead of surgical resection. Emerging techniques such as endoscopic full-thickness resection or natural orifice transmural endoscopic surgery can also be considered, but attention should be paid to avoid tumor spillage.

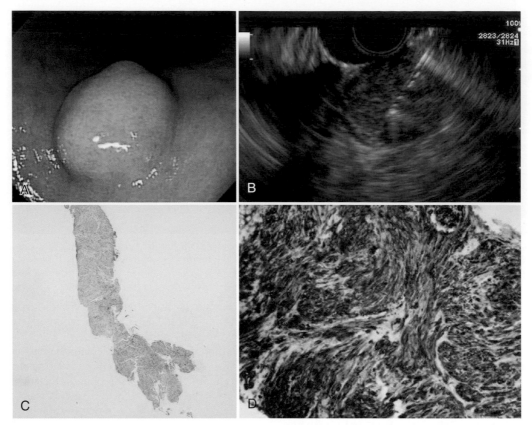

FIGURE 11-14 EUS-guided Tru-Cut biopsy of a gastrointestinal stromal tumor in the stomach. **A,** Endoscopic view reveals a round submucosal lesion at lesser curvature side of the gastric body. **B,** Tru-Cut needle is inserted into the mass with a linear echoendoscope. **C,** Gross finding of acquired tissue core. **D,** Immunohistochemical stains show a positive reaction of the tumor cells for CD117 and CD34.

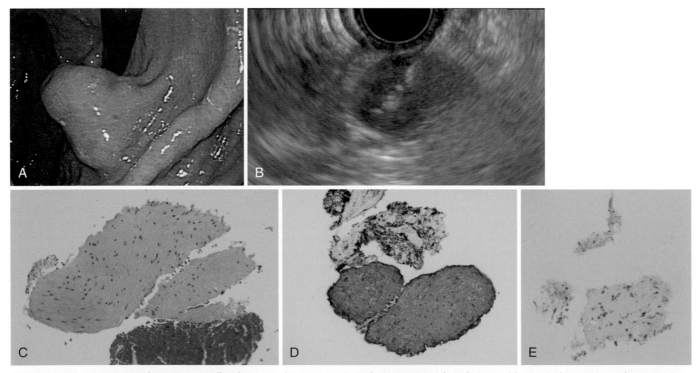

FIGURE 11-15 EUS FNA with ProCore needle of a gastric leiomyoma. **A,** Endoscopic view of a submucosal lesion in the gastric cardia. **B,** ProCore needle was inserted into the mass and the stylet was pulled back slowly as the needle was moved back and forth within the lesion. **C,** Tissue core was obtained. **D** and **E,** Immunohistochemical stains show a positive reaction of the tumor cells for smooth muscle actin and negative for CD117.

TABLE 11-5

DIAGNOSTIC ACCURACY OF EUS-GUIDED FINE-NEEDLE ASPIRATION FOR GASTROINTESTINAL SUBEPITHELIAL LESIONS

Authors (year)	Number of Patients	Accuracy (%)	Diagnostic Method
Çağlar E et al[95] (2013)	67	98	EUS FNA
Rong et al[96] (2012)	46	80	EUS FNA
Suzuki et al[97] (2011)	47	75	EUS FNA
Mekky et al[98] (2010)	69	96	EUS FNA
Hoda et al[99] (2009)	112	84	EUS FNA
Polkowski et al[14] (2009)	49	63	EUS TCB
Akahoshi et al[48] (2007)	51	82	EUS FNA
Chen et al[15] (2005)	42	98	EUS FNA
Vander Noot et al[100] (2004)	51	82	EUS FNA
Arantes et al[101] (2004)	10	80	EUS FNA
Levy et al[89] (2003)	5	80	EUS TCB
Matsui et al[13] (1998)	15	93	EUS FNA

EUS, endoscopic ultrasonography; FNA, fine-needle aspiration; TCB, fine-needle biopsy using a Tru-Cut needle.

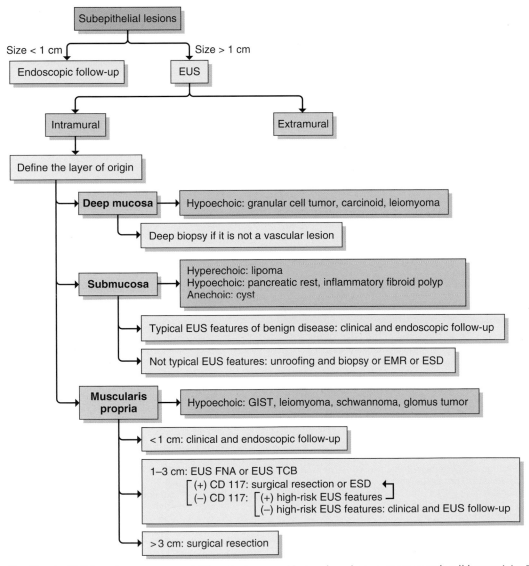

FIGURE 11-16 Algorithm for EUS-based management of different submucosal lesions based on appearance and wall layer origin. EMR, endoscopic mucosal resection; ESD, endoscopic submucosal dissection; FNA, fine-needle aspiration; GIST, gastrointestinal stromal tumor; TCB, Tru-Cut needle biopsy.

Surveillance may be appropriate for subepithelial lesions without definite tissue diagnosis in patients who are at high operative risk. If the lesion is a suspected GIST, changes in size and echogenicity should be monitored. If the size increases or malignant features (echogenic foci, heterogeneity, internal cystic space, irregularity of extraluminal margins, and adjacent lymphadenopathy) develop, resection should be recommended. The follow-up interval depends on the index of suspicion of the examiner and is usually one year. When the characteristics of the lesion do not change on two consecutive follow-up examinations with EUS, a longer follow-up interval may be justified.[102]

Summary

Subepithelial lesions involving the GI tract are difficult to diagnose definitively by conventional imaging methods such as GI radiography, ultrasonography, CT, and MRI. Endoscopic views are limited and standard biopsy techniques have a low yield. EUS is an essential modality in the evaluation of these lesions. Any subepithelial lesion that appears to be larger than 1 cm on endoscopic examination, and is not regarded as a lipoma or cyst, should be referred for EUS evaluation. With the unique ability of EUS to visualize the layers of the GI tract wall, to identify the layer of origin of the subepithelial lesion, and to assess the lesion's size, extent, and sonographic characteristics, a presumptive diagnosis can be made in most cases.

Although a characteristic endosonographic appearance has been described for some subepithelial lesions, EUS cannot reliably distinguish benign from malignant lesions, especially in terms of the malignant potential of GISTs. The addition of EUS FNA or EUS TCB can be helpful to obtain cytologic or histologic samples from subepithelial lesions.

EUS is also helpful in the selection of patients for endoscopic resection because it can enable the examiner to determine the depth and originating wall layer of the lesion. EUS can also be used in the follow-up of subepithelial tumors that are left in situ.

Examination Checklist

Transition zone: Perpendicular imaging at the edge of the lesion produces an image that shows where the normal gut wall layers are merging into the lesion.
Overlying layers: Perpendicular imaging with the transducer positioned on top of the lesion (but not touching it) demonstrates which layers overlie the lesion.

REFERENCES

1. Hedenbro JL, Ekelund M, Wetterberg P. Endoscopic diagnosis of submucosal gastric lesions. The results after routine endoscopy. *Surg Endosc.* 1991;5:20-23.
2. Caletti G, Zani L, Bolondi L, et al. Endoscopic ultrasonography in the diagnosis of gastric submucosal tumor. *Gastrointest Endosc.* 1989;35:413-418.
3. Yasuda K, Nakajima M, Yoshida S, et al. The diagnosis of submucosal tumors of the stomach by endoscopic ultrasonography. *Gastrointest Endosc.* 1989;35:10-15.
4. Boyce GA, Sivak MV Jr, Rosch T, et al. Evaluation of submucosal upper gastrointestinal tract lesions by endoscopic ultrasound. *Gastrointest Endosc.* 1991;37:449-454.
5. Nesje LB, Laerum OD, Svanes K, et al. Subepithelial masses of the gastrointestinal tract evaluated by endoscopic ultrasonography. *Eur J Ultrasound.* 2002;15:45-54.
6. Van Stolk RU. Subepithelial lesions. In: Van Dam J, Sivak MV, eds. *Gastrointestinal Endosonography.* 1st ed. Philadelphia: Saunders; 1999:153-165.
7. Chak A. EUS in submucosal tumors. *Gastrointest Endosc.* 2002;56(suppl):S43-S48.
8. Reddymasu SC, Oropeza-Vail M, Pakseresht K, et al. Are endoscopic ultrasonography imaging characteristics reliable for the diagnosis of small upper gastrointestinal subepithelial lesions? *J Clin Gastroenterol.* 2012;46:42-45.
9. Karaca C, Turner BG, Cizginer S, et al. Accuracy of EUS in the evaluation of small gastric subepithelial lesions. *Gastrointest Endosc.* 2010;71:722-727.
10. Ji F, Wang ZW, Wang LJ, et al. Clinicopathological characteristics of gastrointestinal mesenchymal tumors and diagnostic value of endoscopic ultrasonography. *J Gastroenterol Hepatol.* 2008;23:e318-e324.
11. Kwon JG, Kim EY, Kim YS, et al. Accuracy of endoscopic ultrasonographic impression compared with pathologic diagnosis in gastrointestinal submucosal tumors. *Korean J Gastroenterol.* 2005;45:88-96.
12. Kojima T, Takahashi H, Parra-Blanco A, et al. Diagnosis of submucosal tumor of the upper GI tract by endoscopic resection. *Gastrointest Endosc.* 1999;50:516-522.
13. Matsui M, Goto H, Niwa Y, et al. Preliminary results of fine needle aspiration biopsy histology in upper gastrointestinal submucosal tumors. *Endoscopy.* 1998;30:750-755.
14. Polkowski M, Gerke W, Jarosz D, et al. Diagnostic yield and safety of endoscopic-ultrasound guided trucut biopsy in patients with gastric submucosal tumors: a prospective study. *Endoscopy.* 2009;41:329-334.
15. Chen VK, Eloubeidi MA. Endoscopic ultrasound-guided fine-needle aspiration of intramural and extraintestinal mass lesions: diagnostic accuracy, complication assessment, and impact on management. *Endoscopy.* 2005;37:984-989.
16. Shen EF, Arnott ID, Plevris J, et al. Endoscopic ultrasonography in the diagnosis and management of suspected upper gastrointestinal submucosal tumours. *Br J Surg.* 2002;89:231-235.
17. Nickl NJ, Bhutani MS, Catalano M, et al. Clinical implications of endoscopic ultrasound: the American Endosonography Club Study. *Gastrointest Endosc.* 1996;44:371-377.
18. Park YS, Park SW, Kim TI, et al. Endoscopic enucleation of upper-GI submucosal tumors by using an insulated-tip electrosurgical knife. *Gastrointest Endosc.* 2004;59:409-415.
19. Hoteya S, Iizuka T, Kikuchi D, Yahagi N. Endoscopic submucosal dissection for gastric submucosal tumor, endoscopic sub-tumoral dissection. *Digestive Endoscopy.* 2009;21:266-269.
20. Rosch T, Lorenz R, Dancygier H, et al. Endosonographic diagnosis of submucosal upper gastrointestinal tract tumors. *Scand J Gastroenterol.* 1992;27:1-8.
21. Futagami K, Hata J, Haruma K, et al. Extracorporeal ultrasound is an effective diagnostic alternative to endoscopic ultrasound for gastric submucosal tumours. *Scand J Gastroenterol.* 2001;36:1222-1226.
22. Goto O, Kambe H, Niimi K, et al. Discrepancy in diagnosis of gastric submucosal tumor among esophagogastroduodenoscopy, CT, and endoscopic ultrasonography: a retrospective analysis of 93 consecutive cases. *Abdom Imaging.* 2012;37:1074-1078.
23. Okten RS, Kacar S, Kucukay F, et al. Gastric subepithelial masses: evaluation of multidetector CT (multiplanar reconstruction and virtual gastroscopy) versus endoscopic ultrasonography. *Abdom Imaging.* 2012;37:519-530.
24. Rosch T, Kapfer B, Will U, et al. Accuracy of endoscopic ultrasonography in upper gastrointestinal submucosal lesions: a prospective multicenter study. *Scand J Gastroenterol.* 2002;37:856-862.
25. Motoo Y, Okai T, Ohta H, et al. Endoscopic ultrasonography in the diagnosis of extraluminal compressions mimicking gastric submucosal tumors. *Endoscopy.* 1994;26:239-242.
26. Zhang QL, Nian WD. Endoscopic ultrasonography diagnosis in submucosal tumor of stomach. *Endoscopy.* 1998;30(suppl):A69-A71.
27. Polkowski M, Butruk E. Submucosal lesions. *Gastrointest Endosc Clin N Am.* 2005;15:33-54, viii.
28. Oztas E, Oguz D, Kurt M, et al. Endosonographic evaluation of patients with suspected extraluminal compression or subepithelial lesions during upper gastrointestinal endoscopy. *Eur J Gastroenterol Hepatol.* 2011;23:586-592.

29. Miettinen M, Sobin LH, Lasota J. Gastrointestinal stromal tumors of the stomach: a clinicopathologic, immunohistochemical, and molecular genetic study of 1765 cases with long-term follow-up. *Am J Surg Pathol.* 2005;29:52-68.

30. Miettinen M, Sarlomo-Rikala M, Lasota J. Gastrointestinal stromal tumors: recent advances in understanding of their biology. *Hum Pathol.* 1999;30:1213-1220.

31. Berman J, O'Leary TJ. Gastrointestinal stromal tumor workshop. *Hum Pathol.* 2001;32:578-582.

32. Fletcher CD, Berman JJ, Corless C, et al. Diagnosis of gastrointestinal stromal tumors: a consensus approach. *Hum Pathol.* 2002;33:459-465.

33. Okai T, Minamoto T, Ohtsubo K, et al. Endosonographic evaluation of c-kit-positive gastrointestinal stromal tumor. *Abdom Imaging.* 2003;28:301-307.

34. Kim GH, Park DY, Kim S, et al. Is it possible to differentiate gastric GISTs from gastric leiomyomas by EUS? *World J Gastroenterol.* 2009;15:3376-3381.

35. Jeon SW, Park YD, Chung YJ, et al. Gastrointestinal stromal tumors of the stomach: endosonographic differentiation in relation to histological risk. *J Gastroenterol Hepatol.* 2007;22:2069-2075.

36. Shah P, Gao F, Edmundowicz SA, et al. Predicting malignant potential of gastrointestinal stromal tumors using endoscopic ultrasound. *Dig Dis Sci.* 2009;54:1265-1269.

37. Onishi M, Tominaga K, Sugimori S, et al. Internal hypoechoic feature by EUS as a possible predictive marker for the enlargement potential of gastric GI stromal tumors. *Gastrointest Endosc.* 2012;75:731-738.

38. Chak A, Canto MI, Rosch T, et al. Endosonographic differentiation of benign and malignant stromal cell tumors. *Gastrointest Endosc.* 1997;45:468-473.

39. Palazzo L, Landi B, Cellier C, et al. Endosonographic features predictive of benign and malignant gastrointestinal stromal cell tumours. *Gut.* 2000;46:88-92.

40. Nickl N. Decision analysis of hypoechoic intramural tumor study results. *Gastrointest Endosc.* 2002;56(suppl):S102.

41. Kannengiesser K, Mahlke R, Petersen F, et al. Contrast-enhanced harmonic endoscopic ultrasound is able to discriminate benign submucosal lesions from gastrointestinal stromal tumors. *Scand J Gastroenterol.* 2012;47:1515-1520.

42. Sakamoto H, Kitano M, Matsui S, et al. Estimation of malignant potential of GI stromal tumors by contrast-enhanced harmonic EUS (with videos). *Gastrointest Endosc.* 2011;73:227-237.

43. DeWitt J, Emerson RE, Sherman S, et al. Endoscopic ultrasound-guided Trucut biopsy of gastrointestinal mesenchymal tumor. *Surg Endosc.* 2011;25:2192-2202.

44. Watson RR, Binmoeller KF, Hamerski CM, et al. Yield and performance characteristics of endoscopic ultrasound-guided fine needle aspiration for diagnosing upper GI tract stromal tumors. *Dig Dis Sci.* 2011;56:1757-1762.

45. Fernández-Esparrach G, Sendino O, Solé M, et al. Endoscopic ultrasound-guided fine-needle aspiration and trucut biopsy in the diagnosis of gastric stromal tumors: a randomized crossover study. *Endoscopy.* 2010;42:292-299.

46. Sepe PS, Moparty B, Pitman MB, et al. EUS-guided FNA for the diagnosis of GI stromal cell tumors: sensitivity and cytologic yield. *Gastrointest Endosc.* 2009;70:254-261.

47. Chatzipantelis P, Salla C, Karoumpalis I, et al. Endoscopic ultrasound-guided fine needle aspiration biopsy in the diagnosis of gastrointestinal stromal tumors of the stomach. A study of 17 cases. *J Gastrointestin Liver Dis* 2008;17:15-20.

48. Akahoshi K, Sumida Y, Matsui N, et al. Preoperative diagnosis of gastrointestinal stromal tumor by endoscopic ultrasound-guided fine needle aspiration. *World J Gastroenterol.* 2007;13:2077-2082.

49. Mochizuki Y, Kodera Y, Fujiwara M, et al. Laparoscopic wedge resection for gastrointestinal stromal tumors of the stomach: initial experience. *Surg Today.* 2006;36:341-347.

50. Okubo K, Yamao K, Nakamura T, et al. Endoscopic ultrasound-guided fine-needle aspiration biopsy for the diagnosis of gastrointestinal stromal tumors in the stomach. *J Gastroenterol.* 2004;39:747-753.

51. Ando N, Goto H, Niwa Y, et al. The diagnosis of GI stromal tumors with EUS-guided fine needle aspiration with immunohistochemical analysis. *Gastrointest Endosc.* 2002;55:37-43.

52. Armstrong CP, King PM, Dixon JM, et al. The clinical significance of heterotopic pancreas in the gastrointestinal tract. *Br J Surg.* 1981;68:384-387.

53. Jovanovic I, Knezevic S, Micev M, et al. EUS mini probes in diagnosis of cystic dystrophy of duodenal wall in heterotopic pancreas: a case report. *World J Gastroenterol.* 2004;10:2609-2612.

54. Matsushita M, Hajiro K, Okazaki K, et al. Gastric aberrant pancreas: EUS analysis in comparison with the histology. *Gastrointest Endosc.* 1999;49:493-497.

55. Parmar JH, Lawrence R, Ridley NT. Submucous lipoma of the ileocaecal valve presenting as caecal volvulus. *Int J Clin Pract.* 2004;58:424-425.

56. Watanabe F, Honda S, Kubota H, et al. Preoperative diagnosis of ileal lipoma by endoscopic ultrasonography probe. *J Clin Gastroenterol.* 2000;31:245-247.

57. Zhou PH, Yao LQ, Zhong YS, et al. Role of endoscopic miniprobe ultrasonography in diagnosis of submucosal tumor of large intestine. *World J Gastroenterol.* 2004;10:2444-2446.

58. Garcia M, Buitrago E, Bejarano PA, et al. Large esophageal liposarcoma: a case report and review of the literature. *Arch Pathol Lab Med.* 2004;128:922-925.

59. Nakamura S, Iida M, Yao T, et al. Endoscopic features of gastric carcinoids. *Gastrointest Endosc.* 1991;37:535-538.

60. Ichikawa J, Tanabe S, Koizumi W, et al. Endoscopic mucosal resection in the management of gastric carcinoid tumors. *Endoscopy.* 2003;35:203-206.

61. Matsumoto T, Iida M, Suekane H, et al. Endoscopic ultrasonography in rectal carcinoid tumors: contribution to selection of therapy. *Gastrointest Endosc.* 1991;37:539-542.

62. Yasuda E, Tomita K, Nagura Y, et al. Endoscopic removal of granular cell tumor. *Gastrointest Endosc.* 1995;41:163-167.

63. Nakachi A, Miyazato H, Oshiro T, et al. Granular cell tumor of the rectum: a case report and review of the literature. *J Gastroenterol.* 2000;35:631-634.

64. Love MH, Glaser M, Edmunds SE, et al. Granular cell tumour of the oesophagus: endoscopic ultrasound appearances. *Australas Radiol.* 1999;43:253-255.

65. Palazzo L, Landi B, Cellier C, et al. Endosonographic features of esophageal granular cell tumors. *Endoscopy.* 1997;29:850-853.

66. Kim DU, Kim GH, Ryu DY, et al. Endosonographic features of esophageal granular cell tumors using a high-frequency catheter probe. *Scand J Gastroenterol.* 2011;46:142-147.

67. Hizawa K, Matsumoto T, Kouzuki T, et al. Cystic submucosal tumors in the gastrointestinal tract: endosonographic findings and endoscopic removal. *Endoscopy.* 2000;32:712-714.

68. Wildi SM, Hoda RS, Fickling W, et al. Diagnosis of benign cysts of the mediastinum: the role and risks of EUS and FNA. *Gastrointest Endosc.* 2003;58:362-368.

69. Fazel A, Moezardalan K, Varadarajulu S, et al. The utility and the safety of EUS-guided FNA in the evaluation of duplication cysts. *Gastrointest Endosc.* 2005;62:575-580.

70. Faigel DO, Burke A, Ginsberg GG, et al. The role of endoscopic ultrasound in the evaluation and management of foregut duplications. *Gastrointest Endosc.* 1997;45:99-103.

71. Geller A, Wang KK, DiMagno EP. Diagnosis of foregut duplication cysts by endoscopic ultrasonography. *Gastroenterology.* 1995;109:838-842.

72. Dancygier H, Lightdale CJ. Endoscopic ultrasonography of the upper gastrointestinal tract and colon. In: Stevens PD, ed. *Endosonography in Gastroenterology: Principles, Techniques, Findings.* New York: Thieme; 1999:76-89.

73. Faigel DO, Rosen HR, Sasaki A, et al. EUS in cirrhotic patients with and without prior variceal hemorrhage in comparison with noncirrhotic control subjects. *Gastrointest Endosc.* 2000;52:455-462.

74. Tio TL, Kimmings N, Rauws E, et al. Endosonography of gastroesophageal varices: evaluation and follow-up of 76 cases. *Gastrointest Endosc.* 1995;42:145-150.

75. Lahoti S, Catalano MF, Alcocer E, et al. Obliteration of esophageal varices using EUS-guided sclerotherapy with color Doppler. *Gastrointest Endosc.* 2000;51:331-333.

76. Binmoeller KF, Weilert F, Shah JN, Kim J. EUS-guided transesophageal treatment of gastric fundal varices with combined coiling and cyanoacrylate glue injection (with videos). *Gastrointest Endosc.* 2011;74:1019-1025.

77. Matsushita M, Hajiro K, Okazaki K, et al. Endoscopic features of gastric inflammatory fibroid polyps. *Am J Gastroenterol.* 1996;91:1595-1598.

78. Matsushita M, Hajiro K, Okazaki K, et al. Gastric inflammatory fibroid polyps: endoscopic ultrasonographic analysis in comparison with the histology. *Gastrointest Endosc.* 1997;46:53-57.

79. Imamura A, Tochihara M, Natsui K, et al. Glomus tumor of the stomach: endoscopic ultrasonographic findings. *Am J Gastroenterol.* 1994;89: 271-272.

80. Baek YH, Choi SR, Lee BE, Kim GH. Gastric glomus tumor: analysis of endosonographic characteristics and computed tomographic findings. *Dig Endosc.* 2013;25:80-83.

81. Tang M, Hou J, Wu D, et al. Glomus tumor in the stomach: computed tomography and endoscopic ultrasound findings. *World J Gastroenterol.* 2013;28;19:1327-1329.

82. Kim EY. Diagnosis of subepithelial lesion: still "tissue is the issue". *Clin Endosc.* 2013;46:313-314.

83. Ji JS, Lee BI, Choi KY, et al. Diagnostic yield of tissue sampling using a bite-on-bite technique for incidental subepithelial lesions. *Korean J Intern Med.* 2009;24:101-105.

84. Lee CK, Chung IK, Lee SH, et al. Endoscopic partial resection with the unroofing technique for reliable tissue diagnosis of upper GI subepithelial tumors originating from the muscularis propria on EUS (with video). *Gastrointest Endosc.* 2010;71:188-194.

85. Kim EY. Introduction: value of endoscopic ultrasound-guided fine needle aspiration. *Clin Endosc.* 2012;45:115-116.

86. Moon JS. Endoscopic ultrasound-guided fine needle aspiration in submucosal lesion. *Clin Endosc.* 2012;45:117-123.

87. Giovannini M, Seitz JF, Monges G, et al. Fine-needle aspiration cytology guided by endoscopic ultrasonography: results in 141 patients. *Endoscopy.* 1995;27:171-177.

88. Eckardt AJ, Adler A, Gomes EM, et al. Endosonographic large-bore biopsy of gastric subepithelial tumors: a prospective multicenter study. *Eur J Gastroenterol Hepatol.* 2012;24:1135-1144.

89. Levy MJ, Jondal ML, Clain J, et al. Preliminary experience with an EUS-guided Trucut biopsy needle compared with EUS-guided FNA. *Gastrointest Endosc.* 2003;57:101-106.

90. Varadarajulu S, Fraig M, Schmulewitz N, et al. Comparison of EUS-guided 19-gauge Trucut needle biopsy with EUS-guided fine-needle aspiration. *Endoscopy.* 2004;36:397-401.

91. Săftoiu A, Vilmann P, Guldhammer Skov B, Georgescu CV. Endoscopic ultrasound (EUS)-guided Trucut biopsy adds significant information to EUS-guided fine-needle aspiration in selected patients: a prospective study. *Scand J Gastroenterol.* 2007;42:117-125.

92. Kaffes AJ, Chen RY, Tam W, et al. A prospective multicenter evaluation of a new side-port endoscopic ultrasound-fine-needle aspiration in solid upper gastrointestinal lesions. *Dig Endosc.* 2012;24: 448-451.

93. Kida M, Araki M, Tokunaga S, et al. Role of a forward-viewing echoendoscope in fine-needle aspiration. *Gastrointest Interv.* 2013; 2:12-16.

94. Nguyen-Tang T, Shah JN, Sanchez-Yague A, Binmoeller KF. Use of the front-view forward-array echoendoscope to evaluate right colonic subepithelial lesions. *Gastrointest Endosc.* 2010;72:606-610.

95. Çağlar E, Hatemi İ, Atasoy D, et al. Concordance of endoscopic ultrasonography-guided fine needle aspiration diagnosis with the final diagnosis in subepithelial lesions. *Clin Endosc.* 2013;46:379-383.

96. Rong L, Kida M, Yamauchi H, et al. Factors affecting the diagnostic accuracy of endoscopic ultrasonography-guided fine-needle aspiration (EUS-FNA) for upper gastrointestinal submucosal or extraluminal solid mass lesions. *Dig Endosc* 2012;24:358-363.

97. Suzuki T, Arai M, Matsumura T, et al. Factors associated with inadequate tissue yield in EUS-FNA for gastric SMT. *ISRN Gastroenterol* 2011;2011:619128.

98. Mekky MA, Yamao K, Sawaki A, et al. Diagnostic utility of EUS-guided FNA in patients with gastric submucosal tumors. *Gastrointest Endosc* 2010;71:913-919.

99. Hoda KM, Rodriguez SA, Faigel DO. EUS-guided sampling of suspected GI stromal tumors. *Gastrointest Endosc* 2009;69:1218-1223.

100. Vander Noot MR 3rd, Eloubeidi MA, Chen VK, et al. Diagnosis of gastrointestinal tract lesions by endoscopic ultrasound-guided fine-needle aspiration biopsy. *Cancer.* 2004;102:157-163.

101. Arantes V, Logrono R, Faruqi S, et al. Endoscopic sonographically guided fine-needle aspiration yield in submucosal tumors of the gastrointestinal tract. *J Ultrasound Med.* 2004;23:1141-1150.

102. Hwang JH, Rulyak SD, Kimmey MB. American Gastroenterological Association Institute technical review on the management of gastric subepithelial masses. *Gastroenterology.* 2006;130:2217-2228.

12

EUS in the Evaluation of Gastric Tumors

Bronte Holt • Thomas Rösch • Shajan Peter

Key Points

- EUS is useful for staging gastric cancer but is an ineffective modality for screening.
- In patients without metastasis, EUS enables preoperative assessment of local tumor extent that will determine the choice of treatment.
- Two methods for imaging can be used: water-filled stomach and balloon contact.
- Endoscopic resection can be considered for well-differentiated and intramucosal gastric cancer less than or equal to 2 cm in size.

Endoscopic ultrasonography (EUS) plays an important role in the diagnosis and staging of luminal gastrointestinal tumors. Gastric cancer and other gastrointestinal tumors such as gastric lymphoma are staged using a combination of EUS and computed tomography (CT), with or without positron emission tomography (PET). EUS is the most accurate modality for local regional staging of gastric cancer. EUS evaluates the individual gastric wall layers and can sample lymph nodes distant to the primary tumor by fine-needle aspiration (FNA). This improves the tumor staging accuracy and thereby the best mode of therapy. In addition, EUS plays an important role in evaluating patients with large gastric folds of unclear origin, with the aim of diagnosing infiltrative diseases such as lymphoma or linitis plastica.

Gastric Cancer

Despite decreases in incidence and mortality, gastric cancer remains the second leading cause of cancer-related deaths worldwide.[1] In the United States in 2013, there were an estimated 21,600 new cases and 10,990 deaths from gastric cancer.[2] The treatment algorithm is based on accurate staging that includes determination of tumor extent and nodal involvement.[3,4] Although the 5-year survival rate is greater than 70% for early gastric cancer confined to the mucosa or submucosa (stage IA) following resection, it is less than 50% for patients with stage IIA disease, and 4% in the presence of distal metastases (stage IV).[5] Accurate staging is imperative to ensure appropriate therapy is selected. In general, endoscopic resection may be considered in patients without submucosal invasion.[6] Surgery is the mainstay of curative therapy in patients with locally advanced, resectable disease.

Postoperative chemoradiation[7] or perioperative chemotherapy[8] has additional survival benefits compared to surgery alone. The optimal management of patients with locally advanced unresectable but nonmetastatic gastric cancer is not well defined, and there may be a role for chemotherapy to downstage for potential resection. Patients with metastatic disease are considered for palliative chemotherapy.

Role of EUS

Noninvasive imaging studies such as CT are widely available, but they lack accuracy for assessing the depth of tumor invasion or lymph node involvement.[9,10] EUS is the most reliable nonsurgical method available for evaluating the depth of invasion of primary gastric cancers,[11,12] is relatively low risk, and provides a more accurate prediction of T and N stage than CT imaging.[13–15] Moreover, EUS-guided FNA of both regional and distant lymph nodes adds to the accuracy of nodal staging.[16,17]

The role of EUS in gastric cancer can be categorized as follows:

- Determination of treatment.
- Detection of distant metastasis missed by CT: Small metastatic deposits in the left lobe of the liver or low-volume malignant ascites can be diagnosed by EUS-guided FNA, obviates the need for staging laparoscopy, and establishes nonoperative disease.
- EUS does not add to patient management in patients with metastatic gastric cancer identified by CT.
- The role of EUS in restaging after chemotherapy or radiation therapy is unclear.

Echoendoscopes

The radial echoendoscope is generally preferred for gastric cancer staging because of its ease of manipulation and its ability to evaluate the relationship between the lesion and adjacent organs. The ultrasonic mini-probe is useful for small lesions, as these lesions can be viewed simultaneously by endoscopy and endosonography. In patients with suspected nodal disease where cytology confirmation is required, a curvilinear echoendoscope is used.

A three-dimensional probe-based EUS system (Olympus Medical Systems Corporation, UM-DG20-25R [20 MHz] and UM-DG12-25R [12 MHz]) is commercially available. It generates real-time radial images and computer-reconstructed linear images displayed simultaneously, as in helical CT scanning, and may improve accuracy in determining the depth of invasion and enable measurement of tumor volume.

Examination Techniques for Tumor Staging

Radial echoendoscope examinations commence by instilling de-aerated water into the stomach to submerge the lesion and aspirating all the air to optimize acoustic coupling (Figure 12-1). This maneuver permits ultrasonographic evaluation of the lesion without direct apposition of the echoendoscope balloon or probe tip over the lesion, avoiding compression of tissue planes and inaccurate T staging (Videos 12-1 and 12-2). The patient's position can be changed to completely immerse the lesion. The echoendoscope transducer is maintained perpendicular to the lesion to avoid tangential imaging. Most examinations with the radial echoendoscope are performed at frequencies of 7.5 and 12 MHz, which allow a penetration of approximately 8 and 3 cm, respectively. The depth of penetration is lower at higher frequencies, but the greater resolution is preferred for evaluating early stage gastric cancer.

T Staging

Five distinct layers of the gastric wall are seen with the radial echoendoscope: three hyperechoic and two hypoechoic, visible as alternating bright and dark layers (Figure 12-2). The first two echo layers correspond histologically to the mucosa, the third corresponds to the submucosa, the fourth to the muscularis propria, and the fifth to the serosa. T-stage classification by EUS is as follows:[18]

T1: Tumor involvement of the mucosal (T1a) or both the mucosal and submucosal (T1b) layers.

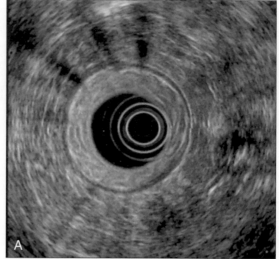
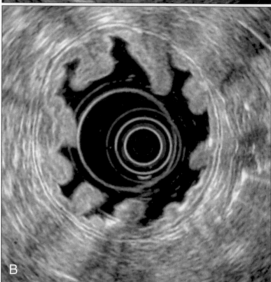

FIGURE 12-1 Evaluation of gastric wall layers. **A,** The gastric wall layers cannot be well evaluated at EUS in the absence of water instillation. **B,** After water instillation, the individual wall layers can be well examined using a radial echoendoscope.

T2: Tumor infiltration into the muscularis propria.
T3: Tumor penetrates subserosal connective tissue without invasion of the visceral peritoneum or adjacent structures.
T4a: Tumor invasion of serosa.
T4b: Tumor invasion of adjacent organs or structures.

Video 12-1. Radial EUS, performed after instillation of water, reveals a T1 gastric cancer confined to the mucosal layer.

Video 12-2. Radial EUS revealing a T3 gastric cancer that abuts the liver but without any invasion.

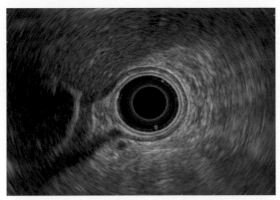

FIGURE 12-2 The five-layer gastric wall as examined using a radial echoendoscope at 7.5 MHz.

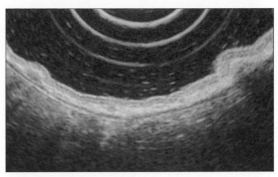

FIGURE 12-3 The nine-layer gastric wall as examined using a 20-MHz high-frequency EUS mini-probe.

Tumors confined to the mucosa can be considered for endoscopic resection; however, submucosal involvement usually obligates surgery due to a nearly 20% risk of nodal metastasis.[19] Therefore accurate staging is imperative before determining treatment.

Small (<2 cm) or sessile lesions are ideally assessed with the high-frequency, high-resolution ultrasonic mini-probe (Video 12-3). Because of their limited depth of penetration, the mini-probe should not be used for evaluating large gastric lesions as staging accuracy decreases.[20] The gastric wall appears as a nine-layer structure (Figure 12-3). In addition to the normal five layers, a border echo (third layer) with the hypoechoic muscularis mucosa (fourth layer), a hypoechoic inner muscle layer (sixth layer), a border echo layer (seventh layer), and a hypoechoic outer muscle layer (eighth layer) are seen (Figure 12-4).

N Staging

Perigastric and regional lymph node stations are surveyed. Lymph nodes on ultrasound, such as low echogenicity (hypoechoic versus others), sharp versus irregular borders, round versus elliptical shape, and large size (>10 mm versus <10 mm), are predictive of tumoral involvement. However, only 25% of malignant lymph nodes have all four features, and no single feature can independently predict nodal metastasis.[21]

M Staging

EUS is limited in the detection of metastatic disease but can provide vital information in a subset of patients that alters

Video 12-3. EUS examination performed using a 20-MHz high-frequency mini-probe (water-fill technique) reveals a T1 gastric cancer confined to the mucosal region. The tumor was subsequently removed by injection-assisted polypectomy.

management. The echoendoscope is advanced to the gastric antrum, and surrounding structures (left lobe of liver, peritoneum, pleural layers of the lung, and mediastinum) are carefully examined on slow withdrawal. Malignant ascites or pleural effusion (Figure 12-5) or metastasis in distant nodes preclude surgical treatment.[22,23] Diagnosis of small metastatic deposits missed by staging CT EUS-guided FNA (Figure 12-6) can change patient management (Video 12-4).[23,24]

Accuracy of EUS in Staging

After endoscopy, EUS is the most important diagnostic procedure for local staging in patients with gastric cancer. Current staging guidelines are based on the American Joint Committee on Cancer (AJCC) staging system (Table 12-1). Several studies have investigated the accuracy of EUS in tumor, node, and metastasis (TNM) staging of gastric cancer (Table 12-2) and include a variety of instrumentations, scanning frequencies, and tumor locations.

T Staging

Changes to the T-stage classification of gastric cancer were made in the 7th Edition of the AJCC classification system in 2010.[5] In the latest edition, T1 (mucosa and submucosa) has been divided into T1a (mucosa) and T1b (submucosa), T2b (subserosa) has been reclassified as T3, and T3 (penetrates serosa) has been reclassified as T4a. The majority of studies evaluating the accuracy of EUS in T staging used the 2002 guidelines.

Early stage gastric cancer is usually defined as lesions confined to the mucosa (Tis and T1a, or T1m) and submucosa (T1b or T1sm) (Figure 12-7). Wall layer irregularity and a "budding sign" larger than 1 mm in depth in the third wall layer are features suggestive of submucosal invasion in early gastric cancer.[42,43]

The overall accuracy of EUS staging using the mini-probe is between 65% and 72%. Overstaging of T1 mucosal lesions as T1 submucosal lesions occurred in 29% to 46% of cases, and T1 submucosal understaging occurred in 6% to 48% of cases.[20,44–46] Kim and colleagues[47] used a high-frequency catheter probe (20 Mhz) and found an overall accuracy of 81% when assessing the depth of invasion. Accuracy for nonulcerated lesions less than 2 cm in size was 83%; however, this declined to 70% for ulcerated lesions and 43% for lesions with superficial (<500 μm) submucosal extension. Accuracy

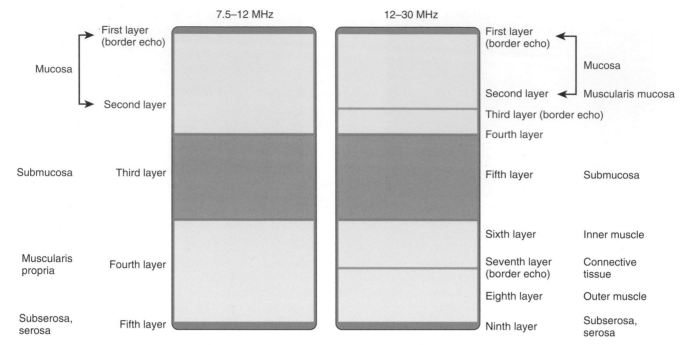

FIGURE 12-4 Schematic representation of the normal gastric wall as examined using a radial echoendoscope and a high-frequency mini-probe.

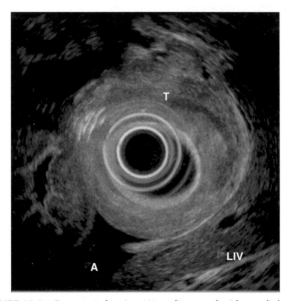

FIGURE 12-5 Presence of ascites (A) as diagnosed with a radial echoendoscope in advanced gastric cancer. LIV, liver; T, tumor.

FIGURE 12-6 Hepatic metastasis of gastric cancer. EUS-guided fine-needle aspiration of a metastatic deposit in the left lobe of the liver in a patient with gastric cancer that was missed on computed tomography imaging.

T stage was 75% with a moderate Kappa value (0.52). EUS was most accurate for T3 cancers (85%), followed by T4 (79%), T1 (77%), and T2 (65%). The meta-analysis by Mocellin and colleagues showed that the pooled sensitivity for T1 cancer was 83%, T2 (65%), T3 (86%), and T4 (66%).[51] These

of high-frequency mini-probes is also affected by gastric folds and protruding lesions.

The overall accuracy of EUS[49] in determining T stage ranges from 71% to 92%, with an average of 83% (see Table 12-2). EUS accuracy is best for T1, T3, and T4 lesions, whereas it is least accurate (range 60% to 70%) for T2 lesions (Table 12-3). In an earlier meta-analysis, the pooled sensitivity was 88% for T1 lesions, 82% for T2, 90% for T3, and 99% for T4 lesions.[49] Two recent meta-analyses have addressed the utility of EUS staging for gastric cancer (see Table 12-5). Cardoso and colleagues[50] showed that the pooled accuracy for

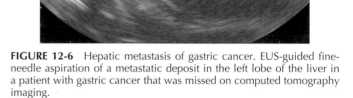

Video 12-4 (with narration). Video demonstrating T3 gastric cancer as imaged with a radial echoendoscope. FNA of a liver mass confirms gastric metastasis in the same patient.

TABLE 12-1

TNM STAGING FOR GASTRIC CANCER

Anatomic Stage/Prognostic Groups

Stage	T	N	M
Stage 0	Tis	N0	M0
Stage IA	T1	N0	M0
Stage IB	T2	N0	M0
	T1	N1	M0
Stage IIA	T3	N0	M0
	T2	N1	M0
	T1	N2	M0
Stage IIB	T4a	N0	M0
	T3	N1	M0
	T2	N2	M0
	T1	N3	M0
Stage IIIA	T4a	N1	M0
	T3	N2	M0
	T2	N3	M0
Stage IIIB	T4b	N0	M0
	T4b	N1	M0
	T4a	N2	M0
	T3	N3	M0
Stage IIIC	T4b	N2	M0
	T4b	N3	M0
	T4a	N3	M0
Stage IV	Any T	Any N	M1

Primary Tumor (T)

TX	Primary tumor cannot be assessed
T0	No evidence of primary tumor
Tis	Carcinoma in situ: intraepithelial tumor without invasion of the lamina propria
T1	Tumor invades lamina propria, muscularis mucosa, or submucosa
T1a	Tumor invades lamina propria or muscularis mucosa
T1b	Tumor invades submucosa
T2	Tumor invades muscularis propria[a]
T3	Tumor penetrates subserosal connective tissue without invasion of visceral peritoneum or adjacent structures[b,c]
T4	Tumor invades serosa (visceral peritoneum) or adjacent structures[b,c]
T4a	Tumor invades serosa (visceral peritoneum)
T4b	Tumor invades adjacent structures

Regional Lymph Nodes (N)

NX	Regional lymph node(s) cannot be assessed
N0	No regional lymph node metastasis[d]
N1	Metastasis in 1-2 regional lymph nodes
N2	Metastasis in 3-6 regional lymph nodes
N3	Metastasis in seven or more regional lymph nodes
N3a	Metastasis in 7-15 regional lymph nodes
N3b	Metastasis in 16 or more regional lymph nodes

Distant Metastatis (M)

M0	No distant metastasis
M1	Distant metastasis

[a]Note: A tumor may penetrate the muscularis propria with extension into the gastrocolic or gastrohepatic ligaments, or into the greater or lesser omentum, without perforation of the visceral peritoneum covering these structures. In this case, the tumor is classified T3. If there is perforation of the visceral peritoneum covering the gastric ligaments or the omentum, the tumor should be classified T4.

[b]The adjacent structures of the stomach include the spleen, transverse colon, liver, diaphragm, pancreas, abdominal wall, adrenal gland, kidney, small intestine, and retroperitoneum.

[c]Intramural extension to the duodenum or esophagus is classified by the depth of the greatest invasion in any of these sites, including the stomach.

[d]Note: A designation of pN0 should be used if all examined lymph nodes are negative, regardless of the total number removed and examined.

(From Edge S, Byrd DR, Compton CC, Fritz AG, Greene FL, Trotti A, eds. AJCC Cancer Staging Manual. 7th ed. New York, NY: Springer; 2010: 117-120.)

TABLE 12-2

ACCURACY OF EUS IN GASTRIC CANCER WITH RESPECT TO OVERALL T STAGING

Authors (year)	Frequency (MHz)	Patients (n)	T-Stage Accuracy (%)
Murata et al[25] (1988)	7.5-10	146	79
Tio et al[26] (1989)	7.5-12	72	81
Akahoshi et al[27] (1991)	7.5-12	74	81
Botet et al[28] (1991)	7.5-12	50	92
Caletti et al[29] (1993)	7.5-12	35	91
Dittler and Siewert[30] (1993)	7.5-12	254	83
Grimm et al[31] (1993)	7.5	147	78
Ziegler et al[32] (1993)	7.5-12	108	86
Massari et al[33] (1996)	7.5-12	65	89
Perng et al[34] (1996)	7.5-12	69	71
Wang et al[22] (1998)	7.5-12	119	70
Tseng et al[35] (2000)	7.5-12	74	85
Willis et al[36] (2000)	7.5-12	116	78
Habermann et al[37] (2004)	7.5-12	51	86
Tsendsuren et al[38] (2006)	5-7.5	41	69
Ganpathi et al[14] (2006)	7.5-20	126	80
Bentrem et al[39] (2007)	7.5-12	225	57
Lok et al[40] (2008)	5-20	123	64
Repiso et al[41] (2010)	7.5-20	46	70

rates reflect the difficulty in differentiating T2 (muscularis propria and subserosal) from T3 (serosal) invasion (Figure 12-8), leading to potential understaging and overstaging. Larger studies consistently showed overstaging of T2 lesions in 12% to 30% of tumors and understaging in 4% to 10% of tumors. Whereas microscopic invasion was the most frequent cause of understaging, overstaging was attributed to peritumoral fibrosis, ulceration, and inflammation. In addition, certain anatomic features can lead to inaccuracy in T staging. In areas such as the lesser curvature and the posterior wall of the fundus, which are not covered with serosa, tumors with complete transmural growth are histologically classified as T3, thus potentially leading to overstaging. In other areas where the stomach is not covered completely by the serosa, such as attachment sites of the gastrocolic ligament, gastrohepatic ligament, and omentum major and minor, tumors invading the fatty plane may appear endosonographically as T3 lesions when in fact histologically they are T2. From the meta-analysis by Mocellin and colleauges, EUS nonetheless could differentiate T1-T2 from T3-T4 gastric cancer with an overall sensitivity of 86% and specificity of 91%.[52] The diagnostic accuracy is only 43.5% for gastric lesions ≥30 mm in size compared to 87.8% for lesions <30 mm.[53]

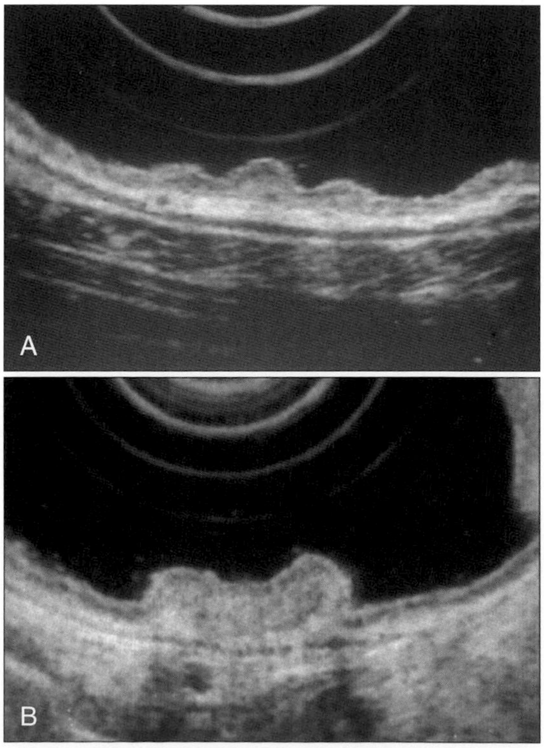

N Staging

The overall accuracy of EUS for N staging ranges from 65% to 90% (Table 12-4). The pooled sensitivity for N1 stage disease is 58.2%, and for N2 it is 64.9%.[49] The meta-analysis by Cardoso and colleagues[50] revealed the accuracy, sensitivity, and specificity of EUS for N staging (N0 versus N+) was 64%, 74%, and 80%, respectively. In their analysis, Mocellin and colleagues[51] showed a sensitivity of 69% and specificity of 84% for N stage (N0 versus N+) (Table 12-5). In general, the accuracy for N staging is low because of the difficulty in differentiating malignant from benign inflammatory lymph nodes. Results among studies vary because of heterogeneity of criteria used to define malignant nodes. In the description by François and colleagues,[54] hypoechoic lymph nodes with well-defined margins and a ratio of largest to smallest diameter of less than 2 were considered to be malignant. Nonetheless, a strong correlation exists between increasing T stage and

FIGURE 12-7 Early stage gastric cancer. **A**, Early stage gastric cancer confined to the mucosal layer. **B**, Early stage gastric cancer extending to the submucosal layer.

TABLE 12-3

ACCURACY OF EUS IN GASTRIC CANCER STAGING IN T CATEGORY

Authors (year)	Frequency (MHz)	Patients (n)	T1 (%)	T2 (%)	T3 (%)	T4 (%)
Murata et al[25] (1988)	7.5-10	146	93	50	41	—
Tio et al[26] (1989)	7.5-12	72	77	93	81	88
Akahoshi et al[27] (1991)	7.5-12	74	93	57	100	60
Botet et al[28] (1991)	7.5-12	50	92	97	86	—
Caletti et al[48] (1993)	7.5-12	35	83	100	86	100
Dittler and Siewert[30] (1993)	7.5-12	254	81	71	87	79
Grimm et al[31] (1993)	7.5	147	74	73	85	85
Ziegler et al[32] (1993)	7.5-12	108	91	81	84	94
Massari et al[33] (1996)	7.5-12	65	100	86	85.7	88.8
Perng et al[34] (1996)	7.5-12	69	58	63	79	83
Wang et al[22] (1998)	7.5-12	119	68	67	81	53
Tseng et al[35] (2000)	7.5-12	74	100	74	87	86
Willis et al[36] (2000)	7.5-12	116	80	63	95	83
Habermann et al[37] (2004)	7.5-12	51	—	90	79	100
Tsendsuren et al[38] (2006)	7.5	41	83	60	100	25
Ganpathi et al[14] (2006)	7.5-20	126	79	74	86	73
Bentrem et al[39] (2007)	7.5-12	225	80	49	—	—
Lok et al[40] (2008)	5-20	123	24	43	97	33
Repiso et al[41] (2010)	7.5-20	46	100	38	82	100

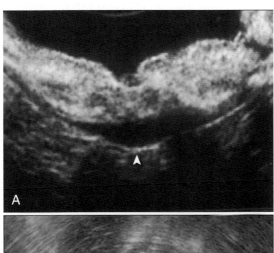
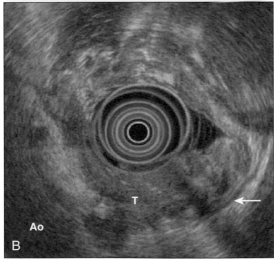

FIGURE 12-8 Staging of T2 and T3 gastric cancer. **A,** Gastric cancer staged as T2 where the tumor invades the subserosa *(arrowhead).* **B,** Gastric cancer staged as T3 where the tumor invades the serosal layer of the stomach *(arrow).* Ao, aorta; T, tumor.

the presence of lymph node metastases, such that the accuracy and sensitivity for diagnosing lymph node metastases are higher for T3 and T4 lesions. Dittler and Siewert[30] observed that when EUS did not show malignant lymph nodes in T1 or T2 stage, stage N0 could be assumed; when lymph nodes were visualized at EUS in stages T3 and T4, these nodes tended to be malignant. However, it is difficult to diagnose lymph node metastases in T1 stage because there are usually very few nodes involved and they are difficult to detect. Another reason for inaccuracy in nodal staging is the inability to visualize distant lymph nodes. Nonetheless, EUS can be clincally informative, as it increases the probability of being classified as node positive from 55% to 84% when positive, and it lowers the probability to 31% when negative.[51]

Detection of lymph node metastasis is easier when the lymph nodes are within 3 cm of the primary lesion and are located around the lesser curvature rather than the greater curvature of the stomach. This is due to the poor depth of penetration beyond 5 to 7 cm and the wider area of visualization required along the greater curvature. The role of FNA in nodal staging has not been well evaluated; however, EUS-guided FNA cytology may improve diagnostic yield when the endosonographic features of malignant involvement are not clear.

M Staging

EUS has a limited role in the detection of metastatic disease such as ascites and peritoneal and liver metastases, with an overall pooled sensitivity of 73.2%.[49] In a recent study involving 234 patients by Hassan and colleagues,[55] 42% of patients had positive EUS-guided FNA when targeting distant metastases based on echo features and location. The majority of sampled lesions were mediastinal nodes. EUS-guided FNA changed the subsequent management by precluding surgery in 15% of these patients. Endosonographic detection and FNA of ascites or pleural effusion also improves tumor staging.[56]

TABLE 12-4

ACCURACY OF EUS IN GASTRIC CANCER STAGING IN N CATEGORY

Authors (year)	Frequency (MHz)	Patients (n)	N (%)	N0 (%)	N1 (%)	N2 (%)	N3 (%)
Tio et al[26] (1989)	7.5-12	72	68	50	62	90	—
Botet et al[28] (1991)	7.5-12	50	78	91	68	82	—
Caletti et al[53] (1993)	7.5-12	35	69	—	—	—	—
Dittler and Siewert[30] (1993)	7.5-12	254	66	93	65	52	—
Grimm et al[31] (1993)	7.5	148	83	79	46	91	—
Ziegler et al[32] (1993)	7.5-12	108	74	71	74	100	—
Massari et al[33] (1996)	7.5-12	56	68	58	65	73	—
Perng et al[34] (1996)	7.5-12	69	65	75	53	60	—
Wang et al[22] (1998)	7.5-12	119	68	73	69	52	—
Willis et al[36] (2000)	7.5-12	116	77	82	75	64	—
Habermann et al[37] (2004)	7.5-12	51	90	100	83	84	—
Tsendsuren et al[38] (2006)	7.5	41	66	100	41	—	—
Ganpathi et al[14] (2006)	7.5-20	126	83	74	78	54	50
Bentrem et al[39] (2007)	7.5-12	225	71	72	69 (N+)	—	—
Lok et al[40] (2008)	5-20	123	75	85	69 (N+)	—	—
Repiso et al[41] (2010)	7.5-20	46	58	—	88 (N+)	—	—

The presence of ascites correlates well with the depth of tumor invasion and lymph node metastases but does not correlate with peritoneal carcinomatosis found at surgery. In a study of 301 patients with gastric cancer that compared the sensitivity of different diagnostic techniques for predicting peritoneal metastases, EUS was more sensitive (87.1%) than combined ultrasound with CT (16.1%) and laparoscopy or laparotomy (40.9%).[57] In a study by Chu and colleagues,[58] 402 consecutive patients with histopathologically confirmed gastric adenocarcinoma underwent mini-probe EUS, and the accuracy of mini-probe EUS for the detection of ascites was compared with findings at laparoscopy or laparotomy. Compared with laparoscopy or laparotomy, EUS was 60.7% sensitive and 99.4% specific for detecting ascites. In addition, EUS-detected peritoneal metastasis in 63.9% of patients with ascites and in 11.3% of patients without ascites. These studies indicate that EUS has a high specificity and moderate sensitivity for the detection of ascites.

Limitations of EUS in Staging

Interpretation of EUS findings is an important factor that restricts staging accuracy. The true accuracy of EUS in staging gastric cancer is still unclear because studies with blinding of the endosonographer have not been performed, and the accuracy of EUS may be overstated. Meining and colleagues[59] videotaped 33 EUS studies performed to stage gastric cancer. The videos were independently reviewed and the tumors staged by proceduralists who were unaware of the clinical history. Tumor staging was compared to the initial, unblinded EUS assessment obtained during routine clinical evaluation. Overall accuracy for T staging was higher from proceduralists who were aware of the clinical history compared to those who were not (66.7% versus 45.5%).

There is substantial interobserver variability in interpretation of EUS findings. Meining and colleagues[60] subsequently assessed interobserver variability among five blinded experienced examiners in determining T and N staging for gastric cancer in 55 patients. Kappa (κ) values for assessing T1, T2, T3, and T4 lesions were 0.47, 0.38, 0.39, and 0.34, respectively, findings consistent with a sizable degree of interobserver variability. Interobserver variability in determining nodal stage was even greater, with κ values of 0.46, 0.34, and 0.34 for N0, N1, and N2 stages, respectively. The learning curve for accurate gastric cancer staging by individual endosonographers has not been assessed.

TABLE 12-5

META-ANALYSIS OF STUDIES FOR EUS AND STAGING OF GASTRIC CANCER

Authors (year)	Studies (n)	Patients (n)	Results	Stage				N (positive vs negative)
				T1	T2	T3	T4	
Mocellin et al[51] (2011)	54	5601	Overall sensitivity (95% CI)	0.83 (0.77-0.88)	0.65 (0.57-0.89)	0.86 (0.83-0.89)	0.66 (0.52-0.77)	0.69 (0.63-0.74)
			Overall specificity (95% CI)	0.96 (0.93-0.97)	0.91 (0.88-0.92)	0.85 (0.80-0.89)	0.98 (0.97-0.98)	0.84 (0.81-0.88)
Cardosa et al[50] (2012)	22	2445	Overall Accuracy (95% CI)	0.74 (0.70-0.84)	0.65 (0.53-0.73)	0.85 (0.82-0.88)	0.79 (0.68-0.90)	0.64 (0.43-0.84)

Clinicopathologic features such as tumor location, size, and histologic type may affect diagnostic performance of EUS. Kim and colleagues[61] found inaccurate T staging was more common with undifferentiated histologic type and larger tumor size. Tumor size larger than 3 cm was associated with overstaging by EUS, and tumors with poorly differentiated histology were associated with understaging. It needs to be determined whether these clinicopathologic features affect the diagnostic performance of EUS in differentiating early from locally advanced gastric cancers.

Microscopic submucosal tumor invasion less than 500 μm can be difficult to diagnose on endoscopic ultrasound. False-positive results may be reduced by using pattern analysis, particularly for tumors with ulceration or surrounding fibrosis.[62] Whereas EUS has a high sensitivity in diagnosis of locally advanced gastric cancer, overstaging of T2 cancers can occur. Kutup and colleagues[63] showed that overstaging occurred at a rate of 45% for T and 43% for N status. The differentiation between T1/2 N0 and T3/4 or any N+ is important, as the latter groups will benefit from neoadjuvant or adjuvant therapy and therefore overstaging can result in incorrect assignment for treatment. Overstaging is more common than understaging, with Meyer and colleagues reporting a rate of 46% versus 11% between both.[64]

Tumor location (cardia, fundus, the lesser curve at the incisura, and the pyloric channel) and vascular pulsation, breathing motion, air bubbles, and mucus can affect tumor staging. Contrast-enhanced harmonic EUS, EUS elastography, or three-dimensional EUS, which is still in evolution, have shown promise in improving the staging accuracy.[65]

Comparison of EUS with Other Imaging Modalities

CT has been the primary method for staging gastric cancer. EUS is superior to CT in its ability to study the gastric wall layers (T stage), but it is not as accurate for the assessment of nodal disease and distant metastasis (Tables 12-6 and 12-7). In an early study by Ziegler and colleagues,[32] CT failed to detect six lesions and overstaged T1 lesions in 12 of 22 patients. Newer studies using multidetector CT (MDCT) yield better results. Hwang and colleagues[66] compared staging with MDCT to EUS and showed comparable overall accuracy of 75% versus 77%, respectively, between these modalities.

A systematic review showed the diagnostic accuracy of T staging with EUS, CT, and magnetic resonance imaging (MRI) was between 65% and 92.1%, 77.1% and 88.9%, and 71.4% and 82.6%, respectively.[71] Sensitivity for assessing T4 (serosal) involvement for EUS, CT, and MRI varied between 77.8% and 100%, 82.8% and 100%, and 89.5% and 93.1%, respectively. Specificity for assessing T4 (serosal) involvement for EUS, CT, and MRI varied between 67.9% and 100%, 80% and 96.8%, and 91.4% and 100%, respectively.[71] The same investigators systematically reviewed the role of imaging in lymph node status (N stage). The median sensitivities and specificities for each modality were as follows: EUS, 71% sensitivity and 49% specificity; MDCT, 80% sensitivity and 78% specificity; and MRI, 68% sensitivity and 75% specificity.[72] Although EUS, MDCT, and MRI achieved similar results in terms of diagnostic accuracy for T and N staging, CT offers a better modality for assessing distant metastases (M stage).

TABLE 12-6

COMPARISON OF T STAGING ACCURACY OF GASTRIC CANCER WITH EUS, COMPUTED TOMOGRAPHY, AND MAGNETIC RESONANCE IMAGING

Authors (year)	Patients (n)	EUS (%)	CT (%)	MRI (%)
Botet et al[9] (1991)	50	92	42	—
Grimm et al[31] (1993)	118	82	11	—
Ziegler et al[32] (1993)	108	86	43	—
Kuntz and Herfarth[67] (1999)	82	73	51	48
Polkowski et al[15] (2004)[a]	88	63	44	—
Bhandari et al[68] (2004)[a]	63	88	83	—
Arocena et al[69] (2006)	17	35	—	53
Hwang et al[66] (2009)[a]	277	75	77	—

[a]Multidetector row CT (MDCT).
CT, computed tomography; EUS, endoscopic ultrasound; MRI, magnetic resonance imaging.

A recent systematic review compared the ability of different imaging modalities for assessing distant metastases.[73] The pooled sensitivity and specificity for detecting "peritoneal" metastases was 34% and 96% for EUS, versus 33% and 99% for CT, versus 28% and 97% for [18]FDG PET, versus 9% and 99% for conventional ultrasound, respectively. In the same study, the pooled sensitivity and specificity for detecting liver metastases was 74% and 99% for CT, versus 70% and 96% for [18]FDG PET, versus 54% and 99% for conventional ultrasound, respectively. There were not enough studies on EUS to do a pooled analysis for the latter parameter.

In summary, the most experience has been with EUS. Fewer studies are available for MDCT and even fewer for MRI or [18]FDG PET. The performance of integrated PET CT scans and functional MRI in gastric cancer still needs to be determined. EUS remains superior in diagnosing the depth of gastric cancer invasion, and CT is preferred for the diagnosis

TABLE 12-7

COMPARISON OF N STAGING ACCURACY OF GASTRIC CANCER WITH EUS, COMPUTED TOMOGRAPHY, AND MAGNETIC RESONANCE IMAGING

Authors (year)	Patients (n)	EUS (%)	CT (%)	MRI (%)
Botet et al[70] (1991)	50	78	48	—
Grimm et al[31] (1993)	118	88	21	—
Ziegler et al[32] (1993)	108	74	51	—
Kuntz and Herfarth[67] (1999)	82	87	65	69
Polkowski et al[15] (2004)[a]	60	30	47	—
Bhandari et al[68] (2004)[a]	48	79	75	—
Arocena et al[69] (2006)	—	54	—	50
Hwang et al[66] (2009)[a]	277	66	63	—

[a]Multidetector row CT (MDCT).
CT, computed tomography; EUS, endoscopic ultrasound; MRI, magnetic resonance imaging.

of distant metastases. Therefore, these technologies are complementary for overall staging.

EUS in the Management of Gastric Cancer

The role of EUS in the management of gastric cancer is outlined in Figure 12-9. In addition to staging, EUS is useful in the following situations.

Selection of Patients for Endoscopic Resection

Endoscopic resection may be suitable for early gastric cancer with low risk of lymph node metastasis and a high likelihood of en bloc resection. Endoscopic resection is minimally invasive, preserves the stomach, is low cost, and has good post-procedural morbidity and quality of life outcomes. It is both a staging procedure and curative for early gastric cancer and does not preclude subsequent gastrectomy if the resection is incomplete or there is unfavorable histology. According to the Japanese Gastric Cancer Treatment Guidelines 2010,[6] endoscopic resection is reserved for intramucosal (T1a) lesions of differentiated (intestinal) type that are 2 cm or less in size. Expanded indications for investigational studies of endoscopic resection have also been proposed. ESD has a number of potential advantages over EMR for early gastric cancer. In a recent meta-analysis,[74] ESD had a higher rate of en bloc resection, histologically complete resection, and lower local

recurrence compared to EMR, but a higher risk of perforation. Given the importance of lesion evaluation and en bloc resection, endoscopic resection should ideally be performed at centers with experience.

Improved Patient Selection for Staging Laparoscopy

Metastatic disease such as peritoneal involvement is not well visualized on CT imaging,[75] and laparoscopy is recommended as a staging procedure for patients with apparent localized gastric cancer.[76] In a prospective study of 94 patients with localized gastric cancer who underwent staging EUS followed by laparoscopy, metastatic disease was noted in 4% of patients with T1 or T2, N0 disease as compared with 25% of patients, T3 or T4 or N+ disease.[11] The negative predictive value for metastatic disease in patients staged T1 or T2, N0 by EUS was 96%. This finding suggests that staging laparoscopy could be used selectively in those with T3 or T4 or N+ disease as staged by EUS.

Predictor of Survival After Neoadjuvant Chemotherapy

In a prospective study of 40 patients with locally advanced gastric cancer, patients underwent CT and EUS before and after neoadjuvant chemotherapy, followed by surgical treatment.[77] After chemotherapy, the accuracy of CT and EUS was 57% versus 47% for T staging and 37% versus 39% for N staging, respectively. The 3-year overall survival rate for patients downstaged with EUS for T or N classification was greater than that for patients who were not downstaged (69% versus 41%). In addition, the 2-year recurrence-free survival rate was better for the EUS-downstaged patients than for the patients who were not downstaged (77% versus 47%). Conversely, there was no difference in survival or recurrence-free survival rates in patients downstaged or not downstaged using CT.

EUS-Detected Low-Volume Ascites as a Predictor of Inoperability

EUS is more sensitive in detecting ascites than transabdominal US, CT, laparoscopy, or laparotomy.[57,78] In a study of 21 patients who underwent staging laparoscopy after detection of low-volume ascites at EUS,[79] the presence of ascites on EUS was indicative of inoperable disease in 76%. Eleven patients were deemed inoperable at laparoscopy, and of the 10 patients who were assessed as suitable for surgery, only 5 underwent curative resection. EUS-guided FNA of low-volume ascites can be performed safely, with a diagnostic accuracy of nearly 80%.[80]

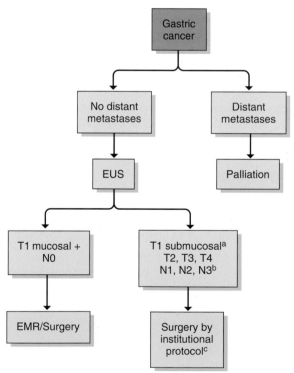

^cNeoadjuvant/adjuvant therapy
^aIn Japan, some patients with T$_1$ submucosal N$_0$ disease undergo endoscopic submucosal dissection.
^bN3 - staged as T4 disease

FIGURE 12-9 EUS-based algorithmic approach to the management of gastric cancer. EMR, endoscopic mucosal resection.

Gastric Cancer: Examination Check List
Primary tumor: depth of penetration
Regional lymph nodes: perigastric region, celiac axis, gastrohepatic ligament
Left lobe of the liver: metastatic deposits
Peritoneum: low-volume malignant ascites
Pleural lining: malignant effusion
Mediastinal lymph nodes: metastatic spread

Primary Gastric Non-Hodgkin Lymphoma

The stomach is the most common extranodal site of non-Hodgkin lymphoma (NHL) and accounts for nearly 70% of all lymphomas that involve the gastrointestinal tract.[81,82] The stomach can harbor primary NHL, or it may be involved secondarily by disseminated nodal disease. Most primary gastric lymphomas are either the extranodal marginal zone B-cell lymphoma of mucosa-associated lymphoid tissue (MALT) type or diffuse large B-cell lymphoma (DLBCL). Other rare types include mantle cell lymphoma, follicular lymphomas, and peripheral T-cell lymphoma. The management of primary NHL is based on tumor staging, and EUS is regarded as the most accurate modality for local staging of gastric lymphoma.[83–87] Secondary gastric NHL, which occurs in 20% to 60% of newly diagnosed cases, reflects disseminated disease that requires extensive diagnostic and systemic treatment strategies. This chapter focuses mainly on the role of EUS in the evaluation of primary gastric NHL.

Diffuse Large B-Cell Lymphoma

DLBCL was previously known as high-grade MALT lymphoma. Patients with DLBCL tend to have a more advanced-stage disease at initial presentation and present with severe systemic symptoms such as abdominal pain, gastric outlet obstruction, bleeding, or perforation.[88,89] Upper endoscopy may reveal large, multiple ulcers or a protruding exophytic mass. Histology reveals confluent sheets or clusters of large cells that resemble centroblasts or immunoblasts.[90] These tumors are cytogenetically, biologically, and clinically different from MALT lymphoma and have a worse prognosis. The term *high-grade MALT lymphoma* should be avoided for DLBCL, because it may lead to inappropriate undertreatment. Although EUS may help to determine the depth of tumor penetration into the gastric wall, local staging alone has a lesser impact, given the extent of disease and the multimodality treatment involved in the care of these patients.

Mucosa-Associated Lymphoid Tissue Lymphoma

MALT lymphoma is a low-grade disease that can occur anywhere in the gastrointestinal tract, but it is most commonly found in the stomach.[91,92] The stomach does not normally contain an appreciable amount of lymphoid tissue. However, stimulation by *Helicobacter pylori* may lead to the development of lymphoid tissue populated by B cells and CD4+ lymphocytes that are recruited to the gastric mucosa. Further stimulation by *H. pylori* leads to the formation of centrocyte-like cells that arise from the marginal zone of the lymphoid tissue and result in a monoclonal population of B cells known as MALT lymphoma.[93,94] More than 90% of patients with MALT lymphoma are infected with *H. pylori*. Although several studies suggested a causative association between *H. pylori* and MALT lymphoma,[95,97,98] the strongest evidence is demonstrated disease regression following eradication of *H. pylori*.[99–101]

Most patients with early stage MALT lymphoma are asymptomatic or present with nonspecific symptoms such as epigastric pain or discomfort, anorexia, weight loss, nausea or vomiting, occult gastrointestinal bleeding, and early satiety.[82,91,92] The diagnosis of gastric lymphoma is usually established by upper endoscopy with biopsy. Findings on upper endoscopy are diverse and may include mucosal erythema, a mass or polypoid lesion with or without ulceration, benign-appearing gastric ulcer and nodularity, or thickened gastric folds.[102,103] In one study, 27 of 51 cases of MALT lymphoma were reported as benign based on biopsy results.[104] Therefore multiple biopsy specimens should be obtained from the stomach, the duodenum, and the gastroesophageal junction, from both normal- and abnormal-appearing gastric mucosa, using large biopsy specimens where possible. Standard biopsy forceps may miss the diagnosis because gastric lymphoma can infiltrate the submucosa without affecting the mucosa; this occurrence is most likely in the absense of an obvious mass. Snare biopsies, biopsies within biopsies, and needle aspiration can increase diagnostic yield in such cases.[105,106]

Endoscopic biopsies determine whether the patient is infected with *H. pylori*. Once a diagnosis of MALT lymphoma is established, further workup includes serologic testing for any underlying viral illness, EUS for tumor local staging, and CT of the chest, abdomen, and pelvis. The disease pattern imaged by EUS may correlate with the type of lymphoma. In one series, for example, superficial spreading or diffuse infiltrating lesions on EUS were seen with MALT lymphoma, whereas mass-forming lesions were typical of DLBCL.[83] The need for PET scan or bone marrow biopsy depends on the disease extent.

In general, patients with early stage (mucosal or submucosal disease without lymph node involvement) *H. pylori*–positive lymphoma are initially treated by *H. pylori* eradication. Patients without *H. pylori* infection and tumors with the t(11;18) translocation are typically treated with local radiation. Patients with more advanced-stage (>T2, N+) disease are treated with *H. pylori* eradication therapy if they are *H. pylori* positive and then are either observed until the development of symptoms or given more aggressive chemotherapy or immunotherapy.[107] Gastric resection is reserved for patients with complications such as perforation or obstruction.[108] The management of MALT lymphoma is stage dependent, and EUS is currently considered the most accurate modality for local staging.

Role of EUS in MALT Lymphoma

The role of EUS in the management of MALT lymphoma can be categorized as follows (Figure 12-10):

- Local staging of disease: EUS evaluates the depth of gastric wall involvement and the presence of perigastric lymphadenopathy. *H. pylori*–positive patients with mucosal or submucosal disease may respond to antimicrobial treatment, and those with T2 to T4 disease may require more aggressive treatment protocols. EUS alone has suboptimal accuracy in distinguishing benign from malignant lymph nodes.[48,109] When combined with FNA, the overall accuracy approaches 90% (versus 66% for EUS alone).[110] Higher accuracy is achieved when flow cytometry is performed on the FNA aspirate.[111]

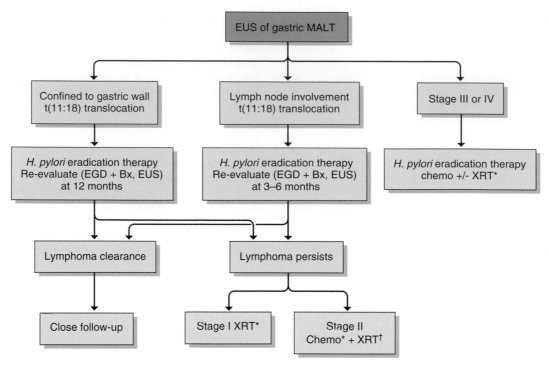

*Chemo: according to institutional protocol
†XRT: external radiation therapy according to institutional protocol

FIGURE 12-10   Algorithmic approach to the management of mucosa-associated lymphoid tissue (MALT) lymphoma. Bx, biopsy; EGD, esophago-gastroduodenoscopy. *(Adapted from Yoon S, Coit D, Portlock C, Karpeh M. The diminishing role of surgery in the treatment of gastric lymphoma. Ann Surg. 2004;240:28-37.)*

- Tissue diagnosis: MALT lymphoma is best diagnosed by endoscopic biopsies. In the rare patient with thickened gastric folds in whom all endoscopic biopsy results are unrevealing, EUS-guided FNA or core tissue sampling of the deeper wall layers may be diagnostic.[112]
- Predicting response to therapy: There is a direct relationship between tumor grading by EUS and response to therapy.[29] Patients with mucosal and submucosal disease have better clinical outcomes compared with patients with deeper wall layer involvement (Table 12-8).
- Post-treatment follow-up: EUS may show restoration of normal gastric wall layers or significant reduction in thickness of the wall layers following successful treatment.[113] Patients with persistently thick gastric wall layers are more likely to have residual disease, even when endoscopic biopsy is negative.

Examination Technique and Disease Correlates

The procedural technique for EUS evaluation of MALT lymphoma is similar to that described for evaluation of gastric cancer. Given the diffuse nature of the disease process, a radial echoendoscope is usually preferred for tumor staging with examinations performed at frequencies of 7.5 and 12 MHz.

T Staging

EUS assessment of the depth of lymphoma infiltration is based on the TNM classification, and the extent of wall layer involvement.[114] The modified Ann Arbor classification has been used to categorize the disease process in multiple studies (Tables 12-9 and 12-10).[115]

T1: Tumor located in the mucosa and/or submucosa (Figure 12-11)

TABLE 12-8

TREATMENT RESPONSE OF MALT LYMPHOMA ACCORDING TO EUS STAGING

Response	T1mN0	T1smN0	T2N0	T1mN1	T1smN1
Complete response	12 (75%)	11 (58%)	1 (25%)	2 (50%)	2 (50%)
Persistent disease or relapse	4 (25%)	8 (42%)	3 (75%)	2 (50%)	2 (50%)

(From Caletti G, Zinzani P, Fusaroli P, et al. The importance of endoscopic ultrasonography in the management of low-grade gastric mucosa-associated lymphoid tissue lymphoma. Aliment Pharmacol Ther. 2002;16:1715-1722.)

TABLE 12-9

ANN ARBOR CLASSIFICATION, MODIFIED BY MUSSHOFF AND SCHMIDT-VOLLMER

Grade	Description
IE	Lymphoma restricted to GI tract on one side of diaphragm
IE1	Infiltration limited to mucosa and submucosa
IE2	Lymphoma extending beyond submucosa
IIE	Lymphoma additionally infiltrating lymph nodes on same side of diaphragm
IIE1	Infiltration of regional lymph nodes
IIE2	Infiltration of lymph nodes beyond regional nodes
IIIE	Lymphoma infiltrating gastrointestinal tract and/or lymph nodes on both sides of diaphragm
IVE	Localized infiltration of associated lymph nodes together with diffuse or disseminated involvement of extragastrointestinal organs

(From Musshoff K, Schmidt-Vollmer H. Proceedings: prognosis of non-Hodgkin's lymphomas with special emphasis on the staging classification. Z Krebsforsch Klin Onkol Cancer Res Clin Oncol. 1975;83:323-341.)

T2: Tumor infiltration into the muscularis propria (Figure 12-12)
T3: Tumor penetration into the subserosa (Figure 12-13)
T4: Tumor infiltration into adjacent structures (Figure 12-14)

N Staging

EUS can detect lymph nodes as small as 3 to 4 mm. However, it is not possible to differentiate benign from malignant lymph nodes by EUS imaging alone, and EUS-guided FNA increases the accuracy of detecting lymph node involvement. Rounded, sharply demarcated, homogeneous, hypoechoic lymph nodes greater than 1 cm in diameter are predictive of malignancy, whereas elongated, heterogeneous, hyperechoic lymph nodes with indistinct borders are more likely to be benign.[70] However, assessment of these features is highly operator dependent, and they may not be present with microscopic disease.

Accuracy of EUS in Staging MALT Lymphoma

EUS features that differentiate it from cancer include the following: (1) infiltrative gastric cancer typically grows vertically (transmural) through the gastric wall and lymphoma grows

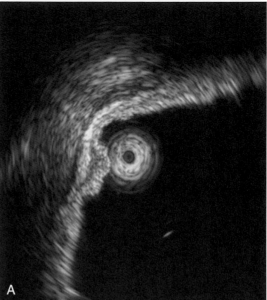
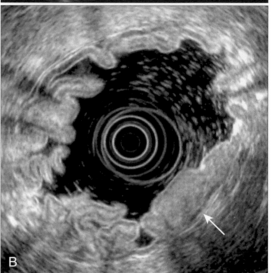

FIGURE 12-11 Staging of lymphoma. **A,** Small sessile lesion confined to the mucosal layer (T1m) as visualized using a 12-MHz mini-probe. **B,** Lymphomatous changes involving the submucosal layer (T1sm) but without infiltration of the muscularis propria *(arrow)*.

horizontally; (2) gastric wall thickening is typically more diffuse and homogeneous in lymphoma than in gastric cancer; (3) lymphoma rarely results in luminal narrowing and obstruction, even in the presence of diffuse infiltration, and it most commonly involves the distal half of the stomach; also, in contrast to gastric adenocarcinoma, lymphoma is often multifocal within the stomach; (4) at an early stage, lymphomas can manifest with thickening of the second layer alone or separately in the second and third layers with preservation of layer architecture; in advanced stages, lymphomas show diffuse thickening with fusion of wall layers; and (5) diffuse and superficial infiltration is more often indicative of a low-grade MALT lymphoma, whereas the presence of masses is more frequently associated with aggressive high-grade lymphomas.[104]

TABLE 12-10

COMPARISON OF MODIFIED ANN ARBOR AND TNM CLASSIFICATIONS

Ann Arbor	TNM	Comment
IE1	T1m-smN0	Mucosa, submucosa
IE2	T2-4N0	Muscularis propria
IIE1	T1-4N1	Perigastric lymph nodes
IIE2	T1-4N2	Regional lymph nodes
IIIE	T1-4N3	Lymph nodes on both sides of diaphragm
IVE	T1-4N0-3M1	Visceral metastases or second extranodal site

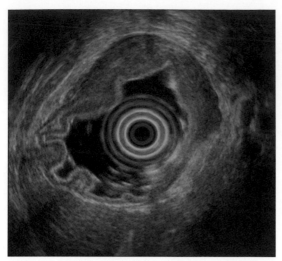

FIGURE 12-12   Radial scanning at 12 MHz revealing lymphoma infiltrating the muscularis propria (T2).

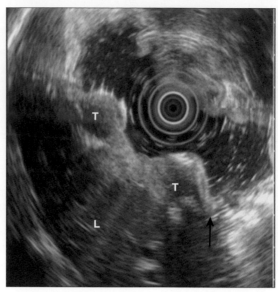

FIGURE 12-14   High-grade gastric lymphoma infiltrating all the wall layers *(arrow)* and into the perigastric structures (liver, L), consistent with T4 disease. T, tumor.

Gastric lymphoma stage is a crucial prognostic factor required for therapeutic planning; however, staging is controversial. As previously described, several staging classifications for MALT lymphomas have been applied (Table 12-11). The commonly used classifications for EUS staging are the TNM and the modified Ann Arbor systems (see Table 12-10). TNM staging differentiates the degree of mural involvement layer by layer, whereas the modified Ann Arbor classification uses only two stages of mural involvement. The TNM staging system was originally developed for gastric cancer and was modified for primary gastrointestinal lymphoma and termed the Paris classification system.[116] This system records the depth of the tumor infiltration into the gastric layers (T category), extent of nodal involvement (N category), and evidence of extranodal metastases (M category). The modified Ann Arbor stage IE$_1$ corresponds to T1a and T1b, and stage

IE$_2$ corresponds to multiple stages including T2, T3, and T4. The Lugano classification system incorporates stage IIE for penetration of serosa involving the adjacent organs into the modified Ann Arbor system.[117] The modified Ann Arbor staging system is generally considered inadequate for prognostic staging, and the TNM system is most commonly used.

EUS is the most accurate imaging modality for the evaluation and staging of gastric lymphomas. Most studies were conducted when surgical resection was standard. The accuracy of EUS T staging is 80% to 90% (Table 12-12). In a single-center experience reported by Caletti and colleagues,[48] the sensitivity and specificity of EUS were 89% and 97%, respectively. In a large study reported by Fischbach and colleagues[100] involving 34 centers using the modified Ann Arbor classification, data from preoperative EUS were compared with the histologic stage at resection. The sensitivities for stages IE1, IE2, and IIE2 were 67%, 83%, and 71%, respectively. The majority of centers had low patient numbers, potentially impacting EUS accuracy.

EUS accuracy of lymph node detection is 77% to 90% (see Table 12-12). The distinction between benign and malignant lymph nodes is challenging. The interpretation is operator dependent, and lymph node micrometastases may be missed; EUS-guided FNA of suspicious lymph nodes may overcome this limitation.[110]

Yasuda and colleagues[121] achieved a positive diagnosis in 96% of lymphomas (48 of 50 cases) by using a 19-G EUS-guided FNA needle. In another study, the overall sensitivity, specificity, and accuracy of EUS-guided FNA for the diagnosis of lymphoma was 74%, 93%, and 81%, respectively, when combined with flow cytometry and immunohistochemistry.[111] However, these studies did not focus on primary gastric MALT, and further studies will be necessary to define the role of these techniques.

CT is preferred to EUS for evaluation of distant metastases. Comparative studies between MRI and PET CT scans and EUS

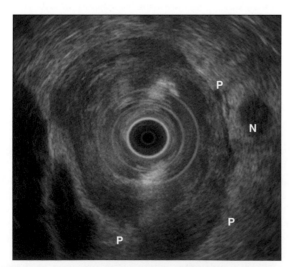

FIGURE 12-13   Radial image revealing infiltration of the subserosal connective tissue (pseudopodia, P) by the lymphoma and the presence of peritumoral lymph nodes (N) (T3N1).

TABLE 12-11

COMPARISON OF STAGING CLASSIFICATIONS FOR MALT LYMPHOMAS

Lymphoma Extension	TNM Modifications in the Paris System[117]	Musshoff Modified Ann Arbor Staging[118]	Lugano Staging[116]
Mucosa	T1mN0M0	IE_1	Stage I: confined to GI tract (single primary or multiple, noncontiguous)
Submucosa	T1smN0M0	IE_2	
Muscularis propria serosa	T2N0M0 T3N0M0		
Perigastric lymph nodes	T1-3N1M0	IIE_1	Stage II: extending into the abdomen (stage II_1: local nodal involvement; stage II_2: distant nodal involvement)
More distant regional nodes	T1-3N2M0	IIE_2	
Extra-abdominal lymph nodes	T1-3N3M0	—	
Invasion of adjacent tissues	—	IE	Stage II_E: penetration of serosa to involving adjacent organs or tissues
Lymph nodes on both sides of the diaphragm, and/or additional extranodal sites with noncontinuous involvement of separate GI sites	T1-4N3M0	IIIE	
Or noncontinuous involvement of non-GI sites	T1-4N0-3M1 T1-4N0-3M2	IVE	Stage I: disseminated extranodal involvement or concomitant supradiaphragmatic nodal involvement
Bone marrow not assessed	T1-4N0-3M0-2 BX	—	
Bone marrow not involved	T1-4N0-3M0-2 B0	—	
Bone marrow involved	T1-4N0-3M2 B1	—	

(Adapted from Ferrucci P, Zucca E. Primary gastric lymphoma pathogenesis and treatment: what has changed over the past 10 years? Br J Haematol. 2007;136:521-538.)
GI, gastrointestinal.

are lacking. High-resolution mini-probes are good for differentiating superficial gastric wall layers and targeting smaller lesions. Lügering and colleagues[122] studied the use of mini-probes (12 MHz) for staging of gastric lymphoma and reported a superior performance when compared with echoendoscopes. These investigators recommended the use of mini-probes in clinical practice, as the examination can be performed as a single-step procedure during diagnostic endoscopy. However, mini-probes are not ideal for lymph node staging.

TABLE 12-12

ACCURACY OF EUS IN STAGING GASTRIC LYMPHOMA

Authors (year)	Patients (n)	T Stage (%)	N Stage (%)
Fujishima et al[109] (1991)	11	91	82
Caletti et al[53] (1993)	44	92	77
Suekane et al[83] (1993)	15	n/a	83
Schüeder et al[119] (1993)	10	80	90
Palazzo et al[84] (1993)	24	91	83
Fischbach et al[120] (2002)	70	59	71

n/a, not applicable.
(Adapted from Fischbach W. Staging role of EUS. Best Pract Res Clin Gastroenterol. 2010;24:13-17.)

Role of EUS in Predicting Response to Therapy

Low-grade MALT lymphomas account for approximately 35% of primary gastric lymphomas, and accurate EUS staging and follow-up is essential to guide treatment. EUS can predict the outcome of treatment of MALT lymphoma by simple eradication of *H. pylori*. Although encouraging results of antibiotic treatment have been reported, many authors have failed either to include EUS in their staging methods or to correlate EUS staging results, when available, with remission rates. EUS shows promise in predicting response to therapy in patients with localized disease, and few patients with deeper infiltration have a lower likelihood of complete response.[100,123] In an early pilot study of 22 patients, Sackmann and colleagues[124] investigated whether staging by EUS predicted the outcome of MALT lymphoma treatment by *H. pylori* eradication. *H. pylori* was eradicated in all patients. After a median follow-up of 10 months, complete remission was achieved in 12 of 14 patients with lymphoma limited to the second or third layer (mucosa or submucosa) at EUS, compared with none of 10 patients with deeper gastric wall involvement. Thus, EUS may help differentiate which patients are suitable for antibiotic therapy alone and who should be referred for additional oncologic treatment.

Ruskoné-Fourmestraux and colleagues[125] evaluated predictive factors for regression of gastric MALT lymphoma following *H. pylori* treatment. A total of 44 consecutive patients with localized gastric MALT lymphoma (Ann Arbor stages IE and IIE) underwent EUS and *H. pylori* eradication. Overall, histologic regression of the lymphoma was seen in only 43% of the patients; median follow-up for these 19 responders was 35 months. The response rate was significantly different between patients with disease restricted to the mucosa and those with deeper lymphoma involvement. The complete response rate increased from 56% for patients with nodal involvement to 79% when no nodal involvement was found at EUS. The investigators concluded that the absence of lymph node involvement was predictive of successful treatment response.

Nakamura and colleagues[126] found that 93% of MALT lymphomas restricted to the mucosa completely regressed after therapy as compared with only 23% of lymphomas involving the submucosa. The presence of a high-grade component or perigastric lymphadenopathy, or clinical staging before eradication therapy, correlated poorly with lymphoma regression. Levy and colleagues[127] noted a 69% overall complete response rate in 48 patients treated for *H. pylori* infection. The response rate did not correlate with endoscopic features or histologic grade. In contrast, when EUS features were taken into account, remission was achieved in 76% of patients who had no detectable perigastric lymph nodes as compared with only 33% of patients with detectable lymph nodes. Remission was achieved with chlorambucil monochemotherapy in 58% of patients who did not respond to *H. pylori* treatment. In the multicenter Italian study by Caletti and colleagues,[128] 51 patients with low-grade MALT lymphomas had successful *H. pylori* eradication in 45 (88%) patients. Two years after therapy, regression of lymphoma was noted in 28 (55%). Complete response was achieved in 12 (75%) of 16 patients with T1aN0 disease and in 11 (58%) of 19 patients with stage T1bN0 disease compared with only 4 (50%) of 8 patients with stage T1aN1 and T1bN1 and 1 of 4 (25%) patients with stage T2N0 disease. No patients with T2N1 disease achieved a complete response (see Table 12-8).

A more recent multicenter trial aimed to determine the long-term outcome in patients undergoing *H. pylori* eradication therapy alone.[100] Ninety patients with a low-grade gastric MALT lymphoma were followed for at least 12 months, and successful *H. pylori* eradication was achieved in 88 (98%) patients using a triple regimen. Long-term outcome was characterized by a complete response in 56 patients (62%), minimal residual disease in 17 (19%), partial remission in 11 (12%), no change in 4 (4%), and progressive disease in 2 patients (2%). The regression rate, as assessed by EUS, was higher in stage IE1 disease compared with stage IE2.

In conclusion, accurate EUS staging of MALT lymphoma is important to optimize treatment. Early stage lesions (T1) may regress following *H. pylori* therapy alone, and more advanced lesions (T2 to T4) may require more aggressive treatment protocols, including combination chemotherapy, radiation therapy, and surgery. In addition, assessment of response to therapy requires long-term follow-up with interval upper endoscopy and mapping biopsies in combination with EUS. When biopsy results remain positive for lymphoma but EUS shows no structural wall changes, it may be appropriate to "wait and watch," as *H. pylori* therapy may take up to 18 months to produce complete remission.[129]

Role of EUS in Clinical Follow-Up

EUS surveillance can determine response to therapy and detect early disease recurrence. Correlation of EUS and histology is important, as EUS may show restoration of normal gastric wall layers before complete histologic remission. In addition, recurrent wall thickening or disruption may indicate recurrent disease in patients previously thought to be in remission. Patients with a persistently thickened gastric wall on EUS despite adequate antibiotic therapy should be considered for other treatment modalities, even if endoscopic biopsy is negative, because the likelihood of persistent or recurrent lymphoma is high.[128]

Most studies on EUS for pretreatment staging of gastric MALT lymphoma agree that EUS can be used for post-treatment surveillance. However, given the relative lack of long-term follow-up series, when and how often to perform EUS, the exact clinical and histologic correlations with EUS, and the role of EUS is still being defined. Püspök and colleagues[130] performed 158 EUS examinations in 33 patients with primary gastric lymphoma before and every 3 to 6 months after nonsurgical treatment. Endosonographic remission was defined as a wall thickness ≤4 mm with preserved five-layer structure and the absence of suspicious lymph nodes. At a median follow-up of 15 months, 82% of patients achieved histologic remission, whereas EUS remission was noted in only 64%. Eighteen patients (55%) achieved both histologic and EUS remission, and EUS remission occurred later than histologic remission (35 versus 18 weeks). Moreover, histologic relapse was demonstrated by EUS in only one of five cases. The investigators concluded that none of the tested endosonographic parameters were able to predict histologic remission. The reason for the lack of EUS concordance could be that the investigators did not use the TNM classification for EUS assessment of disease in the gastric wall, leading to underpowering of EUS parameters in predicting remission.

Yeh and colleagues[113] evaluated the role of EUS in 20 patients with low-grade gastric MALT lymphoma before and after *H. pylori* eradication and reached a different conclusion. Of 17 patients who were *H. pylori* positive, 14 (82%) obtained histologic remission. The investigators found that, although pretreatment EUS performed with a 12-MHz mini-probe showed significantly greater wall thickness in patients with MALT lymphoma than in controls (6.1 mm versus 2.8 mm), follow-up showed a comparative and statistically significant reduction in wall thickness. For patients with a significant reduction in wall thickness shortly after *H. pylori* eradication, the probability of a complete response of the MALT lymphoma was 40% at 12 months and 84% at the end of 24 months. Despite the absence of endoscopic lesions, half the patients in the foregoing study had persistent changes noted on EUS. This finding may be interpreted in few ways: (1) EUS tends to over-stage residual disease because it is unable to differentiate between tumor and fibrosis; (2) EUS is able to detect persistent lymphoma residue that is not evident histologically because the cells are limited to the submucosa or deeper layers; or (3) persistence of a B-cell monoclonal pattern of lymphoma cells in the gastric wall has been documented in roughly half of the patients who have had histologic remission using molecular markers.[131,132] The molecular pattern disappears in the majority of patients during follow-up, although this process can be slow and variable. A persistently abnormal EUS with negative histology may not be clinically relevant in all instances, as the majority of patients do not require further treatment.[133] The EUS abnormality often resolves on prolonged follow-up and correlates with histological remission, unlike that seen in "high-grade" gastric lymphomas.[134] The role of EUS in detecting relapse is still unclear, and long-term follow-up studies are required.

EUS is not an alternative to endoscopic biopsies, and both are required to maximize the diagnostic yield for staging and follow-up of patients with gastric MALT lymphoma.

Limitations of Staging EUS

EUS is an operator-dependent technique. Interobserver agreement in assessing MALT lymphoma staging was studied by Fusaroli and colleagues (Italian MALT Lymphoma Study Group)[135] in a multicenter study involving 10 endosonographers. EUS was performed before and after 6 month of treatment in 54 and 42 patients, respectively. Overall, interobserver agreement for T stage was fair, before and after treatment ($\kappa = 0.38$ and $\kappa = 0.37$, respectively). Interobserver agreement for N stage was substantial before treatment, but only fair after treatment ($\kappa = 0.63$ and $\kappa = 0.34$, respectively). The lowest values of agreement were for T1sm ($\kappa = 0.20$) and T2 lesions ($\kappa = 0.33$). Performance between endosonographers was compared, and interobserver agreement correlated with their level of experience. The investigators suggest a baseline of 100 gastric EUS examinations may be associated with better diagnostic performance.

EUS-Based Workup

Patients with advanced disease usually require more aggressive treatment protocols than *H. pylori* positive patients with T1 disease. EUS determines response to therapy and detects early relapse. EUS may show restoration of normal gastric wall layers before evident histologic remission, and recurrent wall thickening or disruption may represent disease recurrence in individuals previously in remission. Patients with a persistently thickened gastric wall on EUS despite antibiotic therapy should be considered for more aggressive treatment, even if endoscopic biopsies are negative, due to the risk of lymphoma.

Evaluation of Thickened Gastric Folds at EUS

The normal five-layered gastric wall is between 0.8 and 3.6 mm on EUS[136] and is considered thickened when it exceeds 4 mm.[28] There are multiple possible causes of thickened gastric folds observed at endoscopy (Table 12-13), and those commonly encountered in clinical practice are linitis plastica, Ménétrier's disease, and lymphoma.

Linitis Plastica

Limited data are available on the endosonographic features of linitis plastica, also known as scirrhous-type gastric cancer. At endoscopy, the gastric folds are thickened and the stomach

TABLE 12-13

DIFFERENTIAL DIAGNOSIS FOR THICKENED GASTRIC FOLDS NOTED AT ENDOSCOPY

Category	Disorder
Malignant diseases	Adenocarcinoma, linitis plastica, lymphoma, metastases
Infections	Secondary syphilis, tuberculosis, cytomegalovirus infection, herpes simplex virus infection, histoplasmosis, cryptococcosis, aspergillosis, *H. pylori* infection, anisakiasis
Infiltrative disorders	Crohn disease, sarcoidosis, amyloidosis, gastritis diseases (eosinophilic, granulomatous, and lymphocytic)
Vascular disorders	Portal hypertensive gastropathy, gastric varices
Other diseases	Ménétrier's disease, Zollinger-Ellison syndrome, hyperrugosity, gastritis cystica profunda

may distend poorly. Histopathologically, linitis plastica is characterized by the diffuse growth of malignant cells with signet ring features, and is usually associated with marked submucosal fibrosis and gastric wall thickening.[137] The diagnosis is often challenging because of the lack of a distinct, protruding lesion and the difficulty in obtaining deeper diagnostic tissue from standard biopsy forceps. Standard biopsies and brushings are negative in up to 30% of cases, particularly those without mucosal lesions.[138] On EUS, linitis plastica is characterized by diffuse thickening of all gastric wall layers,[138] as well as thickening primarily confined to the second, third, and fourth layers of the gastric wall (Figure 12-15).[139] Thickening of the fourth layer is rarely benign, and should raise the concern of linitis plastica in the setting of large gastric folds. Linitis plastica can be diagnosed by EUS-guided FNA following negative endoscopic biopsies.[137] Cytology shows malignant epithelial cells containing eccentric nuclei with foamy cytoplasm (resembling degenerated histiocytes) and rare cells with intracytoplasmic vacuoles and crescent-shaped, hyperchromatic nuclei, characteristic of signet ring cells.

Ménétrier's Disease

Ménétrier's disease is characterized by epithelial hyperplasia involving the surface and foveolar mucous cells. The pathogenesis of Ménétrier's disease is incompletely understood but may involve transforming growth factor-alpha (TGF-α). TGF-α increases gastric mucus production and inhibits acid secretion,[140] and levels are usually elevated in the gastric mucous cells in patients with Ménétrier's disease. Patients typically present with epigastric pain, asthenia, anorexia, weight loss, edema, and vomiting. The enlarged folds are usually confined to the body and fundus of the stomach. The folds are frequently symmetrically enlarged, although asymmetrical enlargement with a polypoid appearance can occur. Full-thickness biopsy is usually required for diagnosis, which

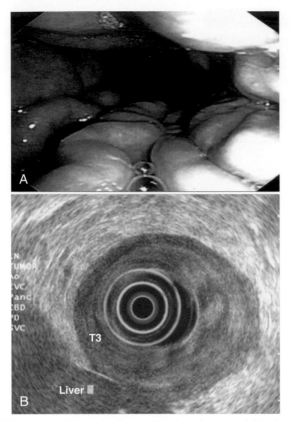

FIGURE 12-15 Linitis plastica. **A**, Thickened gastric folds that are poorly distensible at endoscopy. **B**, At radial scanning, the tumor is seen to involve the upper four layers of the gastric wall, consistent with linitis plastica.

In a prospective study of 61 patients, Gines and colleagues[145] reported that submucosal thickening with or without muscularis propria thickening was the single most important predictor of malignancy. Using this parameter, the probability of having malignancy increased to 95%, whereas it was 5% when only superficial layers were involved. In another study that analyzed the EUS features in 35 patients with giant gastric folds, Ménétrier's disease was suspected when the second layer alone was thickened, and anisakiasis was considered when the third layer alone was thickened. Linitis plastica typically had an abnormally enlarged third and fourth layer. Although the second and third layers could be thickened in healthy subjects with simple hyperrugosity, these layers could also be thickened in patients with gastric lymphoma. Fourth-layer thickening was only seen in malignant conditions. In a study of 21 patients with gastric wall thickening,[147] EUS Tru-Cut biopsy had a sensitivity, specificity, and positive and negative predictive values of 85%, 100%, 100%, and 74%, respectively, for the diagnosis of malignancy. There were no immediate or late complications.

Gastritis cystic profunda is a rare cause of thickened gastric folds in which multiple small cysts are seen in the mucosa and submucosa of the stomach.[148] The diagnosis is usually established by findings at EUS and mucosectomy. EUS should be used in conjunction with endoscopic biopsy and can assist in determining the best site for biopsy to reduce false-negative results.

is established by the demonstration of extreme foveolar hyperplasia with glandular atrophy.[141,142] At EUS (Figure 12-16), Ménétrier's disease displays a more localized thickening, which is hyperechoic rather than hypoechoic, predominantly involving the second gastric layer.[143]

EUS and Large Gastric Folds

The role of EUS in evaluating large gastric folds was assessed in a study of 28 patients, most of whom had endoscopic biopsies inconclusive for malignancy.[144] Biopsies were not performed in four patients because EUS demonstrated gastric varices. Three patients with normal biopsies had wall thickening involving layers 3 and 4 on EUS and were diagnosed with primary gastric carcinoma at laparotomy. In the remaining 21 patients, large-forceps endoscopic biopsy revealed acute or chronic inflammation in 16 (67%), malignancy in 4 (17%), and Ménétrier's disease in 1 (4%). Malignancy did not develop in any of the patients with gastric wall thickening limited to layer 2 during a mean follow-up of 35 months. The investigators concluded that endoscopic biopsies are diagnostic when EUS abnormalities involve the mucosal layer alone. Abnormalities involving the muscularis propria in the absence of ulceration strongly suggest malignancy and should be investigated further if endoscopic biopsies are negative. EUS can also be used to diagnose gastric varices, where biopsies should be avoided.

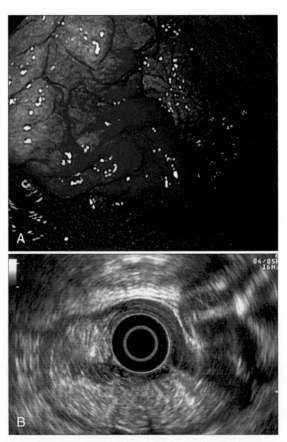

FIGURE 12-16 Ménétrier's disease. **A**, Hypertrophic gastric folds in the fundic region as seen on endoscopy. **B**, On EUS, the second layer of the gastric wall is found to be hyperechoic and thickened, consistent with Ménétrier's disease (proven by surgical resection).

EUS-Based Workup

An algorithmic workup based on EUS findings can be suggested for patients with large gastric folds of unclear origin. For an early diagnosis, when the EUS pattern is normal and endoscopic findings are inconclusive, multiple standard endoscopic biopsies should be performed and large-forceps biopsy or snare biopsy considered. When abnormalities involve layer 2, endoscopic biopsies are diagnostic. When abnormalities involve layers 2 and 3, large-forceps biopsy is appropriate. When abnormalities involve layer 4, malignancy should be strongly suspected even if results of standard biopsies are negative, and EUS-guided FNA or core biopsy should be performed.

REFERENCES

1. Ferlay J, Shin HR, Bray F, et al. GLOBOCAN 2008 v2.0, Cancer Incidence and Mortality Worldwide: IARC CancerBase No. 10 [Internet]. Lyon, France: International Agency for Research on Cancer; 2010 Available from: <http://globocan.iarc.fr>; accessed on 14/09/2013.
2. Siegel R, Naishadham D, Jemal A. Cancer statistics, 2013. CA Cancer J Clin. 2013;63:11-30.
3. Siewert J, Böttcher K, Stein H, Roder J. Relevant prognostic factors in gastric cancer: ten-year results of the German Gastric Cancer Study. Ann Surg. 1998;228:449-461.
4. Nakamura K, Ueyama T, Yao T, et al. Pathology and prognosis of gastric carcinoma. Findings in 10,000 patients who underwent primary gastrectomy. Cancer. 1992;70:1030-1037.
5. Edge SB, Byrd DR, Compton CC, et al., eds. American Joint Committee on Cancer Staging Manual. 7th ed. New York: Springer; 2010:117.
6. Japanese Gastric Cancer Association. Japanese gastric cancer treatement guidelines 2010 (ver. 3). Gastric Cancer. 2011;14:113-123.
7. Macdonald J, Smalley S, Benedetti J, et al. Chemoradiotherapy after surgery compared with surgery alone for adenocarcinoma of the stomach or gastroesophageal junction. N Engl J Med. 2001;345:725-730.
8. Cunningham D, Allum W, Stenning S, et al. Perioperative chemotherapy versus surgery alone for resectable gastroesophageal cancer. N Engl J Med. 2006;355:11-20.
9. Botet J, Lightdale C, Zauber A, et al. Preoperative staging of gastric cancer: comparison of endoscopic US and dynamic CT. Radiology. 1991;181:426-432.
10. Sussman S, Halvorsen RJ, Illescas F, et al. Gastric adenocarcinoma: CT versus surgical staging. Radiology. 1988;167:335-340.
11. Power D, Schattner M, Gerdes H, et al. Endoscopic ultrasound can improve the selection for laparoscopy in patients with localized gastric cancer. J Am Coll Surg. 2009;208:173-178.
12. Mouri R, Yoshida S, Tanaka S, et al. Usefulness of endoscopic ultrasonography in determining the depth of invasion and indication for endoscopic treatment of early gastric cancer. J Clin Gastroenterol. 2009;43:318-322.
13. Blackshaw G, Lewis W, Hopper A, et al. Prospective comparison of endosonography, computed tomography, and histopathological stage of junctional oesophagogastric cancer. Clin Radiol. 2008;63:1092-1098.
14. Ganpathi I, So J, Ho K. Endoscopic ultrasonography for gastric cancer: does it influence treatment? Surg Endosc. 2006;20:559-562.
15. Polkowski M, Palucki J, Wronska E, et al. Endosonography versus helical computed tomography for locoregional staging of gastric cancer. Endoscopy. 2004;36:617-623.
16. Sultan J, Robinson S, Hayes N, et al. Endoscopic ultrasonography-detected low-volume ascites as a predictor of inoperability for oesophagogastric cancer. Br J Surg. 2008;95:1127-1130.
17. Singh P, Mukhopadhyay P, Bhatt B, et al. Endoscopic ultrasound versus CT scan for detection of the metastases to the liver: results of a prospective comparative study. J Clin Gastroenterol. 2009;43:367-373.
18. Edge SB, Byrd DR, Compton CC, et al, eds. AJCC Cancer Staging Manual. 7th ed. New York: Springer; 2010:241-249.
19. Hölscher A, Drebber U, Mönig S, et al. Early gastric cancer: lymph node metastasis starts with deep mucosal infiltration. Ann Surg. 2009;250:791-797.
20. Okamura S, Tsutsui A, Muguruma N, et al. The utility and limitations of an ultrasonic miniprobe in the staging of gastric cancer. J Med Invest. 1999;46:49-53.
21. Bhutani M, Hawes R, Hoffman B. A comparison of the accuracy of echo features during endoscopic ultrasound (EUS) and EUS-guided fine-needle aspiration for diagnosis of malignant lymph node invasion. Gastrointest Endosc. 1997;45:474-479.
22. Wang J, Hsieh J, Huang Y, et al. Endoscopic ultrasonography for preoperative locoregional staging and assessment of resectability in gastric cancer. Clin Imaging. 1998;22:355-359.
23. Prasad P, Schmulewitz N, Patel A, et al. Detection of occult liver metastases during EUS for staging of malignancies. Gastrointest Endosc. 2004;59:49-53.
24. Yoshida S, Tanaka S, Kunihiro K, et al. Diagnostic ability of high-frequency ultrasound probe sonography in staging early gastric cancer, especially for submucosal invasion. Abdom Imaging. 2005;30:518-523.
25. Murata Y, Suzuki S, Hashimoto H. Endoscopic ultrasonography of the upper gastrointestinal tract. Surg Endosc. 1988;2:180-183.
26. Tio T, Schouwink M, Cikot R, Tytgat G. Preoperative TNM classification of gastric carcinoma by endosonography in comparison with the pathological TNM system: a prospective study of 72 cases. Hepatogastroenterology. 1989;36:51-56.
27. Akahoshi K, Misawa T, Fujishima H, et al. Preoperative evaluation of gastric cancer by endoscopic ultrasound. Gut. 1991;32:479-482.
28. Botet J, Lightdale C. Endoscopic sonography of the upper gastrointestinal tract. AJR Am J Roentgenol. 1991;156:63-68.
29. Caletti G, Ferrari A, Bocus P, et al. Endoscopic ultrasonography in gastric lymphoma. Schweiz Med Wochenschr. 1996;126:819-825.
30. Dittler H, Siewert J. Role of endoscopic ultrasonography in esophageal carcinoma. Endoscopy. 1993;25:156-161.
31. Grimm H, Binmoeller K, Hamper K, et al. Endosonography for preoperative locoregional staging of esophageal and gastric cancer. Endoscopy. 1993;25:224-230.
32. Ziegler K, Sanft C, Zimmer T, et al. Comparison of computed tomography, endosonography, and intraoperative assessment in TN staging of gastric carcinoma. Gut. 1993;34:604-610.
33. Massari M, Cioffi U, De Simone M, et al. Endoscopic ultrasonography for preoperative staging of gastric carcinoma. Hepatogastroenterology. 1996;43:542-546.
34. Perng D, Jan C, Wang W, et al. Computed tomography, endoscopic ultrasonography and intraoperative assessment in TN staging of gastric carcinoma. J Formos Med Assoc. 1996;95:378-385.
35. Tseng L, Mo L, Tio T, et al. Video-endoscopic ultrasonography in staging gastric carcinoma. Hepatogastroenterology. 2000;47:897-900.
36. Willis S, Truong S, Gribnitz S, et al. Endoscopic ultrasonography in the preoperative staging of gastric cancer: accuracy and impact on surgical therapy. Surg Endosc. 2000;14:951-954.
37. Habermann C, Weiss F, Riecken R, et al. Preoperative staging of gastric adenocarcinoma: comparison of helical CT and endoscopic US. Radiology. 2004;230:465-471.
38. Tsendsuren T, Jun S, Mian X. Usefulness of endoscopic ultrasonography in preoperative TNM staging of gastric cancer. World J Gastroenterol. 2006;12:43-47.
39. Bentrem D, Gerdes H, Tang L, et al. Clinical correlation of endoscopic ultrasonography with pathologic stage and outcome in patients undergoing curative resection for gastric cancer. Ann Surg Oncol. 2007;14:1853-1859.
40. Lok K, Lee C, Yiu H, et al. Current utilization and performance status of endoscopic ultrasound in a community hospital. J Dig Dis. 2008;9:41-47.
41. Repiso A, Gomez-Rodriguez R, Lopez-Pardo R, et al. Usefulness of endoscopic ultrasonography in preoperative gastric cancer staging: diagnostic yield and therapeutic impact. Rev Esp Enferm Dig. 2010;102:413-420.
42. Yasuda K. Development and clinical use of ultrasonic probes. Endoscopy. 1994;26:816-817.
43. Matsumoto Y, Yanai H, Tokiyama H, et al. Endoscopic ultrasonography for diagnosis of submucosal invasion in early gastric cancer. J Gastroenterol. 2000;35:326-331.
44. Yanai H, Noguchi T, Mizumachi S, et al. A blind comparison of the effectiveness of endoscopic ultrasonography and endoscopy in staging early gastric cancer. Gut. 1999;44:361-365.
45. Yanai H, Matsumoto Y, Harada T, et al. Endoscopic ultrasonography and endoscopy for staging depth of invasion in early gastric cancer: a pilot study. Gastrointest Endosc. 1997;46:212-216.

46. Akahoshi K, Chijiwa Y, Hamada S, et al. Pretreatment staging of endo-scopically early gastric cancer with a 15 MHz ultrasound catheter probe. *Gastrointest Endosc.* 1998;48:470-476.
47. Kim GH, Park do Y, Kida M, et al. Accuracy of high-frequency catheter-based endoscopic ultrasonography according to the indications for endoscopic treatment of early gastric cancer. *J Gastroenterol Hepatol.* 2010;25:506-511.
48. Caletti G, Ferrari A, Brocchi E, Barbara L. Accuracy of endoscopic ultrasonography in the diagnosis and staging of gastric cancer and lymphoma. *Surgery.* 1993;113:14-27.
49. Puli S, Batapati Krishna Reddy J, Bechtold M, et al. How good is endo-scopic ultrasound for TNM staging of gastric cancers? A meta-analysis and systematic review. *World J Gastroenterol.* 2008;14:4011-4019.
50. Cardoso R, Coburn N, Seevaratnam R, et al. A systematic review and meta-analysis of the utility of EUS for preoperative staging for gastric cancer. *Gastric Cancer.* 2012;15(suppl 1):S19-S26.
51. Mocellin S, Marchet A, Nitti D. EUS for the staging of gastric cancer: a meta-analysis. *Gastrointest Endosc.* 2011;73:1122-1134.
52. Choi J, Kim SG, Im JP, et al. Is endoscopic ultrasonography indispens-able in patients with early gastric cancer prior to endoscopic resection? *Surg Endosc.* 2010;24:3177-3185.
53. Okada K, Fujisaki J, Kasuga A, et al. Endoscopic ultrasonography is valuable for identifying early gastric cancers meeting expanded-indication criteria for endoscopic submucosal dissection. *Surg Endosc.* 2011;25:841-848.
54. François E, Peroux J, Mouroux J, et al. Preoperative endosonographic staging of cancer of the cardia. *Abdom Imaging.* 1996;21:483-487.
55. Hassan H, Vilmann P, Sharma V. Impact of EUS-guided FNA on man-agement of gastric carcinoma. *Gastrointest Endosc.* 2010;71:500-504.
56. Chang K, Albers C, Nguyen P. Endoscopic ultrasound-guided fine needle aspiration of pleural and ascitic fluid. *Am J Gastroenterol.* 1995;90:148-150.
57. Lee Y, Ng E, Hung L, et al. Accuracy of endoscopic ultrasonography in diagnosing ascites and predicting peritoneal metastases in gastric cancer patients. *Gut.* 2005;54:1541-1545.
58. Chu K, Kwok K, Law S, Wong K. A prospective evaluation of catheter probe EUS for the detection of ascites in patients with gastric carci-noma. *Gastrointest Endosc.* 2004;59:471-474.
59. Meining A, Dittler H, Wolf A, et al. You get what you expect? A critical appraisal of imaging methodology in endosonographic cancer staging. *Gut.* 2002;50:599-603.
60. Meining A, Rösch T, Wolf A, et al. High interobserver variability in endosonographic staging of upper gastrointestinal cancers. *Z Gastroen-terol.* 2003;41:391-394.
61. Kim J, Song K, Youn Y, et al. Clinicopathologic factors influence accu-rate endosonographic assessment for early gastric cancer. *Gastrointest Endosc.* 2007;66:901-908.
62. Kida M, Tanabe S, Watanabe M, et al. Staging of gastric cancer with endoscopic ultrasonography and endoscopic mucosal resection. *Endos-copy.* 1998;30(suppl 1):A64-A68.
63. Kutup A, Vashist YK, Groth S, et al. Endoscopic ultrasound staging in gastric cancer: does it help management decisions in the era of neoad-juvant treatment? *Endoscopy.* 2012;44:572-576.
64. Meyer L, Meyer F, Schmidt U, et al. Wschodnioniemiecka Grupa na Rzecz Kontroli Jakosci i Rozwoju Regionalnego w C. Endoscopic ultra-sonography (EUS) in preoperative staging of gastric cancer—demand and reality. *Pol Przegl Chir.* 2012;84:152-157.
65. Yoshimoto K. Clinical application of ultrasound 3 D imaging system in lesions of the gastrointestinal tract. *Endoscopy.* 1998;30(suppl 1):A145-A148.
66. Hwang SW, Lee DH, Lee SH, et al. Preoperative staging of gastric cancer by endoscopic ultrasonography and multidetector-row computed tomography. *J Gastroenterol Hepatol.* 2010;25:512-518.
67. Kuntz C, Herfarth C. Imaging diagnosis for staging of gastric cancer. *Semin Surg Oncol.* 1999;17:96-102.
68. Bhandari S, Shim C, Kim J, et al. Usefulness of three-dimensional, multidetector row CT (virtual gastroscopy and multiplanar reconstruc-tion) in the evaluation of gastric cancer: a comparison with conven-tional endoscopy, EUS, and histopathology. *Gastrointest Endosc.* 2004;59:619-626.
69. Arocena M, Barturen A, Bujanda L, et al. MRI and endoscopic ultraso-nography in the staging of gastric cancer. *Rev Esp Enferm Dig.* 2006;98:582-590.
70. Catalano M, Sivak MJ, Rice T, et al. Endosonographic features predictive of lymph node metastasis. *Gastrointest Endosc.* 1994;40:442-446.
71. Kwee R, Kwee T. Imaging in local staging of gastric cancer: a systematic review. *J Clin Oncol.* 2007;25:2107-2116.
72. Kwee R, Kwee T. Imaging in assessing lymph node status in gastric cancer. *Gastric Cancer.* 2009;12:6-22.
73. Wang Z, Chen JQ. Imaging in assessing hepatic and peritoneal metas-tases of gastric cancer: a systematic review. *BMC Gastroenterol.* 2011;11:19.
74. Lian J, Chen S, Zhang Y, Qiu F. A meta-analysis of endoscopic submu-cosal dissection and EMR for early gastric cancer. *Gastrointest Endosc.* 2012;76(4):763-770.
75. Kayaalp C, Arda K, Orug T, Ozcay N. Value of computed tomography in addition to ultrasound for preoperative staging of gastric cancer. *Eur J Surg Oncol.* 2002;28:540-543.
76. Burke E, Karpeh M, Conlon K, Brennan M. Laparoscopy in the management of gastric adenocarcinoma. *Ann Surg.* 1997;225:262-267.
77. Park S, Lee J, Kim C, et al. Endoscopic ultrasound and computed tomography in restaging and predicting prognosis after neoadjuvant chemotherapy in patients with locally advanced gastric cancer. *Cancer.* 2008;112:2368-2376.
78. Chen C, Yang C, Yeh Y. Preoperative staging of gastric cancer by endo-scopic ultrasound: the prognostic usefulness of ascites detected by endoscopic ultrasound. *J Clin Gastroenterol.* 2002;35:321-327.
79. Fritscher-Ravens A, Schirrow L, Atay Z, et al. Endosonographically controlled fine needle aspiration cytology—indications and results in routine diagnosis. *Z Gastroenterol.* 1999;37:343-351.
80. DeWitt J, LeBlanc J, McHenry L, et al. Endoscopic ultrasound-guided fine-needle aspiration of ascites. *Clin Gastroenterol Hepatol.* 2007;5:609-615.
81. Papaxoinis G, Papageorgiou S, Rontogianni D, et al. Primary gastroin-testinal non-Hodgkin's lymphoma: a clinicopathologic study of 128 cases in Greece. A Hellenic Cooperative Oncology Group study (HeCOG). *Leuk Lymphoma.* 2006;47:2140-2146.
82. Koch P, del Valle F, Berdel W, et al. Primary gastrointestinal non-Hodgkin's lymphoma: I. Anatomic and histologic distribution, clinical features, and survival data of 371 patients registered in the German Multicenter Study GIT NHL 01/92. *J Clin Oncol.* 2001;19:3861-3873.
83. Suekane H, Iida M, Yao T, et al. Endoscopic ultrasonography in primary gastric lymphoma: correlation with endoscopic and histologic findings. *Gastrointest Endosc.* 1993;39:139-145.
84. Palazzo L, Roseau G, Ruskone-Fourmestraux A, et al. Endoscopic ultra-sonography in the local staging of primary gastric lymphoma. *Endos-copy.* 1993;25:502-508.
85. Van Dam J. The role of endoscopic ultrasonography in monitoring treatment: response to chemotherapy in lymphoma. *Endoscopy.* 1994;26:772-773.
86. Hordijk M. Restaging after radiotherapy and chemotherapy: value of endoscopic ultrasonography. *Gastrointest Endosc Clin N Am.* 1995;5:601-608.
87. Caletti G, Fusaroli P, Togliani T, et al. Endosonography in gastric lym-phoma and large gastric folds. *Eur J Ultrasound.* 2000;11:31-40.
88. Paryani S, Hoppe R, Burke J, et al. Extralymphatic involvement in diffuse non-Hodgkin's lymphoma. *J Clin Oncol.* 1983;1:682-688.
89. Reddy S, Pellettiere E, Saxena V, Hendrickson F. Extranodal non-Hodgkin's lymphoma. *Cancer.* 1980;46:1925-1931.
90. De Paepe P, Achten R, Verhoef G, et al. Large cleaved and immunoblas-tic lymphoma may represent two distinct clinicopathologic entities within the group of diffuse large B-cell lymphomas. *J Clin Oncol.* 2005;23:7060-7068.
91. Radaszkiewicz T, Dragosics B, Bauer P. Gastrointestinal malignant lym-phomas of the mucosa-associated lymphoid tissue: factors relevant to prognosis. *Gastroenterology.* 1992;102:1628-1638.
92. Cogliatti S, Schmid U, Schumacher U, et al. Primary B-cell gastric lymphoma: a clinicopathological study of 145 patients. *Gastroenterol-ogy.* 1991;101:1159-1170.
93. Clark E, Ledbetter J. How B and T cells talk to each other. *Nature.* 1994;367:425-428.
94. D'Elios M, Amedei A, Manghetti M, et al. Impaired T-cell regulation of B-cell growth in Helicobacter pylori–related gastric low-grade MALT lymphoma. *Gastroenterology.* 1999;117:1105-1112.

95. Parsonnet J, Hansen S, Rodriguez L, et al. *Helicobacter pylori* infection and gastric lymphoma. *N Engl J Med.* 1994;330:1267-1271.
96. REFERENCE DELETED IN PROOFS.
97. Eck M, Schmausser B, Haas R, et al. MALT-type lymphoma of the stomach is associated with Helicobacter pylori strains expressing the CagA protein. *Gastroenterology.* 1997;112:1482-1486.
98. Wotherspoon A, Ortiz-Hidalgo C, Falzon M, Isaacson P. Helicobacter pylori-associated gastritis and primary B-cell gastric lymphoma. *Lancet.* 1991;338:1175-1176.
99. Steinbach G, Ford R, Glober G, et al. Antibiotic treatment of gastric lymphoma of mucosa-associated lymphoid tissue. An uncontrolled trial. *Ann Intern Med.* 1999;131:88-95.
100. Fischbach W, Goebeler-Kolve M, Dragosics B, et al. Long term outcome of patients with gastric marginal zone B cell lymphoma of mucosa associated lymphoid tissue (MALT) following exclusive Helicobacter pylori eradication therapy: experience from a large prospective series. *Gut.* 2004;53:34-37.
101. Carlson S, Yokoo H, Vanagunas A. Progression of gastritis to monoclonal B-cell lymphoma with resolution and recurrence following eradication of Helicobacter pylori. *JAMA.* 1996;275:937-939.
102. Spinelli P, Lo Gullo C, Pizzetti P. Endoscopic diagnosis of gastric lymphomas. *Endoscopy.* 1980;12:211-214.
103. Fork F, Haglund U, Högström H, Wehlin L. Primary gastric lymphoma versus gastric cancer. An endoscopic and radiographic study of differential diagnostic possibilities. *Endoscopy.* 1985;17:5-7.
104. Taal B, Boot H, van Heerde P, et al. Primary non-Hodgkin lymphoma of the stomach: endoscopic pattern and prognosis in low versus high grade malignancy in relation to the MALT concept. *Gut.* 1996;39:556-561.
105. Komorowski R, Caya J, Geenen J. The morphologic spectrum of large gastric folds: utility of the snare biopsy. *Gastrointest Endosc.* 1986;32:190-192.
106. Martin T, Onstad G, Silvis S, Vennes J. Lift and cut biopsy technique for submucosal sampling. *Gastrointest Endosc.* 1976;23:29-30.
107. Kuldau JG, Holman PR, Savides TJ. Diagnosis and management of gastrointestinal lymphoma. In: Faigel DO, Kochman ML, eds. *Endoscopic Oncology: Gastrointestinal Endoscopy and Cancer Management.* ed 1. Toronto, NJ: Humana Press; 2006:139-149 [Chapter 13].
108. Yoon S, Coit D, Portlock C, Karpeh M. The diminishing role of surgery in the treatment of gastric lymphoma. *Ann Surg.* 2004;240:28-37.
109. Fujishima H, Misawa T, Maruoka A, et al. Staging and follow-up of primary gastric lymphoma by endoscopic ultrasonography. *Am J Gastroenterol.* 1991;86:719-724.
110. Harada N, Wiersema M, Wiersema L. Endosonography guided fine needle aspiration biopsy (EUS FNA) in the evaluation of lymphadenopathy: staging accuracy of EUS FNA versus EUS alone. *Gastrointest Endosc.* 1997;45:AB31. (abstract).
111. Wiersema M, Gatzimos K, Nisi R, Wiersema L. Staging of non-Hodgkin's gastric lymphoma with endosonography-guided fine-needle aspiration biopsy and flow cytometry. *Gastrointest Endosc.* 1996;44:734-736.
112. Vander Noot MR 3rd, Eloubeidi MA, Chen VK, et al. Diagnosis of gastrointestinal tract lesions by endoscopic ultrasound-guided fine-needle aspiration biopsy. *Cancer.* 2004;102:157-163.
113. Yeh H, Chen G, Chang W, et al. Long-term follow up of gastric low-grade mucosa-associated lymphoid tissue lymphoma by endosonography emphasizing the application of a miniature ultrasound probe. *J Gastroenterol Hepatol.* 2003;18:162-167.
114. Shimodaira M, Tsukamoto Y, Niwa Y, et al. A proposed staging system for primary gastric lymphoma. *Cancer.* 1994;73:2709-2715.
115. Musshoff K, Schmidt-Vollmer H. Proceedings: Prognosis of non-Hodgkin's lymphomas with special emphasis on the staging classification. *Z Krebsforsch Klin Onkol Cancer Res Clin Oncol.* 1975;83:323-341.
116. Ruskoné-Fourmestraux A, Dragosics B, Morgner A, et al. Paris staging system for primary gastrointestinal lymphomas. *Gut.* 2003;52:912-913.
117. Rohatiner A, d'Amore F, Coiffier B, et al. Report on a workshop convened to discuss the pathological and staging classifications of gastrointestinal tract lymphoma. *Ann Oncol.* 1994;5:397-400.
118. Musshoff K. Clinical staging classification of non-Hodgkin's lymphomas (author's transl). *Strahlentherapie.* 1977;153:218-221.
119. Schüder G, Hildebrandt U, Kreissler-Haag D, et al. Role of endosonography in the surgical management of non-Hodgkin's lymphoma of the stomach. *Endoscopy.* 1993;25:509-512.
120. Fischbach W, Goebeler-Kolve ME, Greiner A. Diagnostic accuracy of EUS in the local staging of primary gastric lymphoma: results of a prospective, multicenter study comparing EUS with histopathologic stage. *Gastrointest Endosc.* 2002;56:696-700.
121. Yasuda I, Tsurumi H, Omar S, et al. Endoscopic ultrasound-guided fine-needle aspiration biopsy for lymphadenopathy of unknown origin. *Endoscopy.* 2006;38:919-924.
122. Lügering N, Menzel J, Kucharzik T, et al. Impact of miniprobes compared to conventional endosonography in the staging of low-grade gastric malt lymphoma. *Endoscopy.* 2001;33:832-837.
123. Pavlick A, Gerdes H, Portlock C. Endoscopic ultrasound in the evaluation of gastric small lymphocytic mucosa-associated lymphoid tumors. *J Clin Oncol.* 1997;15:1761-1766.
124. Sackmann M, Morgner A, Rudolph B, et al. Regression of gastric MALT lymphoma after eradication of Helicobacter pylori is predicted by endosonographic staging. MALT Lymphoma Study Group. *Gastroenterology.* 1997;113:1087-1090.
125. Ruskoné-Fourmestraux A, Lavergne A, Aegerter P, et al. Predictive factors for regression of gastric MALT lymphoma after anti-Helicobacter pylori treatment. *Gut.* 2001;48:297-303.
126. Nakamura S, Matsumoto T, Suekane H, et al. Predictive value of endoscopic ultrasonography for regression of gastric low grade and high grade MALT lymphomas after eradication of Helicobacter pylori. *Gut.* 2001;48:454-460.
127. Levy M, Copie-Bergman C, Traulle C, et al. Conservative treatment of primary gastric low-grade B-cell lymphoma of mucosa-associated lymphoid tissue: predictive factors of response and outcome. *Am J Gastroenterol.* 2002;97:292-297.
128. Caletti G, Zinzani P, Fusaroli P, et al. The importance of endoscopic ultrasonography in the management of low-grade gastric mucosa-associated lymphoid tissue lymphoma. *Aliment Pharmacol Ther.* 2002;16:1715-1722.
129. Zucca E, Cavalli F. Are antibiotics the treatment of choice for gastric lymphoma? *Curr Hematol Rep.* 2004;3:11-16.
130. Püspök A, Raderer M, Chott A, et al. Endoscopic ultrasound in the follow up and response assessment of patients with primary gastric lymphoma. *Gut.* 2002;51:691-694.
131. Thiede C, Wündisch T, Alpen B, et al. Long-term persistence of monoclonal B cells after cure of Helicobacter pylori infection and complete histologic remission in gastric mucosa-associated lymphoid tissue B-cell lymphoma. *J Clin Oncol.* 2001;19:1600-1609.
132. Bertoni F, Conconi A, Capella C, et al. Molecular follow-up in gastric mucosa-associated lymphoid tissue lymphomas: early analysis of the LY03 cooperative trial. *Blood.* 2002;99:2541-2544.
133. Di Raimondo F, Caruso L, Bonanno G, et al. Is endoscopic ultrasound clinically useful for follow-up of gastric lymphoma? *Ann Oncol.* 2007;18:351-356.
134. Vetro C, Romano A, Chiarenza A, et al. Endoscopic ultrasonography in gastric lymphomas: appraisal on reliability in long-term follow-up. *Hematol Oncol.* 2012;30:180-185.
135. Fusaroli P, Buscarini E, Peyre S, et al. Interobserver agreement in staging gastric malt lymphoma by EUS. *Gastrointest Endosc.* 2002;55:662-668.
136. Kimmey M, Martin R, Haggitt R, et al. Histologic correlates of gastrointestinal ultrasound images. *Gastroenterology.* 1989;96:433-441.
137. Feng J, Al-Abbadi M, Kodali U, Dhar R. Cytologic diagnosis of gastric linitis plastica by endoscopic ultrasound guided fine-needle aspiration. *Diagn Cytopathol.* 2006;34:177-179.
138. Levine M, Kong V, Rubesin S, et al. Scirrhous carcinoma of the stomach: radiologic and endoscopic diagnosis. *Radiology.* 1990;175:151-154.
139. Fujishima H, Misawa T, Chijiwa Y, et al. Scirrhous carcinoma of the stomach versus hypertrophic gastritis: findings at endoscopic US. *Radiology.* 1991;181:197-200.
140. Dempsey P, Goldenring J, Soroka C, et al. Possible role of transforming growth factor alpha in the pathogenesis of Ménétrier's disease: supportive evidence form humans and transgenic mice. *Gastroenterology.* 1992;103:1950-1963.
141. Wolfsen H, Carpenter H, Talley N. Menetrier's disease: a form of hypertrophic gastropathy or gastritis? *Gastroenterology.* 1993;104:1310-1319.
142. Sundt TR, Compton C, Malt R. Ménétrier's disease. A trivalent gastropathy. *Ann Surg.* 1988;208:694-701.

143. Hizawa K, Kawasaki M, Yao T, et al. Endoscopic ultrasound features of protein-losing gastropathy with hypertrophic gastric folds. *Endoscopy.* 2000;32:394-397.

144. Mendis R, Gerdes H, Lightdale C, Botet J. Large gastric folds: a diagnostic approach using endoscopic ultrasonography. *Gastrointest Endosc.* 1994;40:437-441.

145. Gines A, Pellise M, Fernandez-Esparrach G, et al. Endoscopic ultrasonography in patients with large gastric folds at endoscopy and biopsies negative for malignancy: predictors of malignant disease and clinical impact. *Am J Gastroenterol.* 2006;101:64-69.

146. Songür Y, Okai T, Watanabe H, et al. Endosonographic evaluation of giant gastric folds. *Gastrointest Endosc.* 1995;41:468-474.

147. Thomas T, Kaye PV, Ragunath K, Aithal GP. Endoscopic-ultrasound-guided mural trucut biopsy in the investigation of unexplained thickening of esophagogastric wall. *Endoscopy.* 2009;41:335-339.

148. Okada M, Iizuka Y, Oh K, et al. Gastritis cystica profunda presenting as giant gastric mucosal folds: the role of endoscopic ultrasonography and mucosectomy in the diagnostic work-up. *Gastrointest Endosc.* 1994;40:640-644.

SECTION IV

Pancreas and Biliary Tree

13

How to Perform EUS in the Pancreas, Bile Duct, and Liver

Robert H. Hawes • Paul Fockens • Shyam Varadarajulu

Pancreas

Successful pancreatic imaging requires the ability to image the entire gland. In general, the body and tail of the pancreas are imaged through the posterior wall of the stomach, and, in most cases, the transgastric approach provides images of the genu (neck) of the pancreas as well. Complete imaging of the pancreatic head, however, requires placement of the transducer in three different positions within the duodenum: the apex of the duodenal bulb (the apical view), directly opposite the papilla ("kissing the papilla"), and distal to the papilla to visualize the uncinate process. This organized, station-based approach to pancreatic imaging is critical for individuals who are just learning or who have limited experience with endoscopic ultrasonography (EUS). Although the stations are the same for radial and linear endosonography, the images produced are different, as are the techniques for maneuvering the echoendoscope. As a result, representative images and illustrations from the various stations are presented for radial and linear echoendoscopes. As the reader is learning these techniques, it is also important for him or her to refer to the corresponding videos. Obtaining complete, accurate, and high-quality images of the pancreas and biliary tree represents the most difficult task facing the endosonographer.

Evaluation of the Body and Tail of the Pancreas

The examination of the body and tail of the pancreas begins by positioning the tip of the echoendoscope just distal to the squamocolumnar junction. From this position, the aorta is easily located and becomes the "arrow" that points the way. When the radial scope is used, the aorta is round and anechoic. With the linear scope, the aorta fills the screen as a long, anechoic structure extending across the entire monitor.

Radial Echoendoscopes

With the tip of the endoscope just distal to the squamocolumnar junction, the endosonographer inflates the balloon and positions the transducer in the center. The aorta is located, and with the endosonographer in a comfortable position (neither body nor scope shaft twisted or torqued), the aorta is electronically rotated to the 6-o'clock position (Video 13-1).

At this point, one usually sees a hypoechoic structure that moves from the esophageal wall and wraps partially around the aorta; this comprises the diaphragmatic crura. From here, one simply advances the echoendoscope while the aorta is kept in its cross-sectional conformation; the aorta must not be allowed to elongate. If the aorta is seen to elongate on advancement, it is an indication that the tip of the echoendoscope is being pushed laterally or is embedding in the gastric wall (often within a hiatal hernia pouch). If this occurs, the tip must be realigned and the maneuver repeated because it is important to keep the aorta in its round configuration. If this maneuver fails repeatedly, the echoendoscope should be advanced beyond the hiatal hernia and withdrawn. This maneuver helps one to visualize first the portal vein confluence (at the 6-o'clock position), and then the pancreas.

With advancement, when the crura disappear, the celiac trunk is seen to emerge from the aorta and tract toward the transducer (Figure 13-1). In some cases with the radial scope, one first sees the splenic artery as a round, anechoic structure adjacent to the transducer. In this case, one just advances 1 to 2 cm, and the splenic artery traces into the celiac trunk. The celiac artery bifurcates into the hepatic and splenic arteries; with the radial scope, the bifurcation can look like a whale's tail (Figure 13-2). Slight advancement of the scope beyond the celiac artery takeoff produces images of the body of the pancreas. The pancreas is seen directly below the transducer. The pancreatic parenchyma is usually slightly hypoechoic relative to surrounding tissue and has a homogeneous "salt and pepper" appearance. From this position, deep to the pancreas is an anechoic structure that looks like the head of a golf club. This is the portal vein confluence and is often referred to as the *club head* (Figure 13-3).

Once the club head has been identified, it becomes relatively straightforward to image the rest of the body and tail of the pancreas. Clockwise torque and withdrawal of the scope will trace the tail of the pancreas. It may also require some "right" adjustment on the left-right knob. During this maneuver, the left kidney comes into the picture as a large, oval structure with a hypoechoic, homogeneous outer "shell" (cortex) and an inhomogeneous, echo-rich central portion (medulla). The kidney roughly marks the body-tail junction of the pancreas (Figure 13-4). On further withdrawal, one sees the splenic artery and vein course right below the transducer, and a homogeneous, echo-poor bean-shaped structure

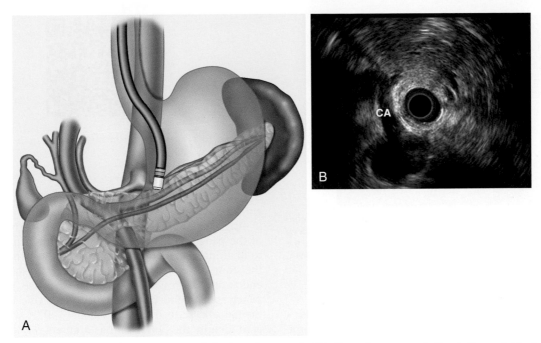

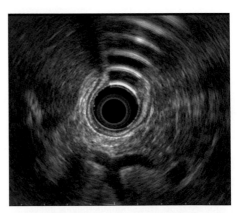

FIGURE 13-1   Pancreatic body and tail examination: radial echoendoscope. **A,** This illustration represents the starting point for imaging the pancreatic body and tail with the radial echoendoscope. The scope is advanced while the aorta is traced, starting at the gastroesophageal junction. The first branch of the aorta is the celiac artery. **B,** By tracing the celiac artery (CA), the pancreatic body and tail can be found.

occupies the right side of the image. This is the spleen, and the splenic vein and artery can be seen to insert into the splenic hilum. Once this image is seen, the examination of the distal body and tail is complete. From the tail of the pancreas, one simply reverses the maneuvers by advancing the scope, torquing counterclockwise, and returning to the portal vein confluence. From here, further advancement and counterclockwise torque allow imaging of the genu (neck) of the pancreas. The pancreatic duct is seen to dive away from the transducer as it courses through the neck. During the movements mentioned earlier, some left and right tip deflection may be required to obtain an elongated view of the pancreas. Once the elongated view of the pancreas is achieved, very slow and purposeful advancement and withdrawal of the scope demonstrate the entire width of the pancreas, including the pancreatic duct.

In the station approach, if one cannot see the typical landmarks that characterize the station during the course of the examination (no matter which station one is working on), one should return immediately to the starting point for that station and repeat the standard maneuvers. In the case of the pancreatic body and tail, this means returning to the gastroesophageal junction, tracing the aorta until the celiac trunk is seen,

and so forth. A particular station should be examined as many times as required until the endosonographer is comfortable that the examination is complete. Sometimes, however, despite repeated attempts, one cannot achieve the imaging goals of a particular station. In this case, the endosonographer can continue the examination by going to other stations and then return later to the difficult station. Often, the return examination is successful.

Linear Echoendoscopes

Examination of the pancreatic body and tail with the linear scope follows the same basic approach as with the radial instrument. The examination begins at the gastroesophageal junction (Video 13-2). In this case, however, the endosonographer must torque the scope shaft in a clockwise direction until the aorta is seen. Using the up-down dial, the aorta should gently slope down from right to left. Just as with

Video 13-1. Evaluation of the body and tail of the pancreas using a radial echoendoscope.

FIGURE 13-2   The celiac artery bifurcates into the hepatic and splenic arteries, which on endosonography can look like a whale's tail.

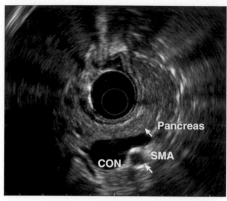

FIGURE 13-3 The portal vein confluence (CON) is referred to as a *club head* because it looks like the head of a golf club and is located deep to the pancreas. In this view, the pancreas is located directly below the transducer and has a homogeneous "salt and pepper" pattern. SMA, superior mesenteric artery.

the radial scope, the diaphragmatic crura is seen as a hypoechoic structure between the transducer and the aorta. This landmark is important because, as one advances the scope, the celiac trunk takes off soon after the crura disappear (Figure 13-5).

Unlike the radial scope, with which scope advancement is a passive maneuver (because of its 360-degree image), the linear scope must be gently torqued clockwise and counterclockwise to visualize the side of the aorta. Not uncommonly, the celiac trunk comes off the side of the aorta, and one can pass right by it if not systematically scanning back and forth. Once the celiac artery has been identified, it is traced until it bifurcates. Once the bifurcation is identified, and with 1 to 2 cm of further advancement combined with a gentle "down" on the up-down dial ("big dial away from you"), the pancreas and portal vein confluence come into view. From here, clockwise torque and withdrawal image the pancreatic body and tail (Figure 13-6), and counterclockwise rotation and advancement provide images of the genu (Figure 13-7). As with a radial echoendoscope, the pancreas should be traced all the way to the tail, which is confirmed when the splenic hilum is seen. As with all aspects of linear array imaging, gentle clockwise and counterclockwise torquing is mandatory throughout the examination to obtain complete imaging. Left and right

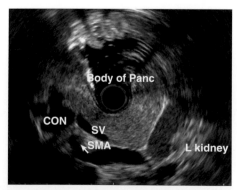

FIGURE 13-4 The left kidney has a hypoechoic outer cortex and an echo-rich medullary zone. This landmark roughly indicates the body-tail junction of the pancreas. CON, portal vein confluence; Panc, pancreas; SMA, superior mesenteric artery; SV, superior mesenteric vein.

Video 13-2. Evaluation of the body and tail of the pancreas using a curvilinear echoendoscope.

tip deflection is of minimal importance when the linear echoendoscope is used.

An alternative technique used to examine the body and tail of the pancreas when using a linear array echoendoscope is to first differentiate the left lobe of the liver from the body of the stomach. From this position, when the shaft of the echoendoscope is torqued 180 degrees clockwise, the body of the pancreas can be identified and the gland traced all the way to the tail as described earlier (Video 13-3). A similar approach is to identify the portal vein as it enters the liver. Advancing the scope combined with clockwise torque enables one to follow the portal vein until the confluence is reached. Once the "club head" is identified, the pancreas will be between the portal vein confluence and the transducer (Video 13-3).

Evaluation of the Head and Uncinate Regions of the Pancreas

To examine the entire head of the pancreas confidently, all three positions (the apex, papilla, and distal to the papilla) should be achieved. The most efficient position is the apex of the duodenal bulb, because from this position most of the pancreatic head, distal bile duct, and portal vein can be seen together. As with other stations, positioning is the same with radial and linear scopes, but the subtle maneuvers to optimize imaging and the pictures produced are different.

Head of the Pancreas

Radial Echoendoscopes. This position allows imaging of the entire head of the pancreas (sometimes with the exception of the uncinate process) and also includes efficient imaging of the distal common bile duct. The radial echoendoscope should be slowly advanced through the stomach and allowed to bow along the greater curve. Once the pylorus has been visualized, the tip is advanced through the pylorus, at which point air is instilled into the duodenal bulb, and some gentle downward deflection is applied to the tip of the echoendoscope (Video 13-4). This maneuver allows direct endoscopic visualization of the apex of the duodenal bulb. Once the apex is visualized, the tip of the echoendoscope should be advanced until it is at the level of the apex. The balloon is then inflated until it gently occludes the lumen of the duodenum (Figure 13-8), and any residual air is aspirated from the duodenal lumen (all done under endoscopic control). At this point, EUS imaging commences, and the endosonographer turns his or her attention to the EUS image, first looking for the liver. Once the liver has been identified, the image should be electronically rotated (*do not torque the scope*) such that the liver is positioned in the upper left-hand corner of the screen.

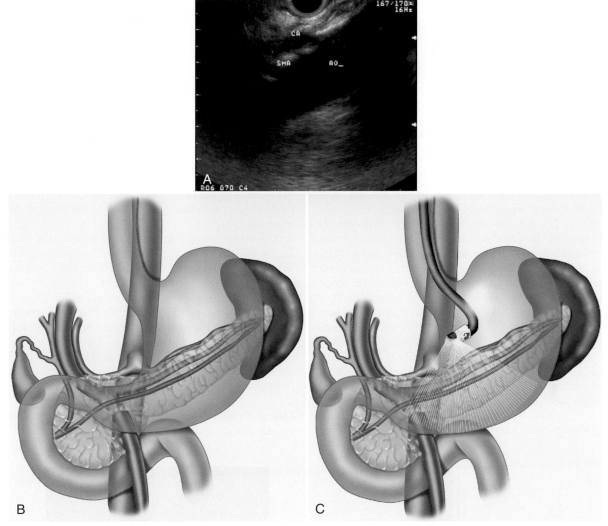

FIGURE 13-5 Pancreatic body and tail examination: linear echoendoscope. **A**, EUS image and **B, C,** illustrations represent the starting point for imaging the pancreatic body and tail using the curvilinear echoendoscope. The transducer is advanced while the aorta is traced, starting at the gastroesophageal junction. The first branch of the aorta represents the celiac axis; by tracing along the celiac axis, the pancreatic body can be found.

This technique provides uniform orientation and allows the endosonographer to identify the normal and abnormal structures more easily. When the liver is in the upper left-hand corner, the head of the pancreas is at the 6-o'clock position, and the bile duct is seen as an anechoic tube lying close to the transducer and coursing from the liver down to the 6-o'clock area.

From this position, one should look for four landmarks (Figure 13-9). The most important is the *duodenal falloff.* This is a hypoechoic line that represents the muscularis propria of the duodenal wall. It is seen to course down and away from the transducer. To the right of this line, the image

FIGURE 13-6 Clockwise torque from the portal confluence coupled with gradual scope withdrawal enables imaging of the body and tail regions of the pancreas. PD, pancreatic duct; SA, splenic artery; SV, splenic vein.

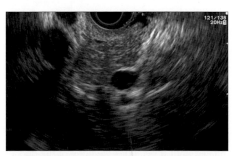

FIGURE 13-7 Counterclockwise rotation coupled with scope advancement enables visualization of the pancreatic genu.

Video 13-3. Evaluation of the body and tail of the pancreas using a curvilinear echoendoscope by adopting alternative techniques.

Video 13-4. Evaluation of the head of the pancreas using a radial echoendoscope.

is chaotic because it represents a mixture of air and fluid within the duodenal lumen. The second landmark is the *common bile duct*, a tubular anechoic structure that extends from at or near the duodenal wall toward the liver and courses closest to the transducer. This structure typically has a three-layer echo appearance. To trace the bile duct, the examiner uses counterclockwise torque and withdrawal of the scope toward the hilum and clockwise torque and advancement of the scope toward the papilla. The third landmark is the *pancreatic duct*. This may or may not be seen in the same plane of imaging as the bile duct. Often, gentle advancement of the scope combined with upward or downward tip deflection is required to see the pancreatic duct. During the entire process of imaging from the apical position, the endosonographer should be prepared to use some gentle upward or downward tip deflection to achieve complete imaging. The fourth landmark is the *portal vein*, which is seen to course in the far left

of the imaging field and is the biggest tubular structure visible. One can use color Doppler imaging to identify the portal vein more easily.

Color Doppler imaging may also be required to differentiate the bile duct from the hepatic and gastroduodenal arteries. When the common bile duct, pancreatic duct, and portal vein are aligned in one view, they appear to be stacked on the top of each other. This image is known as the *stack sign*. Once the apical position is achieved, multiple small movements, which can include clockwise and counterclockwise torquing, forward advancement and withdrawal of the scope, upward and downward tip deflection, and left and right positioning of the tip, are all required to define the anatomic features thoroughly from this position.

Linear Echoendoscopes. Positioning the linear scope for apical imaging is the same as with the radial scope. The scope

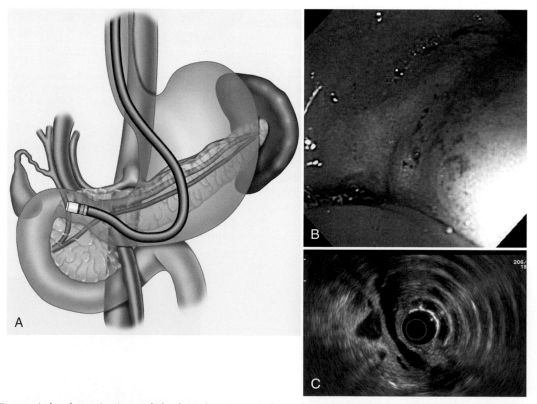

FIGURE 13-8 Pancreatic head examination: radial echoendoscope. **A,** Schema for evaluating the pancreatic head from the duodenal bulb. **B,** The balloon is inflated until it occludes the apex of the duodenal bulb. **C,** The liver is visualized at the left upper corner, the head of the pancreas is at the 6-o'clock position, and the bile duct will be seen as an anechoic tube closer to the transducer and coursing from the liver down to the 6-o'clock area.

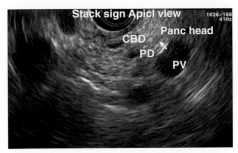

FIGURE 13-9 The stack sign. The stack sign is elicited during evaluation of the pancreatic head and is characterized by the common bile duct (CBD), main pancreatic duct (PD), and the portal vein (PV), which all appear "stacked" on top of each other. Also note the duodenal falloff, which represents the muscularis propria of the duodenal wall.

Video 13-5. Evaluation of the head of the pancreas using a curvilinear echoendoscope.

should be advanced along the greater curve and through the pylorus, where air is instilled and gentle downward tip deflection is applied. Once the apex has been identified, the tip of the linear scope is nestled into the apex of the bulb, and gentle upward deflection is applied to the tip (Video 13-5). The balloon is less important with linear imaging, but some endosonographers like to inflate the balloon in the apex as described with the radial scope. At this point, however, torquing is required, generally in a counterclockwise direction.

From this position, examination of the entire head of the pancreas (perhaps minus the uncinate process) can be achieved (Figure 13-10). The most recognizable structure with the linear scope in this position is the portal vein. Color Doppler imaging can be used to confirm visualization. The bile duct courses along the portal vein (closer to the transducer). The bile duct can be traced to the liver and then down to the papilla through the pancreatic head by simply torquing the scope, with little to no need for advance or withdrawal of

the instrument. The pancreatic duct runs parallel to the bile duct in the pancreatic head, but gentle torquing may be required to see it because it may not be in the exact same plane as the bile duct (Figure 13-11). It is critical for the endosonographer to become very comfortable with this position with the linear scope. This position provides the best imaging to assess the relationship between a pancreatic head mass and the portal vein. It is also the position of choice for performing EUS-guided fine-needle aspiration of pancreatic head masses because the mass is close to the transducer, and the back wall of the duodenum prevents the scope from pushing away from the mass when the needle is inserted (especially important if the mass is very firm).

Papilla

Radial Echoendoscopes. The second position for pancreatic head imaging is from the level of the papilla. This position is best achieved by first using endoscopic visualization to localize the ampulla of Vater. Once that structure is seen, the balloon is inflated until it "kisses" the papilla (Figure 13-12). It is best to try to orient the transducer perpendicular to the papilla and to position it so that upward tip deflection will

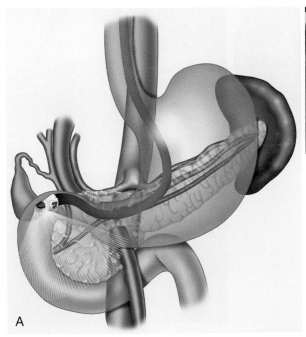

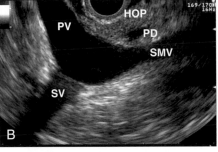

FIGURE 13-10 This is perhaps the most important station for viewing and performing fine-needle aspiration of the pancreatic head (HOP). **A**, The transducer is placed at the level of the apex of the duodenal bulb. **B**, After some manipulation of the scope tip, the neck of the pancreas can be viewed with the portal vein confluence deep to the pancreas. PD, pancreatic duct; PV, portal vein; SMV, superior mesenteric vein; SV, splenic vein.

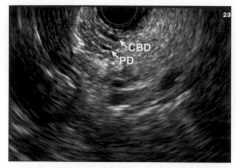

FIGURE 13-11 The pancreatic duct (PD) runs parallel to the common bile duct (CBD) in the head region of the pancreas. Gentle torquing may be required to identify and trace the ductal structures.

Video 13-6. Evaluation of the papilla of Vater using a radial echoendoscope.

cause the balloon to press against the papilla (Video 13-6). Once this position has been achieved, ultrasound imaging begins. The ultrasound image is rotated so that the papilla is located at the 6-o'clock position on the EUS image. From this point, the head of the pancreas is a crescent-shaped structure. As the transducer is moved gently in and out, one looks to see the bile duct and pancreatic duct coursing to the duodenal wall. The pancreatic duct is deep to the bile duct relative to the position of the transducer. Because of the usual appearance of the two ducts from this position, this image is termed *snake eyes*. From this position, it is easiest to see the differentiation between the ventral and the dorsal anlage. The ventral anlage is hypoechoic and has heterogeneous echo architecture when compared with the dorsal pancreas (Figure 13-13). The ventral anlage is triangular and occupies the left portion of the crescent-shaped pancreatic head, whereas the dorsal portion occupies the right portion. This position allows the endosonographer to see the superior mesenteric vein (closest to the pancreas) and the superior mesenteric artery (deeper and thicker wall when compared with the superior mesenteric vein), in addition to the ventral and dorsal anlage.

This is also the position required for detailed imaging of the ampulla of Vater, either to assess an ampullary adenoma or cancer or to look for an impacted stone (in the case of gallstone pancreatitis). To image the papilla itself, the duodenum should be paralyzed with hyoscine butylbromide (Buscopan) or glucagon. Once the duodenum is paralyzed, water should be infused into the duodenum to achieve coupling of the ultrasound waves with the papilla without risking compression from the balloon. Exquisite views of the ampulla can be obtained if one can achieve perpendicular positioning

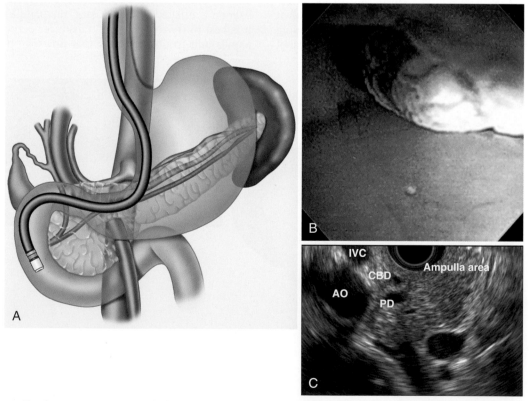

FIGURE 13-12 Papilla of Vater examination: radial echoendoscope. **A,** The position required for evaluating the papilla of Vater. **B,** The balloon is inflated so that it "kisses" the papilla but without causing mechanical compression. **C,** Gentle movement of the transducer enables visualization of the common bile duct (CBD) and the pancreatic duct (PD) coursing through the duodenal wall to the papilla. The presence of two ducts as imaged in this view is termed *snake eyes*. AO, aorta; IVC, inferior vena cava.

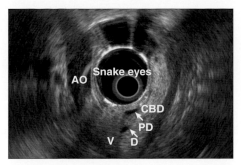

FIGURE 13-13 The ventral anlage is hypoechoic, triangular, and heterogeneous in echo architecture. It occupies the left portion of the crescent-shaped pancreatic head as compared with the dorsal pancreas, which occupies the right portion. AO, aorta; CBD, common bile duct; D, dorsal; PD, pancreatic duct; V, ventral.

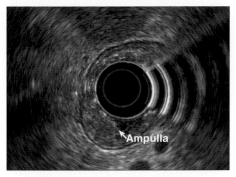

FIGURE 13-14 The ampulla is imaged best by perpendicular positioning of the transducer relative to the papilla coupled with water insufflation and a motionless duodenum.

of the transducer relative to the papilla, obtain adequate water coupling, and keep the duodenum motionless (Figure 13-14). The critical anatomic landmark when staging ampullary neoplasms is the muscularis propria of the duodenal wall. If the process disrupts this layer, tumor invasion can be predicted.

Linear Echoendoscopes. The ampullary position is exactly the same with the linear as with the radial echoendoscope. The papilla is visualized endoscopically, and then the transducer should be positioned perpendicular to the ampulla (Figure 13-15). The orientation should be such that upward tip deflection should press the transducer against the papilla (Video 13-7). If detailed images of the papilla are required, the duodenum should be paralyzed and water infused into the duodenal lumen, just as with the radial instrument. In some circumstances, however, when either the radial or the linear echoendoscope is used, the curvature of the duodenum may be too acute to obtain perpendicular orientation between the transducer and the papilla despite maximal upward

deflection of the endoscope tip. In this circumstance, imaging of the ampulla is somewhat tangential; this degrades the overall image quality and precision of interpretation. The pancreatic head appears crescent shaped, but unlike the radial scope, with which the bile and pancreatic ducts are seen in cross section (snake eyes), the bile and pancreatic ducts are seen in their linear confirmation, with the bile duct more superficial and the pancreatic duct deep. Imaging is carried out by slow withdrawal and continuous gentle torquing clockwise and counterclockwise until the portal vein confluence is seen. This landmark signifies the completion of this station.

Uncinate

Radial Echoendoscopes. The uncinate process can be imaged by positioning the transducer distal to the ampulla of Vater. The critical anatomic structure in this position is the aorta. The up-down dial should be turned maximally "up," and the right-left control should be locked in the "right" position. Very gentle counterclockwise torque allows visualization

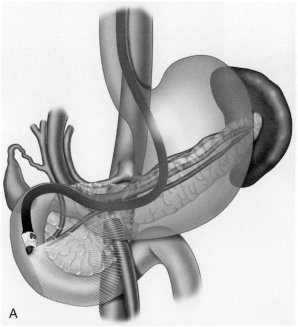

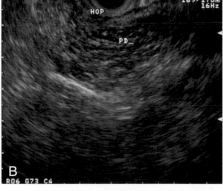

FIGURE 13-15 Papilla of Vater examination: linear echoendoscope. **A,** The transducer is placed at a perpendicular angle to the papilla of Vater. **B,** From this position, the pancreas has a crescent shape, and the bile duct and pancreatic duct can be seen to emerge from the papilla.

Video 13-7. Evaluation of the papilla of Vater using a curvilinear echoendoscope.

Video 13-8. Evaluation of the uncinate region of the pancreas using a radial echoendoscope.

of the aorta, which, if the transducer is deep enough in the duodenum, is seen initially in its longitudinal confirmation. At this point, electronic rotation is used to position the aorta so that it courses top to bottom on the left side of the screen (Video 13-8). Slow withdrawal is then commenced. As the scope is withdrawn, the aorta slowly goes from linear to oval and ultimately to a cross-sectional (round) configuration. From this position, the inferior vena cava is usually visible as well and is typically superior to the aorta. At this point, if one looks to the right of the aorta, the uncinate process will emerge (Figure 13-16). The pancreas is initially triangular but changes to a crescent shape as one withdraws to the level of the papilla. The aorta is critical for this position because if one does not see the pancreas adjacent to the aorta, one cannot be sure that the uncinate process has been visualized.

One problem that can be encountered with withdrawal from this position is that the echoendoscope can suddenly flip back into the duodenal bulb. This problem can be avoided by manipulating the echoendoscope as one would a colonoscope; instead of slow, steady withdrawal, the echoendoscope

is withdrawn a slight amount and then advanced a slight amount. If one can maintain one-to-one reaction of the echoendoscope to the manipulation of the shaft, then rapid uncontrolled withdrawal can be avoided.

Linear Echoendoscopes. The transducer should be passed just distal to the ampulla, and the instrument shaft should be rotated clockwise or counterclockwise, as necessary, to locate the aorta. Once the aorta has been visualized, the echoendoscope should be torqued (usually clockwise) and slowly withdrawn (Video 13-9). With this maneuver, the uncinate process comes into the image adjacent to the transducer and to the right of the aorta (Figure 13-17). The endosonographer simply withdraws the scope slowly while gently torquing back and forth.

It is not possible to read a book and translate the reading to successful imaging of the pancreas. Successful imaging has innumerable nuances, and each patient's anatomy is different. Each case presents its own unique challenges, and no endosonographer, no matter how experienced, achieves successful and complete imaging in all patients. One is always limited

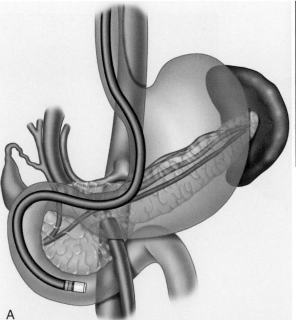

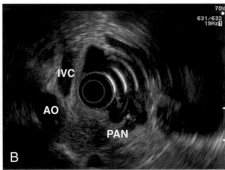

FIGURE 13-16 Uncinate examination: radial echoendoscope. **A,** This illustration reveals the echoendoscope in the second portion of the duodenum. **B,** At this station, by gradual scope withdrawal, the uncinate portion of the pancreas (PAN) is visualized to the right of the aorta (AO). IVC, inferior vena cava.

Video 13-9. Evaluation of the uncinate region of the pancreas using a linear echoendoscope.

by the patient's individual anatomic features, and these limitations must be accepted by the endosonographer.

Bile Duct

EUS imaging of the bile duct is relatively straightforward, but overall it is easier and more efficiently performed with a radial scanning echoendoscope. Basically, two positions must be achieved to evaluate the extrahepatic portion of the bile duct fully. The first position, mentioned earlier, is the apical position. The second position, which is important for achieving full visualization of the bile duct, is one in which the transducer "kisses" the papilla. With a radial scanning echoendoscope, the apical position usually permits a very broad section of the bile duct to be visualized at one time.

Achieving the apical position begins with the tip of the instrument in the stomach. The echoendoscope is advanced along the greater curve of the stomach with a little downward tip deflection to enable visualization of the pylorus. Slight upward tip deflection is applied just before entering the pylorus, and, once within the duodenal bulb, air is instilled along with slight downward tip deflection to visualize the apex of the duodenal bulb (see Video 13-4). The tip of the scope is then positioned in the area of the apex, the balloon is inflated until it occludes the lumen, and slight clockwise torque is then applied to the instrument shaft. Ultrasound imaging then begins. The first structure to look for is the liver. The image should be rotated such that the liver is positioned in the upper left-hand portion of the screen. From this position at least a portion of the bile duct can usually be visualized, although slight advancement or withdrawal of the echoendoscope may be required. The bile duct is seen as an anechoic tubular structure coursing right, adjacent to the transducer (see Figure 13-9; Figure 13-18).

The most important landmark of the apical position is the duodenal falloff. This represents the muscularis propria of the duodenum and is seen to course just adjacent to the transducer and then to fall away directly from it in the 6-o'clock position of the screen. Once the bile duct is visualized, one should recognize that it typically has three layers. Withdrawal and counterclockwise torque of the echoendoscope allow visualization of the bile duct toward the hilum, and clockwise torque and insertion of the endoscope shaft allow visualization of the distal bile duct as it enters the papilla.

The most common mistake made with apical imaging is that the endosonographer allows the transducer to slip back into the duodenal bulb. Some gentle pressure should be kept against the shaft of the instrument to prevent this problem. It is also possible that if too much pressure is applied, the tip will slip around the apex into the second portion of the duodenum. If there is a tendency for this to occur, the balloon should be further inflated on the bulb side of the apex. Once one begins imaging from the apical position, if the bile duct is not recognized within 30 seconds, endoscopic control should be used to reposition the transducer in the apex, and

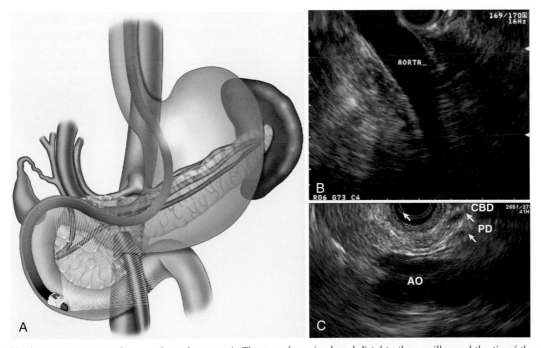

FIGURE 13-17 Uncinate examination: linear echoendoscope. **A,** The transducer is placed distal to the papilla, and the tip of the echoendoscope is moved upward. **B,** From this position, the aorta can be sought; the pancreas is viewed adjacent to it. **C,** Gradual withdrawal and torquing of the echoendoscope reveal the uncinate portion of the pancreas. AO, aorta; CBD, common bile duct; PD, pancreatic duct.

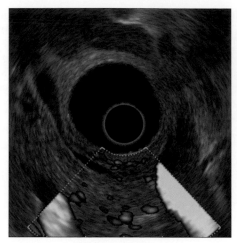

FIGURE 13-18 The use of color Doppler imaging distinguishes the bile duct from the surrounding vasculature.

ultrasound imaging should be restabilized. Three to four repositionings within the apex may sometimes be required to achieve proper imaging of the bile duct.

In some cases, a stone is impacted in the distal bile duct. In this circumstance, the only way to detect the stone may be to position the transducer directly perpendicular to the papilla (see Video 13-6). This is achieved by advancing the echoendoscope into the second portion of the duodenum and then pulling back as one would during an endoscopic retrograde cholangiopancreatography to achieve the straight scope position. The papilla should be visualized endoscopically, the duodenum paralyzed, and water instilled within the duodenal lumen. The balloon is then slightly inflated, but not enough to press firmly against the papilla. One then scans back and forth across the papilla and looks for the bile duct to emerge from the papilla (see Figure 13-12C). One must look carefully because, if a small stone is impacted in the ampulla, only shadowing may be seen, without the intensely echogenic rim typically observed with stones in the bile duct or gallbladder. As always, complete imaging of the bile duct may require multiple attempts at each position.

The technique for imaging the bile duct with the linear echoendoscope is the same as that described for the radial instrument. The two positions remain the same: apical and opposite the papilla. Because the plane of imaging for the linear scope is more restricted than that of the radial scope, it may be difficult to obtain long views of the bile duct. The linear instrument should be positioned in the apex of the duodenal bulb, but usually counterclockwise torque is required to image the bile duct, and some left-right tip deflection may be required (see Videos 13-5 and 13-7). The principle remains the same; that is, withdrawal of the instrument from this position generally gives views toward the hilum, whereas advancing the echoendoscope obtains views toward the papilla (see Figure 13-11). Use of the linear scope for biliary imaging requires much more careful tracing because one single position provides only a small section of the bile duct. Sometimes it is easier to obtain perpendicular views of the papilla with the linear scope than with the radial scope. Of course, color Doppler imaging can be used to help differentiate the bile duct from surrounding vascular structures (see Figure 13-18).

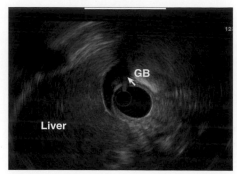

FIGURE 13-19 The echoendoscope is "locked" in the duodenal bulb, and the tip is deflected for obtaining images of the liver and gallbladder (GB).

Liver

There are basically three positions for EUS imaging of the liver. No matter how diligent the endosonographer, the extent to which the liver can be imaged depends largely on the patient's anatomy. In general, one should use the lowest frequency available with the instrument to maximize penetration, and the various liver imaging positions should be repeated several times before the examination is declared complete. Electronic scanning echoendoscopes, whether radial or linear, generally have deeper penetration in liver tissue than do mechanical rotating echoendoscopes.

The first liver position is in the duodenal bulb (see Figure 13-8; Figure 13-19). If one is using the radial scope, the balloon should be overinflated so that one is "locked" in the bulb (Video 13-10). From this position, the tip should be deflected so that it presses as firmly as possible against the liver. The echoendoscope is then advanced and withdrawn to its fullest extent, and at the same time clockwise and counterclockwise torquing is used. The instrument should be advanced until the liver disappears and withdrawn until firm pressure is felt against the pylorus. The duodenal bulb is also the best position for imaging the gallbladder, and the technique of balloon overinflation should be used to obtain full views of the gallbladder. Once imaging from this position has been exhausted, the balloon should be deflated and the transducer repositioned in the antrum. With the tip of the scope in the antrum and the balloon inflated (Figure 13-20), the echoendoscope tip again should be pressed as firmly as possible against the wall of the stomach that lies next to the liver (Video 13-11). Once again, the scope should be advanced and withdrawn to its fullest extent during continuous imaging of the left lobe of the liver. The third position is from the fundus

Video 13-10. Video demonstrating imaging of the liver from the duodenal bulb.

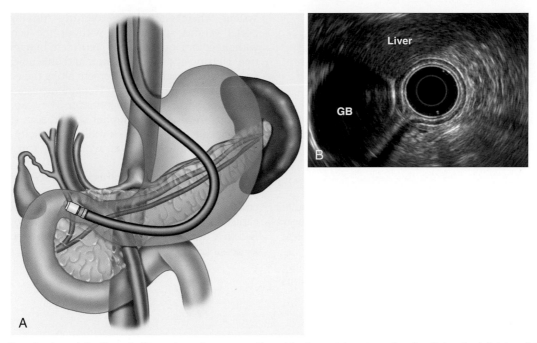

FIGURE 13-20 Examination of the liver. **A,** The echoendoscope positioned in the gastric antrum for visualizing the left lobe of the liver. **B,** The echoendoscope tip should be firmly against the gastric wall to image the liver. GB, gallbladder.

Video 13-11. Video demonstrating imaging of the left lobe of the liver from the gastric antrum.

of the stomach (Figure 13-21). Beginning at the gastroesophageal junction, the transducer is pressed against the gut wall in the direction of the left lobe of the liver (Video 13-12). From this position, the scope is slowly advanced, and at the same time the endosonographer applies clockwise and counterclockwise torque to sweep across the extent of the liver. The scope should be advanced until no further imaging of the liver can be achieved.

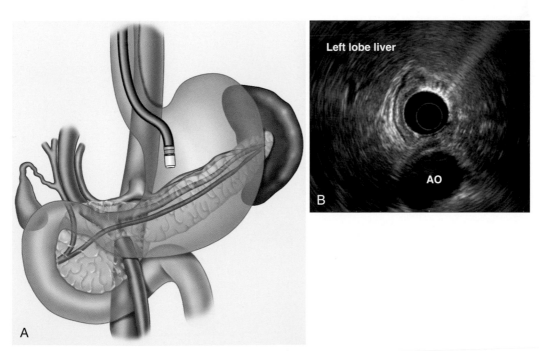

FIGURE 13-21 Examination of the liver. **A,** The echoendoscope in the proximal stomach. **B,** The scope is pressed firmly against the gut wall to image the left lobe of the liver. AO, aorta.

Video 13-12. Video demonstrating imaging of the left lobe of the liver from the fundus of the stomach.

The technique and positions are the same whether a radial or a linear instrument is used. It takes more effort with linear scopes to torque the scope shaft to accomplish as complete an examination as possible.

The anatomy of the liver is relatively simple. Branching structures with echogenic walls represent the portal venous system, whereas anechoic structures running alongside the portal venous system and without the echogenicity (and without color Doppler signal) represent branches of the biliary tree. Hepatic cysts are common and anechoic, and they have a characteristic echo enhancement along the border of the cyst further from the transducer. Hepatic metastases are generally echo poor, without a distinct border. They can be quite subtle, and thus the endosonographer should scan slowly and carefully. Hepatic veins also lack wall echogenicity and run toward the cranial part of the liver, where they can usually be seen entering the caval vein.

Liver imaging can be a frustrating aspect of endosonography because one cannot be sure that the liver has been imaged completely. As a result, the various positions mentioned earlier should be repeated until the endosonographer is satisfied that the extent of the examination has been as complete as possible.

14

EUS in Inflammatory Disease of the Pancreas

Joseph Romagnuolo

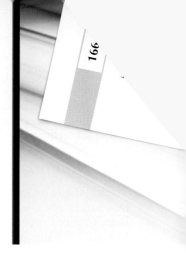

Key Points

- EUS is highly accurate in the diagnosis of chronic pancreatitis when calcifications, or five or more of nine criteria, are present; finding two or fewer criteria has high negative predictive value; the finding of three or four criteria lands right on the borderline of a positive test and so does not change the pretest suspicion of disease.
- Fine-needle aspiration does not appear to add helpful information to the diagnosis of chronic pancreatitis, with added risks of post-FNA pancreatitis.
- MRCP appears to have modest accuracy for chronic pancreatitis but, even with quantitative secretin flow dynamics, remains insensitive for mild disease.
- Although not perfect, EUS is very useful in distinguishing inflammatory pseudotumors from neoplastic masses, even without FNA; PET is also promising.
- Autoimmune pancreatitis should be considered in unexplained inflammatory masses; serum IgG4 is the test of choice, although in selected equivocal cases Tru-Cut biopsy may be helpful.
- EUS in the diagnosis or staging of acute pancreatitis has had limited study.
- EUS appears to be accurate in the diagnosis of gallbladder sludge, tumors, and other causes of apparently "idiopathic" acute pancreatitis; it is most helpful in patients with a gallbladder still in place and in older patients for whom a tumor is unlikely.
- EUS has good accuracy for pancreas divisum—at least as well as MRCP—but specificity is better than sensitivity; attempting to follow the duct from the major papilla to the dorsal gland is most reliable.

Introduction

Endoscopic ultrasound (EUS) is well suited to examine the pancreas because of the proximity of the probe to the pancreatic parenchyma and was originally developed for this purpose in the early 1980s.[1–3] EUS boasts dynamic imaging, together with the fine resolution of parenchyma that real-time ultrasound is capable of, resulting in a huge advantage over static cross-sectional imaging. At the same time, EUS avoids the intervening air and fat that degrade the quality of transabdominal ultrasound. Because higher frequency means lower depth of penetration, transabdominal ultrasound is restricted to a lower frequency (with associated lower resolution) to overcome the distance between the skin and the retroperitoneum. Because of its noninvasive nature, it avoids the risk of pancreatitis associated with ERCP, except when fine-needle aspiration (FNA) is added. The literature regarding chronic pancreatitis, which will be detailed later in the chapter, suggests that EUS is likely to be at least as sensitive as the conventional imaging reference standard, endoscopic retrograde cholangiopancreatography (ERCP), and may identify patients with earlier stages of disease that evade non-EUS testing.

Grading of acute pancreatitis with EUS has not yet been studied. However, EUS appears to have a role in otherwise idiopathic recurrent pancreatitis, identifying unrecognized chronic pancreatitis, biliary sludge, or pancreas divisum. Acute inflammatory masses can be distinguished from neoplasia with greater accuracy than other imaging options. The addition of FNA to EUS, in order to sample equivocal masses and lymph nodes, adds an invaluable dimension to the assessment of the pancreas that other imaging cannot match; however, it appears neither safe nor accurate for the overall diagnosis of chronic pancreatitis, except perhaps when autoimmune disease is suspected. Novel adjuncts to EUS (elastography and contrast-enhanced harmonic ultrasound) may help to distinguish normal from abnormal tissue using variations in tissue stiffness and perfusion, respectively; this is discussed in more detail in Chapter 5.

This systematic study was derived from review of the existing literature. A PubMed search using the MESH terms endosonography" and "pancreatitis" revealed well over 500 abstracts; these abstracts were individually reviewed for relevance, and pertinent complete manuscripts were then reviewed. Multiple topic reviews were also examined,[4-24] including bibliographies, to identify missing articles.

The Noninflamed Pancreas on EUS

The technique for examining the pancreas by EUS is outlined in Chapter 13. Once good position and clear images have been obtained, one needs to be able to recognize what is "normal." Briefly, the normal noninflamed pancreas appears to be a homogeneous structure with a single anechoic (Doppler negative) smooth ductular structure running within it that represents the main pancreatic duct. The body and tail have a fine, diffusely speckled (so-called "salt and pepper") pattern that is, on average, more echogenic (brighter) than the liver; a small amount of fine, diffuse heterogeneity is normal. Caution should be exercised to avoid overcalling of small echogenic foci or short echogenic strands when a high degree of magnification is used (as might be needed in an atrophic gland or a gland with a very small duct). The normal gland contour is generally smooth, but some lobularity of the margin is within normal limits, and this is accentuated when the pancreas is much more echogenic compared with adjacent tissue. The duct wall is barely perceptible, with similar echotexture to surrounding pancreatic tissue.

Although some practitioners have said that "visible side branches" are abnormal, with current technology, side branches can be seen in many normal patients. Even with older equipment, studies noted visible branches in half of control subjects,[25] with mean sizes of 0.7 mm, 0.5 mm, and 0.4 mm in the head, body, and tail, respectively.[26] Only side branches larger than 1 mm should be considered abnormal.[15] The main duct's course can be mildly tortuous, but beading (alternating sizes) should not be present. The duct should taper from the head to the tail, with 3 mm, 2 mm, and 1 mm being normal duct sizes in the head, body, and tail, respectively.[27,28] Above the age of 60 years, an extra 1 mm for the main duct in each section is generally allowed due to expected atrophy of surrounding parenchyma. However, control groups[26] comprising young individuals have exceeded the above duct diameters by up to a 1 mm in each site category. As such, a recent consensus group defined dilation as greater than 3.5 mm in the body, or 1.5 mm in the tail.[15]

The anterior-posterior thickness of the pancreas is approximately 10 to 15 mm;[25,26] the importance of "atrophy" in the diagnosis of chronic pancreatitis, however, is unclear. The dorsal pancreas is generally more echogenic (brighter) than the embryological ventral pancreas (the ventral anlage); the ventral anlage, and the transition zone from darker ventral (head) to brighter dorsal (uncinate, body/tail), can be seen in 45% to 75% of people examined with EUS,[25,26,29] which is more than twice as often as with computed tomography (CT).[30,31] Finally, the head is generally more heterogeneous than the body and tail.

Chronic Pancreatitis Diagnosis and Staging

The diagnosis of chronic pancreatitis can be difficult. CT and magnetic resonance imaging (MRI) must rely on main pancreatic duct dilatation, moderate-sized cysts, and calcifications for the diagnosis, all of which are markers of severe disease by the ERCP Cambridge criteria.[32] Magnetic resonance cholangiopancreatography (MRCP) can make some further inferences regarding main duct irregularity and the presence of dilated or irregular side branches; unfortunately, the resolution is often too poor to be accurate in this assessment when the ducts are not dilated. Adding secretin can allow better ductal imaging and functional assessments; atrophy and changes in parenchymal signal can also be seen.[24,33,34] ERCP carries the risk of causing further pancreatic damage, especially when filling both the pancreas to the tail and the side branches.[35] Furthermore, other than stones in the parenchyma large enough to be radiopaque on plain radiographs, an assessment of parenchyma outside the ducts is not possible with ERCP.

In contrast, EUS can use parenchymal criteria in addition to ductal criteria to make a diagnosis of chronic pancreatitis. Smaller cysts and more subtly dilated or clubbed side branches can also be more reliably identified. Even calcifications a few millimeters in size can be readily identified as shadowing hyperechoic reflections.

Defining the Criteria and Identifying Them Reliably

The difficulty with interpreting the EUS literature regarding chronic pancreatitis is that, conventionally, the EUS diagnosis relied on tallying the number of criteria present. This generally assumed equal weighting to those criteria. Denominators (number of criteria sought) and criteria definitions were also somewhat variable (Table 14-1). There are generally now felt to be nine accepted criteria,[36] including four parenchymal criteria (hyperechoic foci, hyperechoic strands, hypoechoic lobules, and cysts) and five ductal criteria (dilatation, dilated side branches, main duct irregularity, hyperechoic duct margins, and stones).

One should note that hypoechoic lobules, in different publications, have also been referred to as "reduced echogenicity foci," "hypoechoic foci," or "pseudolobularity." An American Society of Gastrointestinal Endoscopy (ASGE)-endorsed consensus conference of an international representation of expert endosonographers was convened in April of 2007 in Rosemont, Illinois, to attempt weighting some criteria as major and minor criteria; the results are summarized briefly in Tables 14-2 and 14-3.[15] Studies are lacking that confirm the Rosemont system performs at least as well as the conventional criteria and has sufficient advantages to justify adopting the added complexity of this new system; interobserver reliability may be no better[44] or may be even poorer with the new system.[45]

Figure 14-1 shows a few examples of the normal pancreas body, with linear and radial views, and of the conventional criteria. The actual histological correlates of these criteria are unknown,[15] but hypothetical correlations have been proposed (Table 14-4). Figure 14-2 provides examples of normal pancreas, periductal fibrosis (likely explaining thickened hyperechoic duct walls), interlobular fibrosis (likely explaining hyperechoic strands), hyperechoic foci (likely explaining focal fibrosis or representing cross-sectional views of the strands), and clustered islands of (anatomic) lobules separated from others by fibrotic strands (likely explaining hypoechoic

TABLE 14-1

CRITERIA AND THRESHOLDS USED BY STUDIES IN DIAGNOSING CHRONIC PANCREATITIS

Study	Threshold Number of Criteria	Parenchymal Criteria					Cyst	Duct Criteria				
		Hyperechoic Foci	Hyperechoic Strands	Hypoechoic Lobules, Foci, or Areas	Accentuation of Lobular Pattern	Irregular Gland Margin or Increased Size		Irregular Duct Contour	Visible Side Branches	Hyperechoic Duct Margin	Dilated Main Duct	Stone
Chong 2007[37]	Calcification; 3 or more, if no calcification (by ROC)	x	x	x			x	x	x	x	x	x
Varadarajulu 2007[38]	4 or more (noncalcific) (by ROC)	x	x	x			x	x	x	x	x	x
Pungpapong 2007[39]	4 or more (by ROC)	x	x	x			x	x	x	x	x	x
Kahl 2002[40]	1 or more	x > 3 mm	x[e]	x	[e]	x increased gland size	x	x	x	x	x	x
Hollerbach 2001[41]	2 or more	x hyperechoic lobules	x septa				x	x	x	x	x	x
Hastier 1999[42]	Unclear (possibly 1 or more)	x		x			x	x	x	x	x	x
Catalano 1998[25]	1-2 called "mild," but ≥3 used in comparisons with ERCP	x[d]	x septa	[c]	[c]	x irregular margin	x	x	x "ectatic"	x	x	x
Sahai 1998[36]	<3 criteria rules out disease; >4 criteria rules in disease	x 1-2 mm	x	x 2-5 mm			x >2 mm	x	x	x	x[f]	x
Buscail 1995[43]	Not reported	[b]	[b]	x	[b]			x	x	x[b]	x	x
Wiersema 1993[26]	3 or more by ROC	x[a] > 3 mm	x	x[a]	x		x	x[a]	x[a]	x	x[a]	x

x indicates that this criterion was sought.

ROC, receiver-operator characteristic curve analysis.

[a]Significant in multivariate analysis.

[b]Diffusely heterogeneous, diffusely hyperechoic, and hypertrophic were other parenchymal criteria used in this study, and heterogeneous appears to refer to hyperechoic strands and foci; echogenic duct wall was considered normal but hyperechogenic duct wall was recorded as abnormal.

[c]Heterogeneous parenchyma was an additional criteria, separate from strands and foci.

[d]Foci were called "calcifications" parenthetically in the paper, but it is not clear if acoustic shadowing was required or not.

[e]Hypoechoic areas and hyperechoic areas surrounded by septae were considered two different criteria.

[f]>3 mm in the head, >2 mm in the body, >1 mm in the tail.

TABLE 14-2

CONVENTIONAL AND ROSEMONT[15] EUS CRITERIA FOR DIAGNOSIS OF CHRONIC PANCREATITIS

Conventional Criteria	Rosemont Criteria
Parenchymal Criteria	***Major Criteria A***
Hyperechoic foci	Hyperechoic foci (>2 mm in length/width with shadowing)
Hyperechoic strands	Major duct calculi (echogenic structure(s) within the MPD with acoustic shadowing)
Hypoechoic lobules, foci, or areas	***Major Criteria B***
Cyst	Lobularity (≥3 contiguous lobules = "honeycombing")
Duct Criteria	***Minor Criteria***
Irregular duct contour	Cyst (anechoic, round/elliptical with or without septations)[a]
Visible side branches	Dilated duct (≥3.5 mm in body or >1.5 mm in tail)[a]
Hyperchoic duct margin	Irregular duct contour (uneven or irregular outline and ectatic course)
Dilated main duct	Dilated side branch (>3 tubular anechoic structures each measuring ≥1 mm in width, budding
Stone	from the MPD)[a]
	Hyperechoic duct wall (echogenic, distinct structure >50% of entire MPD in the body and tail)
	Hyperechoic strands (≥3 mm in at least two different directions with respect to the imaged plane)
	Hyperechoic foci (>2 mm in length/width that are nonshadowing)[a]
	Lobularity (>5 mm, noncontiguous lobules)

MPD, main pancreatic duct
[a]If any of these minor criteria are present, patient cannot be classified as "normal."
(Data from: Catalano MF, Sahai A, Levy M, et al. EUS-based criteria for the diagnosis of chronic pancreatitis: the Rosemont classification. Gastrointest Endosc. 2009;69(7):1251-1261.)

"lobules," where each single EUS "lobule" is really a cluster of multiple anatomic lobules). A very hyperechoic pancreas (so-called snowstorm pancreas or sometimes called "fatty pancreas") can hide a few of the more subtle features of chronic pancreatitis (Figure 14-1C and D) but is not in itself associated with chronic pancreatitis; it may be associated with body mass index and metabolic syndrome, though.[46]

The earliest comparative study of paid volunteers and patients with pancreatic pain,[26] after excluding 1 patient with calcifications, found 5 of 11 tentative criteria to be significant independent predictors of abnormal ERCP: (1) areas of reduced echogenicity; (2) irregular duct contour; (3) main duct dilatation; (4) dilated side branches; and (5) echogenic

foci (>3 mm). Interestingly, three other criteria, some of which are commonly used today, were not predictive in multivariate analysis (echogenic duct wall, "accentuated lobular pattern," and cysts). Echogenic strands were not assessed in this analysis.

Some endosonographers believe gland contour ("lobular" versus smooth) may be important, but many do not.[15] Either way, the term "lobularity" is best avoided in a report, as a lobular outer gland margin and hypoechoic lobules could get confused.[25] Loss of a distinct ventral anlage is usually not listed as a separate criterion and has not been tested as such, but this phenomenon does seem to occur more often in inflammatory disorders of the pancreas than in controls (71% versus 25%).[29]

Minimal standard terminology (MST) has been developed for these criteria and other EUS findings in the pancreas and other organs and is periodically updated by the World Organisation of Digestive Endoscopy (OMED) committee of documentation and standardization (Table 14-5).[47,48]

Reproducibility and Interobserver Agreement

The first assessment of a diagnostic test, after pilot studies defining what is normal and what is abnormal, involves measurement of reproducibility and interobserver reliability of the assessment for the criteria.[49] In the study by Wiersema and colleagues,[26] concordance (for the five criteria that achieved significance in multivariate analysis) was 83% to 94% among three reviewers.

Beyond reporting the proportion of observers agreeing, one can measure agreement using the kappa (κ) statistic, as a measure of agreement beyond chance. A κ < 0 is agreement that is less often than by chance, 0 is no more than chance agreement, and 1 is perfect agreement;[49] the minimum threshold for "fair" agreement varies from 0.20 to 0.40.[50–52] Using

TABLE 14-3

CLASSIFICATION OF PATIENTS BASED ON EUS CRITERIA

Conventional Criteria	Rosemont Criteria[15]
Normal (or Low Probability)	***Consistent with***
0-2 Criteria	2 major A
	1 major A + 1 major B
Indeterminate or Intermediate Probability	1 major A + ≥3 minor
3-4 Criteria	***Suggestive***
	Major A + <3 minor
High Probability	Major B + ≥3 minor
5-9 Criteria	≥5 minor, no major
Calcifications/stones	***Indeterminant***
	Major B alone + <3 minor
	Normal
	<3 minor, no major

(Data from: Catalano MF, Sahai A, Levy M, et al. EUS-based criteria for the diagnosis of chronic pancreatitis: the Rosemont classification. Gastrointest Endosc. 2009;69(7):1251-1261.)

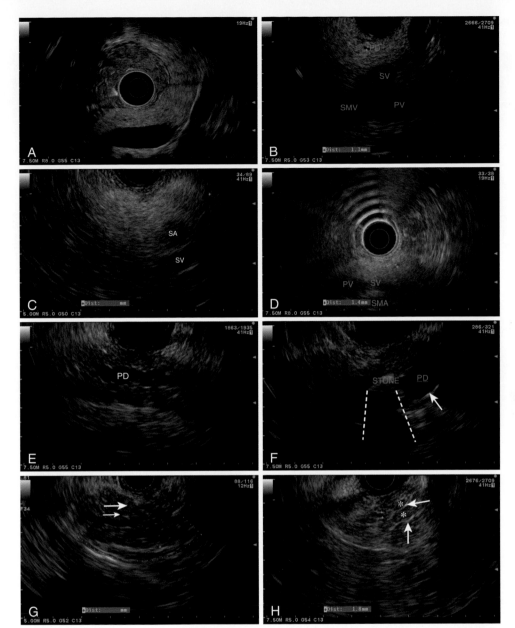

FIGURE 14-1 **A**, Normal pancreas (electronic radial EUS). **B**, Normal pancreas: linear EUS. **C**, Fatty/snowstorm body of pancreas (BOP) on L-EUS and **D**, electronic radial EUS. The splenic artery (SA), splenic vein (SV) and portal vein (PV) are blurry and barely discernible due to marked attenuation by the pancreas above them; a duct is difficult to see. **E**, Linear EUS of an irregular pancreatic duct (PD) in BOP. **F**, Obstructing stone in the PD in the head of the pancreas on linear EUS, with a wedge of acoustic shadowing (*dotted lines*), and upstream PD dilation (*arrow*). **G**, Dilated side branch (*thin arrow*) with small power color Doppler positive vessels (thick arrow) mimicking branches in BOP on linear EUS. **H**, Hypoechoic (dark) lobules (*) surrounded by bright hyperechoic strands (*arrows*), with an echogenic duct wall (+calipers) in BOP on L-EUS. SMV, superior mesenteric vein.

TABLE 14-4

HYPOTHESIZED HISTOLOGIC CORRELATES OF EUS CRITERIA FOR CHRONIC PANCREATITIS AND THEIR ALTERNATE EXPLANATIONS

EUS Finding	Proposed Histologic Correlate (and Alternative Non-chronic Pancreatitis Explanations)
Hyperechoic/thickened duct margin	Periductal fibrosis (this "interface" can be accentuated [brighter/thicker] when changes in tissue density result in a more abrupt change in acoustic impedance between tissue and duct)
Dilated duct and/or side branches	Dilated duct and/or side branches (small vessels can mimic side branches; obstructed ducts)
Irregular duct contour	Irregularity due to fibrosis
Stones	Stones (pneumopancreatica and calcifications in splenic vessel walls can be mistaken as stones)
Cysts	Cysts and/or cystic side branches (cysts and cystic side branches can represent cystic neoplasms)
Hyperechoic foci and strands	Focal or linear areas of interlobular fibrosis; round foci may also represent strands cut in cross section or small calcifications or protein plugs that are not dense enough to cause an acoustic shadow (changes in acoustic impedance will cause linear reflections/strands—this artifact is less likely to explain strands that are not parallel to the probe)
Hypoechoic lobules	Groupings of anatomic lobules with focal edema/inflammation or atrophy, often encapsulated by interlobular fibrosis (EUS "lobules," especially in pancreatic cancer kindreds, can represent nodules of dysplasia or neoplasia)

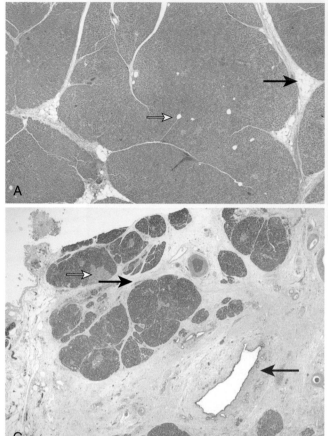
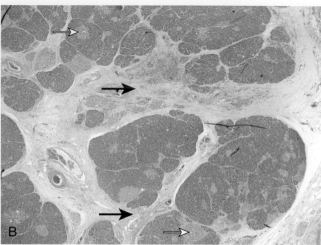

FIGURE 14-2 **A**, Normal pancreas histology. Low power (2× objective) H&E stain of pancreas. Pancreatic acinar tissue is the predominant cellular component. There is limited fat (round clear spaces within the lobule, *white arrow*) and a limited perilobular fibrous component (*black arrow*). **B**, Mild chronic pancreatitis. Low power (2× objective) H&E stain of pancreas. Lobular atrophy with interlobular fibrosis is apparent (*black arrow*). Prominent Islets of Langerhans are present (*white arrow*). **C**, Moderate chronic pancreatitis. Low power (2× objective) H&E stain of pancreas. Lobular atrophy with interlobular fibrosis is apparent (*black arrow*), causing the "honeycombing" appearance of multiple adjacent "hypoechoic lobules" (multiple anatomic lobules in clusters, surrounded by strands of fibrosis). Prominent Islets of Langerhans are present (*white arrow*). A large pancreatic duct with periductal fibrosis is present in the lower right of the image (*red arrow*).

κ, Wallace and colleagues measured the interobserver reliability of 11 experienced endosonographers for the overall diagnosis of chronic pancreatitis, estimating a κ of 0.45; there was poorer reliability for individual criteria.[27] Neither advanced training nor experience (>1000 procedures) improved agreement.[27] Only two of the nine criteria had κ of >0.40: main duct dilatation (0.61) and "lobularity" (0.51).[27] Ranking of the importance of criteria was variable except for stones, which were felt to be the most important.[27] Perhaps because of some variability in an endosonographer's tolerance for trivial dilation, particularly in older patients, even the more objective duct size criterion[27] did not have complete agreement. Although these values for reliability appear poor at first glance, the authors[27] correctly point out that identification of bleeding ulcer stigmata (κ = 0.34 to 0.66),[53] stroke localization by radiologists using brain CT (κ = 0.56 to 0.62),[54] and heart sounds interpretation (κ = 0.05 to 0.18)[55] have comparable or poorer interobserver reliability. MRCP may have slightly better agreement among experts, but community agreement is not known.[56]

Another dimension to a test's reliability includes its test-retest and *intra*observer reliability. The latter, a measure of how often one agrees with oneself when presented with the same images at a later time, was recently studied across multiple institutions and was excellent (90% agreement; average kappa 0.75)[57] and at least as good as the ERCP intraobserver reliability of only 61% to 78%.[58] In another study, test-retest

agreement using back-to-back EUS by two endosonographers was poorer for most individual criteria.[38]

How Many Criteria Should Be Sought? How Many Is Too Many?

A summary of the different criteria sought and the thresholds recommended for use is presented in Table 14-1. Unfortunately, the thresholds for how many criteria are enough for the "abnormal" categorization vary in studies from one to six, and the denominator of criteria sought also varies from five to more than ten. The criteria with the most consistent use across studies are the ductal ones. Of the parenchymal criteria, the most consistently used are hyperechoic foci (although the size criterion is not consistent), cysts, and hypoechoic lobules (also called hypoechoic "areas" or hypoechoic "foci" by some).

Calcific Disease

Calcifications or ductal stones are considered diagnostic for chronic pancreatitis (Video 14-1). Because of this, and because patients with calcifications were largely excluded from threshold-seeking studies, this is not a criterion to be "counted"; it stands on its own. Our group showed that 30 of 71 patients in our surgical series had calcifications by EUS, but only 16 (58%) were picked up by CT or MR.[37] Another

TABLE 14-5

DEFINITION OF INFLAMMATORY PANCREATIC EUS CRITERIA USING SELECTED MINIMUM STANDARD TERMS

Term	Definition	Comment
Cyst	Abnormal anechoic (i.e., without echoes) round or oval structure	Specify size, septations, wall thickening or mural nodules, debris, connection with main duct or side branch, and associated solid mass Inflammatory cysts are generally thin walled, have single or no septations, often contain debris, and are often in communication with the main pancreatic duct
Calcification	Hyperechoic lesion with acoustic shadowing (reduction in echo due to a strongly attenuating or reflecting structure) within a parenchymal organ or a mass	Generally not recommended for describing the pancreas, unless describing components of a cyst or mass
Stone	Hyperechoic lesion with acoustic shadowing (reduction in echo due to a strongly attenuating or reflecting structure) within a duct or gallbladder	All calcifications in the pancreas (excluding masses and cysts) are by definition intraductal, although the side branch duct in which they reside may be too small to appreciate Generally stones and pancreatic "calcifications" are both considered "ductal" features Size measurement may be inaccurate because typically only the hyperechoic proximal part of the lesion is seen as echogenic Specify number, approximate size, location in gland (head/body/tail), and whether present within main duct
Hyperechoic Foci	Small distinct reflectors	Some studies separate <3 mm and ≥3 mm sizes, but relative significance is not known Generally do not have acoustic shadowing Specify extent, location
Hyperechoic Strands	Small, string-like, hyperechoic (echoes are brighter than normal and/or brighter than surrounding tissues) structures	Specify extent, location
Hypoechoic Lobules	Rounded homogeneous areas separated by strands of another echogenicity	Almost by definition, lobules and strands coexist, and foci also frequently coexist "Lobulated" can be used to describe a gland with lobules but is sometimes confused with a "lobular gland margin" and is probably a term that is best avoided Care must be taken to ensure that lobules >1 cm are not in fact masses Specify extent, location
Irregular Duct Contour	Coarse, uneven outline of the duct	Specify extent, location
Tortuous Duct	Duct with numerous twists and bends	To be distinguished from "irregular." Not necessarily abnormal
Hyperechoic Duct Wall	Region of the duct where the echoes are brighter than normal and/or brighter than surrounding tissues	A normal pancreatic duct wall surrounded by normal tissue is barely perceptible on ultrasound and is essentially isoechoic to surrounding parenchyma
Dilated Duct	Abnormal increase in caliber	Duct size should be measured from the closest echo of the wall closest to the probe to the closest echo of the wall furthest from the probe Size and location, beading (alternating small and large calibers), and localized narrowings (strictures) should be noted

(Data from: The International Working Group for Minimum Standard Terminology for Gastrointestinal E. Reproduction of minimum standard terminology in gastrointestinal endosonography. Digestive Endoscopy. 1998;10:158-184.; World Organisation of Digestive Endoscopy (OMED) committee of documentation and standardization. Minimum Standard Terminology (MST v 3.0)- http://www.omed.org/index.php/resources/re_mst/. 3.0 ed; 2009.)
"Hypoechoic foci" and "accentuation of lobular pattern" are terms not listed in the MST paper.

small study recently showed that 7 of 16 patients being evaluated were found to have small calcifications missed on other imaging.[59] Therefore EUS is arguably the most sensitive test for calcifications or stones, a finding that is very specific for chronic pancreatitis.

Although highly specific, because calcifications can rarely have other causes, some supporting findings should be sought, as suggested in the Rosemont study.[15] Care should be taken to ensure that the calcifications are not just due to atherosclerosis of a nearby vessel or a calcified node. Air

Video 14-1. Video segment of EUS showing calcifications (shadowing hyperechoic foci).

artifact (pneumopancreatica) can also mimic a ductal stone in patients who have had a pancreatic sphincterotomy, so extra caution is needed after sphincterotomy.

Noncalcific Disease

In patients *without calcifications*, the number of criteria (out of the remaining eight) then becomes critical (Video 14-2). Wiersema and colleagues[26] used receiver-operator characteristic (ROC) curve analysis and found three or more criteria to be best. Sahai and colleauges[36] informally looked at different thresholds and showed that finding less than three criteria effectively excluded patients with moderate or severe chronic pancreatitis on ERCP; five or more criteria strongly suggested at least mild chronic pancreatitis on ERCP. Both of these studies did not include calcifications as a criterion, as those patients were excluded from analysis. Supporting these cutoffs, symptomatic controls had a mean of 1.9 ± 1.8 criteria in a Medical University of South Carolina (MUSC) study looking at the prevalence of findings in dyspepsia; no controls had more than six criteria[28] and 67% had less than four criteria. This would have likely been even more striking if the controls with a history of alcohol abuse (which doubles the number of criteria on average, perhaps from subclinical chronic pancreatitis) had been excluded. Our group also compared EUS findings with surgical pathology in 71 patients.[37] In patients without calcifications ($n = 41$), ROC curve analysis revealed that three or more EUS criteria provided the best balance of sensitivity and specificity. Using a higher histologic fibrosis score threshold, another similar study found four or more EUS criteria to be the best ROC-derived cutoff ($n = 21$).[60]

Interpreting Degree of Certainty of Chronic Pancreatitis

Diagnostic tests that result in an array of values or use continuous measures often have extreme levels on one end of the spectrum that are considered diagnostic (e.g., lipase more than three times the upper limit of normal) and extreme levels

Video 14-2. Video segment showing an example of "high-probability" noncalcific (so-called "minimal change") chronic pancreatitis.

on the other end that are considered very reassuring (e.g., cyst fluid carcinoembryonic antigen less than 5); values near or at the "best cutoff" are generally less helpful or considered indeterminate.

The interpretation of the number of EUS criteria for chronic pancreatitis is no exception: having three or four criteria is considered equivocal because that result lands on or near the best cutoffs. This essentially leaves the pretest suspicion of disease unchanged (i.e., a likelihood ratio of near 1). Therefore in the presence of risk factors that increase the pretest likelihood of disease, such as alcohol abuse, smoking, family history, or symptoms suggestive of pancreatic disease,[40] this value may still indicate chronic pancreatitis. Similar to other continuous measures, a low result (less than three criteria) is very reassuring, and a high result (five or more criteria) is very specific for disease. Of note, these levels are meant to represent *probability*, not *severity*.[15] There is only a modest correlation between increasing number of criteria and more severe fibrosis[37,60] or more severe ERCP Cambridge score.

Adjusting Thresholds for Demographics

Making *special adjustments or allowances* for different age, gender, and risk factor groups is not supported by the literature, other than perhaps duct size for advanced age.[15] Rajan and colleagues[61] showed some relationship between age and number of criteria, but this was not significant in multivariate analysis when corrected for other factors;[62] even this relationship may have disappeared if they had allowed a higher duct size threshold for older patients. Yusoff and colleagues[63] did not find an age association either.

Another study showed a significantly higher number of findings in alcoholic subjects versus nonalcoholic subjects, and EUS criteria for chronic pancreatitis could predict their alcohol history. This is not surprising and is in keeping with probable subclinical pancreas and liver damage in alcoholic subjects.[64] Both smoking and alcohol were significant predictors of finding more criteria,[63] but because these are both known risk factors for chronic pancreatitis, the higher number of criteria likely represents actual subclinical pancreatic disease in asymptomatic patients. As such, it does not seem logical that allowances should be made. This would be analogous to allowing a higher threshold for calling an abnormal cardiac stress test in an asymptomatic smoker, rather than simply labeling it as subclinical coronary disease.

Male gender was independently associated with more EUS features in both studies.[61,63] It is not clear why that is. It could be that alcohol and smoking exposures were higher in men than in women and/or were more likely to be underreported in men; or there could be a true gender-specific risk factor. In the end, based on the literature, no criteria threshold adjustments are recommended for these groups after adjustment is made for duct size in older patients.

Accuracy and Test Performance

Reference Standards and Competing Technologies

After one is confident with the reliability of a test, the next step is to assess its accuracy against a reference standard.[49] Unfortunately, for chronic pancreatitis, the reference standard is also a problem. Although complex advanced statistical techniques exist to try to account for imperfect reference standards,[65] they have not been used in the literature to date. Even for *histology*, grading and diagnosis is unfortunately not standardized and limited to small series.[41,66] The number of histologic criteria required is arbitrary and differs from study to study.[37,60] Disease can be patchy just as it can be in cirrhosis,[67] FNA appears unreliable and does not increase accuracy significantly,[41] and it is not clear if both chronic inflammation *and* fibrosis need to be present for the diagnosis (often, fibrosis is all that is seen even histologically). ERCP and secretin-stimulated pancreatic juice analysis have historically been considered the nonhistologic reference standard, but it is clear that both techniques likely miss disease that is at an early stage, yet is bad enough to be causing pain.

Not all chronic pancreatitis results in ductal disease sufficient to be seen at ERCP, and the pancreas has tremendous functional reserve that results in false-negative secretin tests until late in the disease process. ERCP relies on ductal (main and side branch) irregularity and dilation, intraductal filling defects or stones, and inflammatory cysts that communicate with the main pancreatic duct, graded using the widely accepted, albeit consensus-derived, Cambridge classification (Table 14-6).[32] Fibrotic or inflammatory parenchymal changes are not able to be assessed with ERCP until they cause ductal irregularity and/or obstruction.

There are multiple types of noninvasive pancreatic *function testing*, including measurement of stool enzymes (e.g., fecal elastase)[16] and assessing the cleavage of promarkers by proteases by measuring the markers in urine, blood, or breath.[16,68] Invasive tests involve measuring bicarbonate/fluid (hydraletic) or enzymes (ecbolic) output after food or hormonal stimulation (e.g., secretin test). Although pancreatic function testing is viewed by some practitioners as the most sensitive and reliable test for chronic pancreatitis and pancreatic insufficiency (accuracy reported as 80% to 90%),[16] sensitivity frequently drops to under 40% in early disease.[6] One recent moderately sized study from Japan comparing the secretin test to histology (consensus-derived histology scoring system

[grades 0 to 4] from the Japanese Society of Gastroenterology) in 108 patients (39 of which had abnormal histology) showed a sensitivity of under 70%.[69,70] Other older comparisons with histology have found similarly modest sensitivity.[71,72] Fecal elastase has a sensitivity of 45% to 63% for mild disease but 73% to 100% for severe disease[73–75] compared with ERCP[73] or invasive pancreatic function tests[74,75] as reference standards.

Studies[76,77] of MRCP have shown that the main pancreatic duct is seen well, especially with secretin, although resolution of side branches is inferior to ERCP. Calvo and colleagues[78] showed an 86% sensitivity and 94% specificity compared with ERCP for ductal abnormalities in 78 patients. In contrast, Alcaraz and colleagues[79] studied 81 patients undergoing both MRCP and ERCP but only showed a 50% sensitivity (with 99% specificity) for MRCP in chronic pancreatitis. Another study found only 25% sensitivity of MRCP for mild disease versus 82% to 100% for severe disease.[24] Other adjuncts to MRCP that need further study and validation include noting gland atrophy, lower T2 gland signal intensity,[80] secretory response (duct dilation and/or duodenal filling) to a test (Lundh) meal or secretin,[33,80] lower T1 (perfusion) intensity, (virtual) pancreatoscopy,[81] and secretin-MRCP with diffusion-weighting (which assesses water molecule movement to identify diffusion and microcirculation changes that occur in inflamed and fibrotic tissue).[24]

The comparative literature regarding MRCP in chronic pancreatitis is far less voluminous than that for EUS. One study compared secretin-MRCP to pancreatic function tests (urinary pancreolauryl and fecal elastase-1). It was abnormal in steatorrhea patients, but many false-positive (4% to 18%) and false-negative (16% to 25%) results were noted compared with function tests.[33] Another study showed that although secretin-stimulated flow was reduced in severe pancreatitis (5.6 mL/min), it was actually similar for control subjects, mild disease patients, and moderate disease patients (7.4, 7.5, and 7.0 mL/min, respectively).[34] Other features such as T1/T2 intensity and atrophy have been proposed (and used by some) but need further validation. In contrast to EUS, the MRCP literature does not propose a scoring system for counting or weighting features, so disease may be reported as "suspected" when *any* of these features are found.

Test Performance and Study Limitations

Fortunately, EUS has been compared to ERCP and/or secretin-stimulated pancreatic function testing as the best available reference standards for chronic pancreatitis, notwithstanding the above limitations, in multiple studies. The studies with and without clinical follow-up are summarized in Tables 14-7 and 14-8 and in Figure 14-3.

Pilot and Retrospective Studies

In 1993, Wiersema and colleagues[26] compared a sample of 20 healthy volunteers with 69 patients with pancreaticobiliary pain. Thirty had chronic pancreatitis by various definitions: ERCP (n = 19), ERCP and PPJ (secretin-stimulated "pure pancreatic juice" collection) (n = 3), PPJ alone (n = 6), and clinical (n = 2) criteria. Three or more criteria was defined as abnormal, based on ROC analysis of a composite reference standard. The sensitivity and specificity of EUS for chronic pancreatitis was 100% and 79%, respectively, compared with ERCP, and 80% and 86%, respectively, compared with the

---

TABLE 14-6

CAMBRIDGE CLASSIFICATION OF CHRONIC PANCREATITIS BY ERCP

Class	Definition
0: Normal	Visualization of entire duct system with uniform filling of side branches without acinar opacification, with a normal main duct and normal side branches
1: Equivocal	Normal main duct One to three abnormal branches
2: Mild	Normal main duct More than three abnormal side branches
3: Moderate	Dilated main duct with irregularity More than three abnormal side branches Small cysts (<10 mm)
4: Marked/Severe	Large cysts (>10 mm) Gross irregularity of main pancreatic duct Intraductal calculus/calculi Stricture(s) Obstruction with severe dilation

(From: Axon AT, Classen M, Cotton PB, et al. Pancreatography in chronic pancreatitis: international definitions. Gut. 1984;25:1107-1112.)

TABLE 14-7

REVIEW OF LITERATURE *WITHOUT CLINICAL FOLLOW-UP* REGARDING DIAGNOSTIC TEST PERFORMANCE OF EUS IN CHRONIC PANCREATITIS

Reference	Number of Patients	Design	Results	Comments
Wiersema 1993[26]	69	20 controls examined 69 patients with pancreatic or biliary pain studied All 69 had ERCP, 16 had PPJ testing	30 had chronic pancreatitis by ERCP (19), ERCP and PPJ (3), PPJ alone (6), and clinical (2) SN 80%; SP 86% if ≥3 criteria of 11 used, as per ROC curve analysis SN 100%; SP 79% vs ERCP SN 67%; SP 29% vs PPJ for EUS SN 33%; SP 86% vs PPJ for ERCP	11 total criteria, 5 significant in logistic regression Called foci >3 mm 20 controls not used in accuracy calculation
Buscail 1995[43]	44	81 consecutive patients, 44 had ERCP, plus 18 controls	SN 88%; SP 100%	Nonconsecutive enrollment "Hand-picked" controls Called echogenic duct wall normal Nonstandard terms and criteria No threshold reported
Catalano 1998[25]	80	Consecutive patients with recurrent pancreatitis	SN 86%; SP 95% vs ERCP SN 84%; SP 98% vs ERCP and PPJ testing 0 criteria: 100% NPV ≥6 criteria: 100% PPV 3-5 criteria: 92% positive ERCP, 50% positive PPJ 1-2 criteria: 17% positive ERCP, 13% positive PPJ	Even 1 criterion was considered abnormal (mild), but only moderate/severe considered positive for analysis (≥3 criteria) Waited 6 weeks since last attack Blinded EUS (not ERCP)
Sahai 1998[36]	126	Double-blind prospective Patients with unexplained pain or suspected pancreatitis referred for ERCP	<3 criteria: "NPV >85%" ≥6 criteria: "PPV >85%" No actual SN/SP specified	9 criteria used Head ignored Called foci <3 mm Size criteria for most criteria
Hollerbach 2001[41]	37	Suspicion of chronic pancreatitis, with FNA in 27 patients	SN 97%; SP 60% vs ERCP, without FNA SN 100%; SP 67% vs. ERCP, with FNA (n = 27) SN 52%; SP 75% vs indirect pancreatic function tests	5 criteria total Weighted criteria 7% post-FNA pancreatitis
Chowdhury 2005[43]	21	Retrospective review of patients undergoing EUS and secretin stimulation test	≥4 criteria ideal on ROC SN 57%, SP 64% for ≥4 criteria ≥6 criteria had SP 92%	9 EUS criteria Abnormal peak stimulated duodenal (bicarbonate) ≥80 mEq/L
Chong 2007[57]	71	Retrospective review of patients undergoing surgery for pancreatic pain with preoperative EUS on record	Only 58% of 30 with calcifications had these seen on pre-EUS imaging 41 of 71 did not have calcifications ≥3 criteria ideal on ROC (noncalcific) SN 83%; SP 80% for ≥3 criteria ≥5 criteria: 100% SP 2 or fewer: 90% SN $r = 0.40$ for criteria vs histologic severity	9 EUS criteria 12 histologic criteria (≥2 abnormal) Blinded GI pathologist Mass lesions excluded
Varadarajulu 2007[38]	42	Prospective study patients undergoing preoperative EUS, without calcifications, before pancreatic surgery for variety of indications	≥4 criteria ideal on ROC SN 91%; SP 86% for ≥4 criteria $r = 0.85$ for criteria vs histologic severity	9 EUS criteria 12 histologic criteria (≥6 abnormal) Blinded GI pathologist Patients with resectable masses were included, examining pancreas "furthest from the mass"

ERCP, endoscopic retrograde cholangiopancreatography; FNA, fine-needle aspiration; GI, gastrointestinal; NPV, negative predictive value; PPJ, secretin-stimulated bicarbonate testing on pure pancreatic juice; PPV, positive predictive value; ROC, receiver-operator characteristic; SN, sensitivity; SP, specificity.

REVIEW OF LITERATURE *WITH CLINICAL FOLLOW-UP* REGARDING DIAGNOSTIC TEST PERFORMANCE OF EUS IN CHRONIC PANCREATITIS

Reference	Number of Patients	Design	Results	Comments
Hastier 1999[42]	18	72 patients with alcoholic cirrhosis without pancreatic symptoms 32 controls with abdominal pain and normal ERCP, without history of pancreatitis or alcohol 18 had EUS parenchymal criteria only and either follow-up EUS or ERCP	None of patients with parenchymal criteria only on EUS had progression on follow-up EUS or new abnormalities on ERCP (n = 10)	8 criteria sought Denominator was 104 patients Selection bias likely due to confounding by the clinical factors leading to repeat EUS or ERCP Kasugai ERCP grading No blinding
Chen 2002 (abstract)[82]	19	Retrospective study of normal EUS and ERCP repeated >12 months later	5 (83%) of 6 patients with normal ERCP, but abnormal EUS, had abnormal ERCP 1 (7%) of 13 with normal EUS and ERCP had abnormal ERCP in follow-up	Denominator was 299 patients Selection bias likely due to confounding by the clinical factors leading to repeat ERCP
Kahl 2002[40]	38	Symptomatic with suspected chronic pancreatitis but normal ERCP 32 had abnormal EUS 22 of the 22 who had follow-up ERCP were abnormal on 2nd ERCP	Half of abnormal second ERCPs were Cambridge 1, half were Cambridge 2 Using second ERCP as a gold standard in those with abnormal EUS, ERCP had an 81% SN EUS had 100% SN; 16% SP (74% SP using 2nd ERCP as gold standard)	10 criteria sought, ≥1 called abnormal Cambridge ERCP grading No blinding Most ERCP progression was subtle Most common criterion (lobular pattern = strands, foci) was really 2 criteria
Singh 2004 (abstract)[83]	39	Retrospective study EUS patients with ≤3 criteria	18% developed diabetes over a mean of 5 years follow-up, many times higher than the age-sex expected rate	No data on whether ERCP was normal at baseline Suggests 1-3 criteria may mean structural damage

ERCP, endoscopic retrograde cholangiopancreatography; SN, sensitivity; SP, specificity.

"final diagnosis" (ERCP, secretin testing, and/or "clinical criteria"). In the 16 that had PPJ (including 9 abnormal), EUS had a sensitivity and specificity of 67% and 29%, respectively. ERCP, in contrast, compared to function testing and clinical criteria had sensitivity of 33% and 86%, respectively. The cutoff determination and test performance characteristics could be biased because of the lack of external validation.[49]

Buscail and colleagues[43] reviewed 81 consecutive patients referred for suspected pancreatic disease. The results of the 44 patients that had ERCP were compared with 18 control subjects. EUS definitions were somewhat nonstandard (e.g., an "echogenic wall" was considered normal, and nonstandard terms such as "diffusely heterogeneous," "diffusely hyperechoic," "hypoechoic areas," and "hypertrophic" were used to describe abnormalities). The threshold number of criteria for diagnosis was vague, but a sensitivity and specificity of 88% and 100%, respectively, was reported. Although common and acceptable for pilot study designs, comparing "cases" to "controls" to assess diagnostic test performance is prone to so-called spectrum bias (i.e., it is generally easier to separate frankly normal [control] patients from frankly abnormal [case] patients than it is to separate normal and abnormal patients in a series of consecutive real-life patients with clinical suspicion of disease).[49,84,85]

Another retrospective study by Chowdhury and colleagues,[86] performed at the University of Florida, examined how EUS compared to invasive pancreatic function testing (secretin test, normal peak stimulated duodenal bicarbonate concentration ≥80 mEq/L). Using data from the 21 patients studied with both tests, ROC curve analysis showed that the best balance of sensitivity and specificity was using a cutoff of four or more criteria (sensitivity 57%, specificity 64%).[86] A threshold of six or more criteria (out of nine) had 92% specificity.

Prospective and Consecutive Series

Catalano[25] compared 80 consecutive patients with recurrent pancreatitis in a prospective comparative trial. Patients waited at least 6 weeks after their last acute pancreatitis attack before undergoing EUS with ERCP and a secretin test. "Mild" chronic pancreatitis by EUS was defined as 1 to 2, "moderate" as 3 to 5, and "severe" as >5 criteria of 10 criteria, including one termed "heterogeneity." Normal was therefore defined as having no criteria. Fortunately, in the analysis of test performance, only "moderate/severe" EUS was considered positive (≥3 criteria). EUS had 86% sensitivity and 95% specificity compared with ERCP and had 84% sensitivity and 98% specificity when compared with ERCP plus secretin test. Both

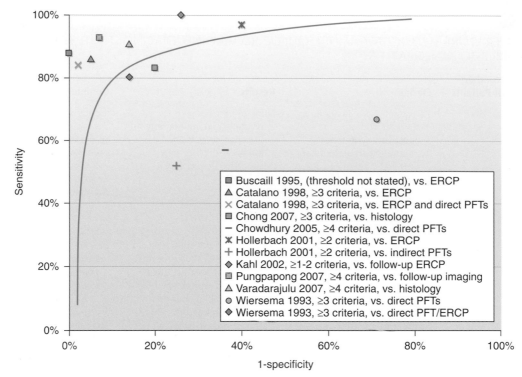

FIGURE 14-3   Test performance (receiver-operator characteristics) of various studies of EUS in chronic pancreatitis, plotted as sensitivity against 1-specificity (false-positive rate). EUS, endoscopic ultrasound; ERCP, endoscopic retrograde cholangiopancreatography; PFT, pancreatic function test. *Most studies either did not include calcific pancreatitis or had a very small number of patients with calcifications. A rough qualitative summary curve is provided. A quantitative curve is not calculated due to the inhomogeneity of the reference standard of the studies.

normal EUS and "severe"-disease EUS had 100% agreement with normality or abnormality on ERCP and a secretin test, respectively; the grades also often agreed ($\kappa = 0.82$). Three to five criteria ("moderate" disease) by EUS still had 92% agreement with ERCP but only 50% with the secretin test. "Mild pancreatitis" (1 to 2 criteria) had a 17% rate of abnormal ERCP and 13% of abnormal secretin test (i.e., a small percentage of "low-probability" EUS patients likely still have chronic pancreatitis). The terms "mild," "moderate," and "severe" imply *grading* rather than *probability* of disease and are best avoided, as supported by the recent consensus document lead-authored by the same group.[15] A source of bias in this study was that ERCP endoscopists were not necessarily blinded to the EUS result.

The largest prospective study is from MUSC by Sahai and colleagues.[36] in 1998. In this study, 126 patients with unexplained abdominal pain or suspected pancreatitis referred for ERCP underwent EUS first, and then ERCP blinded to EUS results. Nine criteria were used, and size definitions for echogenic foci (1 to 2 mm), hypoechoic lobules (2 to 5 mm), ductal size (>3 mm in head, >2 mm in body, >1 mm in tail), and cysts (>2 mm) were given. Abnormal ERCP was defined as Cambridge 3 (25%) or higher (21%); as such, normal/equivocal (Cambridge <2) (24%) findings and "mild" chronic pancreatitis (Cambridge 2) (29%) on ERCP were considered normal (see Table 14-7). Interestingly, neither individual criteria nor the number of criteria were apparently significant in multivariate analysis, although when they changed the ERCP threshold to Cambridge 2 or higher, the number of parenchymal criteria became a significant predictor. Less than three criteria had a negative predictive value ">85%," and more

than six criteria (i.e., seven or more) had a positive predictive value ">85%"; unfortunately, other more specific performance numbers were not mentioned in the paper.

Studies Involving FNA or Biopsy

In 2001, Hollerbach and colleagues[41] studied 37 German patients suspected clinically of having chronic pancreatitis[31] (84% had abnormal ERCP). Patients underwent EUS with (n = 27) or without FNA, ERCP, and noninvasive pancreatic function testing (fecal chymotrypsin and elastase-1 and urinary pancreolauryl testing). Only five criteria were sought (hyperechoic lobules [foci], "septae" (hyperechoic strands), ductal irregularity, calcifications, and cysts) and were weighted into three grades: (1) lobularity and strands; (2) grade 1 plus ductal irregularities; or (3) grade 1 or 2 plus stones or cysts. EUS had a sensitivity of 97% (100% with FNA) and a specificity of 60% (67% with FNA) compared with ERCP; sensitivity and specificity were 52% and 75%, respectively, when compared with pancreatic function tests. Two (7%) of 27 patients had complications of post-FNA pancreatitis requiring fluids and analgesia for 1 day.

Dewitt and colleagues[87] attempted EUS-guided Tru-Cut biopsies in 16 patients with suspected (three or more criteria) chronic pancreatitis on EUS. Results were compared to ERCP in 13 patients. The agreement between the biopsy result and either the EUS or the ERCP was poor ($\kappa = 0$ and 0.25, respectively). Of the five patients with a normal ERCP, none had a normal Tru-Cut biopsy (four patients had an abnormal Tru-Cut result [i.e., 80% false-positive rate] and one patient was nondiagnostic). Of the eight patients with an abnormal ERCP, only one had an abnormal Tru-Cut biopsy (three patients had a normal Tru-Cut result and four patients were nondiagnostic; sensitivity 13%). Two patients (13%) had pain requiring overnight admission.

It therefore seems that neither FNA nor Tru-Cut biopsy adds information to the EUS-derived diagnosis and often may be misleading; the maneuver adds a 5% to 15% adverse event (unanticipated hospital stay) rate to EUS. An ASGE practice guideline supports the position that its limited value is not worth its risk.[17]

Studies with Comparison to Surgical Pathology

An animal study in dogs using a pancreatic stent-induced pancreatitis model showed some correlation between EUS findings and necropsy findings.[88] Two groups,[37,60] including one at MUSC, compared EUS findings with surgical pathology in humans. The MUSC study had 71 patients who had undergone surgery for suspected chronic pancreatitis or pancreatic pain from refractory sphincter stenosis or pancreas divisum.[37] In patients without calcifications ($n = 41$), three or more EUS criteria (cutoff based on ROC curve analysis) had a sensitivity of 83% and specificity of 80%. A cutoff of five or more criteria had 100% specificity; two or fewer criteria had a false-negative rate of less than 10% (sensitivity 90%). In the subgroup without calcifications, positive histology ranged from 8 (67%) of 12 if a core/wedge biopsy was the sample to 28 (97%) of 29 if a block of tissue (e.g., Whipple procedures, distal pancreatectomy) was available to the pathologist, highlighting the sampling error even with surgical core biopsies.

A group at the University of Alabama also studied the correlation between EUS and surgical pathology prospectively in 42 patients operated on for a variety of indications, including resectable neoplastic cysts and masses. They found four or more EUS criteria (cutoff based on ROC curve analysis) to have 91% sensitivity and 86% specificity.[60] Correlation between the number of EUS criteria and histological fibrosis severity score was higher ($r = 0.85$) than it was in the MUSC study ($r = 0.40$), although both were statistically significant. Of note, the MUSC investigators used a more conservative minimum fibrosis score threshold (2 of 12 on Ammann classification[39]) than did Alabama investigators (6 of 12).

Studies with Clinical or Radiologic Follow-up

Because our "gold" reference standards are somewhat "tarnished," a few studies have aimed to follow-up patients with so-called "false-positive EUS" to see if early chronic pancreatitis (i.e., those patients that may have been missed on the traditional gold standards) progresses to more overt disease. The results are conflicting (see Table 14-8 and Figure 14-3).

In a 2002 study from MUSC by Chen and colleagues,[82] 6 of 51 patients with normal ERCP but abnormal EUS underwent repeat ERCP more than 1 year later, and 5 (83%) ERCP results became abnormal (i.e., a positive predictive value >80% despite normal initial ERCP). In contrast, 13 of 248 patients with both normal EUS and normal ERCP underwent ERCP more than 1 year later, and only 1 (7%) became abnormal (i.e., a negative predictive value of 93%).

Hastier and colleagues[42] studied 72 French patients with alcoholic cirrhosis (without symptoms of pancreatitis) and 32 age-sex-matched control subjects with abdominal pain and a normal ERCP, without history of pancreatitis or alcohol abuse. Eight criteria (five ductal and three parenchymal) were sought. Of these patients, 18 with one or more parenchymal criteria

on EUS, and also successfully underwent a normal ($n = 18$) ERCP and a repeat EUS 12 to 38 months later. Ten of these had a repeat ERCP. In all 18 patients, EUS findings were unchanged; in all 10 of those who underwent repeat ERCP, ERCP remained normal.

A second German study by Kahl and colleagues[40] studied 32 symptomatic patients with suspected chronic pancreatitis and a normal ERCP yet abnormal EUS (more than one criterion); 92 patients had abnormal ERCP. Of note, over half (57%) of these patients drank alcohol during the follow-up period of 6 to 25 months. Ten criteria (five parenchymal [including "gland size"] and five ductal) were sought; all patients had lobules and "septations." Twenty-two (69%) of the 32 patients had an ERCP in follow-up and all were abnormal (approximately half Cambridge group 1 and half Cambridge group 2). If the abnormal second ERCP is used as a reference standard, the first ERCP was 81% sensitive, and the EUS was 100% sensitive. Of note, although only one or more criterion was needed for an EUS to be called positive in this study, accentuation of the lobular pattern was the most common finding and really represents two conventional criteria (i.e., strands and lobules).

A study from the Mayo Clinic by Pungpapong and colleagues[89] used a combination of nonblinded ERCP, imaging (at least two negative imaging tests if ERCP was normal [i.e. Cambridge group 0 or 1]), and clinical impression after a minimum 7-month follow-up (median 15 months) as a composite reference standard to assess the diagnostic performance of EUS showing four or more of nine criteria (cutoff derived by ROC curve analysis) in 99 symptomatic patients. Sensitivity and specificity were 93% and 93%, respectively. In comparison, MRI and MRCP, using one or more criteria, had a sensitivity and specificity of 65% and 90%, respectively.

These study results conflict with one another, possibly due to different diagnostic criteria for chronic pancreatitis by EUS, different ERCP classifications (Kasugai[42] versus Cambridge[40,89]), asymptomatic[42] versus symptomatic[40,89] patient cohorts, varying proportions of ongoing alcohol in the study groups, and relatively subtle findings on some ERCPs considered positive.[40,89] A critical source of bias in all three studies is that the physicians interpreting the follow-up imaging were not blinded to the original assessments.[49,84]

Comparison and follow-up with respect to endocrine pancreatic function has generally not been reported, mainly because endocrine insufficiency (impaired glucose tolerance or diabetes) is a late finding due to the tremendous endocrine reserve of the gland. However, an interesting study has described the follow-up of 39 patients with a low probability of chronic pancreatitis by EUS (three or less criteria) and found that seven patients (18%) developed diabetes over 5 years,[83] which was higher than the 5-year age-sex-matched standardized incidence.

Summarizing Performance

Summarizing test performance has been difficult for EUS in chronic pancreatitis for several reasons: meta-analysis of diagnostic tests requires a unique set of statistical skills; the literature is very heterogeneous; and the "gold" or reference standards are far from perfect. Our group and a Bayesian statistics group at McGill University collaborated to use Bayesian methods to adjust for the imperfection in the reference standards to summarize test performance, after assessing the quality and risk of bias with published (QUADAS) scores.[90] We asked the Bayesian model to consider what we know about the limitations of the reference standards ("prior information"). In lay terms, the model considers that some discrepancies between EUS and the reference standard could be due to the reference standard being wrong (i.e., a "false-positive" EUS could really be a "false-negative" reference test). Adjusting for the imperfect reference standard yielded higher test performance characteristics for EUS than if perfection in the reference standard was assumed. Median pooled sensitivity and specificity were 87% and 93% for the three or more criteria cutoff. Adjusted sensitivities and specificities for the reference standards ranged from 74% to 95% and 85% to 95% for minimal change disease where histology was most accurate (>90%) and function tests least sensitive (<80%) but specific (>90%).[90]

Staging versus Probability of Disease

EUS criteria thresholds and ranges have *not* been generally validated to "stage" chronic pancreatitis *severity* but rather to assess the *probability* of disease. That being true, EUS can detect the features (stones, strictures, and duct and side branch dilation) that comprise the ERCP Cambridge classification.[32] As such, one can use EUS effectively to anticipate the Cambridge severity class. However, high-probability disease (i.e., more than five criteria) does not necessarily mean severe disease; it can range between normal/equivocal and severe Cambridge severity.

Low, intermediate, and high numbers of criteria of chronic pancreatitis only loosely correlate with advancing histology[37,60] or advancing Cambridge class, and so those cutoffs should generally not be used to stage severity of disease. That is, low probability should not be called "mild" and intermediate probability should not be called "moderate," and so on. A recent consensus conference agreed with this principle,[15] but some publications have (in the author's opinion, incorrectly) used number of criteria to define categories of "severity."

Differentiating Inflammatory Pseudotumors from Neoplastic Masses

Acute inflammatory exacerbations of chronic pancreatitis can result in focal edema. This focal edema on CT can be indistinguishable from a neoplastic mass; a 16% to 23% error rate has been reported in this setting.[91,92] Although the coexisting chronic pancreatitis features raise the suspicion of something inflammatory, cancer can still be present because 2% to 4% of patients with nonfamilial chronic pancreatitis develop pancreatic cancer after 10 to 20 years.[93] False-negative results can have serious consequences (missed opportunities to remove a resectable cancer), as can false-positive results (unnecessary Whipple's pancreatoduodenectomy).

Painless (versus painful) presentations, weight loss, frank jaundice, persistent or progressive (versus fluctuating) cholestasis, recent onset or worsening of diabetes, or vascular invasion on cross-sectional imaging can all be helpful in distinguishing benign and malignant causes of the mass. Absence of risk factors for pancreatitis, such as alcohol, is another red flag. Unfortunately, the presentation in benign cases can uncommonly be accompanied by weight loss, particularly in

smoldering acute pancreatitis or in chronic pancreatitis associated with decreased intake, meal-induced nausea/pain, and/or pancreatic insufficiency. Diabetes can also worsen abruptly in someone with benign, acute-on-chronic inflammation or can newly present if endocrine function was already borderline. CA 19-9 has tremendous overlap between benign and malignant disease, especially when biliary obstruction is present. Lymph nodes, including celiac nodes, can occur in both benign and neoplastic pancreatic diseases. Biliary and/or pancreatic duct dilation (including the "double duct sign") is unfortunately common in both benign and malignant disease. Pancreatic duct irregularity is common in both scenarios.[94] Benign pancreatic duct strictures can be tight and irregular in both conditions, and pancreatic duct cytology is low yield in neoplasia.[95,96] Because of this overlap, management decisions can be very difficult.

The accuracy of EUS, with or without FNA, for pancreatic cancer has been well studied[97] and is detailed in Chapter 15, but most of those studies, unfortunately, do not have a good mix of neoplastic and non-neoplastic cases. As a typical example, the study by Mallery and colleagues[98] had a 92% prevalence of malignancy.

EUS is uniquely able to see parenchymal detail in pancreatic tissue and does not solely rely on size, asymmetry of the gland, or upstream ductal dilation to assess pseudotumors. The usual parenchymal features and ducts are generally focally missing in neoplastic masses, which are generally more homogeneous and distinctly hypoechoic compared with surrounding tissue. Neoplastic masses are seldom calcified, and so masses with internal calcification are more likely to be benign; malignancies within a calcified pancreas often push the calcified parenchyma aside, toward the periphery. One significant limitation to EUS in calcific chronic pancreatitis is that acoustic shadowing from the calcifications can obscure variable proportions of the gland from assessment. Signs of vascular invasion are generally highly suggestive of malignancy; however, in some cases, inflammation-related compression/adherence of vascular structures (Figure 14-4) and/or thrombosis can be misleading.

Barthet and colleagues[99] claimed 100% sensitivity for EUS, based on the workup of 5 of 85 patients with 2- to 3.5-cm masses in calcific chronic pancreatitis, all of whom had jaundice and weight loss. However, they only "verified" (i.e., gathered follow-up on) the positive EUS patients, introducing a verification bias.[84,100] Kaufman and Sivak[101] studied 25 patients (10 malignant); there was one false-negative result (90% sensitivity) and two false-positive results (87% specificity). Nattermann and colleagues[102] studied 130 consecutive patients (61 with malignancies) and found several features that had different frequencies in cancer versus focal inflammation (7% versus 23% hyperechoic foci, 30% versus 7% loss of demarcation with the luminal wall, 28% versus 9% loss of separation between vascular structures, and 11% versus 0% frank invasion of a vessel); however, none was significant, and tremendous overlap was evident by these numbers. Glasbrenner and colleagues[103] studied 95 consecutive patients (50 malignant); EUS (not blinded to history) without FNA had a 78% sensitivity and 93% specificity. A study by Varadarajulu and colleagues[104] showed that the sensitivity of EUS FNA was significantly lower in the 25% of "mass" patients who had chronic pancreatitis (74% versus 91%; $p = 0.02$), required

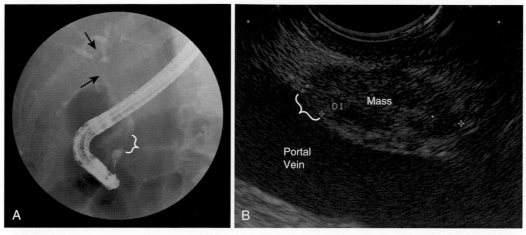

FIGURE 14-4 **A** and **B**, Endoscopic retrograde cholangiopancreatography (ERCP) and linear EUS of a 70-year-old Asian man with painless jaundice, mild weight loss, and no past history of alcohol or pancreatitis. **A**, ERCP showed a tight-shouldered distal biliary stricture (curved brackets), but cytology from biliary brushings were negative. Intrahepatic irregularities are also noted (*arrows*). CT scan of the pancreas was normal. **B**, A 5 × 25 mm hypoechoic mass, distinct from adjacent noninflamed parenchyma, is seen in the head, abutting the portal vein with a short loss of the interface (curved bracket). The rest of the pancreas appeared normal (no chronic pancreatitis criteria). Fine-needle aspiration showed benign cells without plasma cells. Serum IgG4 was not requested preoperatively, but surgical pathology was consistent with focal chronic pancreatitis of the head, likely autoimmune.

more EUS FNA passes (median, 5 versus 2; $p < 0.001$), and had lower predictive value when negative (46% versus 89%). Given that some genes are overexpressed in pancreatic cancer[105–114] and others are differentially expressed in chronic pancreatitis,[115–119] there is potential for reverse transcription polymerase chain reaction[120] to complement cytology on FNA-acquired specimens in these diagnostic dilemmas as well. However, this situation requires further study given conflicting results in brush cytology literature—one study showed great results with k-*ras*,[121] but another showed performance (sensitivity 42%) no better than brush cytology.[122] Similarly, p53 immunostain results were promising, but results have been conflicting, with yields that may be as low as 51%.[123]

Digital image analysis (DIA) and fluorescence in situ hybridization (FISH), analyzing nuclear DNA content, and the presence of aneuploidy have also been piloted to enhance diagnostic accuracy of EUS FNA, with slightly lower sensitivity (87% versus 97%) but comparable specificity to routine cytology in one small study (19 pancreatic FNA patients).[124] "Enhanced EUS" with contrast harmonic imaging or with elastography is discussed in a separate chapter (see Chapter 5).[125]

Other competing imaging methods have been studied in this area. Intraductal ultrasound may be a helpful adjunct in some cases because of its high-imaging resolution, but results are conflicting and poor overall. Fluoro-deoxyglucose positron-emission tomography (FDG-PET) appears promising, with a reported sensitivity as high as 88%; however, it uses metabolic activity to distinguish inflammatory and neoplastic lesions, and there is marked overlap in metabolic activity between inflammation and cancer.[126–129] False-negative PET is also an issue; in one study ($n = 200$ pancreatic masses), there were 8 false-negative results,[129] and up to 20% of cancers had decreased delayed uptake (a benign PET feature).[130] In another small ($n = 6$ cancers in chronic pancreatitis) study, sensitivity was 83% and there was a 13% false-positive rate.[131]

Finally, it is also often misleadingly positive in autoimmune pancreatitis.[132]

Autoimmune Pancreatitis

Autoimmune pancreatitis (AIP) is a steroid-responsive inflammatory condition of the pancreas, accounting for less than 5% of patients investigated for acute and chronic pancreatitis,[133] which can produce focal inflammatory masses that mimic cancers.[14] AIP is found in about 2% of pancreatoduodenectomy specimens for suspected pancreatic cancer. AIP can present with pancreatic insufficiency and weight loss, with minimal pain, and can be associated with jaundice and malignant-looking biliary strictures.

Several publications exist detailing diagnostic criteria, including reports from Asia,[19] the United States (Mayo Clinic),[134] and, most recently, Japan.[20] In the United States and Europe, type I AIP (lymphoplasmacytic sclerosing pancreatitis) is more common than type 2 (idiopathic duct-centric chronic pancreatitis, or AIP with granulocytic epithelial lesions).[18] Type 1 is more clearly an autoimmune disease, likely a pancreatic manifestation of systemic disease (including biliary strictures, retroperitoneal fibrosis, renal involvement, and salivary gland enlargement), with elevated serum IgG4. It typically affects males over age 50. Sensitivity and specificity of elevated serum IgG4 (>140 mg/dL) for diagnosing AIP were 73% to 76% and 93%, respectively.[135,136] The specificity rose to 99% when IgG4 was twice the upper limit of normal (>280 mg/dL).[135] Another serologic marker of AIP (antibody to plasminogen-binding protein) was recently tested and was found to be about 95% sensitive and specific; it may be more accurate than IgG4.[137] Type 2 patients have wider age and gender spectra and more often do not have elevated serum IgG4 levels. Therefore type 2 AIP is more likely to need a histologic diagnosis. However, both types can be associated with biliary strictures. When clinical suspicion is high, even a mildly elevated IgG4 level may be sufficient for diagnosis. In other cases, a negative FNA of the mass and a more elevated (>2 times upper limit) IgG4 level may be needed.[18] IgG4-associated disease present elsewhere is also supportive evidence, including ampullary involvement (ampullary biopsy staining positive for IgG4).[138,139]

Tissue biopsy and ERCP have controversial roles in AIP. EUS-FNA cytology is often nondiagnostic, showing non-specific chronic inflammation, although high cellularity of stromal fragments may be suggestive.[140,141] The usefulness of EUS-guided Tru-Cut biopsy is unclear and has a known risk of postprocedural pain and pancreatitis. The Mayo Clinic group[142] and others[143] have found Tru-Cut biopsy to be very helpful (and better than FNA) in small series (Figure 14-5); however, others[144] have not. One study showed that only one quarter were diagnosed histologically with ultrasound-guided cores; IgG4-positive cells were also noted in 25% of alcoholic pancreatitis and 10% of cancers.[144] Although the Asian and Japanese consensus papers require ERCP for diagnosis, North Americans generally avoid diagnostic pancreatography and rely on *h*istology, *i*maging, *s*erology, *o*ther *o*rgan involvement, and *r*esponse to steroid *t*reatment (HISORt). ERCP was recently shown to have poor reliability in preliminary results of a multicenter trial.[145]

Classically, on cross-sectional imaging, diffuse pancreatic enlargement with delayed enhancement is noted, without pancreatic duct dilation, with or without a focal mass; the mass may demonstrate peripheral hypoattenuation, appearing as a so-called "halo."[14] Similar features are seen on EUS, with a diffusely enlarged, somewhat lobular, sausage-shaped gland with hypoechoic margins, sometimes with a focal enlargement or hypoechoic mass, without pancreatic duct dilation.[141,146] Pancreatic strictures (generally without upstream dilation) and biliary wall thickening and strictures can also be seen on EUS (Video 14-3).

It has been recently shown in a multicenter study of over 500 patients that, although generally treated with steroids, up to 74% of patients treated without steroids go into remission spontaneously, compared with 98% of those treated with steroids.[147] Response, generally seen in 2 to 4 weeks, is reassuring for the diagnosis; however, one must keep in mind that adenocarcinomas and lymphomas can respond partially to steroids, too. Although some have suggested prolonged

Video 14-3. Video demonstrating a case of autoimmune pancreatitis with FNA being undertaken.

steroid treatments, tapering over 3 to 6 months,[147] North American centers more commonly treat with 30 to 40 mg/day for 4 to 6 weeks, reassess clinical and radiologic response, and then taper over the next 1 to 2 months.[148] Unfortunately, relapses occur in 30% to 40% of cases; initial steroids may be associated with lower relapse rates, as may normalization in IgG4 and absence of proximal biliary involvement.[147,149] Most Japanese patients are treated with maintenance therapy (usually with low-dose steroids), whereas North American patients are usually only given maintenance therapy (e.g., an immunomodulator such as azathioprine) if remission is not sustained throughout the taper.

Infectious Pancreatitis

Infection is an unusual cause of acute or subacute pancreatitis or of an inflammatory pancreatic mass. One case report showed that EUS FNA can detect *Giardia lamblia* infection.[150] Peripancreatic tuberculous lymphadenopathy has also been described.[151,152]

Chronic Pancreatitis Criteria in Kindreds at High Risk for Pancreatic Cancer

The interpretation of "chronic pancreatitis criteria" in kindreds of familial pancreatic cancer and Peutz-Jeghers should be cautious. These endosonographic findings may have very different histologic correlates in this patient group. Canto and colleagues[153] highlight that in this group of patients, criteria for chronic pancreatitis are common and may be associated with dysplasia rather than with inflammation and fibrosis, with 45% (of 38 patients) having three or more criteria, including 35% of the subgroup that did not drink any alcohol. Another Hopkins study showed that pancreatic intraepithelial neoplasia (PanIN) and intraductal papillary mucinous neoplasm (IPMN) lesions can be associated with so-called "lobular pancreatic atrophy," mimicking chronic pancreatitis.[154] Brentnall and colleagues[155] from Seattle found PanIN in these high-risk patients when ERCP and/or EUS had findings of "chronic pancreatitis." Therefore discrete "lobules," cysts, or nodules in these high-risk patients likely require FNA (in contrast to all-comers with these features) or, at a minimum, close surveillance, with possibly even selective resection in some patients.

Acute Pancreatitis

Acute Pancreatitis Diagnosis and Staging

Except for calcifications, all of the criteria used to detect and grade chronic pancreatitis can also be seen in acute pancreatitis (including cysts and mild ductal dilatation). This is why

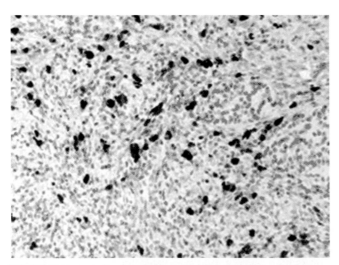

FIGURE 14-5 Lymphoplasmacytic infiltrate with positive IgG4 immunostaining (>30 positive cells per high-power field) from an EUS-guided Tru-Cut biopsy specimen in autoimmune pancreatitis.

it is generally recommended to wait at least 4 to 6 weeks after attacks of acute pancreatitis before looking for evidence of chronic pancreatitis. Identification of fluid collections and estimating the proportion of gland with necrosis are important predictors of outcome in acute pancreatitis and are generally performed by contrast-enhanced CT.[21] There is essentially no other published data on the ability of EUS to detect or stage acute pancreatitis, including with contrast-enhanced EUS (although this could in theory be possible). Assessing perfusion and detecting fluid collections appear feasible with MRI.[156,157] Therefore, MRI and EUS may have a limited role in those with renal failure and/or diabetes in whom intravenous contrast at CT may be harmful, but both remain under-studied.

Idiopathic (Recurrent) Acute Pancreatitis (IRAP) and Pancreas Divisum

Acute pancreatitis is most commonly due to either alcohol abuse or sludge/stones obstructing the common bile duct; these together make up the etiology in 80% of cases. The high accuracy of EUS in choledocholithiasis is discussed in Chapter 17. The other 20% are generally considered idiopathic. Because about 80% of "idiopathic" cases do not recur, after ruling out obvious causes (medications, metabolic causes, and, in older patients, tumors), more extensive workup is generally not needed unless the problem recurs.[158] In up to half of recurrent (IRAP) cases, attacks can be explained by a variety of causes, including medications, microlithiasis, tumors (rare, but especially of concern in those over age 60), sphincter dysfunction (biliary and/or pancreatic), pancreas divisum, metabolic causes (hypercalcemia, hypertriglyceridemia), autoimmune disease, genetic causes, rare infections, and others. Chronic pancreatitis is also present in up to half of IRAP patients but is more likely a sequela of damage from their intermittent acute attacks rather than an "etiology."

EUS is comparable to MRCP in detection of most etiologies, so they can be used interchangeably for this purpose. However, EUS likely has a higher detection rate for tumors (in older patients) and for missed biliary lithiasis (in those

that still have a gallbladder). Figure 14-6 shows an example of gallbladder sludge on EUS, missed by CT and MRCP.

Yusoff and colleagues[159] studied 370 patients in Montreal with idiopathic pancreatitis referred for EUS: 46% (n = 169) had recurrent pancreatitis and 54% (n = 201) a single attack, 34% (n = 124) were postcholecystectomy patients, and 24% to 32% of patients had a possible explanation on EUS (20% higher if considering chronic pancreatitis as an "explanation"). Occult biliary stones were not found in any of the recurrent pancreatitis postcholecystectomy patients but were found as often as 9% in single-attack patients with a gallbladder. Of those who still had a gallbladder, 11% had gallbladder sludge missed on prior imaging. The rate of finding pancreas divisum also varied from 5% if the gallbladder was still present to up to 11% if postcholecystectomy. Neoplasms were seen in 3% to 5% of cases. The allowance of small waits from the last attack (4 weeks) and up to 12 alcoholic drinks per day may have inflated the rate of finding "idiopathic" chronic pancreatitis. Tandon and Topazian[160] reviewed their experience of EUS in 31 patients with idiopathic acute pancreatitis (half recurrent, 10% postcholecystectomy). Findings included microlithiasis (16%), pancreas divisum (7%), and cancer (3%). Chronic pancreatitis was found in 45% of patients; the large group of single-attack patients with a gallbladder still in place (almost 10% had not even had an ultrasound), absence of any prior advanced imaging in some, 52% rate of moderate-to-heavy alcohol use, and only 2 to 3 weeks delay required since the last attack may account for the high rate of chronic pancreatitis findings. Norton and Alderson[161] (n = 44 consecutive patients with idiopathic pancreatitis [23% recurrent, 18% postcholecystectomy]) found an unusually high rate of missed gallbladder stones (50%) but similar rates of other findings to these other studies: choledocholithiasis (9%), pancreas divisum (2%), tumor (2%), and chronic pancreatitis (9%).

A few studies have concentrated on occult biliary lithiasis in recurrent pancreatitis. Liu and colleagues[162] prospectively evaluated 89 idiopathic pancreatitis patients and found cholelithiasis in 14 of 18 patients (78%) with a gallbladder and choledocholithiasis in 17% (confirmed surgically or by ERCP), despite repeated ultrasounds in 50% and even ERCP in 72%

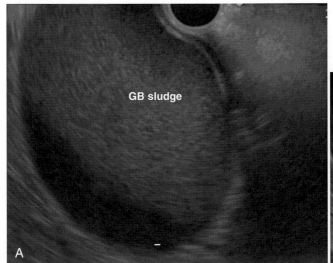
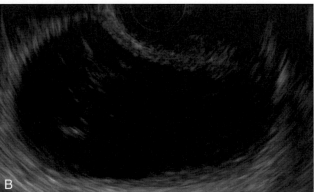

FIGURE 14-6   A, Extensive sludge in the gallbladder (GB) on linear EUS (7.5 MHz) in a patient with acute idiopathic pancreatitis missed on CT scan and MRI. **B,** Mobile nonshadowing 1-mm reflections, seen on linear EUS (7.5 mhz), appreciated only after external palpation and shaking of the gallbladder (by pressing on the right upper quadrant of the abdomen).

prior to the EUS. Another study also showed a relatively high rate of cholelithiasis and/or choledocholithiasis at EUS (35%) in 42 patients with IRAP.[163] The accuracy of duodenal sampling at EUS, with or without cholecystokinin (CCK), is theoretically easy to do but is not well studied, and the infrastructure and experience in centrifuging and detecting bile crystals does not exist in most institutions. Lee and colleagues[164] and Ros and colleagues[165] showed that crystals or sludge were seen in duodenal aspirates in 73% to 74% of patients with unexplained pancreatitis, but it appears that EUS itself may be more sensitive than duodenal fluid crystal analysis (96% versus 67%).[166] A series of 90 patients seen at MUSC with idiopathic pancreatitis[167] had 56 who had EUS with CCK-stimulated duodenal sampling and ERCP with manometry and selective bile sampling; however, the concordance between CCK-stimulated duodenal sampling and direct biliary sampling for bile crystals was not reported. More study is needed to determine if this is a useful adjunct to EUS for idiopathic pancreatitis when sludge and stones are not seen.

The cost-effectiveness of EUS in unexplained pancreatitis is unclear. One study[168] showed lower costs with EUS in patients with a gallbladder in place, but the cost saving is likely to be overestimated given that the 50% missed cholelithiasis and 5% missed bile duct stone assumptions are much higher than figures seen in three studies.[159,160,167] A systematic review supported the usefulness of EUS in older patients (although the age cutoff is unclear) and in those with a gallbladder still in but agreed that younger postcholecystectomy patients with recurrent pancreatitis are probably better served by an ERCP with manometry or pancreas divisum-based therapy where applicable.[22]

Detection of Pancreas Divisum

EUS appears to have modest to high accuracy for pancreas divisum (Video 14-4). Early MRCP studies,[169] suffering from selection and verification biases, show high accuracy; however, the accuracy of MRCP is probably modest as well. The inability to get a "stack sign" at EUS (see Chapter 13 on normal pancreatobiliary examination) because of a rudimentary ventral duct raises the possibility of pancreas divisum. This included a small MUSC study,[170] although it was only based on 6 patients with pancreas divisum with no stack sign; of note, 17% of 30 of patients who did not have pancreas divisum also showed no stack sign. Chen and colleagues[171] showed the inability to obtain a stack sign in 49% of patients with pancreas divisum versus only 6% of patients without pancreas divisum. The above studies, however, clearly show that a stack sign is still able to be obtained in one third to one half of patients with pancreas divisum, unfortunately. Other

Video 14-4. Video segment illustrating pancreas divisum and its assessment on EUS.

features that can be used include a prominent dorsal duct (16% versus 0%) and a "cross-duct" sign (8% versus 0%), which are not sensitive but fairly specific. The latter represents seeing the Santorini cross the plane of the bile duct as the pancreatic duct heads toward the minor papilla. Even this can have false-positive results when a prominent Santorini is seen in otherwise normal patients. Following the pancreatic duct from ampulla and ventral pancreas to the dorsal pancreas is probably the maneuver with the highest negative predictive value. Pancreatic strictures, very small ducts, and ansa pancreatica anatomy can make this difficult.

A prospective study of 162 patients from Minneapolis, with a high (14%) prevalence of pancreas divisum, showed that linear EUS had a high accuracy (95% sensitivity) for pancreas divisum.[172] However, 35 (8%) examinations with incomplete visualization were excluded from analysis, falsely elevating the performance numbers. Classifying those cases as "negative examinations," the sensitivity, specificity, positive predictive value, and negative predictive value were 82%, 98%, 86%, and 97%, respectively. In comparison, 41 patients had MRCP, and the sensitivity and specificity of MRCP were only 60% and 89%, respectively. Our group found a much lower sensitivity and specificity for EUS and MRCP, retrospectively reviewing all-comers for EUS checked for this diagnosis.[173] Reviewing 111 patients who underwent MRCP, we found a 32% sensitivity when read in the community and 67% (whether with or without secretin) when read in a tertiary center.[174]

In addition to diagnosing pancreas divisum, Catalano and colleagues[175] could predict who would respond to minor papilla pancreatic duct stenting by assessing response to secretin at EUS, with over 80% sensitivity and specificity. Interobserver reliability was modest ($\kappa = 0.58$), and their definition of an abnormal response was not clear, but this remains an interesting area for further study.

Summary

EUS is highly accurate in the diagnosis of chronic pancreatitis: calcifications or five or more criteria correlate well with both ERCP and pancreatic exocrine function testing; less than three criteria (especially zero criteria) effectively rules out chronic pancreatitis. Three or four criteria are the best overall cutoffs; studies landing on or near these cutoffs are essentially indeterminate and do not change one's pretest suspicion of disease. Obtaining histology by FNA/Tru-Cut biopsy is not recommended. Using the number of criteria to stage *severity* (i.e., mild/moderate/severe) of chronic pancreatitis is not recommended. Functional MRCP, a competing technology, does not appear to be nearly as accurate for early disease.

EUS is useful for the identification of possible etiologies for idiopathic recurrent pancreatitis, and its yield is highest in older patients, and those with a gallbladder in place, and may even be helpful in addition to MRCP in these patients; yield is more limited in young patients without a gallbladder. Coexisting chronic pancreatitis can also be reliably diagnosed and may be especially relevant in those with chronic pain between attacks. Although more study is needed, the diagnosis of pancreas divisum by EUS appears specific and possibly more sensitive than MRCP (especially MRCP read in the community setting). An inability to achieve a "stack sign" raises suspicion of pancreas divisum but is nonspecific, whereas a cross-duct sign is fairly specific; one's ability to follow the pancreatic duct from the major ampulla to the genu (or from ventral to dorsal) likely has the best negative predictive value.

Although not perfect, EUS is one of the best tests available to distinguish inflammatory (pseudotumors) from neoplastic masses in the pancreas. Often FNA is not required because the EUS appearance of inflammatory changes alone or bulkiness without any perceptible mass has good negative predictive value. In indeterminate masses, FNA for cytology is definitely helpful; DIA/FISH/immunostaining for oncogene products need further study. Most cases in this category require some type of follow-up imaging in approximately a month's time to pick up the rare EUS false-negative results and confirm resolution or stability of benign masses. Autoimmune pancreatitis can be suspected on EUS. Secretin-stimulated EUS, EUS with image analysis, contrast-enhanced EUS, and EUS with elastography are promising adjuncts to EUS that require further study (see Chapter 5).

ACKNOWLEDGEMENTS

The author would like to acknowledge Dr. David Lewin (Professor, Department of Pathology, Medical University of South Carolina) for his help in obtaining histologic figures displaying possible pathologic correlates of the EUS findings.

REFERENCES

1. Hisanaga K, Hisanaga A, Nagata K, Ichie Y. High speed rotating scanner for transgastric sonography. *Am J Radiol.* 1980;135:627-639.
2. DiMagno EP, Buxton JL, Regan PT, et al. Ultrasonic endoscope. *Lancet.* 1980;22:629-631.
3. DiMagno EP, Regan PT, Clain JE, et al. Human endoscopic ultrasonography. *Gastroenterology.* 1982;1982:824-829.
4. Snady H. Endoscopic ultrasonography in benign pancreatic disease. *Surg Clin North Am.* 2001;81(2):329-344.
5. Inui K, Nakazawa S, Yoshino J, et al. Endoluminal ultrasonography for pancreatic diseases. *Gastroenterol Clin North Am.* 1999;28(3):771-781.
6. Clain JE, Pearson RK. Diagnosis of chronic pancreatitis. Is a gold standard necessary? *Surg Clin North Am.* 1999;79:829-845.
7. Raimondo M, Wallace MB. Diagnosis of early chronic pancreatitis by endoscopic ultrasound. Are we there yet? *JOP.* [Electronic Resource] 2004;5(1):1-7.
8. Etemab B, Whitcomb DC. Chronic pancreatitis: diagnosis, classifiction, and new genetic developments. *Gastroenterology.* 2001;120:682-707.
9. Bhutani MS. Endoscopic ultrasound in pancreatic diseases: indications, limitations and the future. *Gastroenterol Clin.* 1999;28:747-770.
10. Wallace MB, Hawes RH. Endoscopic ultrasound in the evaluation and treatment of chronic pancreatitis. *Pancreas.* 2001;23(1):26-35.
11. Dancygier H. Endoscopic ultrasonography in chronic pancreatitis. *Gastrointest Endosc Clin N Am.* 1995;5:795-804.
12. Wiersema MJ, Wiersema LM. Endosonography of the pancreas: normal variation versus changes of early chronic pancreatitis. *Gastrointest Endosc Clin N Am.* 1995;5:487-496.
13. Kahl S, Glasbrenner B, Zimmerman S, Malfertheiner P. Endoscopic ultrasound in pancreatic diseases. *Dig Dis.* 2002;20:120-126.
14. Finkelberg DL, Sahani D, Deshpande V, Brugge WR. Autoimmune pancreatitis. *N Engl J Med.* 2006;355(25):2670-2676.
15. Catalano MF, Sahai A, Levy M, et al. EUS-based criteria for the diagnosis of chronic pancreatitis: the Rosemont classification. *Gastrointest Endosc.* 2009;69(7):1251-1261.
16. Forsmark CE. Chapter 49—Chronic pancreatitis. In: Feldman M, Tschumy WOJ, Friedman LS, Sleisenger MH, eds. *Sleisenger & Fordtran's Gastrointestinal and Liver Disease.* 7th ed. Philadelphia: Elsevier; 2002: 943–969.
17. Adler DG, Lichtenstein D, Baron TH, et al. The role of endoscopy in patients with chronic pancreatitis. *Gastrointest Endosc.* 2006; 63(7):933-937.
18. Chari ST, Longnecker DS, Kloppel G. The diagnosis of autoimmune pancreatitis: a Western perspective. *Pancreas.* 2009;38(8):846-848.
19. Otsuki M, Chung JB, Okazaki K, et al. Asian diagnostic criteria for autoimmune pancreatitis: consensus of the Japan-Korea Symposium on Autoimmune Pancreatitis. *J Gastroenterol.* 2008;43(6):403-408.
20. Okazaki K, Kawa S, Kamisawa T, et al. Japanese clinical guidelines for autoimmune pancreatitis. *Pancreas.* 2009;38(8):849-866.
21. DiMagno EP, Chari S. Chapter 48—Acute pancreatitis. In: Feldman M, Tschumy WOJ, Friedman LS, Sleisenger MH, eds. *Sleisenger & Fordtran's Gastrointestinal and Liver Disease.* 7th ed. Philadelphia: Elsevier Science; 2002:913–942.
22. Wilcox CM, Varadarajulu S, Eloubeidi M. Role of endoscopic evaluation in idiopathic pancreatitis: a systematic review. *Gastrointest Endosc.* 2006; 63(7):1037-1045.
23. Burns PN, Wilson SR. Microbubble contrast for radiological imaging: 1. Principles. *Ultrasound Q.* 2006;22(1):5-13.
24. Sugiyama M, Haradome H, Atomi Y. Magnetic resonance imaging for diagnosing chronic pancreatitis. *J Gastroenterol.* 2007;42(suppl 17):108-112.
25. Catalano MF, Lahoti S, Geenen JE, Hogan WJ. Prospective evaluation of endoscopic ultrasonography, endoscopic retrograde pancreatography, and secretin test in the diagnosis of chronic pancreatitis. *Gastrointest Endosc.* 1998;48(1):11-17.
26. Wiersema MJ, Hawes RH, Lehman G, et al. Prospective evaluation of endoscopic ultrasonography and endoscopic retrograde cholangiopancreatography in patients with chronic abdominal pain of suspected pancreatic origin. *Endoscopy.* 1993;25:555-564.
27. Wallace MB, Hawes RH, Durkalski V, et al. The reliability of EUS for the diagnosis of chronic pancreatitis: interobserver agreement among experienced endosonographers. *Gastrointest Endosc.* 2001;53(3): 294-299.
28. Sahai AV, Mishra G, Penman ID, et al. EUS to detect evidence of pancreatic disase in patients with persistent or nonspecific dyspepsia. *Gastrointest Endosc.* 2000;52:153-159.
29. Savides TJ, Gress FG, Zaidi SA, et al. Detection of embryologic ventral pancreatic parenchyma with endoscopic ultrasound. *Gastrointest Endosc.* 1996;43:14-19.
30. Donald JJ, Shorvon PJ, Lees WR. A hypoechoic area within the head of the pancreas–a normal variant. *Clin Radiol.* 1990;41:337-338.
31. Atri M, Nazarnia S, Mehio A, et al. Hypoechogenic embryologic ventral aspect of the head and uncinate process of the pancreas: in vitro correlation of US with histopathologic findings. *Radiology.* 1994; 190:441-444.
32. Axon AT, Classen M, Cotton PB, et al. Pancreatography in chronic pancreatitis: international definitions. *Gut.* 1984;25:1107-1112.
33. Gillams A, Pereira S, Webster G, Lees W. Correlation of MRCP quantification (MRCPQ) with conventional non-invasive pancreatic exocrine function tests. *Abdom Imaging.* 2008;33(4):469-473.
34. Gillams AR, Lees WR. Quantitative secretin MRCP (MRCPQ): results in 215 patients with known or suspected pancreatic pathology. *Eur Radiol.* 2007;17(11):2984-2990.
35. Cheon YK, Cho KB, Watkins JL, et al. Frequency and severity of post-ERCP pancreatitis correlated with extent of pancreatic ductal opacifiation. *Gastrointest Endosc.* 2007;65(3):385-393.
36. Sahai AV, Zimmerman M, Aabakken L, et al. Prospective assessment of the ability of endoscopic ultrasound to diagnose, exclude, or establish the severity of chronic pancreatitis found by endoscopic retrograde cholangiopancreatography. [see comment]. *Gastrointest Endosc.* 1998; 48(1):18-25.
37. Chong AK, Hawes RH, Hoffman BJ, et al. Diagnostic performance of EUS for chronic pancreatitis: a comparison with histopathology. *Gastrointest Endosc.* 2007;65(6):808-814.
38. Gardner TB, Gordon SR. Interobserver agreement for pancreatic endoscopic ultrasonography determined by same day back-to-back examinations. *J Clin Gastroenterol.* 2011;45(6):542-545.
39. Ammann RW, Heitz PU, Kloppel G. Course of alcoholic chronic pancreatitis: a prospective clinicomorphological long-term study. *Gastroenterology.* 1996;111(1):224-231.
40. Kahl S, Glasbrenner B, Leodolter A, et al. EUS in the diagnosis of early chronic pancreatitis: a prospective follow-up study. *Gastrointest Endosc.* 2002;55(4):507-511.
41. Hollerbach S, Klamann A, Topalidis T, Schmiegel WH. Endoscopic ultrasonography (EUS) and fine-needle aspiration (FNA) cytology for diagnosis of chronic pancreatitis. *Endoscopy.* 2001;33(10):824-831.
42. Hastier P, Buckley MJ, Francois E, et al. A prospective study of pancreatic diseases in patients with alcoholic cirrhosis: comparative diagnostic value of ERCP and EUS and long-term significance of isolated parenchymal abnormalities. *Gastrointest Endosc.* 1999;49:705-709.

43. Buscail L, Escourrou J, Moreau J, et al. Endoscopic ultrasonography in chronic pancreatitis: a comparative prospective study with conventional ultrasonography, computed tomography, and ERCP. *Pancreas*. 1995; 10:251-257.

44. Stevens T, Lopez R, Adler DG, et al. Multicenter comparison of the interobserver agreement of standard EUS scoring and Rosemont classification scoring for diagnosis of chronic pancreatitis. *Gastrointest Endosc*. 2010;71(3):519-526.

45. Kalmin B, Hoffman B, Hawes R, Romagnuolo J. Conventional versus Rosemont endoscopic ultrasound criteria for chronic pancreatitis: comparing interobserver reliability and intertest agreement. *Can J Gastroenterol*. 2011;25(5):261-264.

46. Sepe PS, Ohri A, Sanaka S, et al. A prospective evaluation of fatty pancreas by using EUS. *Gastrointest Endosc*. 2011;73(5):987-993.

47. The International Working Group for Minimum Standard Terminology for Gastrointestinal Endosonography. Reproduction of minimum standard terminology in gastrointestinal endosonography. *Digestive Endoscopy*. 1998;10:158-184.

48. Aabacken L, Rembacken B, LeMoine O, et al. for the OMED committee for standardization and terminology. *Minimum Standard Terminology for Gastrointestinal Endoscopy*. MST 3.0. Available from: http://www.worldendo.org/mst.htm.

49. Romagnuolo J, Joseph L, Barkun AN. Interpretation of diagnostic tests (Chapter 3). In: Rosenberg L, Joseph L, Barkun AN, eds. *Surgical Arithmetic: Epidemiological, Statistical, and Outcome-Based Approach to Surgical Practice*. Georgetown, Texas: Landes Bioscience; 2000:64–83.

50. Altman DG. *Practical Statistics for Medical Students*. London: Chapman and Hall; 1991.

51. Landis JR, Koch GG. An application of hierarchical kappa-type statistics in the assessment of majority agreement among multiple observers. *Biometrics*. 1977;33(2):363-374.

52. Fleiss JL. *Statistical Methods for Rates and Proportions*. 2nd ed. New York: John Wiley & Sons; 1981.

53. Lau JY, Sung JJ, Chan AC, et al. Stigmata of hemorrhage in bleeding peptic ulcers: an interobserver agreement study among international experts. *Gastrointest Endosc*. 1997;46:33-36.

54. von Kummer R, Holle R, Gizyska U, et al. Interobserver agreement in assessing early CT signs of middle cerebral artery infarction. *Am J Neuroradiol*. 1996;17:1743-1748.

55. Lok CE, Moragan CD, Ranganathan N. The accuracy and interobserver agreement in detecting the 'gallop sounds' by cardiac auscultation. *Chest*. 1998;114:1283-1288.

56. Takehara Y, Ichijo K, Tooyama N, et al. Breath-hold MR cholangiopancreatography with a long-echo-train fast spin-echo sequence and a surface coil in chronic pancreatitis. [see comment]. *Radiology*. 1994; 192(1):73-78.

57. Lieb JG 2nd, Palma DT, Garvan CW, et al. Intraobserver agreement among endosonographers for endoscopic ultrasound features of chronic pancreatitis: a blinded multicenter study. *Pancreas*. 2011;40(2):177-180.

58. Reuben A, Johnson AL, Cotton PB. Is pancreatogram interpretation reliable?–a study of observer variation and error. *Br J Radiol*. 1978; 51(612):956-962.

59. Morris-Stiff G, Webster P, Frost B, et al. Endoscopic ultrasound reliably identifies chronic pancreatitis when other imaging modalities have been non-diagnostic. *JOP*. 2009;10(3):280-283.

60. Varadarajulu S, Eltoum I, Tamhane A, Eloubeidi MA. Histopathologic correlates of noncalcific chronic pancreatitis by EUS: a prospective tissue characterization study. *Gastrointest Endosc*. 2007;66(3):501-509.

61. Rajan E, Clain JE, Levy MJ, et al. Age-related changes in the pancreas identified by EUS: a prospective evaluation. *Gastrointest Endosc*. 2005;61(3):401-406.

62. Chong AK, Romagnuolo J. Gender-related changes in the pancreas detected by EUS. *Gastrointest Endosc*. 2005;62(3):475.

63. Yusoff IF, Sahai AV. A prospective, quantitative assessment of the effect of ethanol and other variables on the endosonographic appearance of the pancreas. *Clin Gastroenterol Hepatol*. 2004;2(5):405-409.

64. Thuler FP, Costa PP, Paulo GA, et al. Endoscopic ultrasonography and alcoholic patients: can one predict early pancreatic tissue abnormalities? *JOP*. 2005;6(6):568-574.

65. Joseph L, Gyorkos TW, Coupal L. Bayesian estimation of disease prevalence and the parameters of diagnostic tests in the absence of a gold standard. *Am J Epidemiol*. 1995;141:263-272.

66. Fekete PS, Nunez C, Pitlik DA. Fine-needle aspiration biopsy of the pancreas: a study of 61 cases. *Diagn Cytopathol*. 1986;2:301-306.

67. Regev A, Berho M, Jeffers LJ, et al. Sampling error and intraobserver variation in liver biopsy in patients with chronic HCV infection. *Am J Gastroenterol*. 2002;97(10):2614-2618.

68. Romagnuolo J, Schiller D, Bailey RJ. Using breath tests wisely in a gastroenterology practice: an evidence-based review of indications and pitfalls in interpretation. *Am J Gastroenterol*. 2002;97:1113-1126.

69. Hayakawa T, Kondo T, Shibata T, et al. Relationship between pancreatic exocrine function and histological changes in chronic pancreatitis. *Am J Gastroenterol*. 1992;87:1170-1174.

70. Research committee for chronic pancreatitis in Japanese Society of Gastroenterology. In: Yamagata S, ed. *Clinical diagnostic criteria for chronic pancreatitis*. Tokyo: Igakutosho; 1984.

71. Heij HA, Obertop H, van Blankenstein M, et al. Relationship between functional and histological changes in chronic pancreatitis. *Dig Dis Sci*. 1986;31:1009-1013.

72. Heij HA, Obertop H, van Blankenstein M, et al. Comparison of endoscopic retrograde pancreatography with functional and histologic changes in chronic pancreatitis. *Acta Radiol*. 1987;28:289-293.

73. Hardt PD, Marzeion AM, Schnell-Kretschmer H, et al. Fecal elastase 1 measurement compared with endoscopic retrograde cholangiopancreatography for the diagnosis of chronic pancreatitis. *Pancreas*. 2002; 25(1):e6-e9.

74. Loser C, Mollgaard A, Folsch UR. Faecal elastase 1: a novel, highly sensitive, and specific tubeless pancreatic function test. *Gut*. 1996; 39(4):580-586.

75. Lankisch PG, Schmidt I, Konig H, et al. Faecal elastase 1: not helpful in diagnosing chronic pancreatitis associated with mild to moderate exocrine pancreatic insufficiency. *Gut*. 1998;42(4):551-554.

76. Lomas DJ, Bearcroft PW, Gimson AE. MR cholangiopancreatography: prospective comparison of a breath-hold 2D projection technique with diagnostic ERCP. *Eur Radiol*. 1999;9(7):1411-1417.

77. Manfredi R, Costamagna G, Brizi MG, et al. Severe chronic pancreatitis versus suspected pancreatic disease: dynamic MR cholangiopancreatography after secretin stimulation. *Radiology*. 2000;214(3):849-855.

78. Calvo MM, Bujanda L, Calderon A, et al. Comparison between magnetic resonance cholangiopancreatography and ERCP for evaluation of the pancreatic duct. *Am J Gastroenterol*. 2002;97:347-353.

79. Alcaraz MJ, De la Morena EJ, Polo A, et al. A comparative study of magnetic resonance cholangiography and direct cholangiography. [see comment]. *Rev Esp Enferm Dig*. 2000;92(7):427-438.

80. Czako L, Endes J, Takacs T, et al. Evaluation of pancreatic exocrine function by secretin-enhanced magnetic resonance cholangiopancreatography. *Pancreas*. 2001;23(3):323-328.

81. Kalapala R, Sunitha L, Nageshwar RD, et al. Virtual MR pancreatoscopy in the evaluation of the pancreatic duct in chronic pancreatitis. *JOP*. 2008;9(2):220-225.

82. Chen RYM, Hino S, Aithal GP, et al. Endoscopic ultrasound (EUS) features of chronic pancreatitis predate subsequent development of abnormal endoscopic retrograde pancreatogram (ERP) (abstract). *Gastrointest Endosc*. 2002;55:AB242.

83. Singh P, Vela S, Agrawal D, et al. Long term outcome in patients with endosonographic findings suggestive of mild chronic pancreatitis. (abstract). *Gastrointest Endosc*. 2004;59:AB231.

84. Begg CB. Biases in the assessment of diagnostic tests. *Stat Med*. 1987;6:411-423.

85. Lachs MS, Nachamkin I, Edelstein PH, et al. Spectrum bias in the evaluation of diagnostic tests: lessons from the rapid dipstick test for urinary tract infection. *Ann Intern Med*. 1992;117(2):135-140.

86. Chowdhury R, Bhutani MS, Mishra G, et al. Comparative analysis of direct pancreatic function testing versus morphological assessment by endoscopic ultrasonography for the evaluation of chronic unexplained abdominal pain of presumed pancreatic origin. *Pancreas*. 2005; 31(1):63-68.

87. DeWitt J, McGreevy K, LeBlanc J, et al. EUS-guided Trucut biopsy of suspected nonfocal chronic pancreatitis. *Gastrointest Endosc*. 2005; 62(1):76-84.

88. Bhutani MS, Ahmed I, Verma D, et al. An animal model for studying endoscopic ultrasound changes of early chronic pancreatitis with histologic correlation: a pilot study. *Endoscopy*. 2009;41(4):352-356.

89. Pungpapong S, Wallace MB, Woodward TA, et al. Accuracy of endoscopic ultrasonography and magnetic resonance cholangiopancreatography for the diagnosis of chronic pancreatitis: a prospective comparison study. *J Clin Gastroenterol*. 2007;41(1):88-93.

90. Romagnuolo J, Dendukuri N, Schiller I, Joseph L. Test performance of EUS for chronic pancreatitis: novel meta-analysis using Bayesian tech-

niques designed for imperfect reference standards. *Gastrointest Endosc.* 2012;75(4):AB204-AB205.

91. Delhaze M, Jonard P, Gigot JF, et al. [Chronic pancreatitis and pancreatic cancer. An often difficult differential diagnosis] (French). *Acta Gastroenterol Belg.* 1989;52:458-466.

92. DelMaschio A, Vanzulli A, Sironi S, et al. Pancreatic cancer versus chronic pancreatitis: diagnosis with CA 19-9 assessment, US, CT, and CT-guided fine-needle biopsy. *Radiology.* 1991;178:95-99.

93. Lowenfels AB, Maisonneuve P, Cavallini G, et al. Pancreatitis and the risk of cancer. *NEJM.* 1993;328:1433-1437.

94. Becker D, Strobel D, Bernatik T, Hahn EG. Echo-enhanced color- and power-Doppler EUS for the discrimination between focal pancreatitis and pancreatic carcinoma. *Gastrointest Endosc.* 2001;53(7):784-789.

95. McGuire DE, Venu RP, Brown RD, et al. Brush cytology for pancreatic carcinoma: an analysis of factors influencing results. *Gastrointest Endosc.* 1996;44(3):300-304.

96. Vandervoort J, Soetikno RM, Montes H, et al. Accuracy and complication rate of brush cytology from bile duct versus pancreatic duct. *Gastrointest Endosc.* 1999;49(3 Pt 1):322-327.

97. Kochman ML. EUS in pancreatic cancer. *Gastrointest Endosc.* 2002;56:S6-S12.

98. Mallery JS, Centeno BA, Hahn PF, et al. Pancreatic tissue sampling guided by EUS, CT/US, and surgery: a comparison of sensitivity and specificity. *Gastrointest Endosc.* 2002;56:218-224.

99. Barthet M, Portal I, Boujaoude J, et al. Endoscopic ultrasonographic diagnosis of pancreatic cancer complicating chronic pancreatitis. *Endoscopy.* 1996;28(6):487-491.

100. Sackett DL, Haynes RB, Guyatt GH, Tugwell P. *Clinical Epidmiology: a Basic Science for Clinical Medicine.* 2nd ed. Boston, MA: Little Brown; 1991.

101. Kaufman AR, Sivak MV Jr. Endoscopic ultrasonography in the differential diagnosis of pancreatic disease. *Gastrointest Endosc.* 1989;35:214-219.

102. Nattermann C, Goldschmidt AJ, Dancygier H. [Endosonography in the assessment of pancreatic tumors. A comparison of the endosonographic findings of carcinomas and segmental inflammatory changes] (German). *Dtsch Med Wochenschr.* 1995;120:1571-1576.

103. Glasbrenner B, Schwartz M, Pauls S, et al.. Prospective comparison of endoscopic ultrasound and endoscopic retrograde cholangiopancreatography in the preoperative assessment of masses in the pancreatic head. *Dig Surg.* 2000;17:468-474.

104. Varadarajulu S, Tamhane A, Eloubeidi MA. Yield of EUS-guided FNA of pancreatic masses in the presence or the absence of chronic pancreatitis. *Gastrointest Endosc.* 2005;62(5):728-736, quiz 51, 53.

105. Yu XJ, Long J, Fu DL, et al. Analysis of gene expression profiles in pancreatic carcinoma by using cDNA microarray. *Hepatobiliary Pancreat Dis Int.* 2003;2(3):467-470.

106. Chhieng DC, Benson E, Eltoum I, et al. MUC1 and MUC2 expression in pancreatic ductal carcinoma obtained by fine-needle aspiration. *Cancer.* 2003;99(6):365-371.

107. Crnogorac-Jurcevic T, Missiaglia E, Blaveri E, et al. Molecular alterations in pancreatic carcinoma: expression profiling shows that dysregulated expression of S100 genes is highly prevalent. *J Pathol.* 2003;201(1):63-74.

108. Iacobuzio-Donahue CA, Ashfaq R, Maitra A, et al. Highly expressed genes in pancreatic ductal adenocarcinomas: a comprehensive characterization and comparison of the transcription profiles obtained from three major technologies. *Cancer Res.* 2003;63(24):8614-8622.

109. Jonckheere N, Perrais M, Mariette C, et al. A role for human MUC4 mucin gene, as the ErbB2 ligand, as a target of TGF-beta in pancreatic carcinogenesis. *Oncogene.* 2004;23(34):5729-5738.

110. Juuti A, Nordling S, Louhimo J, et al. Loss of p27 expression is associated with poor prognosis in stage I-II pancreatic cancer. *Oncology.* 2003;65(4):371-377.

111. Missiaglia E, Blaveri E, Terris B, et al. Analysis of gene expression in cancer cell lines identifies candidate markers for pancreatic tumorigenesis and metastasis. *Int J Cancer.* 2004;112(1):100-112.

112. Su SB, Motoo Y, Iovanna JL, et al. Expression of p8 in human pancreatic cancer. *Clin Cancer Res.* 2001;7(2):309-313.

113. Maacke H, Jost K, Opitz S, et al. DNA repair and recombination factor Rad51 is over-expressed in human pancreatic adenocarcinoma. *Oncogene.* 2000;19(23):2791-2795.

114. Biankin AV, Morey AL, Lee CS, et al. DPC4/Smad4 expression and outcome in pancreatic ductal adenocarcinoma. *J Clin Oncol.* 2002;20(23):4531-4542.

115. Boltze C, Schneider-Stock R, Aust G, et al. CD97, CD95 and Fas-L clearly discriminate between chronic pancreatitis and pancreatic ductal adenocarcinoma in perioperative evaluation of cryocut sections. *Pathol Int.* 2002;52(2):83-88.

116. Casey G, Yamanaka Y, Friess H, et al. p53 mutations are common in pancreatic cancer and are absent in chronic pancreatitis. *Cancer Lett.* 1993;69(3):151-160.

117. Di Sebastiano P, di Mola FF, Di Febbo C, et al. Expression of interleukin 8 (IL-8) and substance P in human chronic pancreatitis. *Gut.* 2000;47(3):423-428.

118. Liao Q, Kleeff J, Xiao Y, et al. Preferential expression of cystein-rich secretory protein-3 (CRISP-3) in chronic pancreatitis. *Histol Histopathol.* 2003;18(2):425-433.

119. Logsdon CD, Simeone DM, Binkley C, et al. Molecular profiling of pancreatic adenocarcinoma and chronic pancreatitis identifies multiple genes differentially regulated in pancreatic cancer. [erratum appears in Cancer Res. 2003 Jun 15;63(12):3445]. *Cancer Res.* 2003;63(10):2649-2657.

120. Mitas M, Cole DJ, Hoover L, et al. Real-time reverse transcription-PCR detects KS1/4 mRNA in mediastinal lymph nodes from patients with non–small-cell lung cancer. *Clin Chem.* 2003;49:312-315.

121. Yamaguchi Y, Watanabe H, Yrdiran S, et al. Detection of mutations of p53 tumor suppressor gene in pancreatic juice and its application to diagnosis of patients with pancreatic cancer: comparison with K-ras mutation. *Clin Cancer Res.* 1999;5(5):1147-1153.

122. Sturm PD, Rauws EA, Hruban RH, et al. Clinical value of K-ras codon 12 analysis and endobiliary brush cytology for the diagnosis of malignant extrahepatic bile duct stenosis. *Clin Cancer Res.* 1999;5(3):629-635.

123. Stewart CJ, Burke GM. Value of p53 immunostaining in pancreaticobiliary brush cytology specimens. *Diagn Cytopathol.* 2000;23(5):308-313.

124. Levy MJ, Clain JE, Clayton A, et al. Preliminary experience comparing routine cytology results with the composite results of digital image analysis and fluorescence in situ hybridization in patients undergoing EUS-guided FNA. *Gastrointest Endosc.* 2007;66(3):483-490.

125. Chari ST, Takahashi N, Levy MJ, et al. A diagnostic strategy to distinguish autoimmune pancreatitis from pancreatic cancer. *Clin Gastroenterol Hepatol.* 2009;7(10):1097-1103.

126. Keogan MT, Tyler D, Clark L, et al. Diagnosis of pancreatic carcinoma: role of FDG PET. *AJR Am J Roentgenol.* 1565;171(6):1565-1570.

127. Rajput A, Stellato TA, Faulhaber PF, et al. The role of fluorodeoxyglucose and positron emission tomography in the evaluation of pancreatic disease. *Surgery.* 1998;124(4):793-797.

128. Bares R, Klever P, Hauptmann S, et al. F-18 fluorodeoxyglucose PET in vivo evaluation of pancreatic glucose metabolism for detection of pancreatic cancer. *Radiology.* 1994;192(1):79-86.

129. Higashi T, Saga T, Nakamoto Y, et al. Diagnosis of pancreatic cancer using fluorine-18 fluorodeoxyglucose positron emission tomography (FDG PET) –usefulness and limitations in "clinical reality". *Ann Nucl Med.* 2003;17:261-279.

130. Nakamoto Y, Higashi T, Sakahara H, et al. Delayed (18)F-fluoro-2-deoxy-D-glucose positron emission tomography scan for differentiation between malignant and benign lesions in the pancreas. *Cancer.* 2000;89:2547-2554.

131. van Kouwen MC, Jansen JB, van Goor H, et al. FDG-PET is able to detect pancreatic carcinoma in chronic pancreatitis. *Eur J Nucl Med Mol Imaging.* 2005;32(4):399-404.

132. Kajiwara M, Kojima M, Konishi M, et al. Autoimmune pancreatitis with multifocal lesions. *J Hepatobiliary Pancreat Surg.* 2008;15(4):449-452.

133. Sah RP, Pannala R, Chari ST, et al. Prevalence, diagnosis, and profile of autoimmune pancreatitis presenting with features of acute or chronic pancreatitis. *Clin Gastroenterol Hepatol.* 2009.

134. Chari ST, Smyrk TC, Levy MJ, et al. Diagnosis of autoimmune pancreatitis: the Mayo Clinic experience. *Clin Gastroenterol Hepatol.* 2006;4(8):1010-1016, quiz 934.

135. Ghazale A, Chari ST, Smyrk TC, et al. Value of serum IgG4 in the diagnosis of autoimmune pancreatitis and in distinguishing it from pancreatic cancer. *Am J Gastroenterol.* 2007;102(8):1646-1653.

136. Choi EK, Kim MH, Lee TY, et al. The sensitivity and specificity of serum immunoglobulin G and immunoglobulin G4 levels in the diagnosis of autoimmune chronic pancreatitis: Korean experience. *Pancreas.* 2007;35(2):156-161.

137. Frulloni L, Lunardi C, Simone R, et al. Identification of a novel antibody associated with autoimmune pancreatitis. *N Engl J Med.* 2009;361(22):2135-2142.

138. Kubota K, Kato S, Akiyama T, et al. Differentiating sclerosing cholangitis caused by autoimmune pancreatitis and primary sclerosing cholangitis according to endoscopic duodenal papillary features. *Gastrointest Endosc.* 2008;68(6):1204-1208.

139. Kamisawa T, Tu Y, Egawa N, et al. A new diagnostic endoscopic tool for autoimmune pancreatitis. *Gastrointest Endosc.* 2008;68(2):358-361.

140. Deshpande V, Mino-Kenudson M, Brugge WR, et al. Endoscopic ultrasound guided fine needle aspiration biopsy of autoimmune pancreatitis: diagnostic criteria and pitfalls. *Am J Surg Pathol.* 2005;29(11):1464-1471.

141. Farrell JJ, Garber J, Sahani D, Brugge WR. EUS findings in patients with autoimmune pancreatitis. *Gastrointest Endosc.* 2004;60(6):927-936.

142. Levy MJ, Reddy RP, Wiersema MJ, et al. EUS-guided trucut biopsy in establishing autoimmune pancreatitis as the cause of obstructive jaundice. *Gastrointest Endosc.* 2005;61(3):467-472.

143. Mizuno N, Bhatia V, Hosoda W, et al. Histological diagnosis of autoimmune pancreatitis using EUS-guided trucut biopsy: a comparison study with EUS-FNA. *J Gastroenterol.* 2009;44(7):742-750.

144. Bang SJ, Kim MH, Kim do H, et al. Is pancreatic core biopsy sufficient to diagnose autoimmune chronic pancreatitis? *Pancreas.* 2008;36(1):84-89.

145. Sugumar A, Levy MJ, Kamisawa T, et al. Utility of endoscopic retrograde pancreatogram (ERP) to diagnose autoimmune pancreatitis (AIP): an international, double blind randomized, multicenter study (Abstract). *Gastrointest Endosc.* 2009;69:AB124.

146. Hoki N, Mizuno N, Sawaki A, et al. Diagnosis of autoimmune pancreatitis using endoscopic ultrasonography. *J Gastroenterol.* 2009;44(2):154-159.

147. Kamisawa T, Shimosegawa T, Okazaki K, et al. Standard steroid treatment for autoimmune pancreatitis. *Gut.* 2009;58(11):1504-1507.

148. Pannala R, Chari ST. Corticosteroid treatment for autoimmune pancreatitis. *Gut.* 2009;58(11):1438-1439.

149. Ghazale A, Chari ST, Zhang L, et al. Immunoglobulin G4-associated cholangitis: clinical profile and response to therapy. *Gastroenterology.* 2008;134(3):706-715.

150. Carter JE, Nelson JJ, Eves M, Boudreaux C. *Giardia lamblia* infection diagnosed by endoscopic ultrasound-guided fine-needle aspiration. *Diagn Cytopathol.* 2007;35(6):363-365.

151. Cherian JV, Somasundaram A, Ponnusamy RP, Venkataraman J. Peripancreatic tuberculous lymphadenopathy. An impostor posing diagnostic difficulty. *JOP.* 2007;8(3):326-329.

152. Boujaoude JD, Honein K, Yaghi C, et al. Diagnosis by endoscopic ultrasound guided fine needle aspiration of tuberculous lymphadenitis involving the peripancreatic lymph nodes: a case report. *World J Gastroenterol.* 2007;13(3):474-477.

153. Canto MI, Goggins M, Yeo CJ, et al. Screening for pancreatic neoplasia in high-risk individuals: an EUS-based approach. *Clin Gastroenterol Hepatol.* 2004;2:606-621.

154. Brune K, Abe T, Canto M, et al. Multifocal neoplastic precursor lesions associated with lobular atrophy of the pancreas in patients having a strong family history of pancreatic cancer. *Am J Surg Pathol.* 2006;30(9):1067-1076.

155. Brentnall TA, Bronner MP, Byrd DR, et al. Early diagnosis and treatment of pancreatic dysplasia in patients with a family history of pancreatic cancer. *Ann Intern Med.* 1999;131:247-255.

156. Lecesne R, Taourel P, Bret PM, et al. Acute pancreatitis: interobserver agreement and correlation of CT and MR cholangiopancreatography with outcome. *Radiology.* 1999;211:727-735.

157. Arvanitakis M, Delhaye M, De Maertelaere V, et al. Computed tomography and magnetic resonance imaging in the assessment of acute pancreatitis. *Gastroenterology.* 2004;126:715-723.

158. Ballinger AB, Barnes E, Alstead EM, Fairclough PD. Is intervention necessary after a first episode of acute idiopathic pancreatitis? *Gut.* 1996;38:293-295.

159. Yusoff IF, Raymond G, Sahai AV. A prospective comparison of the yield of EUS in primary vs. recurrent idiopathic acute pancreatitis. *Gastrointest Endosc.* 2004;60:673-678.

160. Tandon M, Topazian M. Endoscopic ultrasound in idiopathic acute pancreatitis. *Am J Gastroenterol.* 2001;96(3):705-709.

161. Norton SA, Alderson D. Endoscopic ultrasonography in the evaluation of idiopathic acute pancreatitis. [see comment]. *Br J Surg.* 2000;87(12):1650-1655.

162. Liu CL, Lo CM, Chan JK, et al. EUS for detection of occult cholelithiasis in patients with idiopathic pancreatitis. *Gastrointest Endosc.* 2000;51(1):28-32.

163. Morris-Stiff G, Al-Allak A, Frost B, et al. Does endoscopic ultrasound have anything to offer in the diagnosis of idiopathic acute pancreatitis? *JOP.* 2009;10(2):143-146.

164. Lee SP, Nicholls JF, Park HZ. Biliary sludge as a cause of acute pancreatitis. *NEJM.* 1992;326:589-593.

165. Ros E, Navarro S, Bru C, et al. Occult microlithiasis in "idiopathic" acute pancreatitis: prevention of relapses by cholecystectomy or ursodeoxycholic acid therapy. *Gastroenterology.* 1991;101:1701-1709.

166. Dahan P, Andant C, Levy P, et al. Prospective evaluation of endoscopic ultrasonography and microscopic examination of duodenal bile in the diagnosis of cholecystolithiasis in 45 patients with normal conventional ultrasonography. *Gut.* 1996;38:277-281.

167. Coyle WJ, Pineau BC, Tarnasky PR, et al. Evaluation of unexplained acute and acute recurrent pancreatitis using endoscopic retrograde cholangiopancreatography, sphincter of Oddi manometry and endoscopic ultrasound. *Endoscopy.* 2002;34(8):617-623.

168. Wilcox CM, Kilgore M. Cost minimization analysis comparing diagnostic strategies in unexplained pancreatitis. *Pancreas.* 2009;38(2):117-121.

169. Bret PM, Reinhold C, Taourel P, et al. Pancreas divisum: evaluation with MR cholangiopancreatography. *Radiology.* 1996;199(1):99-103.

170. Bhutani MS, Hoffman B, Hawes RH. Diagnosis of pancreas divisum by endoscopic ultrasonography. *Endoscopy.* 1999;31:167-169.

171. Chen RYM, Hawes RH, Wallace MB, Hoffman BJ. Diagnosing pancreas divisum in patients with abdominal pain and pancreatitis: is endoscopic ultrasound (EUS) accurate enough? (abstract). *Gastrointest Endosc.* 2002;55:AB96.

172. Lai R, Freeman ML, Cass OW, Mallery S. Accurate diagnosis of pancreas divisum by linear-array endosonography. *Endoscopy.* 2004;36:705-709.

173. Vaughan R, Mainie I, Hawes RH, et al. Accuracy of endoscopic ultrasound in the diagnosis of pancreas divisum in a busy clinical setting (abstract). *Gastrointest Endosc.* 2006;63:AB263.

174. Carnes ML, Romagnuolo J, Cotton PB. Miss rate of pancreas divisum by magnetic resonance cholangiopancreatography in clinical practice. *Pancreas.* 2008;37(2):151-153.

175. Catalano MF, Lahoti S, Alcocer E, et al. Dynamic imaging of the pancreas using real-time endoscopic ultrasonography with secretin stimulation. *Gastrointest Endosc.* 1998;48:580-587.

EUS and Pancreatic Tumors

Leticia Perondi Luz • Mohammad Al-Haddad • John DeWitt

Key Points

- EUS is the most sensitive imaging modality for the detection of pancreatic masses. It is particularly useful for identification of tumors undetected by other tests such as CT.
- EUS is superior to CT and angiography for detection of tumor invasion of the portal vein or confluence. CT appears to be superior to EUS for invasion of the superior mesenteric vessels and major arteries of the upper abdomen.
- Due to anatomical and equipment limitations, CT and MRI are superior to EUS for detection of metastatic cancer. EUS FNA of liver metastases, ascites, or celiac adenopathy may prevent surgical exploration.
- EUS FNA of pancreatic tumors has a sensitivity of 85% with a specificity approaching 100%. Diagnostic yield appears to be maximized by the presence of on-site cytopathology interpretation.
- Most studies demonstrate that EUS, CT, and MRI are equivalent for the determination of surgical resectability of pancreatic cancer. However, EUS is usually used preoperatively in combination with CT or MRI to evaluate for vascular invasion or previously undetected metastases.
- EUS is the most accurate test for detection of PNETs, particularly tumors smaller than 2 cm in diameter. Optimal workup of suspected PNETs should incorporate EUS, EUS FNA with immunostaining, and somatostatin receptor scintigraphy.

Examination of the pancreas and other upper abdominal retroperitoneal structures by endoscopic ultrasound (EUS) is considered the most technically challenging anatomical region to master and reproducibly visualize. However, once these skills are learned, EUS permits the most detailed nonoperative view of the pancreas that is available. This chapter summarizes the role of EUS for the evaluation of solid pancreatic neoplasms.

Detection of Pancreatic Tumors

EUS is the most sensitive nonoperative imaging test for the detection of benign or malignant pancreatic lesions (Figures 15-1 and 15-2). When summarizing the results of 23 studies containing 1096 patients over a 21-year period, the sensitivity of EUS for detection of a pancreatic mass was 95% with a range of 85% to 100%.[1-23] Some of these studies, however, included benign pancreatic disease and ampullary tumors,[1-4,11,12,17-19] which may bias the analysis of tumor detection in favor of EUS. Therefore caution must be exercised when extrapolating this data to pancreatic malignancy. In 16 studies that compared EUS and computed tomography

(CT) over the same time period,* the sensitivity of EUS (98%) for mass detection was superior to CT (77%; Table 15-1). EUS is clearly superior to conventional CT[3,4,6,16] and transabdominal ultrasound (US)[2-4,6,12] for pancreatic tumor detection. Compared to single-detector helical CT, however, EUS has been reported to be either equivalent[13] or superior.[11,17-19] Currently available CT scanners utilize a 32- or 64-row detector that enables acquisition of multiple images with very thin collimation and three-dimensional reconstruction of ductal and parenchymal anatomy.[24,25] Comparative studies between EUS and multidetector-row CT (MDCT) for pancreatic tumors have demonstrated the superiority of EUS for tumor detection compared to 4-row CT. Agarwal and colleagues[21] reported an EUS sensitivity of 100% for the diagnosis of cancer compared to 86% for MDCT. Similarly, DeWitt and colleagues[22] reported that the sensitivity of EUS (98%) was statistically superior to MDCT (86%) for a cohort of 80 patients with pancreatic cancer. There are relatively sparse comparative data between EUS and magnetic resonance imaging (MRI) for tumor detection. EUS has been reported to be either superior[7] or inferior[20]

---

*3,4,6–13,16–19,21,22

Examination Checklist for Evaluation of a Suspected Pancreatic Tumor

1. **Lymph nodes**: Examination of the following stations for possible metastatic disease: celiac axis, peripancreatic (including head, body, and tail), porta hepatis, gastrohepatic ligament, aortocaval, and possibly posterior mediastinal stations. Metastatic lymph nodes will usually be round, well defined, hypoechoic, and at least 5 mm in diameter. However, not all malignant lymph nodes will have all of these features. If a suspected lymph node is identified, its characteristics and distance from the tumor should be noted. EUS FNA should be performed on suspected distant metastatic lymph nodes.

2. **Liver:** Transgastric and limited transduodenal examination of the liver for metastatic lesions. Liver metastases from primary pancreatic cancer are usually hypoechoic and well defined. There may be one or more than one lesion identified. EUS FNA of any suspected lesion should be performed when accessible.

3. **Ascites:** This usually appears as a triangular or irregularly shaped anechoic region just outside the duodenal or gastric wall. This may be seen from peritoneal metastases or chronic venous occlusion. Omental nodules may also be visualized. EUS-guided fluid aspiration or biopsy of a nodule should be performed when possible.

4. **Vascular invasion:** For tumors in the pancreatic head, the relationship of the tumor to the portal vein, portosplenic confluence, superior mesenteric vessels, hepatic artery, and gastroduodenal artery should be noted. For tumors in the body, its relationship to the celiac artery, superior mesenteric artery, portal confluence, hepatic artery, and

splenic vessels should be defined. For tumors in the pancreatic tail, the splenic vessels also should be interrogated. The relationship of the vessel and the tumor should be carefully examined. Notation may be stated as: intact hyperechoic tumor/vessel interface, adherent to vessel wall without irregular interface, irregular tumor/vessel interface, tumor invasion, or occlusion of the vessel. For occlusion of the portal or superior mesenteric vein, venous collaterals in the liver hilum or periduodenal region may be seen. For splenic vein occlusion, collaterals in the splenic hilum or gastric fundus may occur.

5. **Tumor:** The following characteristics of all visualized masses should be noted: maximal dimensions, irregular or well-defined borders, isoechoic or hypoechoic or hyperechoic characteristics, and any solid or cystic structures.

6. **EUS FNA:** Tissue sampling should be performed from the most distant metastatic site first. If ascites, a distant metastatic lymph node, omental nodule, or a suspicious liver lesion is present, one of these should be biopsied first. If these test negative for malignancy, either the suspected tumor or a regional lymph node may be sampled. The following information should be noted from each site biopsied: numbers of passes required, whether suction is used, and if preliminary interpretation of any specimen obtained is available.

7. **Staging:** All suspected malignant tumors of the pancreas should be assigned a TNM staging based on the most current American Joint Committee on Cancer (AJCC) staging classification.

to MRI. Future studies between EUS to 3.0 or higher Tesla MRI are needed to define the roles of each in the diagnosis of pancreatic masses.

EUS is particularly useful for identification of small tumors that have been undetected by other imaging modalities.* For

*1,3,7,13,17,21,22,26

tumors ≤20 mm in diameter, EUS was found to have a sensitivity of 90% to 100% compared to 40% to 67% for CT and 33% for MRI.[7,13] With thinner slice imaging and precisely timed contrast administration coupled with multiplanar reconstruction,[24,27] CT may now be able to identify small pancreatic masses that previously went undetected by conventional or even single-detector dual-phase imaging.[22] We recommend that EUS should be performed in all patients with

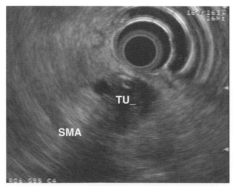

FIGURE 15-1 Linear EUS image (5 MHz) of a poorly defined, hypoechoic 22 mm × 21 mm ductal adenocarcinoma (TU) in the head of the pancreas adjacent to but not involving the superior mesenteric artery (SMA) and vein. A plastic biliary stent is present. Multidetector CT with dual-phase imaging did not visualize any tumor.

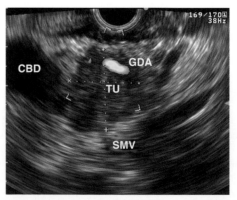

FIGURE 15-2 Linear EUS image (6 MHz) of a 2.5-cm mass (TU) in the head of the pancreas occluding the gastroduodenal artery (GDA). Doppler imaging demonstrates preserved blood flow within the vessel. The mass does not invade the duodenal wall or the superior mesenteric vein (SMV) on this image. The common bile duct (CBD) is obstructed and dilated above the mass.

TABLE 15-1

SENSITIVITY OF EUS COMPARED TO OTHER IMAGING TESTS FOR DETECTION OF PANCREATIC MASSES

Author (year)	Number of Patients	Sensitivity (%)					
		EUS	CT	MRI	US	PET	ERCP
Lin et al[2] (1989)	33	94	—	—	91	—	—
Rosch et al[3] (1991)	102	99	77	—	67	—	90
Rosch et al[4] (1992)	60	98	85	—	78	—	—
Palazzo et al[6] (1993)	49	91	66	—	64	—	—
Muller et al[7] (1994)	33	94	69	83	—	—	—
Marty et al[8] (1995)	37	92	63	—	—	—	—
Melzer et al[9] (1996)	12	100	83	—	—	—	—
Dufour et al[10] (1997)	24	92	88	—	—	—	—
Howard et al[11] (1997)	21	100	67	—	—	—	—
Sugiyama et al[12] (1997)	73	96	86	—	81	—	—
Legmann et al[13] (1998)	30	100	92	—	—	—	—
Gress et al[16] (1999)	81	100	74	—	—	—	—
Midwinter et al[17] (1999)	34	97	76	—	—	—	—
Mertz et al[18] (2000)	31	93	53	—	—	87	—
Rivadeneira et al[19] (2003)	44	100	68	—	—	—	—
Ainsworth et al[20] (2003)	22	87	—	96	—	—	—
Agarwal et al[21] (2004)	71	100	86	—	—	—	—
Dewitt et al[22] (2004)	80	98	86	—	—	—	—
Total Subjects	837	837	782	55	317	31	102
Overall Sensitivity	—	98	77	88	76	87	90

CT, computed tomography; ERCP, endoscopic retrograde cholangiopancreatography; MRI, magnetic resonance imaging; PET, positron emission tomography; US, ultrasonography.

obstructive jaundice in whom CT or MRI do not definitively identify a pancreatic lesion both to detect any tumor and to exclude non-neoplastic diseases. In a recent study by Wang and colleagues,[26] EUS had a sensitivity, specificity, positive predictive value (PPV), and accuracy of 87%, 98%, 98%, and 92%, respectively, in diagnosing pancreatic malignancy in patients where CT was indeterminate.

EUS may fail to identify true pancreatic masses in patients with chronic pancreatitis, a diffusely infiltrating carcinoma, a prominent ventral/dorsal split, or a recent episode (<4 weeks) of acute pancreatitis.[28] In a study of 80 patients with clinical suspicion of pancreatic cancer and a normal EUS, Catanzaro and colleagues[29] found no patient with a normal pancreatic EUS developed cancer during a follow-up period of 24 months. Therefore a normal pancreas by EUS examination essentially rules out pancreatic cancer, but follow-up EUS or other study should be undertaken when EUS demonstrates chronic pancreatitis without a definite mass. It is important to remember that acoustic shadowing caused by an indwelling biliary or pancreatic stent may impede visualization of a small pancreatic mass.

Several studies evaluated the accuracy of endosonographic findings of the pancreas for the diagnosis or exclusion of pancreatic malignancy. Lee and colleagues[30] demonstrated that the periductal hypoechoic sign (defined as patchy hypoechoic areas adjacent to a dilated pancreatic duct) had a sensitivity of 74%, a specificity of 86%, and an accuracy of 80% for the diagnosis of pancreatic malignancy. Pancreatic duct diameter or dilation of both bile and pancreatic ducts were not predictive of malignancy in this study. Nevertheless, Rodriguez and colleagues[31] showed that in the setting of negative fine-needle aspiration (FNA), pancreatic duct dilation and

vascular invasion were significantly associated with cancer. In the same study, the absence of pancreatic duct dilation and a negative FNA had a negative predictive value (NPV) of 100%.[31] Eloubeidi and colleagues[32] demonstrated that EUS measurement of a pancreatic duct diameter to pancreatic gland width ratio greater or equal to 0.34 at the level of the portosplenic confluence had a PPV, NPV, sensitivity, specificity, and accuracy of 87%, 99%, 94%, 97%, and 97%, respectively. The accuracy and PPV of pancreatic duct dilation alone for diagnosing pancreatic cancer were 83% and 50%, respectively.

Owing to the ability of EUS to provide high-resolution images, there has been interest in using this technique to screen asymptomatic high-risk cohorts for early cancer detection. Canto and colleagues[33] evaluated an EUS-based screening approach in a prospective cohort of 38 asymptomatic individuals with Peutz-Jeghers syndrome or two affected relatives with pancreatic cancer. Six pancreatic benign and malignant masses were found by EUS. The diagnostic yield for detecting clinically significant pancreatic neoplasms was 5.3% (2 of 38). A study by Langer and colleagues[34] found that EUS is superior to MRI among high-risk asymptomatic patients and may disclose adenocarcinoma and side branch intraductal papillary mucinous neoplasia (IPMN) during index screening in individuals with family history of pancreatic cancer or other familial cancer syndromes.[35] A recent cohort study by Zubarik and colleagues[36] utilized serum CA19-9 to screen 546 patients with at least one first-degree relative with pancreatic cancer. Of those, 5% (27 patients) had elevated CA19-9 levels and subsequently underwent EUS. Neoplastic or malignant findings were detected in five patients, including one with pancreatic adenocarcinoma. The cost to detect one pancreatic neoplasia and one pancreatic adenocarcinoma was $8431 and $41,133, respectively.

A recent multicenter study by Canto and colleagues[37] screened 225 asymptomatic high-risk individuals with: (1) Peutz-Jeghers syndrome, (2) familial breast-ovarian cancer who had at least one first- or second-degree relative affected with pancreatic cancer, and (3) relatives of patients with familial pancreatic cancer with at least one affected first-degree relative. In this study, imaging studies including CT, MRI, and EUS were blindly compared. Ninety-two of 216 (42%) individuals were found to have at least one pancreatic mass or a dilated pancreatic duct by any of the imaging modalities. Fifty-one of the 84 patients with a cyst (60%) had multiple lesions, typically small and in multiple locations. CT, MRI, and EUS detected a pancreatic abnormality in 11%, 33%, and 42% of the patients, respectively. Among these abnormalities, proven or suspected neoplasms were identified in 85 patients, and three of five patients who underwent pancreatic resection had high-grade dysplastic lesions.

The recently published International Cancer of the Pancreas Screening (CAPS) Consortium summit[38] agreed that screening is recommended for high-risk individuals; however, more evidence is needed, particularly in regard to long-term management of patients with detected lesions. There was agreement that candidates for screening include first-degree relatives of patients with pancreatic cancer with a familial kindred with at least two affected first-degree relatives, patients with Peutz-Jeghers syndrome, and p16, BRCA2, and hereditary nonpolyposis colorectal cancer mutation carriers with one or more affected first-degree relatives. Consensus was not reached for the age to initiate screening or stop surveillance. It was agreed that initial screening should include EUS and MRI and not CT or endoscopic retrograde cholangiopancreatography (ERCP). Surgery, if needed, should be performed in a high-volume center, but it remains unclear which abnormalities would justify a surgical resection.

Both autoimmune pancreatitis (AIP) and primary pancreatic lymphoma (PPL) may mimic primary pancreatic cancer, and accurate preoperative detection may avoid unnecessary surgery. AIP most commonly presents with obstructive jaundice, abdominal pain, and weight loss.[39,40] EUS morphology of AIP may include diffuse pancreatic enlargement, a focal mass, focal hypoechoic areas, bile duct wall thickening, or peripancreatic lymphadenopathy.[39-42] EUS FNA with small caliber 22-G or 25-G needles may demonstrate a nonspecific plasmacytic predominant chronic inflammatory infiltrate but overall has variable sensitivity and poor specificity. Diagnosis is probably easier to make by EUS-guided Tru-Cut biopsy (EUS TCB) or FNA with 19-G needles.[42,43] PPL may result in a mass lesion indistinguishable from adenocarcinoma (Figure 15-3). Whereas EUS and radiographic imaging alone may not be helpful to confirm the diagnosis of PPL, EUS FNA with flow cytometry is able to accurately diagnose this condition.[44] PPL should be suspected based on clinical appearance, absence of standard malignant cytology, and abundance of abnormal lymphocytes on rapid cytologic review.

Imaging-based technologies such as contrast-enhanced EUS (CE EUS) may be used to differentiate pancreatic adenocarcinomas from other benign or malignant lesions. During CE EUS, an intravenous contrast agent is administered and microbubbles are detected in the microvasculature of

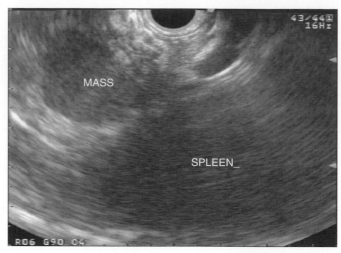

FIGURE 15-3 Linear image (7.5 MHz) of a 1.9-cm lymphoma in the tail of the pancreas adjacent to the spleen.

pancreatic tumors during real-time evaluation. Adenocarcinomas show hypoenhancement whereas neuroendocrine tumors and pseudotumoral chronic pancreatitis are isoenhancing or hyperenhancing. Numerous contrast agents are available including first-generation contrast agents such as Levovist and second-generation agents such as SonoVue and Sonazoid. In a recent meta-analysis including 1139 patients, the pooled sensitivity and specificity of CE EUS for the differential diagnosis of pancreatic adenocarcinoma were 94% and 89%, respectively.[45] This study found that a hypoenhanced lesion by CE EUS was a sensitive and accurate predictor of adenocarcinoma. In the United States, routine use of CE EUS is limited by its high cost and the lack of both agent availability and expertise with this technique.

Another emerging technology used to differentiate benign from malignant masses is EUS elastography. This technology provides real-time evaluation of tissue stiffness and is based on the premise that there is less strain when hard tissues are compressed compared to soft tissues.[46,47] As malignant lesions are generally harder than normal adjacent tissue, measuring strain might aid classification of pancreatic masses. Results from two recent meta-analyses[47,48] demonstrated a high-pooled sensitivity of 95% to 97% but a low-pooled specificity of 67% to 76%, respectively, for differential diagnosis of solid pancreatic masses. Elastography might provide complementary information to EUS, potentially increasing the yield of EUS FNA, and assist endosonographers to improve targeting of FNA.[47] Limitations of this technique include limited availability, difficulty controlling tissue compression by the endosonographer, presence of motion artifacts, and unclear stiffness cutoff values for pancreatic masses.[48]

Saftoiu and colleagues[49] sequentially combined CE power Doppler with real-time elastography in 21 patients with chronic pancreatitis and 33 patients with pancreatic adenocarcinoma undergoing EUS examination. The sensitivity, specificity, and accuracy of combined information provided by both tests to differentiate hypovascular hard masses suggestive of pancreatic carcinoma were 75.8%, 95.2%, and 83.3%, respectively, with a PPV and NPV of 96.2% and 71.4%, respectively.

TABLE 15-2

ACCURACY OF EUS FOR TUMOR (T) AND NODAL (N) STAGING OF PANCREATIC CANCER

Author (year)	Number of Enrolled Patients	Number of Patients to Surgery with Pancreatic Cancer	Accuracy (%) T Stage	N Stage
Tio et al[59] (1990)	43	36	92	74
Grimm et al[53] (1990)	NA	26	85	72
Mukai et al[54] (1991)	26	26	NR	65
Rosch et al[4] (1992)	60	40	NR	72
Rosch et al[56] (1992)	46	35	94	80
Palazzo et al[6] (1993)	64	49	82	64
Yasuda et al[60] (1993)	NA	29	NR	66
Muller et al[7] (1994)	49	16	82	50
Giovannini et al[52] (1994)	90	26	NR	80
Tio et al[58] (1996)	70	52	84	69
Akahoshi et al[14] (1998)	96	37	64	50
Legmann et al[13] (1998)	30	22	90	86
Buscail et al[51] (1999)	73	26	73	69
Midwinter et al[17] (1999)	48	23	NR	74
Gress et al[16] (1999)	151	75	85	72
Ahmad et al[50] (2000)	NA	89	69	54
Rivadeneira et al[19] (2003)	NA	44	NR	84
Soriano et al[57] (2004)	127	62	62	65
Ramsay et al[55] (2004)	27	22	63	69
DeWitt et al[22] (2004)	104	53	67	41

NA, not applicable; NR, not reported.

Staging of Pancreatic Tumors

Staging of pancreatic malignancy is done according to the American Joint Committee for Cancer (AJCC) Staging TNM Classification, which describes the tumor extension (T), lymph node (N), and distant metastases (M) of tumors. Reported accuracies of T staging by EUS range from 63% to 94% (Table 15-2).* This wide variation may be due to improved detection of distant metastasis or vascular invasion by MDCT, resulting in less operative management for suspected locally advanced or metastatic disease. The exclusion of such patients may have resulted in the decreased T staging accuracy of some recent studies compared to earlier ones. For the last 15 years, some tertiary referral centers have attempted to achieve negative surgical margins by surgical reconstruction of the portal and/or superior mesenteric vein in patients with venous invasion but without thrombosis or occlusion (Figures 15-4 to 15-6).[61,62] To better reflect such surgical trends, the 1997 staging criteria were updated in the 2003 AJCC manual (6th edition) to better distinguish potentially resectable (T3) from unresectable (T4) tumors. The AJCC 2003 and the current AJCC 2010 staging criteria classify only vascular invasion of the celiac or superior mesenteric arteries as T4 cancer (Table 15-3). The AJCC was updated again in 2010 (7th edition) with no significant changes in staging of pancreatic malignancy.

Despite the variations of T-staging criteria described for pancreatic cancer, nodal (N) metastases have uniformly been classified as absent (N0) or present (N1) across all AJCC

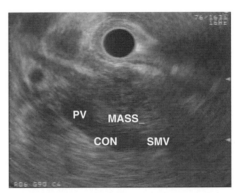

FIGURE 15-4 Radial image (7.5 MHz) of a large pancreatic head mass with adherence and invasion into the superior mesenteric vein (SMV) just below the portal vein confluence. A malignant-appearing lymph node is seen adjacent to the mass. Invasion into the SMV was confirmed at surgery.

editions, including the latest 7th edition. The accuracy of EUS for N staging of pancreatic tumors ranges from 41% to 86%.* Various criteria have been proposed for endosonographic detection of metastatic lymph nodes including size greater than 1 cm, hypoechoic echogenicity, distinct margins, and round shape. When all four features are present within a lymph node, there is an 80% to 100% chance of malignant invasion.[64,65] The sensitivity of EUS alone for the diagnosis of metastatic adenopathy in pancreatic cancer is 28% to 92%;[†] however, most report sensitivities under 65%. This low

---

*4,6,7,13,14,16,17,19,22,50–60

*4,6,7,13,14,16,17,19,22,51–60,63
†6,7,14,17,19,55,57,58

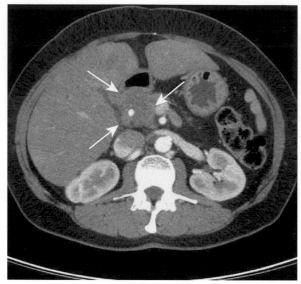

FIGURE 15-5 Axial CT image of the same patient as in Figure 15-4 demonstrating probable invasion into the SMV by the pancreatic head mass *(arrows)*.

sensitivity presumably occurs for two reasons. First, most metastatic lymph nodes do not have all four endosonographic features described previously[64] and may therefore be incorrectly assumed to be benign. Second, peritumoral inflammation and large tumor size may contribute to poor detection of adenopathy.[66] The specificity of EUS alone for the diagnosis of metastatic adenopathy in pancreatic cancer is 26% to 100%;* however, most report specificities above 70%. It is presumed that the addition of EUS FNA of suspicious lymph nodes may increase specificity; however, there are little data that describe the impact of the addition of EUS FNA to EUS alone. Cahn and colleagues[67] reported that EUS FNA diagnosed lymph node metastasis in 7 of 13 patients (62%) with pancreatic cancer in whom sampling was performed. For tumors involving the head of the pancreas, malignant lymph nodes are removed en-bloc with the surgical specimen. Therefore accurate detection of these lymph nodes is not essential[22] and routine EUS FNA of peritumoral lymph nodes with pancreatic head cancers may not be necessary. Because preoperative identification and EUS FNA of celiac nodes may preclude surgery, meticulous survey of this region is critical during staging of all pancreatic tumors. In one series, mediastinal lymph node metastases were reported to occur in 7% of patients undergoing EUS evaluation of pancreatic masses.[68]

*6,7,14,17,19,55,57,58

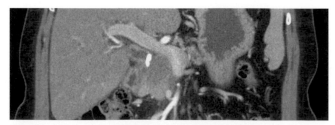

FIGURE 15-6 Multiplanar reconstruction of the axial CT image in the same patient as Figure 15-4 along the portal vein and superior mesenteric vein. Invasion of the SMV below the portal vein is seen.

---

*13,17,19,22,55,57

TABLE 15-3

AMERICAN JOINT COMMITTEE ON CANCER 2010 TNM STAGING CLASSIFICATION FOR PANCREATIC CANCER

Anatomic Stage/Prognostic Groups

Stage 0	Tis, N0, M0
Stage IA	T1, N0, M0
Stage IB	T2, N0, M0
Stage IIA	T3, N0, M0
Stage IIB	T1, N1, M0
	T2, N1, M0
	T3, N1, M0
Stage III	T4, any N, M0
Stage IV	Any T, Any N, M1

Primary Tumor (T)

TX	Primary tumor cannot be assessed
T0	No evidence of primary tumor
Tis	Carcinoma in situ[a]
T1	Tumor limited to the pancreas, 2 cm or less in greatest dimension
T2	Tumor limited to the pancreas, more than 2 cm in greatest dimension
T3	Tumor extends beyond the pancreas but without involvement of the celiac axis or the superior mesenteric artery
T4	Tumor involves the celiac axis or the superior mesenteric artery (unresectable primary tumor)

Regional Lymph Nodes (N)

NX	Regional lymph nodes cannot be assessed
N0	No regional lymph node metastasis
N1	Regional lymph node metastasis

Distant Metastasis (M)

M0	No distant metastasis
M1	Distant metastasis

[a]This also includes the 'PanInIII' classification.
(From Edge S, Byrd DR, Compton CC, Fritz AG, Greene FL, Trotti A eds. AJCC Cancer Staging Manual. 7th ed. New York, NY: Springer; 2010:245-247.)

Therefore a brief survey of this region may be helpful during staging of pancreatic lesions.

Early studies found that EUS was superior to conventional CT for tumor[6,7] and nodal[4,6,7,54] staging of pancreatic cancer (Table 15-4). Whereas one study has reported that EUS is superior to CT for T staging,[22] most found that the two are equivalent for both tumor[17,55,57] or nodal staging.* Soriano and colleagues,[57] on the other hand, found that helical CT was superior to EUS in the assessment of locoregional extension among 62 patients with pancreatic cancer. Similar to CT, early studies showed that EUS was superior to MRI for staging of pancreatic tumors.[6,7] However, two studies[55,57] found no difference between EUS and MRI for both T and N staging. Clearly, the initial advantage demonstrated by EUS over other imaging modalities for the staging of pancreatic tumors was not confirmed in subsequent studies. Future research comparing EUS to MDCT and 3.0 Tesla MRI is needed to confirm these findings and further define the role of EUS for the locoregional staging of pancreatic tumors.

For detection of non-nodal metastatic cancer, CT and MRI are superior to EUS due to both anatomic limitations of

TABLE 15-4

COMPARISON OF THE ACCURACY OF EUS WITH CT, MRI, AND US FOR TUMOR (T) AND NODAL (N) STAGING OF PANCREATIC CANCER

Author (year)	Number of Patients	Accuracy of EUS (%) T	N	Accuracy of CT (%) T	N	Accuracy of MRI (%) T	N	Accuracy of US (%) T	N
Mukai et al[54] (1991)	26	—	65	—	38	—	—	—	58
Rosch et al[4] (1992)	40	—	72	—	38	—	—	—	53
Palazzo et al[6] (1993)	64	82	64	45	50	50	56	—	37
Muller et al[7] (1994)	16	82	50	56	38	57	50	—	—
Legmann et al[13] (1998)	22	90	86	86	77	—	—	—	—
Midwinter et al[17] (1999)	23	—	74	—	65	—	—	—	—
Rivadeneira et al[19] (2003)	44	—	84	—	68	—	—	—	—
Soriano et al[57] (2004)	62	63	67	73	56	62	60	—	—
Ramsay et al[55] (2004)	27	63	69	76	63	83	56	—	—
DeWitt et al[22] (2004)	53	67	44	41	47	—	—	—	—

normal upper gastrointestinal anatomy and the limited range of EUS imaging. Although the entire left and caudate lobes of the liver may be seen by transgastric imaging in most patients, a portion of the right lobe may not be visualized by EUS. Therefore EUS clearly cannot replace but may supplement other modalities for staging of hepatic metastases. The principal advantages of EUS for evaluation of the liver metastases are detection of small lesions missed by other imaging modalities[69,70] and the ability to sample visualized accessible masses by EUS FNA.[69-71] The sensitivity of EUS FNA for benign and malignant liver masses reportedly ranges from 82% to 94%,[71,72] and the diagnosis of liver metastases from pancreatic cancer generally precludes surgical resection.[72] EUS may also identify and sample ascites either previously detected or undetected by other imaging studies (Figures 15-7 to 15-9).[73,74] Identification of malignant ascites and liver metastases (Figure 15-10) by EUS FNA is associated with poor survival following diagnosis.[75] Therefore routine examination of the perigastric and duodenal spaces for ascites should be incorporated in the staging of every pancreatic mass.

Vascular Invasion by Pancreatic Tumors

Interpretation of data regarding the accuracy of EUS for vascular invasion is difficult for several reasons. First, there is little histologic correlation with intraoperative findings regarding vascular invasion in most studies. True vascular invasion may be overestimated or underestimated by intraoperative findings[76,77] and therefore give false information regarding the accuracy of EUS staging. Second, there is no established consensus among endosonographers on the optimal criteria that should be utilized for EUS assessment of vascular invasion by pancreatic or other tumors. Consequently, multiple criteria have been proposed by various authors for this indication.

For overall vascular invasion, the accuracy of EUS ranges from 40% to 100% (Table 15-5).* Sensitivity and specificity of EUS for malignant vascular invasion range from 42% to 91% and 89% to 100%, respectively.[16,51,55,57,78] Although some studies demonstrate that EUS is more accurate[9,16,18,19,54] than CT for vascular invasion, some authors have reported that the accuracy of CT is superior[10,55,57] to that of EUS. Overall

---

*9,10,16,18,19,51,54,55,57

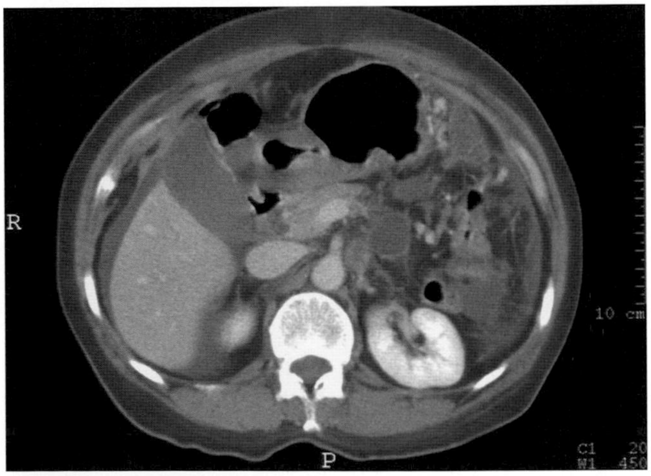

FIGURE 15-7 Axial CT image demonstrating a 3-cm cystic pancreatic body mass and perihepatic ascites.

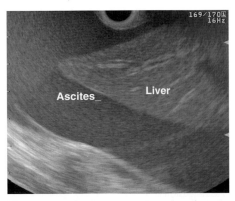

FIGURE 15-8 Linear EUS image (6.0 MHz) of perihepatic ascites.

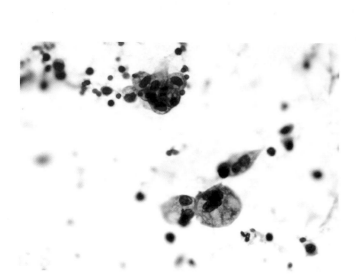

FIGURE 15-9 Cytology specimen from ascites fluid demonstrating metastatic adenocarcinoma (Diff-Quik stain; 100×).

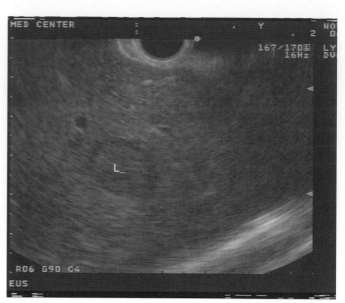

FIGURE 15-10 Linear EUS image (7.5 MHz) of a 15-mm hypoechoic mass in the caudate lobe of the liver in a patient with a mass in the head of the pancreas. The liver lesion was not seen on CT scan.

TABLE 15-5

COMPARISON OF THE OVERALL ACCURACY OF EUS WITH CT, US, ANGIOGRAPHY, AND MRI FOR VASCULAR INVASION BY PANCREATIC CANCER

Author (year)	No. Patients	Test	Sensitivity (%)	Specificity (%)	PPV(%)	NPV(%)	Accuracy (%)
Mukai et al[54] (1991)[a]	26	EUS	—	—	—	—	77
		CT	—	—	—	—	38
		US	—	—	—	—	50
		Angiography	—	—	—	—	56
Melzer et al[9] (1996)	13	EUS	—	—	—	—	92
		CT	—	—	—	—	61
Dufour et al[10] (1997)	24	EUS	—	—	—	—	40
		CT	—	—	—	—	90
Buscail et al[51] (1999)[b]	32	EUS	67	100	100	83	88
Gress et al[16] (1999)	75	EUS	91	96	94	93	93
		CT	15	100	100	60	62
Mertz et al[18] (2000)	6	EUS	—	—	—	—	100
		CT	—	—	—	—	50
Tierney et al[78] (2001)	45	EUS	87	—	—	—	—
		CT	33	—	—	—	—
Rivadeneira et al[19] (2003)	9	EUS	—	—	—	—	100
		CT	—	—	—	—	45
Ramsay et al[55] (2004)	19	EUS	56	89	—	—	68
		CT	80	78	—	—	89
		MRI	56	100	—	—	78
Soriano et al[57] (2004)	62	EUS	42	97	89	74	76
		CT	67	94	89	80	83
		MRI	59	84	72	74	74
		Angiography	21	100	100	64	67
Tellez-Avila et al[79] (2012)	50	EUS	61	90	78	80	80
		CT	55	93	83	77	74

NPV, negative predictive value; PPV, positive predictive value
[a]Retroperitoneal vasculature.
[b]Includes some patients with ampullary cancer.

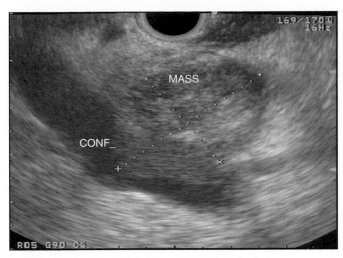

FIGURE 15-11 Linear EUS image (7.5 MHz) of a 2.8-cm pancreatic mass that is invading the portal vein confluence.

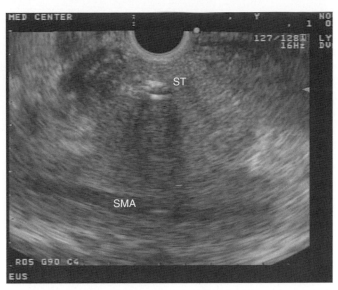

FIGURE 15-13 Linear EUS image (7.5 MHz) of a 31-mm hypoechoic mass in the head of a pancreas with a long segment of the superior mesenteric artery (SMA) encasement. A biliary stent (ST) is also seen.

accuracy of MRI is reportedly equivalent[57] or superior[55] to EUS. For overall venous invasion, EUS is reportedly superior[6] or equivalent to CT.[8] Overall sensitivity and accuracy of EUS for arterial invasion is 56%[8] and 50%,[6] respectively. Angiography is consistently inferior to EUS and CT for assessment of vascular infiltration by tumor and therefore has no current role in the staging of pancreatic tumors.[4,54,57]

The sensitivity of EUS for tumor invasion of the portal vein or portal vein confluence is 60% to 100%,* with most studies demonstrating sensitivities over 80% (Figure 15-11). The sensitivity of EUS for portal vein invasion is also consistently superior to that of CT[4,12,17,56] and angiography.[4,12,56,80] For the superior mesenteric vein (SMV), superior mesenteric artery (SMA), and celiac artery the sensitivity of EUS is only 17% to 83%,[51] 17%,[18] and about 50%,[4,56] respectively (Figures 15-12 and 15-13). The sensitivity of CT for staging of the SMA[17,18] and celiac artery[4,56] appears to be better than EUS. EUS staging of the superior mesenteric vessels may be difficult due to either the inability to visualize the entire course of the vessel or obscuring of these vessels by a large tumor in the uncinate

_____

*1,4,12,17,56,80,81

or inferior portion of the pancreatic head.[81] This is in contrast to the splenic artery and vein, which are generally easily seen and staged well by EUS (Figure 15-14).[1,56,80,81] However, one recent study by Tellez-Avilla and colleagues showed that the PPV of EUS for arterial invasion was 100%, compared to 60% for CT.[79] Until further conclusive data becomes available, assessment of tumor resectability should be done by both EUS and CT (or MRI) rather than by EUS alone.

Several authors have attempted to describe the accuracy of various endosonographic findings to assess vascular invasion by malignant pancreatic tumors. Using the criteria "rough-edged vessel with compression," Yasuda and colleagues[1] found a sensitivity, specificity, and accuracy of 79%, 87%, and 81%, respectively, for malignant invasion of the portal venous system. Rosch and colleagues[4] found a sensitivity, specificity, and accuracy of 91%, 96%, and 94%, respectively, for invasion of the portal vein using the criteria "abnormal contour, loss of hyperechoic interface, and close contact." In further blinded videotape review,[81] these same authors found that no single criterion was able to predict venous invasion with a sensitivity and specificity exceeding 80% each. However, they

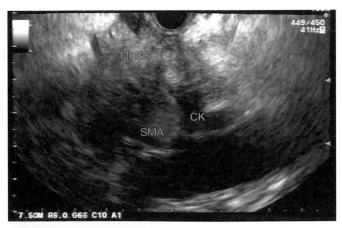

FIGURE 15-12 Linear EUS image (7.5 MHz) of a 45-mm hypoechoic mass invading the celiac trunk (CK) and the superior mesenteric artery (SMA).

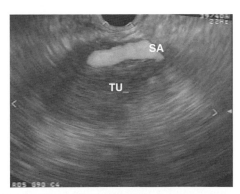

FIGURE 15-14 Linear EUS image (6.0 MHz) of a 3-cm pancreatic body mass (TU) invading the splenic artery (SA). Doppler imaging demonstrates preserved flow in the vessel.

TABLE 15-6

TEST CHARACTERISTICS OF EUS FOR RESECTABILITY OF PANCREATIC CANCER

Author (year)	Number of Patients	Sensitivity (%)	Specificity (%)	PPV (%)	NPV (%)	Accuracy (%)
Howard et al[11] (1997)[a]	21	75	77	67	83	76
Legmann et al[13] (1998)	27	90	83	95	75	92
Buscail et al[51] (1999)	26	47	100	100	50	65
Gress et al[16] (1999)	75	95	92	93	94	93
Ahmad et al[50] (2000)	63	61	63	69	55	62
Tierney et al[78] (2001)	24	93	67	82	83	83
Soriano et al[57] (2004)	62	23	100	100	64	67
Ramsay et al[55] (2004)	26	56	83	91	38	63
DeWitt et al[22] (2004)	53	88	68	71	86	77
Total	377	69	82	86	72	77

NPV, negative predictive value; PPV, positive predictive value.
[a]Includes six patients with ampullary cancer.

found that both complete vascular obstruction and the presence of collaterals demonstrated a specificity of 94% for vascular invasion. Similarly, Snady and colleagues[82] reported 100% specificity for presence of venous collaterals, tumor in the lumen, and loss of hyperechoic interface. Depending on the EUS criteria chosen, Brugge and colleagues[80] found a sensitivity and specificity ranging from 40% to 80% and 23% to 100%, respectively, for malignant invasion of the portal vein. There exists a trade-off between various criteria for sensitivity and specificity for vascular invasion. However, criteria with the highest specificity are needed in order to optimize selection of those most likely to benefit from surgical exploration. Therefore the findings of an irregular vascular wall, venous collaterals, and visible tumor within the vessel are the preferred criteria for assessment of vascular invasion.

Resectability of Pancreatic Tumors

Complete surgical removal of pancreatic cancer with negative histopathologic margins (R0 resection) is the only potential curative treatment and is an independent predictor of postoperative survival.[83,84] Therefore the principal role of preoperative evaluation is to accurately identify patients with resectable disease who may benefit from surgery while avoiding surgery in patients with suspected unresectable disease.

In a pooled analysis of nine studies involving 377 patients (Table 15-6), the sensitivity and specificity of EUS for resectability of pancreatic cancer was 69% and 82%, respectively.* Ranges of reported sensitivities and specificities were 23% to 91% and 63% to 100%, respectively. Overall EUS accuracy for tumor resectability is 77%. Eight of these nine studies also compared the accuracy of EUS to one or more imaging modalities.

Because most studies have reported that EUS is similar to both CT and MRI for assessment of resectability, some authors have proposed that optimal preoperative imaging of pancreatic cancer requires the use of multiple modalities. Using a decision analysis, Soriano and colleagues[57] found that accuracy for tumor resectability was maximized and costs were minimized when CT or EUS was performed initially followed by the other test in those with potentially resectable neoplasms. Ahmad and colleagues[50] proposed that although

---

*11,13,16,22,50,51,55,57,78

individually EUS and MRI are not sensitive for tumor resectability, the use may increase PPV of resectability compared to either test alone. Tierney and colleagues[78] suggest that CT should be performed initially, but EUS should also be utilized in most patients because of its improved detection of vascular invasion. When surgery is performed only when MDCT and EUS agree on tumor resectability, DeWitt and colleagues[22] reported that there is a nonsignificant trend toward improved accuracy of resectability compared to either test alone. Other studies have suggested that EUS should be incorporated into preoperative imaging to prevent unnecessary surgery[51] and to aid detection and staging of tumors missed by CT.[13,22] Clearly, there is no consensus on the best test or tests necessary for preoperative staging of suspected pancreatic tumors (Table 15-7). We propose an EUS-based management algorithm for evaluation of suspected pancreatic cancer (Figure 15-15); however, in reality the role of EUS in these patients depends on its availability, referral patterns, and local expertise. Further cost and decision analysis and comparative studies with EUS to state-of-the-art CT and MRI are required to optimize surgical exploration in appropriate patients.

EUS FNA of Pancreatic Cancer

Prior to the advent of EUS, FNA or core biopsy of pancreatic masses was performed either intraoperatively[85,86] or percutaneously under CT or ultrasound (US) guidance.[87–90] Intraoperative FNA of pancreatic tumors is an accurate, safe technique[88] but may increase intraoperative time considerably, especially with on-site interpretation of specimens. Previous enthusiasm over the use of percutaneous FNA, however, has decreased by both reports of needle-track seeding[91–94] and the development of EUS FNA.

EUS FNA is performed using a linear array echoendoscope under conscious sedation and appropriate cardiorespiratory monitoring. Placement of a transducer on the distal tip of the echoendoscope permits visualization of needle advancement into the target lesion under real-time ultrasound guidance. A variety of commercially available FNA needles is available that range in size from 19 to 25 G. It is recommended that Doppler be used to examine the projected path of the needle to avoid puncturing intervening blood vessels while trying to minimize the amount of normal pancreatic tissue that has to be traversed. Once the target lesion is accessed through the

TABLE 15-7

COMPARISON OF EUS TO CT, MRI, AND ANGIOGRAPHY FOR RESECTABILITY OF PANCREATIC CANCER

Author (year)	Number of Patients	Modality	Sensitivity (%)	Specificity (%)	PPV (%)	NPV (%)	Accuracy (%)
Howard et al[11] (1997)[a]	22	EUS	75	77	67	83	76
		CT	63	100	100	80	86
		Angio	38	92	75	71	71
Legmann et al[13] (1998)	27	EUS	90	83	95	75	92
		CT	90	100	100	77	93
Gress et al[16] (1999)	75	EUS	95	92	93	94	93
	58	CT	97	19	58	83	60
Ahmad et al[50] (2000)	63	EUS	61	63	69	55	62
		MRI	73	72	77	68	73
Tierney et al[78] (2001)	24	EUS	93	67	82	83	83
		CT	100	33	71	100	75
Ramsay et al[55] (2004)	26	EUS	56	83	91	38	63
		CT	79	67	88	50	76
		MRI	81	83	93	67	83
Soriano et al[57] (2004)	62	EUS	23	100	100	64	67
		CT	67	97	95	77	83
		MRI	57	90	81	73	75
		Angio	37	100	65	71	
DeWitt et al[42] (2004)	53	EUS	88	68	71	86	77
		CT	92	64	70	90	77

NPV, negative predictive value; PPV, positive predictive value.
[a]Includes six patients with ampullary cancer.

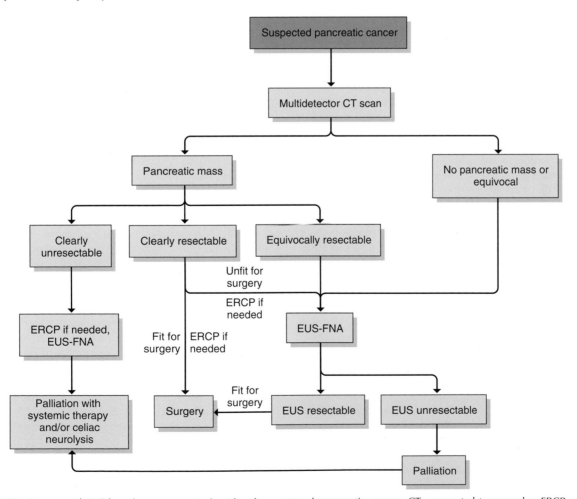

FIGURE 15-15 A proposed EUS-based management algorithm for suspected pancreatic cancer. CT, computed tomography; ERCP, endoscopic retrograde cholangiopancreatography; FNA, fine-needle aspiration.

gastric or duodenal wall, the stylet is withdrawn. The use of suction may be considered but is not required. A to-and-fro rapid jabbing movement within the pancreatic tumor is performed for 30 to 45 seconds. The echogenic tip of the needle should be kept in view at all times to avoid deeper tissue penetration. The needle is then withdrawn into the sheath, and the entire system is removed all together. The material within the needle lumen is then expressed onto two glass slides: one is air dried for rapid staining and on-site review (if possible) and the other is alcohol fixed for future review. The use of suction in subsequent passes depends on the cellularity of the initial few passes; suction should be applied if the specimens are too scant and avoided if they are too bloody.

Advancement of the EUS FNA needle through the biopsy channel can be challenging for lesions in the uncinate process. A "short" scope position (similar to that used for ERCP) may be helpful and is obtained by slow withdrawal of the scope from the second and/or third portions of the duodenum while endosonographically maintaining the lesion in view. However, this position is generally unstable, and the scope occasionally slips back into the stomach. Fine movements of the endoscope, maximal elevation of the distal tip, and insufflation of the balloon may help keep this position. Biopsy of uncinate lesions may also be accomplished by advancement of the endoscope into a "long" position and is obtained by pushing the scope into the apex of the duodenal bulb or proximal second portion, allowing a loop to form against the greater curvature of the stomach. This position is more stable compared to the short position; however, needle advancement can be difficult. Once the lesion is visualized in either position, the scope tip is deflected upward against the lesion and the air is aspirated from the lumen to minimize the distance between the lesion and the scope tip. The shortest distance between the scope and the target lesion is always sought to minimize the amount of normal tissue that the needle is required to traverse. Once the scope is in this position, it is still not uncommon to face difficulty passing the needle out of the channel due to the angulation. In this situation, the endosonographer may be required to reorient the endoscope within the stomach or duodenum and to deflect the tip of the scope downward. This reorientation may then permit gentle advancement of the needle out of the biopsy channel. Once the needle is outside the channel, the distal tip of the scope may then be deflected upward again to bring the lesion back in view. For biopsy of pancreatic tail lesions, the scope is typically in a short position with maximal upward deflection. If vascular structures are found between the transducer and the target lesion, slight reorientation of the scope tip position usually permits location of a safe window for biopsy without intervening vessels.

The first reported use of EUS FNA of a pancreatic mass was described by Villman and colleagues[94] in 1992. Since then, multiple studies have documented the utility of EUS FNA for this indication. Two recently published meta-analyses totaling more than 8400 patients and 67 studies reported a pooled sensitivity for the diagnosis of malignancy based on cytology of 85% and 89% and a pooled specificity of 98% and 99%, respectively (Figure 15-16).[95,96] Some authors have even reported a sensitivity of EUS FNA for pancreatic cancer exceeding 90% in patients following negative or nondiagnostic sampling from previous ERCP or percutaneous

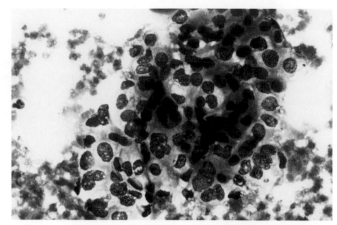

FIGURE 15-16 Cytology from EUS fine-needle aspiration in the same patient as in Figure 15-4 (H&E; 20×). Pleomorphic, overlapping cells with increased nuclear to cytoplasmic ratio are present, consistent with adenocarcinoma.

approach.[97,98] Despite excellent sensitivity, the NPV of EUS FNA for pancreatic tumors remains somewhat limited at 55%.[21,98–105] Therefore a negative or nondiagnostic biopsy does not completely exclude the possibility of malignancy. Fritscher-Ravens and colleagues[106] found that in a series of 207 consecutive patients with focal pancreatic lesions, the sensitivity of EUS FNA for the diagnosis of malignancy in patients with normal parenchyma (89%) was superior to those with parenchymal evidence of chronic pancreatitis (54%). The presence of chronic pancreatitis may also hinder cytologic interpretation of pancreatic biopsy, thus decreasing sensitivity of EUS FNA of pancreatic masses.[107] In addition, in a recent study by Siddiqui and colleagues[108] the false-positive rate for EUS FNA was 4 of 247 (1.1%), and all four patients falsely diagnosed with pancreatic tumors had chronic pancreatitis on surgical pathology.

Because most studies document an overall sensitivity of EUS FNA for pancreatic tumors above 80%, most endosonographers should expect to eventually achieve this level of competency. At least 40 EUS FNA procedures are required for a novice endosonographer to achieve at least 80% sensitivity for the diagnosis of pancreatic cancer.[109] Short mentored training of EUS FNA appears to permit significant improvements in EUS FNA accuracy principally by decreasing the number of inadequate specimens.[110] American Society of Gastrointestinal Endoscopy (ASGE) guidelines for credentialing in EUS[111] and the current ASGE EUS Core Curriculum[112] recommend that at least 50 supervised EUS FNA procedures during monitored training and at least 75 pancreatobiliary cases be performed before competency in EUS can be evaluated. We believe that training for EUS FNA is best accomplished by expert formal instruction in a high-volume referral practice.

At most tertiary referral centers, on-site cytopathology assistance is provided to offer immediate feedback to the endosonographer about the quality of EUS FNA specimens obtained. On-site review correlates highly with the final diagnosis[113] and can both improve diagnostic certainty and minimize diagnostic uncertainty.[114] A recent systematic review by Schmidt and colleagues[115] included five studies that reported head-to-head comparison of sample adequacy and diagnostic accuracy between cases with and without on-site cytologic evaluation during pancreatic EUS FNA. On-site cytopathology was associated with an average 10% improved adequacy rate but had no impact on the diagnostic yield. In a recent meta-analysis by Hebert-Magee and colleagues[96] that evaluated the accuracy of EUS FNA including 34 studies and 3644 patients, rapid on-site evaluation was a significant determinant of EUS FNA accuracy. The optimal number of passes has been evaluated by two studies,[116,117] which reported that at least five to seven EUS FNA passes for pancreatic masses should be performed to maximize diagnostic yield. This information may prove helpful to endosonographers performing EUS FNA when rapid pathology interpretation is not available.

Occasionally, on-site cytology review of a suspected pancreatic cancer demonstrates insufficient tissue to confirm malignancy. This may be due to tumor necrosis (particularly seen with larger tumors), fibrosis, or hypervascularity. Yield may be increased by "fanning the lesion," using different angles of scope deflection in order to sample the peripheral parts of the lesion. In a recent randomized study by Bang and colleagues,[118] "fanning technique" was superior to standard approach, with fewer passes being required to establish a diagnosis. Increasing the number of passes may also overcome the problem of an insufficient sample but may also increase the amount of blood in the sample. In this situation, avoiding suction and switching to a smaller-gauge needle could help limit the amount of blood in the specimen. Finally, EUS-guided core biopsy may be considered in these cases. When on-site cytopathology is unavailable, dynamic telecytopathology, with evaluation of slides by a cytopathologist in a remote location with immediate feedback to the endosonographer, appears to be a promising alternative.[119–121] In addition, cyto-technologist on-site evaluation of FNA sample adequacy was shown in one study[122] to have comparable accuracy to on-site evaluation by cytopathologist.

The most commonly used commercially available EUS FNA needle sizes are 19, 22, and 25 G. Recent studies indicate equivalence of 25-G and 22-G needles for adequate tissue acquisition.[123,124] In a recent meta-analysis by Madhoun and colleagues,[125] 25-G needles were associated with a higher sensitivity but comparable specificity to 22-G needles in 1292 patients. In another meta-analysis by Affolter and colleagues,[126] 25-G needles appeared to confer an advantage in adequacy of passes as compared to 22-G needles, but there was no differences with respect to accuracy, number of passes, or complications. Nevertheless, 25-G needles were associated with less technical failures compared to 22-G needles when sampling pancreatic head and uncinate process lesions in some studies and therefore should be considered first in this case.[127,128]

Traditionally, and due to their inherent rigidity, 19-G needles have been rarely used in the duodenum. Recently, a needle made of nitinol has been developed with enhanced flexibility to overcome the limitations of the currently available 19-G needle (Flex 19, Boston Scientific, Natick, MA). Varadarajulu and colleagues[129] were the first to report on the use of this needle in 38 patients, including 32 pancreatic head/uncinate lesions. Transduodenal FNA yielded samples adequate for cytologic analysis in all 32 patients. There were no technical failures or procedure-related complications reported.

Major complications following EUS FNA of solid pancreatic masses occur in 0.5% to 2.5% of patients.[105,130–134] Due to this exceedingly small risk, antibiotics are not usually required following EUS FNA of solid lesions. Gress and colleagues[130] reported a 1.2% (2 of 121) risk of pancreatitis and 1% (1 of 121) risk of severe bleeding following EUS FNA of solid pancreatic masses. Another prospective trial reported 2 of 100 (2%) patients developing acute pancreatitis following EUS FNA of a pancreatic mass; both patients had a history of recent pancreatitis.[133] Therefore caution should be exercised when performing EUS FNA in these patients. Following EUS FNA of the pancreas, Eloubeidi and colleagues[105] reported self-limited immediate postprocedure complications in 10 of 158 (6.3%) patients including hypoxia, abdominal pain, excessive but inconsequential bleeding at the biopsy site, and sore throat. During the first 3 days after the procedure, 20 of 78 patients contacted reported at least one minor symptom, one patient with mild acute pancreatitis and two with emergency room visits, one of whom was admitted with dehydration. In another prospective study, Al-Haddad and colleagues reported no delayed complications following EUS FNA of 127 patients with solid pancreatic masses followed for 30 days.[132] In a series of 248 patients, including 134 patients who underwent EUS FNA of solid lesions, O'Toole and colleagues[134] reported no complications in any patient. A recent systematic review by Wang and colleagues[135] included 8246 patients with pancreatic lesions, 7337 of those being solid masses, and reported complications occurring in 60 patients (0.82%). Pancreatitis occurred in 36 of 8246 patients with pancreatic lesions, of which 75% where mild; however, one patient with severe pancreatitis died (estimated pancreatitis-related mortality rate of 2.78%). The overall rate of pain, bleeding, fever, and infection were 0.38%, 0.10%, 0.08%, and 0.02%, respectively.

Peritoneal seeding of tumor cells following EUS FNA has been reported in up to 2.2% of patients but appears to be less than CT-guided FNA (16.3%).[136] Ikezawa and colleagues[137] demonstrated that EUS FNA did not increase the risk of peritoneal carcinomatosis in pancreatic cancer, comparing 161 patients who underwent ERCP alone with 56 who underwent EUS FNA. To assess risk of transgastric FNA of pancreatic body and tail tumors, Beane and colleagues[138] evaluated the overall and recurrence-free survival of pancreatic cancer patients who underwent distal pancreatectomy for this indication. In the 179 patients included who underwent preoperative FNA, the overall and recurrence-free survival were no different from the 59 patients who did not undergo preoperative FNA. In addition, recently Ngamruengphong and colleagues[139] evaluated the risk of stomach/peritoneal recurrence after preoperative EUS FNA in 256 patients diagnosed with malignant solid and cystic neoplasms who underwent surgery with curative intent and found that EUS FNA was not associated with increased needle-track seeding.

To date, there have been no large prospective trials comparing the accuracy of EUS FNA to percutaneous FNA of pancreatic masses. Qian and Hecht reported that CT FNA was superior to EUS FNA of pancreatic masses.[140] However, Mallery and colleagues[141] found no significant difference between the accuracy of surgically directed, CT FNA, and EUS FNA of pancreatic masses. Nevertheless, the results of those two studies are difficult to generalize due to selection bias in that tumors sampled by EUS FNA were more difficult compared to those sampled by CT or other imaging studies. It appears that percutaneous FNA is an acceptable option for sampling of pancreatic tumors that are visible, accessible, and clearly inoperable based on imaging findings. For all other lesions, EUS FNA is preferable to percutaneous FNA. Furthermore, the initial use of EUS and EUS FNA appears to be a more cost-effective initial strategy for the initial workup of patients with suspected pancreatic malignancy.[142,143]

Despite excellent accuracy and a low incidence of major complications, EUS FNA of pancreatic masses has several limitations. First, an on-site cytopathologist during EUS FNA is recommended for assessment of specimen adequacy. Second, PPLs and well-differentiated ductal adenocarcinomas are often difficult to diagnose by use of cytology alone. Finally, the low NPV of EUS FNA does not permit exclusion of malignancy in negative specimens. To overcome these limitations, a spring-loaded 19-G Tru-Cut core biopsy needle (Quick-Core; Wilson-Cook, Winston-Salem, NC, USA) was developed to obtain histologic tissue samples using a standard linear array echoendoscope.[144] Larghi and colleagues[145] reported an overall success rate of 74% in obtaining pancreatic tissue using EUS TCB in 23 consecutive patients with solid pancreatic masses. When using a transduodenal compared to transgastric approach, the success rate decreased from 100% to 41%. The authors reported that transduodenal biopsy was difficult when upward deflection of the echoendoscope was required to bring the target lesion into appropriate position as it precluded extension of the needle from the accessory channel. Another study by Varadarajulu and colleagues compared EUS TCB to EUS FNA for multiple sites and found no difference in diagnostic accuracy between the two devices.[146] Another large series of 113 patients undergoing pancreatic EUS TCB among other sites included lesions in the pancreatic head, neck, body, and tail.[147] Overall, 90 of 113 (80%) patients were eventually diagnosed as having malignancy. The sensitivity and diagnostic accuracy of EUS TCB were 62% and 68%, respectively. No significant difference was found in diagnostic yield for lesions in the head or uncinate process compared to neck, body, or tail. The use of TCB is recommended in a few situations where studies have demonstrated better diagnostic yield, including autoimmune pancreatitis[42] and lymphoma.[148] In addition, TCB could be used as a rescue technique when on-site FNA results are inconclusive or if this service is not available. As the use of TCB is technically challenging in the duodenum due to inherent rigidity of the 19-G caliber needle and mechanical friction of the firing mechanism with the torched echoendoscope, a new 19-G fine-needle biopsy (FNB) device was developed (ProCore, Cook Endoscopy, Winston-Salem, NC) with reverse bevel technology to acquire core biopsies. In a study by Iglesias-Garcia and colleagues,[149] which included 114 lesions, EUS FNB was technically feasible in 112 lesions (98%), with adequate histological samples being procured in 102 (89%) and with an overall diagnostic accuracy of over 85%. In this study, puncturing from a duodenal position was successful in 33 of 35 cases and was not negatively associated with the sample quality. The authors reported, however, that transduodenal FNB was technically more difficult and, in many cases, the ProCore needle needed to be pushed out of the endoscope in the stomach before advancing the endoscope into the duodenum.

In a recent series by Larghi and colleagues[150] including 61 pancreatic masses, FNB using a newly developed 22-G ProCore needle was technically feasible and allowed a suitable sample for histologic evaluation in 88% of patients with one single pass. In another randomized trial by Bang and

colleagues[151] including 56 patients with pancreatic masses, there was no difference in the technical performance or diagnostic yield between 22-G FNA needles and 22-G FNB.

Some investigators have evaluated whether analysis of genetic mutations may increase the diagnostic yield of EUS FNA of pancreatic masses. Ogura and colleagues[152] in a recent prospective series including 394 pancreatic masses found that the combination of k-*ras* mutation analysis with cytopathology increased the sensitivity of EUS FNA from 87% to 93% and the accuracy from 89% to 94% for the diagnosis of pancreatic masses. In a recent meta-analysis,[153] which included eight studies with 931 patients undergoing EUS FNA of pancreatic masses, the pooled sensitivity and specificity of EUS FNA were 80% and 97%, respectively; the estimated sensitivity and specificity of k-*ras* mutation analysis were 76.8% and 93.3%, respectively, and 88.7% and 92% for combination of cytology and k-*ras* mutation analysis, respectively. Overall, k-*ras* mutation testing applied to cases that were inconclusive by EUS FNA reduced the false-negative rate by 55.6%, with a false-positive rate of 10.7%. The addition of other somatic mutations such as p53 and p16 to k-*ras* has been shown to increase the sensitivity of cancer detection to up to 100% in cases where FNA was inconclusive.[154] Due to the relative high-diagnostic accuracy of standard EUS FNA, as well as the relatively high cost and limited availability of these genetic tests, the use of genetic testing on EUS FNA samples should be limited to research protocols and inconclusive specimens.

Pancreatic Neuroendocrine Tumors

Pancreatic neuroendocrine tumors (PNETs) represent less than 10% of pancreatic tumors. They are rare neoplasms with an overall prevalence of 10 per 1 million.[155] About 10% to 20% of these tumors are classified as functional PNETs (FPNETs) in which excessive tumor hormone production produces a distinct clinical syndrome. The two most clinically important FPNETs are gastrinomas and insulinomas. When a distinct series of symptoms is present (i.e., refractory hypoglycemia for insulinoma or abdominal pain, diarrhea, and peptic ulcer disease for gastrinoma) and imaging reveals a pancreatic mass, the clinical suspicion of PNET is relatively straightforward. Excessive secretory products are then easily measured to confirm the suspected diagnosis. When PNETs do not produce a clinical syndrome, they are classified as nonfunctional (NFPNETs).[156] Due to a lack of characteristic symptoms related to hormone excess, NFPNETs are usually recognized later with larger tumors and produce nonspecific symptoms such as jaundice, weight loss, abdominal pain, or pancreatitis.[157,158] Differentiation between benign and malignant PNETs is difficult with surgical pathology alone.[159] Therefore malignancy is usually confirmed by the presence of distant metastases, and benign disease is confirmed by clinical follow-up.[160] Similar to primary ductal adenocarcinoma, surgical resection is the only cure for these tumors.[161,162] Therefore a high index of suspicion coupled with a stepwise preoperative evaluation for localization may optimize patient selection for potentially curative surgery.

In a series of studies that compared EUS to other imaging modalities (Table 15-8), the sensitivity of EUS for detection of PNETs was 77% to 94% (Figure 15-17).[163–170] EUS appears especially useful for detection of small PNETs (<2.5 cm)

TABLE 15-8

COMPARISON OF EUS WITH CT, US, MRI, SRS, AND ANGIOGRAPHY FOR EVALUATION OF PANCREATIC NEUROENDOCRINE TUMORS

Author (year)	Number of Patients	Tumor (n)	Test	Sensitivity (%)	Specificity (%)	PPV (%)	NPV (%)	Accuracy (%)
Rosch et al[163] (1992)	37	Insulinomas (31)	EUS	82	95			
		Gastrinomas (7)	CT	0				
		Glucagonoma (1)	US	0				
			Angio	27				
Palazzo et al[164] (1993)	30	Insulinoma (13)	EUS	79				
			CT	14				
		Gastrinoma (17)	US	7				
			EUS	79				
Zimmer et al[170] (1996)	20	Gastrinoma (10)	EUS	79				
			CT	29				
			MRI	29				
			US	29				
			SRS	86				
		Insulinoma (10)	EUS	93				
			CT	21				
			MRI	7				
			US	7				
			SRS	14				
Proye et al[169] (1998)[a]	41	All PNETs	EUS	77		94		
		Insulinoma (20)	SRS	60		100		
		Gastrinoma (21)	SRS	25		100		
		Insulinoma (9)	EUS + SRS	89				
		Gastrinoma (14)		93				
De Angelis et al[166] (1999)	23	Insulinoma (12)	EUS	87				
			CT	30				
			MRI	25				
			US	17				
			SRS	15				
			Angio	27				
Ardengh et al[166] (2000)	12	Insulinoma (12)	EUS	83				
			CT	17				
Anderson et al[165] (2000)	75	Gastrinoma (36)	EUS	100	94	95	100	97
	14	Insulinoma (36)	EUS	88	100	100	43	89
			Angio	44				
Gouya et al[168] (2003)[b]	38	Insulinoma (38)	EUS	94				
			CT	29-94				
Khashab et al[171] (2011)	217	All PNETs (231)	EUS	91				
		Nonfunctional PNET (173)	CT	63				
		Insulinoma (35)						
		Gastrinoma (10)						
		Glucagonoma (7)						
		Vipoma (5)						
		Carcinoid (1)						

Angio, angiography; CT, computed tomography; MRI, magnetic resonance imaging; PNET, pancreatic neuroendocrine tumor; SRS, somatostatin receptor scintigraphy; US, ultrasound.

[a]Overall sensitivity of combined EUS and SRS was 89% for insulinoma (n = 9) and 93% for gastrinoma (n = 14).

[b]Sensitivity of CT for nonhelical CT, thick section MDCT, and thin section MDCT were 29%, 57%, and 94%, respectively.

missed by other imaging studies (Figure 15-18). The sensitivity of transabdominal ultrasound detection of PETs is between 7% and 29%.[164,167,170] Similarly, early studies with CT demonstrated poor detection with reported sensitivities of 14% to 30%.[164,167,170] Gouya and colleagues[168] studied a group of 30 patients with 32 insulinomas over 13 years. The sensitivity of EUS was 94% compared to 29% for nonhelical CT and 57% for dual-phase MDCT. More recently, in a retrospective series with 217 patients, Khashab and colleagues[171] also found that

CT is more likely than EUS to miss insulinomas and PNETs <2 cm. These authors also found that the overall sensitivity of EUS (91%) was greater than CT (63%).

Early studies that compared EUS with MRI[167,170] demonstrated a sensitivity of MRI for PNET detection at 25% to 29%. Recent studies, however, demonstrate a sensitivity of 85% to 100%[172,173] and a PPV of 96%[174] for PNET detection. Because PNETs are hypervascular tumors, angiography will sometimes demonstrate a "blushing" pattern in the pancreas in suspected

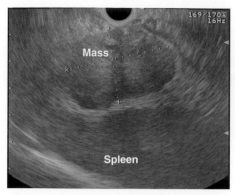

FIGURE 15-17 Linear EUS image (6.0 MHz) of a 4.5-cm well-defined hypoechoic mass in the tail of the pancreas. This patient was asymptomatic.

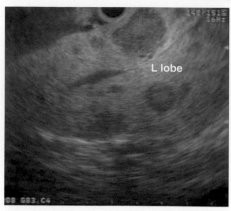

FIGURE 15-19 Examination of the liver in the same patient in Figure 15-17 demonstrates a multiple hyperechoic masses in the left lobe (L lobe) of the liver suggestive of metastases.

PNET. The sensitivity of diagnostic angiography for tumor detection is under 30%.[163,167] The clinical utility of somatostatin receptor scintigraphy (SRS) for identification of insulinomas is limited, with sensitivities ranging from 14% to 60%.[167,169,170] For other PNETs, SRS has a reported sensitivity of 58% to 86% for tumor detection.[170,175,176] Proye and colleagues[169] found that for a series of patients with a histologically proven insulinoma ($n = 20$) or gastrinoma ($n = 21$), the sensitivity and PPV of EUS were 77% and 94%, respectively, for pancreatic tumors. For the same patients, the sensitivity and PPV of SRS for insulinoma and gastrinoma were 60% and 100%, and 25% and 100%, respectively. When both tests were combined for patients with an insulinoma ($n = 9$) and for gastrinoma ($n = 14$), the overall sensitivity of combined EUS and SRS was 89% and 93%, respectively. It appears that the combination of EUS and SRS may optimize preoperative identification of PNETs and limit the need for more invasive tests such as angiography. Similar to pancreatic adenocarcinoma,[142,143] the early incorporation of EUS into the preoperative localization of PNETs appears to be cost effective, principally by decreasing the need for more invasive tests and their attendant morbidity.[177]

The use of EUS FNA permits tissue confirmation of a suspected primary or metastatic PNET (Figures 15-19 to 15-21). In a retrospective study of 30 patients, Ardengh and colleagues[178] reported a sensitivity, specificity, PPV, NPV, and accuracy of EUS-guided FNA of 82.6%, 85.7%, 95%, 60%,

and 83.3%, respectively, for tumor diagnosis. EUS FNA also appears useful for small tumors. Ginès and colleagues[179] demonstrated a sensitivity of 90% for EUS FNA of 10 patients with FPNETs with a mean tumor size of 12 mm. More recently, Pais and colleagues[180] in a retrospective series of 92 patients showed that the sensitivity of EUS FNA for diagnosis of PNETs was 87%. The sensitivity was similar for FPNETs and NFPNETs but higher for malignant compared to benign tumors. In addition, Atiq and colleagues[181] in a retrospective series of 81 patients showed that EUS FNA has a diagnostic accuracy of 90.1% for detection of PNETs. A recent meta-analysis by Puli and colleagues[182] including 13 studies and 456 patients demonstrated that the pooled sensitivity of EUS for detecting a PNET was 87% and the pooled specificity was 98%. These studies demonstrate that EUS may not only identify but also accurately sample PETs. The recent advent of immunohistochemistry has facilitated the diagnosis of neuroendocrine tumors.[183-186] For example, neuron-specific enolase, synaptophysin, and chromogranin A were found to have sensitivity and specificity exceeding 90%. Such high accuracy makes immunohistochemistry invaluable if adequate tissue is available.

Small tumors identified by CT or EUS are sometimes difficult to localize during surgery. Preoperative EUS-guided injection of India ink may aid intraoperative localization.[187]

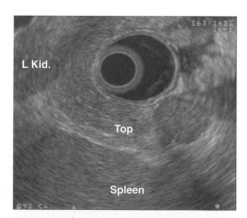

FIGURE 15-18 One subcentimeter hypoechoic pancreatic tail mass in a patient with multiple endocrine neoplasia type 1 (MEN-1). CT of the pancreas demonstrated no masses in the pancreas. L kid., left kidney.

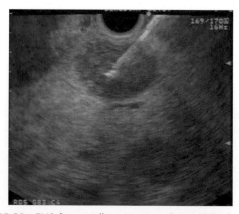

FIGURE 15-20 EUS fine-needle aspiration of one of the hyperechoic masses in the left lobe of the liver in the patient in Figure 15-19.

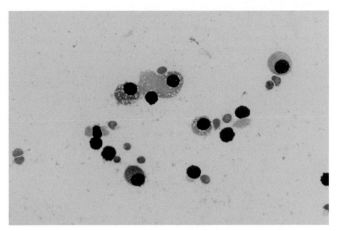

FIGURE 15-21 Cytology from the EUS fine-needle aspiration demonstrating plasmacytoid cells with eccentric nuclei consistent with a metastatic neuroendocrine tumor. Because the patient was without symptoms, this was classified as a nonfunctional pancreatic neuroendocrine tumor with liver metastases.

This information may confirm clinically suspected tumors and aid in the appropriate planning of surgical management. Recently a retrospective series with 30 patients including 10 PNETs showed that EUS-guided tattooing before a laparoscopic distal pancreatic resection is feasible and safe and can assist localization of tumors.[188] The same authors also found that EUS-guided tattooing of pancreatic lesions before laparoscopic distal pancreatectomy decreased operative time as compared with nontattooed patients.[189] Alternatively, EUS-guided fiducial placement may help operative localization of small PETs.[190]

Recently, commercial assays have allowed genetic markers to be reliably assessed on FNA specimens. A recent study of 29 patients with PNETs followed for an average of 33 months showed that the presence of allelic microsatellite loss was associated with increased PNET recurrence, progression, and mortality.[191] Moreover, preoperative determination of Ki-67 expression, an important prognostic factor for grading NFPNETs, is possible in tissue core samples obtained with a 19-G needle. A Ki-67 index obtained with EUS FNA might assist further therapeutic decisions in the management of these tumors.[192]

Intrapancreatic accessory spleen (pancreatic splenosis) is a rare benign condition that can mimic a PNET. In a retrospective series including 2060 patients with pancreatic solid tumors undergoing EUS FNA, pancreatic splenosis was found in 14 (0.6%) patients. Most patients were young asymptomatic males.[193] Common features of an accessory spleen in the pancreas were round, hypoechoic, homogeneous lesions with regular borders and localized most commonly in the tail. The average diameter of these nodules in this series was 2.2 cm. EUS FNA with positive CD8 staining can be helpful to confirm the diagnosis;[194,195] however, the value of this technique in the clinical setting still needs to be determined.

Pancreatic Metastases

Isolated pancreatic masses usually are due to either focal chronic pancreatitis or benign or malignant primary pancreatic tumors. Rarely, secondary involvement of the pancreas by systemic malignancy may occur and has been reported in 2% to 3% of pancreatic resections.[196-198] Accurate identification of isolated pancreatic metastases is clinically important because aggressive surgical resection in selected patients may permit long-term survival.[199-201] In other patients, however, proper diagnosis may avoid unnecessary surgery and permit triage to more appropriate nonoperative therapy.

EUS features of pancreatic metastases appear to be different than those observed in cases of primary pancreatic cancer. In seven patients with metastatic pancreatic lesions, Palazzo and colleagues[202] described homogeneous, round, well-circumscribed lesions in 15 out of 16 masses observed. Compared to patients with primary cancer ($n = 80$), DeWitt and colleagues[203] found that pancreatic metastases ($n = 24$) were more likely to have well-defined than irregular margins. In a report of 11 patients with metastatic renal cell carcinoma (RCC) of the pancreas, Bechade and colleagues[204] found that 10 had well-defined borders. More recently, Hijioka and colleagues[205] demonstrated similar findings in a retrospective study comparing 28 patients with pancreatic metastasis with 60 control patients with pancreatic ductal adenocarcinoma. The absence of main pancreatic duct dilation and the presence of retention cysts were more predictive of pancreatic metastasis than primary malignancy.[205] Therefore EUS visualization of a pancreatic mass with well-defined margins in a patient with a history of malignancy should raise suspicion for a metastatic lesion.

EUS FNA permits an accurate cytologic diagnosis of metastatic lesions to the pancreas (Video 15-1). DeWitt and colleagues[203] reported the use of EUS FNA for the diagnosis of metastasis from primary kidney ($n = 10$), skin ($n = 6$), lung ($n = 4$), colon ($n = 2$), liver ($n = 1$), and stomach ($n = 1$) cancer in 24 patients. Metastasis to the pancreas may occur many years (especially for RCC) after diagnosis of the primary tumor (Figures 15-22 and 15-23). In a recent series of 49 patients, El Hajj and colleagues[206] reported the use of EUS FNA and Tru-Cut biopsy for the diagnosis of metastatic lesions from various primaries, including the kidney, lung, skin, colon, and other organs. EUS FNA had a significant clinical impact in most patients, as it established a diagnosis of recurrent malignancy in 90% after radiographic and/or clinical remission and also enabled initial diagnosis of synchronous or metastatic disease in five patients. Obtaining a detailed medical history of previous malignancy may raise suspicion for this diagnosis. In patients with a remote history of malignancy, obtaining additional cytologic material for cell block and the use of immunocytochemistry may be helpful to confirm the diagnosis of pancreatic metastases and recurrent malignancy.[203]

Video 15-1. EUS fine-needle aspiration of a 2-cm hypoechoic mass in the tail of the pancreas in an asymptomatic patient with history of renal cell carcinoma resected 3 years earlier.

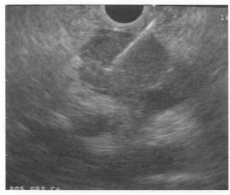

FIGURE 15-22 Linear EUS view (5.0 MHz) demonstrating EUS fine-needle aspiration of a well-defined, hypoechoic 1.5-cm mass in the head of the pancreas in a patient with a remote history of renal cell carcinoma removed 12 years ago.

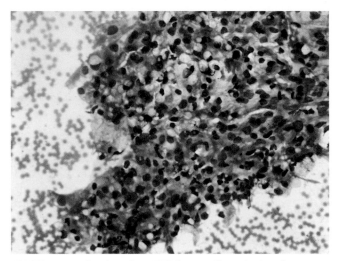

FIGURE 15-23 Cytology from EUS fine-needle aspiration demonstrating clear cells consistent with metastatic, recurrent renal cell carcinoma. These findings were confirmed with surgical resection.

REFERENCES

1. Yasuda K, Mukai H, Fujimoto S, et al. The diagnosis of pancreatic cancer by endoscopic ultrasonography. *Gastrointest Endosc.* 1988; 34:1-8.
2. Lin JT, Wang JT, Wang TH. The diagnostic value of endoscopic ultrasonography in pancreatic disorders. *Taiwan Yi Xue Hui Za Zhi.* 1989; 88:483-487.
3. Rosch T, Lorenz R, Braig C, et al. Endoscopic ultrasound in pancreatic tumor diagnosis. *Gastrointest Endosc.* 1991;37:347-352.
4. Rosch T, Braig C, Gain T, et al. Staging of pancreatic and ampullary carcinoma by endoscopic ultrasonography. Comparison with conventional sonography, computed tomography, and angiography. *Gastroenterology.* 1992;102:188-199.
5. Snady H, Cooperman A, Siegel J. Endoscopic ultrasonography compared with computed tomography with ERCP in patients with obstructive jaundice or small peri-pancreatic mass. *Gastrointest Endosc.* 1992;38:27-34.
6. Palazzo L, Roseau G, Gayet B, et al. Endoscopic ultrasonography in the diagnosis and staging of pancreatic adenocarcinoma. Results of a prospective study with comparison to ultrasonography and CT scan. *Endoscopy.* 1993;25:143-150.
7. Muller MF, Meyenberger C, Bertschinger P, et al. Pancreatic tumors: evaluation with endoscopic US, CT, and MR imaging. *Radiology.* 1994;190:745-751.
8. Marty O, Aubertin JM, Bouillot JL, et al. [Prospective comparison of ultrasound endoscopy and computed tomography in the assessment of locoregional invasiveness of malignant ampullar and pancreatic tumors verified surgically]. *Gastroenterol Clin Biol.* 1995;19:197-203.
9. Melzer E, Avidan B, Heyman Z, et al. Preoperative assessment of blood vessel involvement in patients with pancreatic cancer. *Isr J Med Sci.* 1996;32:1086-1088.
10. Dufour B, Zins M, Vilgrain V, et al. [Comparison between spiral x-ray computed tomography and endosonography in the diagnosis and staging of adenocarcinoma of the pancreas. Clinical preliminary study]. *Gastroenterol Clin Biol.* 1997;21:124-130.
11. Howard TJ, Chin AC, Streib EW, et al. Value of helical computed tomography, angiography, and endoscopic ultrasound in determining resectability of periampullary carcinoma. *Am J Surg.* 1997;174: 237-241.
12. Sugiyama M, Hagi H, Atomi Y, et al. Diagnosis of portal venous invasion by pancreatobiliary carcinoma: value of endoscopic ultrasonography. *Abdom Imaging.* 1997;22:434-438.
13. Legmann P, Vignaux O, Dousset B, et al. Pancreatic tumors: comparison of dual-phase helical CT and endoscopic sonography. *AJR Am J Roentgenol.* 1998;170:1315-1322.
14. Akahoshi K, Chijiiwa Y, Nakano I, et al. Diagnosis and staging of pancreatic cancer by endoscopic ultrasound. *Br J Radiol.* 1998;71: 492-496.
15. Harrison JL, Millikan KW, Prinz RA, et al. Endoscopic ultrasound for diagnosis and staging of pancreatic tumors. *Am Surg.* 1999;65:659-664, discussion 664-655.
16. Gress FG, Hawes RH, Savides TJ, et al. Role of EUS in the preoperative staging of pancreatic cancer: a large single-center experience. *Gastrointest Endosc.* 1999;50:786-791.
17. Midwinter MJ, Beveridge CJ, Wilsdon JB, et al. Correlation between spiral computed tomography, endoscopic ultrasonography and findings at operation in pancreatic and ampullary tumours. *Br J Surg.* 1999; 86:189-193.
18. Mertz HR, Sechopoulos P, Delbeke D, et al. EUS, PET, and CT scanning for evaluation of pancreatic adenocarcinoma. *Gastrointest Endosc.* 2000;52:367-371.
19. Rivadeneira DE, Pochapin M, Grobmyer SR, et al. Comparison of linear array endoscopic ultrasound and helical computed tomography for the staging of periampullary malignancies. *Ann Surg Oncol.* 2003;10: 890-897.
20. Ainsworth AP, Rafaelsen SR, Wamberg PA, et al. Is there a difference in diagnostic accuracy and clinical impact between endoscopic ultrasonography and magnetic resonance cholangiopancreatography? *Endoscopy.* 2003;35:1029-1032.
21. Agarwal B, Abu-Hamda E, Molke KL, et al. Endoscopic ultrasound-guided fine needle aspiration and multidetector spiral CT in the diagnosis of pancreatic cancer. *Am J Gastroenterol.* 2004;99:844-850.
22. DeWitt J, Devereaux B, Chriswell M, et al. Comparison of endoscopic ultrasonography and multidetector computed tomography for detecting and staging pancreatic cancer. *Ann Intern Med.* 2004;141: 753-763.
23. Fisher L, Segarajasingam DS, Stewart C, et al. Endoscopic ultrasound guided fine needle aspiration of solid pancreatic lesions: performance and outcomes. *J Gastroenterol Hepatol.* 2009;24:90-96.
24. Rafique A, Freeman S, Carroll N. A clinical algorithm for the assessment of pancreatic lesions: utilization of 16- and 64-section multidetector CT and endoscopic ultrasound. *Clin Radiol.* 2007;62:1142-1153.
25. Prokesch RW, Schima W, Chow LC, et al. Multidetector CT of pancreatic adenocarcinoma: diagnostic advances and therapeutic relevance. *Eur Radiol.* 2003;13:2147-2154.
26. Wang W, Shpaner A, Krishna SG, et al. Use of EUS-FNA in diagnosing pancreatic neoplasm without a definitive mass on CT. *Gastrointest Endosc.* 2013;doi:10.1016/j.gie.2013.01.040.
27. Bronstein YL, Loyer EM, Kaur H, et al. Detection of small pancreatic tumors with multiphasic helical CT. *AJR Am J Roentgenol.* 2004;182: 619-623.
28. Bhutani MS, Gress FG, Giovannini M, et al. The No Endosonographic Detection of Tumor (NEST) study: a case series of pancreatic cancers missed on endoscopic ultrasonography. *Endoscopy.* 2004;36:385-389.
29. Catanzaro A, Richardson S, Veloso H, et al. Long-term follow-up of patients with clinically indeterminate suspicion of pancreatic cancer and normal EUS. *Gastrointest Endosc.* 2003;58:836-840.
30. Lee SH, Ozden N, Pawa R, et al. Periductal hypoechoic sign: an endosonographic finding associated with pancreatic malignancy. *Gastrointest Endosc.* 2010;71:249-255.

31. Rodriguez S, Faigel D. Absence of a dilated duct predicts benign disease in suspected pancreas cancer: a simple clinical rule. *Dig Dis Sci.* 2010;55:1161-1166.

32. Eloubeidi MA, Luz LP, Tamhane A, et al. Ratio of pancreatic duct caliber to width of pancreatic gland by endosonography is predictive of pancreatic cancer. *Pancreas.* 2013;42:670-679.

33. Canto MI, Goggins M, Yeo CJ, et al. Screening for pancreatic neoplasia in high-risk individuals: an EUS-based approach. *Clin Gastroenterol Hepatol.* 2004;2:606-621.

34. Langer P, Kann PH, Fendrich V, et al. Five years of prospective screening of high-risk individuals from families with familial pancreatic cancer. *Gut.* 2009;58:1410-1418.

35. Poley JW, Kluijt I, Gouma DJ, et al. The yield of first-time endoscopic ultrasonography in screening individuals at a high risk of developing pancreatic cancer. *Am J Gastroenterol.* 2009;104:2175-2181.

36. Zubarik R, Gordon SR, Lidofsky SD, et al. Screening for pancreatic cancer in a high-risk population with serum CA 19-9 and targeted EUS: a feasibility study. *Gastrointest Endosc.* 2011;74:87-95.

37. Canto MI, Hruban RH, Fishman EK, et al. Frequent detection of pancreatic lesions in asymptomatic high-risk individuals. *Gastroenterology.* 2012;142:796-804, quiz e714-795.

38. Canto MI, Harinck F, Hruban RH, et al. International Cancer of the Pancreas Screening (CAPS) Consortium summit on the management of patients with increased risk for familial pancreatic cancer. *Gut.* 2013;62:339-347.

39. Farrell JJ, Garber J, Sahani D, et al. EUS findings in patients with autoimmune pancreatitis. *Gastrointest Endosc.* 2004;60:927-936.

40. Raina A, Yadav D, Krasinskas AM, et al. Evaluation and management of autoimmune pancreatitis: experience at a large US center. *Am J Gastroenterol.* 2009;104:2295-2306.

41. Hoki N, Mizuno N, Sawaki A, et al. Diagnosis of autoimmune pancreatitis using endoscopic ultrasonography. *J Gastroenterol.* 2009;44:154-159.

42. Levy MJ, Reddy RP, Wiersema MJ, et al. EUS-guided trucut biopsy in establishing autoimmune pancreatitis as the cause of obstructive jaundice. *Gastrointest Endosc.* 2005;61:467-472.

43. Iwashita T, Yasuda I, Doi S, et al. Use of samples from endoscopic ultrasound-guided 19-gauge fine-needle aspiration in diagnosis of autoimmune pancreatitis. *Clin Gastroenterol Hepatol.* 2012;10:316-322.

44. Khashab M, Mokadem M, DeWitt J, et al. Endoscopic ultrasound guided fine needle aspiration with or without flow cytometry for the diagnosis of primary pancreatic lymphoma. *Endoscopy* 2010; 42:228-231.

45. Gong TT, Hu DM, Zhu Q. Contrast-enhanced EUS for differential diagnosis of pancreatic mass lesions: a meta-analysis. *Gastrointest Endosc.* 2012;76:301-309.

46. Ophir J, Cespedes I, Ponnekanti H, et al. Elastography: a quantitative method for imaging the elasticity of biological tissues. *Ultrason Imaging.* 1991;13:111-134.

47. Hu DM, Gong TT, Zhu Q. Endoscopic ultrasound elastography for differential diagnosis of pancreatic masses: a meta-analysis. *Dig Dis Sci.* 2013;58:1125-1131.

48. Mei M, Ni J, Liu D, et al. EUS elastography for diagnosis of solid pancreatic masses: a meta-analysis. *Gastrointest Endosc.* 2013;77:578-589.

49. Saftoiu A, Iordache SA, Gheonea DI, et al. Combined contrast-enhanced power Doppler and real-time sonoelastography performed during EUS, used in the differential diagnosis of focal pancreatic masses (with videos). *Gastrointest Endosc.* 2010;72:739-747.

50. Ahmad NA, Lewis JD, Siegelman ES, et al. Role of endoscopic ultrasound and magnetic resonance imaging in the preoperative staging of pancreatic adenocarcinoma. *Am J Gastroenterol.* 2000;95:1926-1931.

51. Buscail L, Pages P, Berthelemy P, et al. Role of EUS in the management of pancreatic and ampullary carcinoma: a prospective study assessing resectability and prognosis. *Gastrointest Endosc.* 1999;50:34-40.

52. Giovannini M, Seitz JF. Endoscopic ultrasonography with a linear-type echoendoscope in the evaluation of 94 patients with pancreatobiliary disease. *Endoscopy.* 1994;26:579-585.

53. Grimm H, Maydeo A, Soehendra N. Endoluminal ultrasound for the diagnosis and staging of pancreatic cancer. *Baillieres Clin Gastroenterol.* 1990;4:869-888.

54. Mukai H, Nakajima M, Yasuda K, et al. [Preoperative diagnosis and staging of pancreatic cancer by endoscopic ultrasonography (EUS)–a comparative study with other diagnostic tools]. *Nippon Shokakibyo Gakkai Zasshi.* 1991;88:2132-2142.

55. Ramsay D, Marshall M, Song S, et al. Identification and staging of pancreatic tumours using computed tomography, endoscopic ultrasound and mangafodipir trisodium-enhanced magnetic resonance imaging. *Australas Radiol.* 2004;48:154-161.

56. Rosch T, Dittler HJ, Lorenz R, et al. [The endosonographic staging of pancreatic carcinoma]. *Dtsch Med Wochenschr.* 1992;117:563-569.

57. Soriano A, Castells A, Ayuso C, et al. Preoperative staging and tumor resectability assessment of pancreatic cancer: prospective study comparing endoscopic ultrasonography, helical computed tomography, magnetic resonance imaging, and angiography. *Am J Gastroenterol.* 2004;99:492-501.

58. Tio TL, Sie LH, Kallimanis G, et al. Staging of ampullary and pancreatic carcinoma: comparison between endosonography and surgery. *Gastrointest Endosc.* 1996;44:706-713.

59. Tio TL, Tytgat GN, Cikot RJ, et al. Ampullopancreatic carcinoma: preoperative TNM classification with endosonography. *Radiology.* 1990;175:455-461.

60. Yasuda K, Mukai H, Nakajima M, et al. Staging of pancreatic carcinoma by endoscopic ultrasonography. *Endoscopy.* 1993;25:151-155.

61. Howard TJ, Villanustre N, Moore SA, et al. Efficacy of venous reconstruction in patients with adenocarcinoma of the pancreatic head. *J Gastrointest Surg.* 2003;7:1089-1095.

62. Al-Haddad M, Martin JK, Nguyen J, et al. Vascular resection and reconstruction for pancreatic malignancy: a single center survival study. *J Gastrointest Surg.* 2007;11:1168-1174.

63. Ahmad NA, Lewis JD, Ginsberg GG, et al. EUS in preoperative staging of pancreatic cancer. *Gastrointest Endosc.* 2000;52:463-468.

64. Bhutani MS, Hawes RH, Hoffman BJ. A comparison of the accuracy of echo features during endoscopic ultrasound (EUS) and EUS-guided fine-needle aspiration for diagnosis of malignant lymph node invasion. *Gastrointest Endosc.* 1997;45:474-479.

65. Catalano MF, Sivak MV Jr, Rice T, et al. Endosonographic features predictive of lymph node metastasis. *Gastrointest Endosc.* 1994;40: 442-446.

66. Nakaizumi A, Uehara H, Iishi H, et al. Endoscopic ultrasonography in diagnosis and staging of pancreatic cancer. *Dig Dis Sci.* 1995;40: 696-700.

67. Cahn M, Chang K, Nguyen P, et al. Impact of endoscopic ultrasound with fine-needle aspiration on the surgical management of pancreatic cancer. *Am J Surg.* 1996;172:470-472.

68. Hahn M, Faigel DO. Frequency of mediastinal lymph node metastases in patients undergoing EUS evaluation of pancreaticobiliary masses. *Gastrointest Endosc.* 2001;54:331-335.

69. Nguyen P, Feng JC, Chang KJ. Endoscopic ultrasound (EUS) and EUS-guided fine-needle aspiration (FNA) of liver lesions. *Gastrointest Endosc.* 1999;50:357-361.

70. tenBerge J, Hoffman BJ, Hawes RH, et al. EUS-guided fine needle aspiration of the liver: indications, yield, and safety based on an international survey of 167 cases. *Gastrointest Endosc.* 2002;55: 859-862.

71. Hollerbach S, Willert J, Topalidis T, et al. Endoscopic ultrasound-guided fine-needle aspiration biopsy of liver lesions: histological and cytological assessment. *Endoscopy.* 2003;35:743-749.

72. DeWitt J, LeBlanc J, McHenry L, et al. Endoscopic ultrasound-guided fine needle aspiration cytology of solid liver lesions: a large single-center experience. *Am J Gastroenterol.* 2003;98:1976-1981.

73. Chang KJ, Albers CG, Nguyen P. Endoscopic ultrasound-guided fine needle aspiration of pleural and ascitic fluid. *Am J Gastroenterol.* 1995;90:148-150.

74. Nguyen PT, Chang KJ. EUS in the detection of ascites and EUS-guided paracentesis. *Gastrointest Endosc.* 2001;54:336-339.

75. DeWitt J, Yu M, Al-Haddad M, et al. Survival in patients with pancreatic cancer following the diagnosis of malignant ascites or liver metastases by EUS-FNA. *Gastrointest Endosc.* 2010;71:260-265.

76. Furukawa H, Kosuge T, Mukai K, et al. Helical computed tomography in the diagnosis of portal vein invasion by pancreatic head carcinoma: usefulness for selecting surgical procedures and predicting the outcome. *Arch Surg.* 1998;133:61-65.

77. Ishikawa O, Ohigashi H, Sasaki Y, et al. Intraoperative cytodiagnosis for detecting a minute invasion of the portal vein during pancreatoduodenectomy for adenocarcinoma of the pancreatic head. *Am J Surg.* 1998;175:477-481.

78. Tierney WM, Francis IR, Eckhauser F, et al. The accuracy of EUS and helical CT in the assessment of vascular invasion by peripapillary malignancy. *Gastrointest Endosc.* 2001;53:182-188.

79. Tellez-Avila FI, Chavez-Tapia NC, Lopez-Arce G, et al. Vascular invasion in pancreatic cancer: predictive values for endoscopic ultrasound and computed tomography imaging. *Pancreas*. 2012;41:636-638.

80. Brugge WR, Lee MJ, Kelsey PB, et al. The use of EUS to diagnose malignant portal venous system invasion by pancreatic cancer. *Gastrointest Endosc*. 1996;43:561-567.

81. Rosch T, Dittler HJ, Strobel K, et al. Endoscopic ultrasound criteria for vascular invasion in the staging of cancer of the head of the pancreas: a blind reevaluation of videotapes. *Gastrointest Endosc*. 2000;52:469-477.

82. Snady H, Bruckner H, Siegel J, et al. Endoscopic ultrasonographic criteria of vascular invasion by potentially resectable pancreatic tumors. *Gastrointest Endosc*. 1994;40:326-333.

83. Benassai G, Mastrorilli M, Quarto G, et al. Factors influencing survival after resection for ductal adenocarcinoma of the head of the pancreas. *J Surg Oncol*. 2000;73:212-218.

84. Richter A, Niedergethmann M, Sturm JW, et al. Long-term results of partial pancreaticoduodenectomy for ductal adenocarcinoma of the pancreatic head: 25-year experience. *World J Surg*. 2003;27:324-329.

85. Saez A, Catala I, Brossa R, et al. Intraoperative fine needle aspiration cytology of pancreatic lesions. A study of 90 cases. *Acta Cytol*. 1995;39:485-488.

86. Schadt ME, Kline TS, Neal HS, et al. Intraoperative pancreatic fine needle aspiration biopsy. Results in 166 patients. *Am Surg*. 1991;57:73-75.

87. Brandt KR, Charboneau JW, Stephens DH, et al. CT- and US-guided biopsy of the pancreas. *Radiology*. 1993;187:99-104.

88. Bret PM, Nicolet V, Labadie M. Percutaneous fine-needle aspiration biopsy of the pancreas. *Diagn Cytopathol*. 1986;2:221-227.

89. Di Stasi M, Lencioni R, Solmi L, et al. Ultrasound-guided fine needle biopsy of pancreatic masses: results of a multicenter study. *Am J Gastroenterol*. 1998;93:1329-1333.

90. Sperti C, Pasquali C, Di Prima F, et al. Percutaneous CT-guided fine needle aspiration cytology in the differential diagnosis of pancreatic lesions. *Ital J Gastroenterol*. 1994;26:126-131.

91. Caturelli E, Rapaccini GL, Anti M, et al. Malignant seeding after fine-needle aspiration biopsy of the pancreas. *Diagn Imaging Clin Med*. 1985;54:88-91.

92. Ferrucci JT, Wittenberg J, Margolies MN, et al. Malignant seeding of the tract after thin-needle aspiration biopsy. *Radiology*. 1979;130:345-346.

93. Smith FP, Macdonald JS, Schein PS, et al. Cutaneous seeding of pancreatic cancer by skinny-needle aspiration biopsy. *Arch Intern Med*. 1980;140:855.

94. Vilmann P, Jacobsen GK, Henriksen FW, et al. Endoscopic ultrasonography with guided fine needle aspiration biopsy in pancreatic disease. *Gastrointest Endosc*. 1992;38:172-173.

95. Hewitt MJ, McPhail MJ, Possamai L, et al. EUS-guided FNA for diagnosis of solid pancreatic neoplasms: a meta-analysis. *Gastrointest Endosc*. 2012;75:319-331.

96. Hebert-Magee S, Bae S, Varadarajulu S, et al. The presence of a cytopathologist increases the diagnostic accuracy of endoscopic ultrasound-guided fine needle aspiration cytology for pancreatic adenocarcinoma: a meta-analysis. *Cytopathology*. 2013;24:159-171.

97. Gress F, Gottlieb K, Sherman S, et al. Endoscopic ultrasonography-guided fine-needle aspiration biopsy of suspected pancreatic cancer. *Ann Intern Med*. 2001;134:459-464.

98. Harewood GC, Wiersema MJ. Endosonography-guided fine needle aspiration biopsy in the evaluation of pancreatic masses. *Am J Gastroenterol*. 2002;97:1386-1391.

99. Voss M, Hammel P, Molas G, et al. Value of endoscopic ultrasound guided fine needle aspiration biopsy in the diagnosis of solid pancreatic masses. *Gut*. 2000;46:244-249.

100. Bhutani MS, Hawes RH, Baron PL, et al. Endoscopic ultrasound guided fine needle aspiration of malignant pancreatic lesions. *Endoscopy*. 1997;29:854-858.

101. Faigel DO, Ginsberg GG, Bentz JS, et al. Endoscopic ultrasound-guided real-time fine-needle aspiration biopsy of the pancreas in cancer patients with pancreatic lesions. *J Clin Oncol*. 1997;15:1439-1443.

102. Wegener M, Pfaffenbach B, Adamek RJ. Endosonographically guided transduodenal and transgastral fine-needle aspiration puncture of focal pancreatic lesions. *Bildgebung*. 1995;62:110-115.

103. Fritscher-Ravens A, Schirrow L, Atay Z, et al. [Endosonographically controlled fine needle aspiration cytology–indications and results in routine diagnosis]. *Z Gastroenterol*. 1999;37:343-351.

104. Ylagan LR, Edmundowicz S, Kasal K, et al. Endoscopic ultrasound guided fine-needle aspiration cytology of pancreatic carcinoma: a 3-year experience and review of the literature. *Cancer*. 2002;96:362-369.

105. Eloubeidi MA, Chen VK, Eltoum IA, et al. Endoscopic ultrasound-guided fine needle aspiration biopsy of patients with suspected pancreatic cancer: diagnostic accuracy and acute and 30-day complications. *Am J Gastroenterol*. 2003;98:2663-2668.

106. Fritscher-Ravens A, Brand L, Knofel WT, et al. Comparison of endoscopic ultrasound-guided fine needle aspiration for focal pancreatic lesions in patients with normal parenchyma and chronic pancreatitis. *Am J Gastroenterol*. 2002;97:2768-2775.

107. Schwartz DA, Unni KK, Levy MJ, et al. The rate of false-positive results with EUS-guided fine-needle aspiration. *Gastrointest Endosc*. 2002;56:868-872.

108. Siddiqui AA, Kowalski TE, Shahid H, et al. False-positive EUS-guided FNA cytology for solid pancreatic lesions. *Gastrointest Endosc*. 2011;74:535-540.

109. Mertz H, Gautam S. The learning curve for EUS-guided FNA of pancreatic cancer. *Gastrointest Endosc*. 2004;59:33-37.

110. Harewood GC, Wiersema LM, Halling AC, et al. Influence of EUS training and pathology interpretation on accuracy of EUS-guided fine needle aspiration of pancreatic masses. *Gastrointest Endosc*. 2002;55:669-673.

111. Eisen GM, Dominitz JA, Faigel DO, et al. Guidelines for credentialing and granting privileges for endoscopic ultrasound. *Gastrointest Endosc*. 2001;54:811-814.

112. Committee AT, DiMaio CJ, Mishra G, et al. EUS core curriculum. *Gastrointest Endosc*. 2012;76:476-481.

113. Eloubeidi MA, Tamhane A, Jhala N, et al. Agreement between rapid onsite and final cytologic interpretations of EUS-guided FNA specimens: implications for the endosonographer and patient management. *Am J Gastroenterol*. 2006;101:2841-2847.

114. Klapman JB, Logrono R, Dye CE, et al. Clinical impact of on-site cytopathology interpretation on endoscopic ultrasound-guided fine needle aspiration. *Am J Gastroenterol*. 2003;98:1289-1294.

115. Schmidt RL, Witt BL, Matynia AP, et al. Rapid on-site evaluation increases endoscopic ultrasound-guided fine-needle aspiration adequacy for pancreatic lesions. *Dig Dis Sci*. 2013;58:872-882.

116. Erickson RA, Sayage-Rabie L, Beissner RS. Factors predicting the number of EUS-guided fine-needle passes for diagnosis of pancreatic malignancies. *Gastrointest Endosc*. 2000;51:184-190.

117. LeBlanc JK, Ciaccia D, Al-Assi MT, et al. Optimal number of EUS-guided fine needle passes needed to obtain a correct diagnosis. *Gastrointest Endosc*. 2004;59:475-481.

118. Bang JY, Magee SH, Ramesh J, et al. Randomized trial comparing fanning with standard technique for endoscopic ultrasound-guided fine-needle aspiration of solid pancreatic mass lesions. *Endoscopy*. 2013;45:445-450.

119. Buxbaum JL, Eloubeidi MA, Lane CJ, et al. Dynamic telecytology compares favorably to rapid onsite evaluation of endoscopic ultrasound fine needle aspirates. *Dig Dis Sci*. 2012;57:3092-3097.

120. Goyal A, Jhala N, Gupta P. TeleCyP (Telecytopathology): real-time fine-needle aspiration interpretation. *Acta Cytol*. 2012;56:669-677.

121. Khurana KK, Rong R, Wang D, et al. Dynamic telecytopathology for on-site preliminary diagnosis of endoscopic ultrasound-guided fine needle aspiration of pancreatic masses. *J Telemed Telecare*. 2012;18:253-259.

122. Olson MT, Ali SZ. Cytotechnologist on-site evaluation of pancreas fine needle aspiration adequacy: comparison with cytopathologists and correlation with the final interpretation. *Acta Cytol*. 2012;56:340-346.

123. Lee JH, Stewart J, Ross WA, et al. Blinded prospective comparison of the performance of 22-gauge and 25-gauge needles in endoscopic ultrasound-guided fine needle aspiration of the pancreas and peripancreatic lesions. *Dig Dis Sci*. 2009;54:2274-2281.

124. Siddiqui UD, Rossi F, Rosenthal LS, et al. EUS-guided FNA of solid pancreatic masses: a prospective, randomized trial comparing 22-gauge and 25-gauge needles. *Gastrointest Endosc*. 2009;70:1093-1097.

125. Madhoun MF, Wani SB, Rastogi A, et al. The diagnostic accuracy of 22-gauge and 25-gauge needles in endoscopic ultrasound-guided fine needle aspiration of solid pancreatic lesions: a meta-analysis. *Endoscopy*. 2013;45:86-92.

126. Affolter KE, Schmidt RL, Matynia AP, et al. Needle size has only a limited effect on outcomes in EUS-guided fine needle aspiration: a systematic review and meta-analysis. *Dig Dis Sci*. 2013;58:1026-1034.

127. Camellini L, Carlinfante G, Azzolini F, et al. A randomized clinical trial comparing 22G and 25G needles in endoscopic ultrasound-guided fine-needle aspiration of solid lesions. *Endoscopy*. 2011;43:709-715.
128. Sakamoto H, Kitano M, Komaki T, et al. Prospective comparative study of the EUS guided 25-gauge FNA needle with the 19-gauge Trucut needle and 22-gauge FNA needle in patients with solid pancreatic masses. *J Gastroenterol Hepatol*. 2009;24:384-390.
129. Varadarajulu S, Bang JY, Hebert-Magee S. Assessment of the technical performance of the flexible 19-gauge EUS-FNA needle. *Gastrointest Endosc*. 2012;76:336-343.
130. Gress FG, Hawes RH, Savides TJ, et al. Endoscopic ultrasound-guided fine-needle aspiration biopsy using linear array and radial scanning endosonography. *Gastrointest Endosc*. 1997;45:243-250.
131. Wiersema MJ, Vilmann P, Giovannini M, et al. Endosonography-guided fine-needle aspiration biopsy: diagnostic accuracy and complication assessment. *Gastroenterology*. 1997;112:1087-1095.
132. Al-Haddad M, Wallace MB, Woodward TA, et al. The safety of fine-needle aspiration guided by endoscopic ultrasound: a prospective study. *Endoscopy*. 2008;40:204-208.
133. Gress F, Michael H, Gelrud D, et al. EUS-guided fine-needle aspiration of the pancreas: evaluation of pancreatitis as a complication. *Gastrointest Endosc*. 2002;56:864-867.
134. O'Toole D, Palazzo L, Arotcarena R, et al. Assessment of complications of EUS-guided fine-needle aspiration. *Gastrointest Endosc*. 2001;53:470-474.
135. Wang KX, Ben QW, Jin ZD, et al. Assessment of morbidity and mortality associated with EUS-guided FNA: a systematic review. *Gastrointest Endosc*. 2011;73:283-290.
136. Micames C, Jowell PS, White R, et al. Lower frequency of peritoneal carcinomatosis in patients with pancreatic cancer diagnosed by EUS-guided FNA vs. percutaneous FNA. *Gastrointest Endosc*. 2003;58:690-695.
137. Ikezawa K, Uehara H, Sakai A, et al. Risk of peritoneal carcinomatosis by endoscopic ultrasound-guided fine needle aspiration for pancreatic cancer. *J Gastroenterol*. 2012;doi:10.1007/s00535-012-0693-x.
138. Beane JD, House MG, Cote GA, et al. Outcomes after preoperative endoscopic ultrasonography and biopsy in patients undergoing distal pancreatectomy. *Surgery*. 2011;150:844-853.
139. Ngamruengphong S, Xu C, Woodward TA, et al. Risk of gastric or peritoneal recurrence, and long-term outcomes, following pancreatic cancer resection with preoperative endosonographically guided fine needle aspiration. *Endoscopy*. 2013;45:619-626.
140. Qian X, Hecht JL. Pancreatic fine needle aspiration. A comparison of computed tomographic and endoscopic ultrasonographic guidance. *Acta Cytol*. 2003;47:723-726.
141. Mallery JS, Centeno BA, Hahn PF, et al. Pancreatic tissue sampling guided by EUS, CT/US, and surgery: a comparison of sensitivity and specificity. *Gastrointest Endosc*. 2002;56:218-224.
142. Harewood GC, Wiersema MJ. A cost analysis of endoscopic ultrasound in the evaluation of pancreatic head adenocarcinoma. *Am J Gastroenterol*. 2001;96:2651-2656.
143. Chen VK, Arguedas MR, Kilgore ML, et al. A cost-minimization analysis of alternative strategies in diagnosing pancreatic cancer. *Am J Gastroenterol*. 2004;99:2223-2234.
144. Levy MJ, Jondal ML, Clain J, et al. Preliminary experience with an EUS-guided trucut biopsy needle compared with EUS-guided FNA. *Gastrointest Endosc*. 2003;57:101-106.
145. Larghi A, Verna EC, Stavropoulos SN, et al. EUS-guided trucut needle biopsies in patients with solid pancreatic masses: a prospective study. *Gastrointest Endosc*. 2004;59:185-190.
146. Varadarajulu S, Fraig M, Schmulewitz N, et al. Comparison of EUS-guided 19-gauge Trucut needle biopsy with EUS-guided fine-needle aspiration. *Endoscopy*. 2004;36:397-401.
147. Thomas T, Kaye PV, Ragunath K, et al. Efficacy, safety, and predictive factors for a positive yield of EUS-guided Trucut biopsy: a large tertiary referral center experience. *Am J Gastroenterol*. 2009;104:584-591.
148. Eloubeidi MA, Mehra M, Bean SM. EUS-guided 19-gauge trucut needle biopsy for diagnosis of lymphoma missed by EUS-guided FNA. *Gastrointest Endosc*. 2007;65:937-939.
149. Iglesias-Garcia J, Poley JW, Larghi A, et al. Feasibility and yield of a new EUS histology needle: results from a multicenter, pooled, cohort study. *Gastrointest Endosc*. 2011;73:1189-1196.
150. Larghi A, Iglesias-Garcia J, Poley JW, et al. Feasibility and yield of a novel 22-gauge histology EUS needle in patients with pancreatic masses: a multicenter prospective cohort study. *Surg Endosc*. 2013; doi:10.1007/s00464-013-2957-9.
151. Bang JY, Hebert-Magee S, Trevino J, et al. Randomized trial comparing the 22-gauge aspiration and 22-gauge biopsy needles for EUS-guided sampling of solid pancreatic mass lesions. *Gastrointest Endosc*. 2012; 76:321-327.
152. Ogura T, Yamao K, Sawaki A, et al. Clinical impact of K-ras mutation analysis in EUS-guided FNA specimens from pancreatic masses. *Gastrointest Endosc*. 2012;75:769-774.
153. Fuccio L, Hassan C, Laterza L, et al. The role of K-ras gene mutation analysis in EUS-guided FNA cytology specimens for the differential diagnosis of pancreatic solid masses: a meta-analysis of prospective studies. *Gastrointest Endosc*. 2013;doi:10.1016/j.gie.2013.04.162.
154. Salek C, Benesova L, Zavoral M, et al. Evaluation of clinical relevance of examining K-ras, p16 and p53 mutations along with allelic losses at 9p and 18q in EUS-guided fine needle aspiration samples of patients with chronic pancreatitis and pancreatic cancer. *World J Gastroenterol*. 2007;13:3714-3720.
155. Jensen RT, Norton JA. Pancreatic endocrine tumors. In: Feldman M, Scharschmidt BF, Sleisenger MH, eds. *Sleisenger and Fordtran's Gastrointestinal and Liver Disease*. 7th ed. Philadelphia: WB Saunders; 2002: 988–1016 2002, DOI.
156. Modlin IM, Tang LH. Approaches to the diagnosis of gut neuroendocrine tumors: the last word (today). *Gastroenterology*. 1997;112: 583-590.
157. Madura JA, Cummings OW, Wiebke EA, et al. Nonfunctioning islet cell tumors of the pancreas: a difficult diagnosis but one worth the effort. *Am Surg*. 1997;63:573-577, discussion 577-578.
158. Lam KY, Lo CY. Pancreatic endocrine tumour: a 22-year clinico-pathological experience with morphological, immunohistochemical observation and a review of the literature. *Eur J Surg Oncol*. 1997; 23:36-42.
159. Kloppel G, Heitz PU. Pancreatic endocrine tumors. *Pathol Res Pract*. 1988;183:155-168.
160. Schindl M, Kaczirek K, Kaserer K, et al. Is the new classification of neuroendocrine pancreatic tumors of clinical help? *World J Surg*. 2000;24:1312-1318.
161. Akerstrom G, Hellman P, Hessman O, et al. Surgical treatment of endocrine pancreatic tumours. *Neuroendocrinology*. 2004;80(suppl 1): 62-66.
162. Azimuddin K, Chamberlain RS. The surgical management of pancreatic neuroendocrine tumors. *Surg Clin North Am*. 2001;81:511-525.
163. Rosch T, Lightdale CJ, Botet JF, et al. Localization of pancreatic endocrine tumors by endoscopic ultrasonography. *N Engl J Med*. 1992;326:1721-1726.
164. Palazzo L, Roseau G, Chaussade S, et al. [Pancreatic endocrine tumors: contribution of ultrasound endoscopy in the diagnosis of localization]. *Ann Chir*. 1993;47:419-424.
165. Anderson MA, Carpenter S, Thompson NW, et al. Endoscopic ultrasound is highly accurate and directs management in patients with neuroendocrine tumors of the pancreas. *Am J Gastroenterol*. 2000; 95:2271-2277.
166. Ardengh JC, Rosenbaum P, Ganc AJ, et al. Role of EUS in the preoperative localization of insulinomas compared with spiral CT. *Gastrointest Endosc*. 2000;51:552-555.
167. De Angelis C, Carucci P, Repici A, et al. Endosonography in decision making and management of gastrointestinal endocrine tumors. *Eur J Ultrasound*. 1999;10:139-150.
168. Gouya H, Vignaux O, Augui J, et al. CT, endoscopic sonography, and a combined protocol for preoperative evaluation of pancreatic insulinomas. *AJR Am J Roentgenol*. 2003;181:987-992.
169. Proye C, Malvaux P, Pattou F, et al. Noninvasive imaging of insulinomas and gastrinomas with endoscopic ultrasonography and somatostatin receptor scintigraphy. *Surgery*. 1998;124:1134-1143, discussion 1143-1134.
170. Zimmer T, Stolzel U, Bader M, et al. Endoscopic ultrasonography and somatostatin receptor scintigraphy in the preoperative localisation of insulinomas and gastrinomas. *Gut*. 1996;39:562-568.
171. Khashab MA, Yong E, Lennon AM, et al. EUS is still superior to multidetector computerized tomography for detection of pancreatic neuroendocrine tumors. *Gastrointest Endosc*. 2011;73:691-696.
172. Semelka RC, Custodio CM, Cem Balci N, et al. Neuroendocrine tumors of the pancreas: spectrum of appearances on MRI. *J Magn Reson Imaging*. 2000;11:141-148.

173. Van Nieuwenhove Y, Vandaele S, Op de Beeck B, et al. Neuroendocrine tumors of the pancreas. *Surg Endosc*. 2003;17:1658-1662.

174. Thoeni RF, Mueller-Lisse UG, Chan R, et al. Detection of small, functional islet cell tumors in the pancreas: selection of MR imaging sequences for optimal sensitivity. *Radiology*. 2000;214:483-490.

175. Gibril F, Reynolds JC, Doppman JL, et al. Somatostatin receptor scintigraphy: its sensitivity compared with that of other imaging methods in detecting primary and metastatic gastrinomas. A prospective study. *Ann Intern Med*. 1996;125:26-34.

176. van Eijck CH, Lamberts SW, Lemaire LC, et al. The use of somatostatin receptor scintigraphy in the differential diagnosis of pancreatic duct cancers and islet cell tumors. *Ann Surg*. 1996;224:119-124.

177. Bansal R, Tierney W, Carpenter S, et al. Cost effectiveness of EUS for preoperative localization of pancreatic endocrine tumors. *Gastrointest Endosc*. 1999;49:19-25.

178. Ardengh JC, de Paulo GA, Ferrari AP. EUS-guided FNA in the diagnosis of pancreatic neuroendocrine tumors before surgery. *Gastrointest Endosc*. 2004;60:378-384.

179. Gines A, Vazquez-Sequeiros E, Soria MT, et al. Usefulness of EUS-guided fine needle aspiration (EUS-FNA) in the diagnosis of functioning neuroendocrine tumors. *Gastrointest Endosc*. 2002;56:291-296.

180. Pais SA, Al-Haddad M, Mohamadnejad M, et al. EUS for pancreatic neuroendocrine tumors: a single-center, 11-year experience. *Gastrointest Endosc*. 2010;71:1185-1193.

181. Atiq M, Bhutani MS, Bektas M, et al. EUS-FNA for pancreatic neuroendocrine tumors: a tertiary cancer center experience. *Dig Dis Sci*. 2012;57:791-800.

182. Puli SR, Kalva N, Bechtold ML, et al. Diagnostic accuracy of endoscopic ultrasound in pancreatic neuroendocrine tumors: a systematic review and meta analysis. *World J Gastroenterol*. 2013;19:3678-3684.

183. Baker MS, Knuth JL, DeWitt J, et al. Pancreatic cystic neuroendocrine tumors: preoperative diagnosis with endoscopic ultrasound and fine-needle immunocytology. *J Gastrointest Surg*. 2008;12:450-456.

184. Chang F, Vu C, Chandra A, et al. Endoscopic ultrasound-guided fine needle aspiration cytology of pancreatic neuroendocrine tumours: cytomorphological and immunocytochemical evaluation. *Cytopathology*. 2006;17:10-17.

185. Collins BT, Cramer HM. Fine-needle aspiration cytology of islet cell tumors. *Diagn Cytopathol*. 1996;15:37-45.

186. Kidd M, Modlin IM, Mane SM, et al. Q RT-PCR detection of chromogranin A: a new standard in the identification of neuroendocrine tumor disease. *Ann Surg*. 2006;243:273-280.

187. Zografos GN, Stathopoulou A, Mitropapas G, et al. Preoperative imaging and localization of small sized insulinoma with EUS-guided fine needle tattoing: a case report. *Hormones (Athens)*. 2005;4:111-116.

188. Lennon AM, Newman N, Makary MA, et al. EUS-guided tattooing before laparoscopic distal pancreatic resection (with video). *Gastrointest Endosc*. 2010;72:1089-1094.

189. Newman NA, Lennon AM, Edil BH, et al. Preoperative endoscopic tattooing of pancreatic body and tail lesions decreases operative time for laparoscopic distal pancreatectomy. *Surgery*. 2010;148:371-377.

190. Law JK, Singh VK, Khashab MA, et al. Endoscopic ultrasound (EUS)-guided fiducial placement allows localization of small neuroendocrine tumors during parenchymal-sparing pancreatic surgery. *Surg Endosc*. 2013;doi:10.1007/s00464-013-2975-7.

191. Fasanella KE, McGrath KM, Sanders M, et al. Pancreatic endocrine tumor EUS-guided FNA DNA microsatellite loss and mortality. *Gastrointest Endosc*. 2009;69:1074-1080.

192. Larghi A, Capurso G, Carnuccio A, et al. Ki-67 grading of nonfunctioning pancreatic neuroendocrine tumors on histologic samples obtained by EUS-guided fine-needle tissue acquisition: a prospective study. *Gastrointest Endosc*. 2012;76:570-577.

193. Ardengh JC, Lopes CV, Kemp R, et al. Pancreatic splenosis mimicking neuroendocrine tumors: microhistological diagnosis by endoscopic ultrasound guided fine needle aspiration. *Arq Gastroenterol*. 2013;50:10-14.

194. Tatsas AD, Owens CL, Siddiqui MT, et al. Fine-needle aspiration of intrapancreatic accessory spleen: cytomorphologic features and differential diagnosis. *Cancer Cytopathol*. 2012;120:261-268.

195. Schreiner AM, Mansoor A, Faigel DO, et al. Intrapancreatic accessory spleen: mimic of pancreatic endocrine tumor diagnosed by endoscopic ultrasound-guided fine-needle aspiration biopsy. *Diagn Cytopathol*. 2008;36:262-265.

196. Roland CF, van Heerden JA. Nonpancreatic primary tumors with metastasis to the pancreas. *Surg Gynecol Obstet*. 1989;168:345-347.

197. Nakeeb A, Lillemoe KD, Cameron JL. The role of pancreaticoduodenectomy for locally recurrent or metastatic carcinoma to the periampullary region. *J Am Coll Surg*. 1995;180:188-192.

198. Sperti C, Pasquali C, Liessi G, et al. Pancreatic resection for metastatic tumors to the pancreas. *J Surg Oncol*. 2003;83:161-166, discussion 166.

199. Z'Graggen K, Fernandez-del Castillo C, Rattner DW, et al. Metastases to the pancreas and their surgical extirpation. *Arch Surg*. 1998;133:413-417, discussion 418-419.

200. Ghavamian R, Klein KA, Stephens DH, et al. Renal cell carcinoma metastatic to the pancreas: clinical and radiological features. *Mayo Clin Proc*. 2000;75:581-585.

201. Faure JP, Tuech JJ, Richer JP, et al. Pancreatic metastasis of renal cell carcinoma: presentation, treatment and survival. *J Urol*. 2001;165:20-22.

202. Palazzo L, Borotto E, Cellier C, et al. Endosonographic features of pancreatic metastases. *Gastrointest Endosc*. 1996;44:433-436.

203. DeWitt J, Jowell P, Leblanc J, et al. EUS-guided FNA of pancreatic metastases: a multicenter experience. *Gastrointest Endosc*. 2005;61:689-696.

204. Bechade D, Palazzo L, Fabre M, et al. EUS-guided FNA of pancreatic metastasis from renal cell carcinoma. *Gastrointest Endosc*. 2003;58:784-788.

205. Hijioka S, Matsuo K, Mizuno N, et al. Role of endoscopic ultrasound and endoscopic ultrasound-guided fine-needle aspiration in diagnosing metastasis to the pancreas: a tertiary center experience. *Pancreatology*. 2011;11:390-398.

206. El H II, LeBlanc JK, Sherman S, et al. Endoscopic ultrasound-guided biopsy of pancreatic metastases: a large single-center experience. *Pancreas*. 2013;42:524-530.

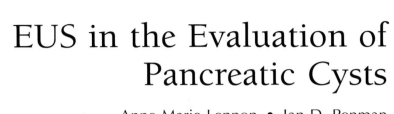

16

EUS in the Evaluation of Pancreatic Cysts

Anne Marie Lennon • Ian D. Penman

Key Points

- The differential diagnosis of pancreatic cystic lesions is wide: the majority of these lesions are benign but detection of mucinous neoplasms (IPMN and MCN) is important because these cysts may be malignant or have malignant potential.
- The diagnostic accuracy of EUS based on morphology alone is limited.
- A combination of EUS features, fluid cytology, carcinoembryonic level, and mucin staining is used to differentiate pancreatic cysts.
- FNA of cystic lesions under antibiotic cover is safe, with low rates of bleeding, infection, and pancreatitis.
- Accurate diagnosis and management of pancreatic cystic lesions require careful evaluation of the clinical setting, other imaging modalities, and multidisciplinary collaboration.

Pancreatic cysts, once thought to be rare, are now detected more frequently as a result of the increased use of high-resolution imaging. Between 2% and 13% of patients undergoing computed tomography (CT)[1] or magnetic resonance imaging (MRI),[2] with no symptoms or history of pancreatic disease, are found to have pancreatic cysts. These lesions represent a broad spectrum of pathologic changes from simple cysts to premalignant and malignant cysts. Pancreatic cysts thus represent an important and increasing disease burden and pose a difficult diagnostic and management problem: how to accurately predict which lesions contain malignancy and require resection versus those that can be followed safely by interval imaging or require no further follow-up.

Despite advances in CT and MRI, the ability of cross-sectional modalities to identify the exact nature of a cyst remains limited. Endoscopic ultrasonography (EUS) is ideally suited to imaging pancreatic lesions because of its high resolution and ability to sample cystic lesions. This chapter discusses the different types of pancreatic cysts, their endosonographic features, and the role of fine-needle aspiration (FNA) for cytologic and tumor marker analysis. A diagnostic approach to patients with pancreatic cysts is also described.

Types of Pancreatic Cysts

The large number of different types of pancreatic cysts include cysts with no or very low malignant potential, those that clearly have the ability to become malignant, and cysts that harbor malignancy (Table 16-1). Pseudocysts are the most common type of pancreatic cyst; however, they account for less than 10% of resected pancreatic cysts. In modern surgical series, the most commonly resected pancreatic cysts are intraductal papillary mucinous neoplasms (IPMN), mucinous cystic neoplasms (MCN), and serous cystadenomas (SCA), which account for 50%, 16%, and 12% of resected cysts, respectively.[3] Solid neoplasms can also undergo cystic degeneration, with pancreatic cystic neuroendocrine tumors, solid pseudopapillary neoplasms (SPN), and cystic pancreatic ductal adenocarcinoma accounting for between 1% and 9% of resected cysts. The clinical presentation, endoscopic features and management of these cysts are discussed later in the chapter.

Diagnostic Approach
Clinical History and Imaging

Acquiring a good clinical history is important. Key questions include: Is there is a history of pancreatitis, jaundice, or recent onset of diabetes? Is there any type of pancreatic abdominal or back pain, anorexia, or weight loss? The presence of any of these features is worrisome for malignant change, and these patients should undergo a careful EUS and be followed closely. Is there a personal or family history of related cancers to suggest multiple endocrine neoplasia type 1, Von Hippel-Lindau syndrome, or any history to suggest an increased risk of pancreatic adenocarcinoma (hereditary nonpolyposis colorectal cancer, Peutz-Jeghers syndrome, BRCA1, BRCA2, familial atypical multiple mole

TABLE 16-1

CLASSIFICATION OF PANCREATIC CYSTS

No or Very Low Malignant Potential	Malignant Potential	Malignant
Pseudocyst	Intraductal papillary mucinous neoplasm	Pancreatic ductal adenocarcinoma
Lymphoepithelial cyst	Mucinous cystic neoplasm	Neuroendocrine tumor
Retention cyst		Solid pseudopapillary neoplasm
Congenital cyst		Pancreatoblastoma
Lymphangioma		Acinar cystadenocarcinoma
Serous cystadenoma		

melanoma)?[4] Does the patient have any risk factors for pancreatitis such as alcohol use?

Most patients have already undergone cross-sectional imaging before they are referred for EUS, but if not, an MRI or pancreatic protocol CT scan is helpful. From the clinical history and cross-sectional imaging, a diagnosis may be apparent. It may also be clear that the patient requires surgical resection. When the diagnosis is not clear, when the patients have worrisome symptoms or features, or if surgery is believed to pose a high risk (e.g., a lesion in the pancreatic head in an older patient of borderline fitness status), EUS is indicated. A pragmatic algorithm for the differential diagnosis and management of pancreatic cysts is shown in Figure 16-1.

Endoscopic Ultrasound

The EUS approach to examining the pancreas and FNA techniques are described in Chapter 21. The general EUS approach to pancreatic cysts is described in this section; the appearances of specific cysts are described later.

When a cystic lesion has been identified, the size, exact location, relation to adjacent vessels and organs, and presence of locoregional or distant metastases should be noted because this information may influence management (Table 16-2). If the lesion is clearly a pseudocyst, it is assessed for the need and suitability for EUS-guided drainage. The cyst itself should be examined to determine the wall thickness, the presence of a mural nodule, or associated mass (see Examination Checklist). The size of the individual cysts (microcystic, macrocystic [>1 cm], or mixed macro- and microcystic), the presence and thickness of any septations (Figure 16-2), and the presence of echo-dense mucus or debris within the cyst should be documented. The size of the main pancreatic duct, whether it communicates with the cyst, the presence of mucin or a mural nodule within the pancreatic duct, or any focal dilation should be noted.

There are several features on EUS that are worrisome for malignant transformation of the cyst. These include the presence of a thick wall or septum, an associated solid mass, or a mural nodule (Figure 16-3). The presence of focal dilation of the main pancreatic duct, a pancreatic duct measuring

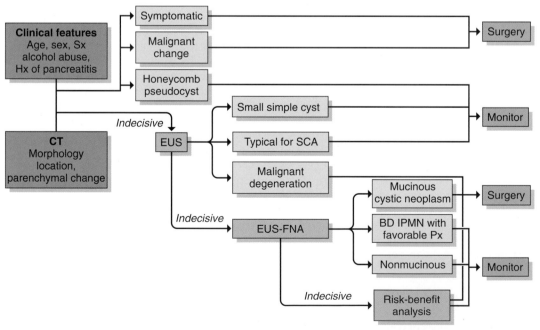

FIGURE 16-1 EUS-based algorithmic approach to the management of pancreatic cystic lesions. BD, branch duct; CT, computed tomography; FNA, fine-needle aspiration; Hx, history; IPMN, intraductal papillary mucinous neoplasia; Px, prognosis; SCA, serous cystadenoma; Sx, symptoms. *(From OH HC, Kim MH, Hwang CY, et al. Cystic lesions of the pancreas: challenging issues in clinical practice. AM J Gastroenterol. 2008;103: 229-239.)*

TABLE 16-2

FEATURES OF CYSTIC PANCREATIC LESIONS

	SCA	MCN	IPMN	SPN	Pseudocyst
Location	Anywhere	Body/tail	Arise from main PD or side branch; head > body/tail	Anywhere	Anywhere
Malignant potential	Very low	Moderate	Moderate High when main PD involved	Moderate	None
EUS features	Multiple small cysts; often microcystic "honeycomb"; central fibrosis or calcification Macrocystic and solid variants also possible	Macrocystic; septations; nodularity or papillary projections	Dilated main PD or dilated side branch. Can have mural nodule or mass	Mixed solid cystic	Unilocular, variable size and wall thickness; echogenic material; features of acute/chronic pancreatitis
Communication with PD	No	Rare	Yes	No	Sometimes
Cytology	Bland glycogen-positive cuboidal cells	Columnar/cuboidal, mucin-positive cells; may show atypia, dysplasia, or malignant features	Columnar/cuboidal mucin-positive cells; may show atypia, dysplasia, or malignant features	Heterogeneous; eosinophilic, papillary cells, PAS-positive deposits, vimentin positivity	Macrophages, inflammatory cells, debris
Cyst fluid	Low viscosity	High viscosity	High viscosity	Low viscosity, bloody and necrotic	Low viscosity, may be blood stained or turbid
Amylase	Low	Variable	Variable	Variable	High
CEA	Low	Usually high	Usually high	Unknown	Low

CEA, carcinoembryonic antigen; IPMN, intraductal papillary mucinous neoplasia; MCN, mucinous cystic neoplasm; PAS, periodic acid–Schiff stain; PD, pancreatic duct; SCA, serous cystadenoma; SPN, solid pseudopapillary neoplasm.

≥10 mm, or a main pancreatic duct measuring between 5 and 9 mm with a mural nodule are concerning and are associated with an increased risk of malignant transformation. One of the EUS features that is most difficult to differentiate in predicting malignant potential is a mural nodule versus a "mucin ball." Several observations can help in differentiating these two lesions (Figure 16-4). Mucin often has a round, well-demarcated outer edge and a hyperechoic edge with hypoechoic center. The presence of all three features is shown to be associated with mucin in 90% of cases in one study (Video 16-1).[5] The existence of vessels is suggestive of a mural nodule and can sometimes be seen with Doppler ultrasound. In addition, mucin can be shown to move within the cyst either by moving the patient's position or by targeting the lesion during EUS FNA, which is then shown to move with the needle (Video 16-1). One group has classified mural nodules into four types: type I, 1- to 2-mm fine, papillary protrusions; type II, a larger polypoid nodule; type III, a larger, protruding component with thickened wall; and type IV, a papillary nodule associated with an ill-defined hypoechoic area within the parenchyma.[6] A study from the same group found that mural nodules increased in size with a mean diameter of 5, 6, 11, and 20 mm for types I to IV, respectively. Furthermore, type III or IV were associated with invasive cancer in almost 90% of the patients.[7] The conclusion is that a mural nodule measuring over 1 cm or those associated with

FIGURE 16-2 Pseudocyst. Thin-walled internal septations (*arrows*) in a patient with a long-standing pseudocyst.

Video 16-1. Video demonstrating the classic appearance of mucin within a cyst.

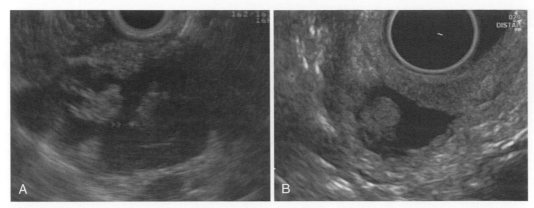

FIGURE 16-3 Main duct intraductal papillary mucinous neoplasia (IPMN). **A,** The main pancreatic duct is markedly dilated, and hyperechoic nodules can be seen arising from the duct wall. **B,** Mural nodule arising from the pancreatic duct wall in a patient with a main duct IPMN.

an ill-defined mass are highly likely to have malignant transformation.

Additional Tools

Contrast-enhanced (CE) endosonography is a technique where microbubbles are injected into a peripheral vein and circulate through the pancreas 30 to 40 seconds later. The technique works on the hypothesis that a malignant tumor has a different vascular pattern compared with either normal pancreatic tissue or mucin. CE EUS has been shown to be helpful for evaluating mural nodules in a small number of studies.[7,8] One prospective study found that CE EUS correctly identified 94% of the mural nodules present on surgical pathology, with high-grade dysplasia or an associated invasive carcinoma identified in 75% of these.[9] Further information about CE EUS can be found in Chapter 5.

EUS-Guided Fine-Needle Aspiration

EUS morphology alone cannot always reliably differentiate benign from malignant pancreatic cystic lesions (PCLs).[10] Interobserver agreement in examining different endoscopic features and in differentiating neoplastic from non-neoplastic pancreatic cysts has been shown to be moderately good in detecting a solid component, fair for the presence of an abnormal pancreatic duct, debris, or septations, and also only fair for the diagnosis of neoplastic versus non-neoplastic lesions.[11] A large prospective multicenter study[12] found that the accuracy of EUS imaging features for diagnosing mucinous lesions (IPMN and MCN) was only 51%, although a more recent study from the Netherlands reported a sensitivity of 78%.[13] Slightly worrisome in the Dutch study was that the sensitivity for detecting malignancy in pancreatic cysts was only 25% for EUS. Other retrospective studies have shown a higher accuracy for the detection of malignant/potentially malignant lesions with a reported sensitivity of 91%.[14] However, despite its high resolution, EUS alone clearly has limitations.

EUS FNA is often performed in patients with pancreatic cysts because it provides additional information that can be helpful in confirming the type of cyst as well as affecting management. No specific type or size of needle is prescribed; the choice is determined by the size of the cyst, its location, and the presence of vessels around the cyst. If possible, a single pass is made into the cyst to minimize the risk of complication, and the fluid in that cyst locule is fully aspirated (Figure 16-5). Aspirating the cyst locule to dryness may decrease the risk of infection, although the evidence for this is slim. For large cysts, it is often helpful to use a large bore needle, such as 19 G, which allows rapid aspiration of fluid.

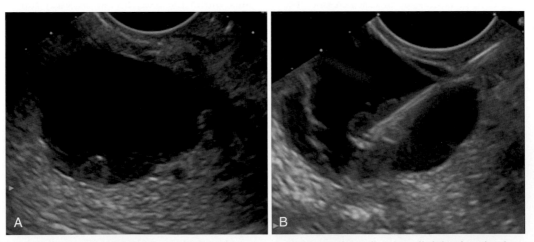

FIGURE 16-4 Mucin. **A,** There is a lesion in the 6-o'clock position that is adjacent to the wall. It is well defined, with a hyperechoic wall and hypoechoic center. These features are suggestive of mucin. **B,** On EUS fine-needle aspiration the lesion was shown to move, confirming that it was mucin and not a mural nodule. *(Copyright AM Lennon.)*

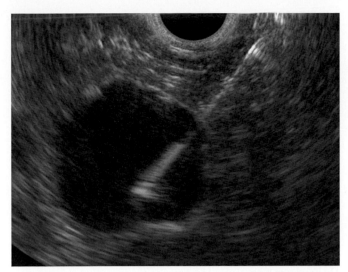

FIGURE 16-5 EUS fine-needle aspiration. A 19-G, 22-G, or 25-G needle can be used. In this case, a 22-G needle was sufficient to aspirate the lesion completely.

Lesions that have a vascular component, such as cystic pancreatic neuroendocrine tumors, often yield bloody samples if large bore needles are used, and often a smaller-gauge needle is helpful. Microcystic SCAs are particularly challenging to FNA. It is often very difficult or impossible to obtain sufficient fluid from these small cysts for analysis. In these cases, a 19-G needle can sometimes be used to obtain a core biopsy of the cyst. The use of core biopsy needles versus regular EUS FNA needles is discussed in detail in Chapter 22. One technique that is helpful is to target the wall of the cyst with a gentle back-and-forth motion to try to aspirate cells from the wall itself. This has been shown to increase the cytologic diagnostic yield for mucinous and malignant cysts.[15]

A 25-G through-the-needle cytologic brush was developed for EUS-guided assessment of PCLs. Studies have shown that use of a cytologic brush is associated with a higher yield of epithelial cells, which appears to be superior in providing diagnostic cells[16] and intracellular mucin[17] compared with direct cyst fluid aspirate. However, other studies have shown no difference in the diagnosis yield between aspiration and brushing (55%).[5] In addition, there are several issues with using a cytologic brush. First, it can only be used with a 19-G EUS FNA needle. These can be difficult to use in head or uncinate lesions, with one study showing that in almost one third of cases the brush could not be used.[16] In addition, the complication rates reported in studies using a cytology brush are significantly higher than would normally be expected for EUS FNA. Rates of up to 18% have been reported, with major complications occurring in up to 8% to 10%, including one fatality.[16,17] We therefore do not recommend routine use of this device.

The risks of complications from EUS FNA are slightly higher than those from FNA of a solid lesion.[9] In a recent systematic review of complications associated with EUS FNA, the most common complication was pancreatitis, which occurred in 1.1% of patients, followed by pain (0.77%), bleeding (0.33%), fever (0.33%), and infection (0.22%).[9] Pancreatitis is usually mild; however, severe cases and one death have been reported.[9] Antibiotic prophylaxis is recommended, usually with intravenous ciprofloxacin before the procedure. The American Society of Gastrointestinal Endoscopy suggest that 3 to 5 days of oral ciprofloxacin may be continued, although the evidence base to support these recommendations is not strong.[18] Malignant seeding following EUS FNA has been reported but is extremely rare.[19] In their practice, the authors perform FNA on cysts that are likely to provide sufficient fluid for serum carcinoembryonic antigen (CEA) analysis or cytology or if there are any suspicious features.

Cyst Fluid Analysis
Cytology

The specificity of cytology in most studies is excellent and approaches 100%, but the sensitivity varies considerably in reported series. This finding reflects the difficulty of interpreting these lesions, especially when the cellularity of samples is low. Brandwein[20] and Brugge and colleagues[12] reported sensitivities of 55% and 59%, respectively, for differentiating benign from malignant or potentially malignant PCLs. In contrast studies by Hernandez[21] and Frossard and colleagues[22] demonstrated sensitivities of 89% and 97%, respectively. The sensitivity of cytology can be affected by several factors. Sampling error may occur. Moreover, the presence of blood or benign epithelial cells from the gastric or duodenal mucosa can make interpretation difficult or can lead to false-positive results. The presence of on-site evaluation for adequacy of samples obtained by EUS FNA can improve results, although results are equally good whether this is performed by a cytotechnologist or cytopathologist.[23] The experience of the operator and/or institution appears to be important, with a recent study showing a trend toward increased accuracy with greater experience.[23] Pancreatic duct fluid can also be analyzed with cytology, with sensitivity varying from 21%[24] to 75%[25] depending on the study.

Tumor Markers

Given the limited sensitivity of cytology, the value of tumor markers in aspirated cyst fluid has been examined. The level of a number of tumor markers in cyst fluid has been studied, including CEA, CA19-9, CA72-4, CA125, and CA15-3.[12,22,26–28] Although some studies have shown interesting results, at present the performance of tumor markers other than CEA is inadequate for diagnostic purposes, and measurement of these other markers, outside of research studies, is not justified.

CEA is found in high levels in mucinous tumors (IPMN and MCN), whereas low levels are found in pseudocysts (unless infected) and SCA[12,22] (see Table 16-2). The sensitivity and specificity of CEA varies depending on the study and the CEA threshold used. The cutoff used by most endoscopists to differentiate a mucinous from a nonmucinous cyst is >192 ng/mL. This is based on a large, prospective, multicenter trial that found this value was associated with an accuracy of 79% for differentiating mucinous from other cyst types and was significantly better than the accuracy of EUS morphology alone (51%) or cytology (59%). In this study, no combination of morphologic features, cytology, and tumor markers was better than CEA alone. However, other studies have found that the optimum cutoff varies anywhere from 100 to 800 ng/mL.[12,22,26,29] One reason for this is that CEA assays are standardized for serum and not cyst fluid, and different assays exist, making comparisons between different studies or centers difficult. A pooled analysis of 12 studies[24] found that a CEA concentration >800 ng/mL strongly suggested a mucinous lesion (sensitivity, 48%; specificity, 98%). Conversely, a low cyst fluid CEA level of <5 ng/mL is very suggestive of a nonmucinous lesion, such as an SCA, with a sensitivity and specificity of between 57% and 100% and 77% and 86%, respectively.[30,31] Another problem with CEA is that laboratories require anywhere from 0.25 to 1 mL of fluid. A recent study from the Netherlands found that sufficient fluid for CEA analysis was obtained in just under 60% of patients.[13] An elevated cyst fluid CEA level has not been shown to be associated with an increased risk of high-grade dysplasia or invasive cancer in the majority of studies and should not be used as a marker of malignant transformation based on the current evidence.[32] Cyst fluid CEA is currently useful in that a very high level is suggestive of a mucinous cyst, whereas a very low level suggests a nonmucinous cyst; however, neither the sensitivity nor specificity is 100%.

Cyst fluid amylase requires approximately 0.5 mL of fluid for analysis in most laboratories and should be sent if a pseudocyst is within the differential diagnosis. A level of <250 U/mL virtually excludes a pseudocyst (sensitivity, 44%; specificity, 98%).[22] The levels of cyst fluid amylase vary in both MCN and IPMN and cannot be used to differentiate between these two entities.[33]

Molecular Markers

Our knowledge of the genes involved in pancreatic cancer and the time over which malignancy develops has increased dramatically over the last 5 years.[34,35] Although not all the genes associated with progression to malignancy in pancreatic cysts are known, several have been identified. An early multicenter study compared the accuracy of cytology, cyst fluid CEA levels, and DNA analysis incorporating DNA quantification, k-*ras* mutations, and multiple allelic loss analysis and found that k-*ras* mutations were highly predictive of a mucinous lesion (odds ratio, 20.9; specificity, 96%), whereas DNA quantity and quality, the presence of k-*ras* mutations, and loss of heterozygosity (LOH) were associated with the presence of malignancy.[36] Subsequent studies have reported that these markers identify mucinous cysts between 33% and 89% of the time.[37-40]

One of the major recent advances was the identification of five genes (*VHL*, *RNF43*, *CTNNB1*, *GNAS*, and k-*ras*) by a group at The Johns Hopkins University, which appear to be able to differentiate the major types of pancreatic cysts.[41] Mutations in the *VHL* and *CTNNB1* genes were able to identify SCA and SPN, respectively, whereas mutations in *GNAS* were found only in patients with IPMN and appear to allow differentiation of patients with MCN from those with IPMN. In a second study, the authors sought to see if they could identify the key mutations in pancreatic cyst fluid.[42] They were able to identify a mutation in either *GNAS* or k-*ras* in 96% of IPMNs. In contrast, none of the patients with SCA had a mutation in either gene. Thus, mutations in these genes could potentially be used to differentiate macrocystic SCA from IPMN and MCN. These markers are currently being validated

in a large, multicenter study, the results of which are expected in 2015.

Types of Pancreatic Cysts

Many different types of pancreatic cysts exist. An overview of rare pancreatic cysts, such as benign epithelial cysts, lymphangioma, hemangioma, acinar cell cystadenoma/adenocarcinoma, pancreaticoblastoma, and others, can be found in the studies of Sakorafas and colleagues.[43] The most commonly seen pancreatic cysts are reviewed in this chapter. One of the most important differentiations to make clinically is between mucinous cysts (i.e., IPMN and MCN) and other types of pancreatic cysts. This differentiation is based on a combination of features including imaging, the presence of a high cyst fluid CEA, and mucin on cytology reports.

Pseudocysts

Pseudocysts are the most common type of pancreatic cyst seen, and they almost always occur in the setting of an episode of acute pancreatitis or in patients with chronic pancreatitis. Knowledge of the clinical presentation is therefore essential in accurately differentiating pseudocysts from cystic neoplasms. Pseudocysts lack a true epithelial lining, with the wall consisting of inflammatory and fibrous tissue. This wall is thin in early pseudocysts but may become thick as they mature. Pseudocysts can be any size and are usually unilocular and anechoic (Video 16-2; Figure 16-6). This appearance may change due to the presence of necrotic debris or infection and may mimic a cystic neoplasm (Figures 16-7 and 16-8). Septations are rare but do occur, and pseudocysts often demonstrate direct communication with the main pancreatic duct. It is often helpful to look for features of acute or chronic pancreatitis elsewhere in the gland, which supports the diagnosis of a pseudocyst. Other features that should be noted are the distance between the intestinal wall and the cyst lumen and the presence of interposed (by Doppler examination) collateral vessels as evidence of segmental portal hypertension secondary to portal or splenic vein thrombosis. These features are important if endoscopic drainage of the pseudocyst is performed. Reactive, inflammatory-looking lymph nodes may also be seen adjacent to the pseudocyst.

Because pseudocysts lack an epithelial lining, no epithelial cells should be present in FNA samples unless there is contamination of the needle with gastric or duodenal epithelium during puncture. Aspirated fluid is of low viscosity, often dark, turbid, or even bloody (Figure 16-9), and contains inflammatory cells such as macrophages and histiocytes. Raised amylase concentrations are present, but levels of other

Video 16-2. Video demonstrating a pseudocyst.

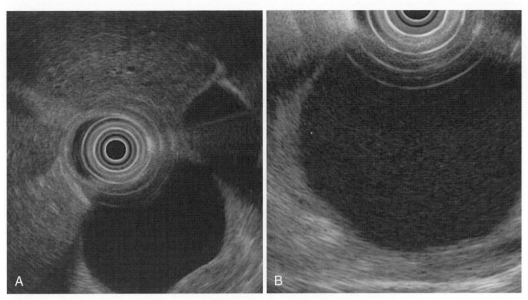

FIGURE 16-6 Pseudocysts. **A**, Radial EUS in a patient with a recent episode of pancreatitis reveals a 3-cm, thin-walled, anechoic cystic lesion in close contact with the gastric wall. **B**, Similar findings in another patient with chronic abdominal pain who presented with chronic pancreatitis and a pseudocyst.

tumor markers should be low, although increased CEA levels have been reported when infection is present. A low amylase level of <250 U/mL virtually excludes a pseudocyst.[30]

Pseudocysts are benign and do not require intervention unless they are infected or are symptomatic. A detailed discussion of the management of pseudocysts is provided in Chapter 24.

Serous Cystadenomas

SCAs are much more common in women. They are single lesions, which can occur anywhere in the pancreas, most commonly occurring in the head or body of the pancreas, and do not communicate with the main pancreatic duct.[44,45] SCA can have four different types of imaging features. The most common presentation, which accounts for approximately 60% of SCAs, is numerous microcystic lesions (Figure 16-10; Video 16-3) with thin septa.[45] However over 35% of SCAs have a macrocystic (>1 cm) (Figure 16-11) or mixed appearance, which is more difficult to differentiate from MCN and branch duct (BD)-IPMN. Finally, a small number present as a solid lesion (Figure 16-12) due to the coalescence of multiple tiny (1- to 2-mm) cysts.[45] Central fibrosis or calcification is a classic appearance in SCA, but they occur in fewer than 20% of cases. The appearance of focal cyst wall nodularity or thickening, intracystic mucin or floating debris, or pancreatic

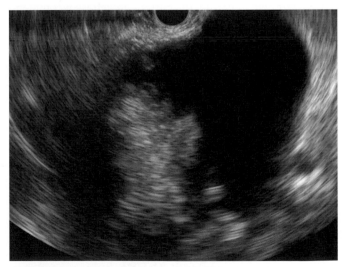

FIGURE 16-7 Atypical appearance of pseudocyst. The patient presented with chronic abdominal pain and weight loss. The EUS appearances were suspicious for a mucinous neoplasm, but fine-needle aspiration revealed old blood-stained fluid with inflammatory cells, low carcinoembryonic antigen levels, and an amylase concentration greater than 66,000 U/mL. Because of ongoing concerns, the lesion was resected, and a pseudocyst was confirmed.

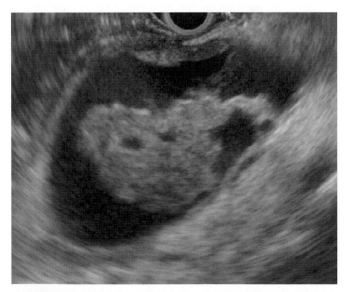

FIGURE 16-8 Infected pseudocyst in a patient with severe acute pancreatitis and fever. The irregular hyperechoic material seen within the cyst raises the suspicion of a cystic neoplasm but it is not murally based. Fine-needle aspiration cytology revealed only macrophages and debris; the amylase concentration was greater than 6000 U/mL.

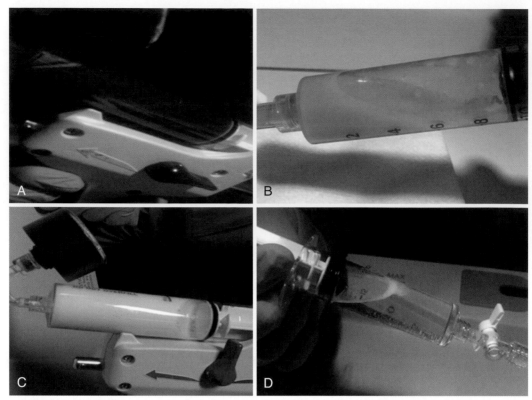

FIGURE 16-9 Cyst fluid. **A,** Hemorrhagic and **B,** turbid fluid from a pseudocyst. **C,** Opaque fluid from a lymphoepithelial cyst. **D,** Clear fluid from a mucinous cyst.

duct dilatation is unusual and suggests that the lesion may be a mucinous tumor.

The morphologic characteristics of serous cystadenomas are often diagnostic of the lesion (see Video 16-3). Nevertheless, cytologic examination may improve the diagnostic accuracy of EUS, particularly in the absence of the classic microcystic appearance. The cytologic appearance is of serous fluid containing small cuboidal cells that stain for glycogen but not mucin. The fluid classically is clear (Video 16-4) and contains low amylase and CEA concentrations; however, obtaining adequate amounts of cyst fluid for CEA analysis can be difficult due to the small size of the cysts. A very low CEA concentration of less than 5 ng/mL virtually

excludes a mucinous lesion and lends support to the diagnosis of an SCA.[30]

SCAs have a very low risk of malignant transformation, with large series reporting a risk of liver metastases of 0.7%, all of which occurred in patients with cysts measuring >10 cm.[44,45] Although not considered malignant by pathological criteria, local invasion into peripancreatic structures or lymph node involvement can occur in up to 5% of patients.[44] Given their benign nature, the current guidelines recommend that SCA should be resected only if symptomatic or where the diagnosis is unclear.[46] Otherwise SCA should be followed, because it can increase in size.[47] The optimum surveillance interval is not known, but we usually follow our patient with SCA with MRI every 2 years.

Mucinous Cystic Neoplasm

MCNs are single cysts, which occur most often in young or middle-aged women and are found in the body or tail of the

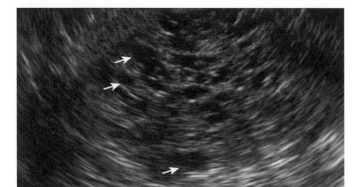

FIGURE 16-10 Serous cystadenoma. Typical appearance of a 2.5-cm microcystic serous cystadenoma. It contains multiple small cysts *(arrows)*. This lesion does not show the central fibrosis or calcification that is sometimes present.

Video 16-3. Video demonstrating EUS examination of a cyst lesion in the pancreas with numerous small septations consistent with serous cystadenoma.

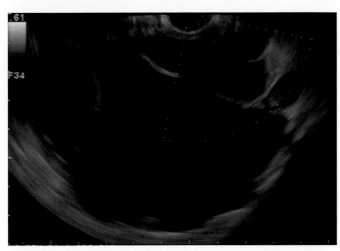

FIGURE 16-11 Macrocystic serous cystadenoma. This is a 9-cm anechoic, well-circumscribed cyst in the tail of the pancreas with thin septations. It was associated with a low CEA and amylase levels; however, the patient was symptomatic and the cyst was therefore removed. Surgical pathology confirmed a serous cystadenoma. *(Copyright AM Lennon.)*

Video 16-4. Video demonstrating clear, thin fluid found in a serous cystadenoma.

pancreatic duct.[48] MCNs are almost always single cysts, and the presence of other cystic lesions elsewhere in the pancreas or a dilated pancreatic duct is unusual, and, if present, a diagnosis of IPMN should be considered. The presence of an irregular or thickened cyst wall, solid regions within the cyst, adjacent solid mass (Figure 16-14), or a strictured, obstructed, or displaced pancreatic duct suggests malignant transformation (Video 16-6). FNA can be useful in confirming the diagnosis. The fluid is usually clear (see Figure 16-9D). The cyst wall and septa should be sampled, in addition to aspirating the fluid. Cytology demonstrates viscous fluid containing mucin and columnar epithelial cells. As discussed earlier in the chapter, cyst fluid amylase levels vary and are not useful for differentiating MCN from IPMN.[33]

Unlike SCA, MCNs have a clear risk of malignant transformation, with large studies showing a risk of either high-grade dysplasia (previously called carcinoma in situ) or invasive cancer of just under 20%.[48,50] Patients who undergo resection have an excellent outcome, with only 6% developing a recurrence. Given these excellent outcomes, the fact that surgery usually involves a distal pancreatectomy rather than a pancreaticoduodenectomy, and the fact that the majority of patients are young and will require long term follow-up, the current guidelines recommend surgical resection in patients who are fit.[46,51] In older patients, or those with multiple comorbidities, observation can be considered.

pancreas in over 90% of cases. They are extremely rare in men, who account for only 2% of cases.[48,49] They are differentiated from IPMN by the presence of ovarian stroma that contains both estrogen and progesterone receptors. On EUS they appear as a macrocystic lesion (Video 16-5) that often contains septations (Figure 16-13). Peripheral calcification, which is found in 15% of patients, is suggestive of MCN but may also be seen in SPN. MCNs classically do not communicate with the main pancreatic duct, a feature used to differentiate them from BD-IPMN. However, a recent multicenter study found that 18% of patients with MCN who underwent an ERCP were found to have a communication with the main

Intraductal Papillary Mucinous Neoplasia

IPMNs were previously thought to be rare but now account for almost 50% of surgically resected pancreatic cysts.[3] Unlike MCN and SCA, IPMNs are equally common in men and women. They can occur at any age but most frequently present in the sixth decade of life. IPMNs can occur throughout the pancreas but have a slight preponderance for the head of the pancreas. In approximately 20% of cases, multiple cysts occur, which can be multifocal (i.e., located in multiple different areas of the pancreas).[52]

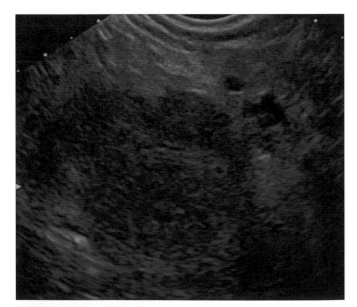

FIGURE 16-12 Solid-appearing serous cystadenoma. A 4-cm hypoechoic lesion in the body of the pancreas. EUS fine-needle aspiration was performed. No cyst fluid was obtained and cytology was nondiagnostic. The lesion was confirmed as a serous cystadenoma at surgery. *(Copyright AM Lennon.)*

Video 16-5. Mucinous cystic neoplasm.

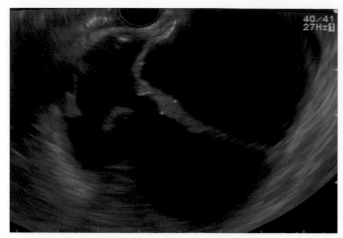

FIGURE 16-13 Mucinous cystadenoma. This shows a 5-cm anechoic lesion that was well circumscribed and contains a slightly thickened (4-mm) septation. EUS fine-needle aspiration was performed, which confirmed a high cyst fluid carcinoembryonic antigen level. Cytology revealed mucin. A mucinous cystadenoma was confirmed on surgical pathology. *(Copyright AM Lennon).*

IPMNs are classified as involving the main pancreatic duct (MD-IPMN), the branch ducts (BD-IPMN), or both, in which case it is termed a mixed-type IPMN (Figure 16-15). Involvement of the main pancreatic duct is defined as focal or diffuse dilation of the main pancreatic duct to >5 mm.[51] This differentiation is very important because it determines the risk of malignant transformation and the management of these patients.

Endoscopic appearances include the presence of focal or diffuse dilation of the main pancreatic duct and/or the presence of dilated side branches. Communication between side and main duct branches is a characteristic feature of BD-IPMN or mixed IPMN (Video 16-7), although this is not always seen because it can be obstructed by mucin. Filling defects can be seen either in the main pancreatic duct or in cysts and can result from either a mural nodule (see Figure 16-3) or mucus plugs (see Figure 16-4 and Video 16-1). Differentiation of these lesions can be difficult and is discussed in detail in the

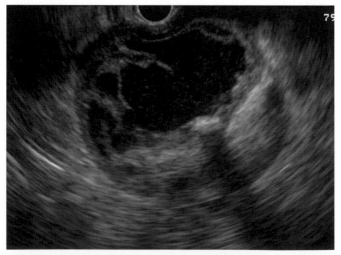

FIGURE 16-14 Mucinous cystadenoma. The cyst wall is irregular and markedly thickened *(asterisk)*.

Video 16-6. Video demonstrating a solid component within a pancreatic cyst lesion consistent with cystadenocarcinoma.

EUS imaging section above. IPMNs have malignant potential (Figure 16-16; Video 16-8). In addition, increasing evidence suggests that patients with IPMN are at greater risk of developing pancreatic ductal adenocarcinoma entirely separate from the cyst (Figure 16-17).[52–57] It is therefore important to inspect not only the cyst but also the entire pancreatic parenchyma, looking for a focal hypoechoic mass. The ampulla of Vater should be inspected, as a gaping "fish mouth" papilla extruding mucus is occasionally seen. The presence of features such as a focal hypoechoic mass or mural nodules (Figures 16-3 and 16-16) is suggestive of malignancy.

EUS FNA allows samples to be obtained for cyst fluid CEA, amylase, and cytology. The fluid is usually clear (Figure 16-9D). IPMNs, similar to MCN, are mucinous cysts and are associated with an elevated cyst fluid CEA. Cyst fluid amylase should be sent for analysis if there is a question as to whether the cyst is an IPMN or a pseudocyst. With this exception, cyst fluid amylase levels are not routinely sent for analysis because they are not helpful in differentiating an MCN from an IPMN. Cytology should be sent because the presence of markedly atypical cytology is one of the criteria for consideration of surgical resection.[51] The presence of mucin is helpful in confirming the diagnosis of either an MCN or IPMN. Psammomatous calcification is uncommon but highly suggestive of IPMN.

Four types of epithelial subtypes have been identified based on the cell morphology and expression patterns of glycoproteins containing mucin (MUC): gastric, intestinal, pancreaticobiliary, and oncocytic. The epithelial subtype has been correlated to degree of dysplasia, with gastric-type cysts more likely to be of low risk for dysplasia (accounting for 91% of all low-risk cysts); pancreatobiliary and intestinal types are

Video 16-7. Video demonstrating EUS evaluation of the pancreas. A large cyst is seen in the pancreatic genu communicating with the main pancreatic duct. In addition, papillary projections are seen in the main pancreatic duct consistent with intraductal papillary mucinous neoplasia. The papillary projections are then aspirated to rule out carcinoma.

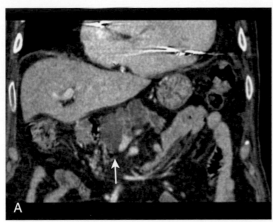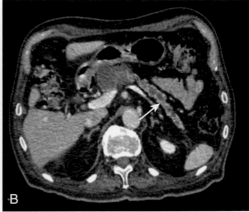

FIGURE 16-15   Mixed intraductal papillary mucinous neoplasia (IPMN). **A,** On this coronal view, a large cystic and solid cyst is seen in the head of the pancreas *(arrow)*. The solid component is suspicious for neoplastic change. **B,** In this view, the dilated main pancreatic duct is clearly seen in the body and tail of the pancreas *(arrow)* with marked atrophy of the parenchyma.

more likely to be high risk for dysplasia (accounting for 79% of all high-risk cysts).[58,59] However, the epithelial subtype usually can be determined only on gross resection specimen.

The risk of malignant transformation, and hence the management of IPMN, is determined by whether or not there is involvement of the main pancreatic duct. MD-IPMN or mixed IPMN have a significantly higher risk than BD-IPMN, with the majority of surgical series reporting a risk of high-grade or invasive cancer of between 45% and 60%.[51] In contrast, 16% to 24% of patients with BD-IPMN who undergo surgical resection are found to have high-grade or invasive cancer. The International Consensus Guidelines for the management of mucinous pancreatic cysts have been recently updated (Figure 16-18).[51] The guidelines recommend surgery for fit patients with an IPMN that is associated with jaundice or an enhancing solid component. Patients who have a recent history of

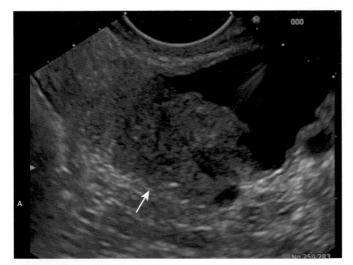

FIGURE 16-16   Branch duct intraductal papillary mucinous neoplasia (IPMN) with solid component. IPMNs have malignant potential. This patient had a cyst that communicated with the main pancreatic duct, which was associated with a high cyst fluid carcinoembryonic antigen, consistent with a branch duct IPMN. As we scan through the cyst, the wall becomes thickened with an irregular edge *(arrow)*. These features are consistent with a type IV mural nodule and are worrisome for malignant transformation of a BD-IPMN. *(Copyright AM Lennon.)*

pancreatitis, a nonenhancing mural nodule, main pancreatic duct dilation measuring between 5 and 9 mm, or where there was an abrupt change in the caliber of the main pancreatic duct should undergo EUS. If there are features suspicious for malignancy on EUS (mural nodule, marked cytologic atypia), surgical resection should be considered. Previous guidelines had recommended surgical resection for all IPMNs greater than 3 cm;[60] however, the most recent guidelines acknowledge the growing body of evidence that size alone is not a predictor of malignancy. Surgery should be considered in young, fit patients with BD-IPMN with cysts >3 cm; however, surveillance can be considered in older patients with cysts >3 cm without suspicious features. Patients without any suspicious features can undergo surveillance alone, with the interval determined by the size of the largest cysts. MRI and EUS are the most commonly used modalities. In the authors' institution, MRI is typically used for surveillance of small cysts, with EUS reserved for larger cysts or if it is believed that the cyst is at higher risk for malignant transformation. The authors await studies to determine the sensitivity and specificity of these new guidelines.

One key difference between IPMN and other types of pancreatic cysts is that IPMN can recur in the remnant pancreas following surgery (see Figure 16-17), with a recent study showing that 15% of patients develop lesions that require surgical intervention. Thus all patients who undergo surgical resection of an IPMN, even if no cysts are apparent within the remnant pancreas, require surveillance. The interval at which they are followed is determined by the pathological grade in the resected specimen and by the size of cysts within the remnant pancreas.[51]

Video 16-8. Video of a pancreatic adenocarcinoma arising within an intraductal papillary mucinous neoplasia.

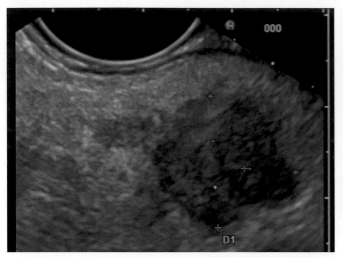

FIGURE 16-17 Adenocarcinoma arising separate to IPMN. This patient had undergone resection of a high-grade IPMN in the head of the pancreas 4 years previously. All the margins were clear. There is an irregular, hypoechoic area, which is separate from any cysts. EUS-FNA was performed of this area, which confirmed adenocarcinoma. *(Copyright AM Lennon.)*

Solid Pseudopapillary Neoplasm

Although PNs were once thought to be rare, this distinctive lesion is now better recognized and accounts for 5% of resected cystic pancreatic tumors.[3] It usually occurs in women, who make up 90% of cases, and has a wide age range, but it typically presents in patients in their mid-20s.[60a] Patients often have vague, nonspecific symptoms, with jaundice and pancreatitis being very rare presentations. With the increased use of cross-sectional imaging, SPNs are increasingly being detected incidentally with almost 40% of patients presenting in this manner.

SPNs are almost always single cysts and can be found in the head, body, or tail of the pancreas. They are usually well circumscribed. The hallmarks of this lesion are central hemorrhagic cystic degeneration creating the classic solid and cystic appearance (Figure 16-19; Video 16-9); however, some can have a mainly solid appearance (Figure 16-20). Only a few case reports and small case series have evaluated the role of EUS and EUS FNA.[61-71] Lesions are usually well demarcated and may appear solid or mixed solid and cystic. Peripheral calcification can occur but is also seen in patients

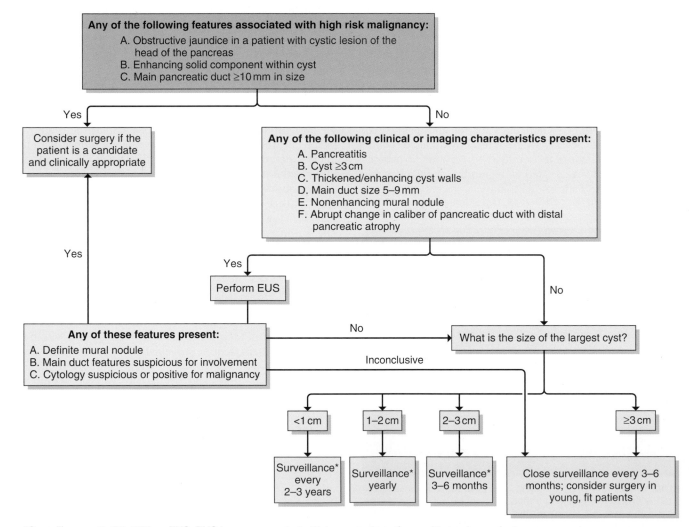

*Surveillance with CT, MRI, or EUS. EUS is recommended with larger cysts or those with worrisome features.

FIGURE 16-18 International Consensus Guidelines for the management of intraductal papillary mucinous neoplasia. CT, computed tomography; MRI, magnetic resonance imaging. *(Adapted from Tanaka M, Fernandez-Del Castillo C, Adsay V, et al. International Consensus Guidelines 2012 for the management of IPMN and MCN of the pancreas. Pancreatology, 2012;12:183-197.)*

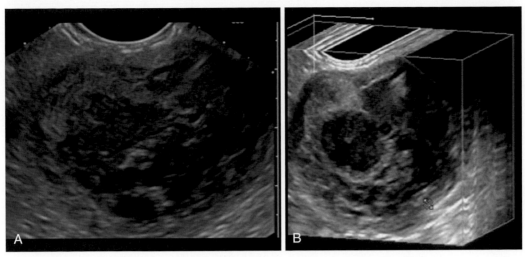

FIGURE 16-19   Solid pseudopapillary neoplasm. **A,** This is the classic appearance of a solid pseudopapillary neoplasm. It is well defined, with both cystic and solid areas. **B,** In the three-dimensional image of the cyst, the hemorrhagic center is clearly seen. *(Copyright AM Lennon.)*

with MCN. The hemorrhagic degeneration often results in a bloody, necrotic FNA sample, which can provide a clue to the diagnosis, although the histologic features are usually characteristic.

SPNs have clear malignant potential with either lymph node involvement or distant metastases found in 8% of patients.[60a] Surgical resection is therefore recommended for all patients with SPN. Patients who have undergone resection of an SPN should be followed for 5 years as 4.4% will develop a recurrence.[60a]

Cystic Neuroendocrine Tumors

Most neuroendocrine tumors of the pancreas are solid, but a small number can present with cystic degeneration (Figures 16-21 and 16-22). They can occur anywhere in the pancreas and are usually single unless they are associated with a syndrome such as multiple endocrine neoplasia or Von Hippel-Lindau syndrome. They are usually well-defined lesions that do not communicate with the main pancreatic duct. Although they can appear as mainly cystic lesions, the majority usually have a thickened wall or solid component. The remaining parenchyma and pancreatic duct are normal. EUS FNA is a helpful diagnosis that can usually be made based on cytology findings. Neither cyst fluid CEA nor amylase are helpful in identifying these cysts.

Cystic Ductal Adenocarcinoma

Ductal adenocarcinoma of the pancreas may occasionally show cystic degeneration. These cysts are different than the

others described earlier in the chapter. They are ill defined and often have an irregular, thickened wall with a solid component (Figure 16-23; Video 16-10). The diagnosis can be confirmed with EUS FNA, which should target the solid component. The evaluation and management of pancreatic ductal adenocarcinoma is discussed in depth in Chapter 15.

Future Developments
Imaging

Confocal laser endomicroscopy (CLE) is a novel imaging technique in which a low-power laser illuminates and scans a single plane of tissue, generating a real-time image or biopsy of the tissue. A probe-based CLE has been developed that can be passed through a 19-G EUS FNA needle and enables imaging of the epithelium to several hundred microns. This process was shown to be feasible in a preliminary in vivo study of pancreatic masses and cysts, with images obtained in over 90% of the patients, 60% of which were high quality.[72] One limitation of this technique is reduced imaging depth. An alternative imaging modality is optical coherence tomography (OCT). OCT can visualize structures up to 2 mm in depth and can image structures that measure several microns in diameter. In preliminary studies of pancreatic cysts ex vivo, OCT was found to have a sensitivity and specificity of between 78% to 100% for differentiating mucinous from nonmucinous lesions.[73] These are interesting preliminary studies. Questions remain about how much of the surface area of the cyst can

Video 16-9. Video of a solid pseudopapillary neoplasm.

Video 16-10. Video demonstrating a solid component within a pancreatic cyst lesion. EUS-guided fine-needle aspiration of the solid component revealed adenocarcinoma.

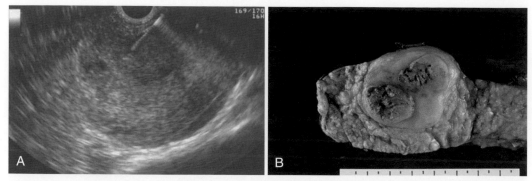

FIGURE 16-20   Solid pseudopapillary neoplasm. **A,** EUS image of a lesion in the body of the pancreas that is mainly solid in appearance. Fine-needle aspiration confirmed a solid cystic pseudopapillary neoplasm. **B,** The corresponding surgical specimen is shown here.

be examined, if all cysts (i.e., those in the uncinate pancreas) can be successfully seen, and what additional information CLE/OCT provides over and above that of standard imaging and cyst fluid analysis.

Molecular Markers

EUS, CEA, and cytology are not without limitations in the evaluation of pancreatic cysts (Table 16-3). It is likely that a panel of molecular markers will be incorporated into a model combining clinical information, imaging characteristics, cytology, and CEA levels that will increase the accuracy with which we can differentiate mucinous from nonmucinous cysts. One interesting development in this area is the analysis of pancreatic juice, which is collected by aspirating it from under the major papilla following secretin stimulation. As discussed previously, *GNAS* mutations appear to be unique to IPMN and have been detected in both pancreatic tissue[41] and pancreatic cyst fluid.[42] In a further development, Kanda and colleagues[74] were able to identify *GNAS* mutations in pancreatic juice from

patients with IPMN. Similar to the prior studies, no *GNAS* mutation was found in patients with other types of cysts. The use of pancreatic juice could be particularly helpful in patients with very small pancreatic cysts where it is impossible to obtain sufficient pancreatic cyst fluid for analysis.

Although *GNAS* and k-*ras* mutations are useful for differentiating the type of pancreatic cyst present, both occur in cystic neoplasms with low- and intermediate-grade dysplasia and thus cannot be used as markers of the degree of dysplasia in a lesion. In contrast, *TP53* mutations are found in IPMNs and MCNs with high-grade dysplasia or an associated invasive adenocarcinoma. A group from The Johns Hopkins University identified *TP53* mutations in pancreatic juice in patients with IPMN and either high-grade dysplasia and invasive pancreatic adenocarcinomas, with only a small number of patients with intermediate-grade and none of the patients with low-grade dysplasia found to have any mutations.[22] Although exciting,

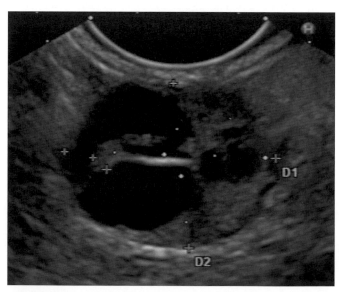

FIGURE 16-21   Pancreatic neuroendocrine tumor. This cyst has a thin septation, however the wall is markedly thickened between the 1-o'clock and 6-o'clock position. The solid component was targeted with EUS fine-needle aspiration and the diagnosis confirmed as a pancreatic neuroendocrine tumor. *(Copyright AM Lennon.)*

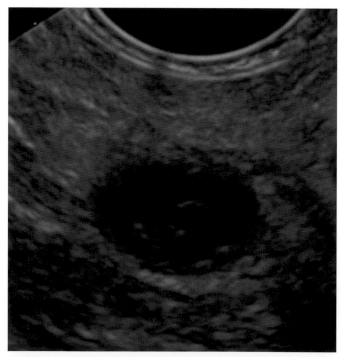

FIGURE 16-22   Pancreatic neuroendocrine tumor. This is a mainly cystic lesion with a small, irregular solid component that can be seen in the 6-o'clock position. *(Copyright AM Lennon.)*

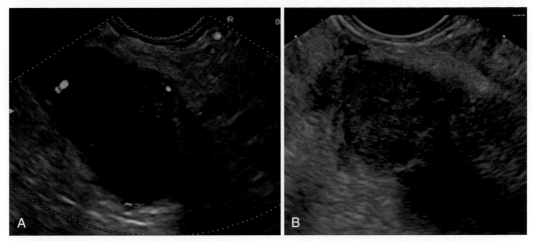

FIGURE 16-23   Cystic pancreatic ductal adenocarcinoma. **A,** There is a cyst with a possible solid component between the 9-o'clock and 12-o'clock position. **B,** On further scanning, an irregular, hypoechoic mass with an irregular edge becomes clear. On fine-needle aspiration (FNA), the cyst fluid carcinoembryonic antigen was low with no mucin on cytology. FNA of the solid component confirmed an adenocarcinoma. *(Copyright AM Lennon.)*

these results need to be validated in large, prospective trials prior to being incorporated into clinical practice.

Cyst Ablation

Pancreatic surgery is associated with significant morbidity and, in the case of pancreaticoduodenectomy, a mortality rate of 1% to 2% in high-volume centers.[3] This has stimulated research into alternative methods of treating cysts. There are now several studies that have examined whether EUS-guided alcohol or alcohol and paclitaxel injection into pancreatic cystic tumors can be used to ablate the epithelium and thus obviate the need for surgery.[75–80] The results have been varied, with cyst resolution reported in 33% to 79% of the cases.[35–40] One of the questions with this type of therapy is how effective is it in ablating all the epithelial lining rather than just decreasing the size of the cyst. In patients who have undergone surgical resection after cyst ablation, the reported success rates range from 0% to 100%. Radiofrequency ablation is an alternative to alcohol or paclitaxel. A multicenter study in patients with both pancreatic neuroendocrine tumors and pancreatic cysts found that cyst size decreased in 75% of patients, with complete resolution on imaging in 25% of

patients.[41] Prospective clinical trials should be performed in patients who undergo surgical resection to determine the exact amount of epithelial ablation of the cyst and also the side effect profile in patients with pancreatic cysts.

Examination Checklist

Localize and describe cyst
- Site and size
- Wall thickness
- Distance from lumen; interposed vessels
- Focal irregularity, papillary projections, or mural nodules and the size of these lesion(s)
- Associated mass lesion
- Central or peripheral calcification
- Presence and size of septation(s)
- Debris or echogenic material in cyst
- Communication and diameter of the pancreatic duct

Examine rest of pancreas, looking in particular for a mass lesion that is not associated with the cyst
Perform EUS-guided FNA of solid lesions
Perform EUS-guided FNA of cyst fluid under antibiotic cover
Send cyst fluid for CEA levels and for cytologic evaluation including mucin staining

---

TABLE 16-3

IMPORTANT LIMITATIONS OF EUS IN THE EVALUATION OF PANCREATIC CYSTIC LESIONS

Procedure Aspect	Limitation
Technical	Attenuation of imaging in large (>6 cm) lesions
EUS imaging	Considerable overlap of morphologic features of lesions
Fine-needle aspiration	Aspiration of viscous fluid with 22-G needles
	Small volumes obtained in microcystic lesions
	Limited accuracy of cytology: contamination with columnar gastroduodenal epithelium; sampling error: dysplasia and malignant change are patchy in mucinous lesions
Amylase concentration	Levels may be variable in lesions that communicate with the main pancreatic duct
Carcinoembryonic antigen level	May be raised in infected pseudocysts and lymphoepithelial cysts
Other tumor markers (e.g., CA19-9, CA72-4)	Unproven value; investigational role

REFERENCES

1. Laffan TA, Horton KM, Klein AP, et al. Prevalence of unsuspected pancreatic cysts on MDCT. *AJR Am J Roentgenol.* 2008;191:802-807.
2. Lee KS, Sekhar A, Rofsky NM, et al. Prevalence of incidental pancreatic cysts in the adult population on MR imaging. *Am J Gastroenterol.* 2010;105:2079-2084.
3. Valsangkar NP, Morales-Oyarvide V, Thayer SP, et al. 851 resected cystic tumors of the pancreas: a 33-year experience at the Massachusetts General Hospital. *Surgery.* 2012;152:S4-S12.
4. Shin EJ, Canto MI. Pancreatic cancer screening. *Gastroenterol Clin North Am.* 2012;41:143-157.
5. Thomas T, Bebb J, Mannath J, et al. EUS-guided pancreatic cyst brushing: a comparative study in a tertiary referral centre. *JOP.* 2010;11:163-169.
6. Ohno E, Hirooka Y, Itoh A, et al. Intraductal papillary mucinous neoplasms of the pancreas: differentiation of malignant and benign tumors by endoscopic ultrasound findings of mural nodules. *Ann Surg.* 2009;249:628-634.
7. Ohno E, Hirooka Y, Itoh A, et al. Intraductal papillary mucinous neoplasms of the pancreas: differentiation of malignant and benign tumors by Endoscopic ultrasonography findings of mural nodules. *Ann Surg.* 2011.
8. Kurihara N, Kawamoto H, Kobayashi Y, et al. Vascular patterns in nodules of intraductal papillary mucinous neoplasms depicted under contrast-enhanced ultrasonography are helpful for evaluating malignant potential. *Eur J Radiol.* 2012;81:66-70.
9. Wang KX, Ben QW, Jin ZD, et al. Assessment of morbidity and mortality associated with EUS-guided FNA: a systematic review. *Gastrointest Endosc.* 2011;73:283-290.
10. Ahmad NA, Kochman ML, Lewis JD, et al. Can EUS alone differentiate between malignant and benign cystic lesions of the pancreas? *Am J Gastroenterol.* 2001;96:3295-3300.
11. Ahmad NA, Kochman ML, Brensinger C, et al. Interobserver agreement among endosonographers for the diagnosis of neoplastic versus non-neoplastic pancreatic cystic lesions. *Gastrointest Endosc.* 2003;58:59-64.
12. Brugge WR, Lewandrowski K, Lee-Lewandrowski E, et al. Diagnosis of pancreatic cystic neoplasms: a report of the cooperative pancreatic cyst study. *Gastroenterology.* 2004;126:1330-1336.
13. de Jong K, van Hooft JE, Nio CY, et al. Accuracy of preoperative workup in a prospective series of surgically resected cystic pancreatic lesions. *Scand J Gastroenterol.* 2012;47:1056-1063.
14. Sedlack R, Affi A, Vazquez-Sequeiros E, et al. Utility of EUS in the evaluation of cystic pancreatic lesions. *Gastrointest Endosc.* 2002;56:543-547.
15. Hong SK, Loren DE, Rogart JN, et al. Targeted cyst wall puncture and aspiration during EUS-FNA increases the diagnostic yield of premalignant and malignant pancreatic cysts. *Gastrointest Endosc.* 2012;75:775-782.
16. Sendino O, Fernandez-Esparrach G, Sole M, et al. Endoscopic ultrasonography-guided brushing increases cellular diagnosis of pancreatic cysts: a prospective study. *Dig Liver Dis.* 2010;42:877-881.
17. Al-Haddad M, Gill KR, Raimondo M, et al. Safety and efficacy of cytology brushings versus standard fine-needle aspiration in evaluating cystic pancreatic lesions: a controlled study. *Endoscopy.* 2010;42:127-132.
18. ASGE Standards Of Practice Committee, Banerjee S, Shen B, et al. Antibiotic prophylaxis for GI endoscopy. *Gastrointest Endosc.* 2008;67:791-798.
19. Hirooka Y, Goto H, Itoh A, et al. Case of intraductal papillary mucinous tumor in which endosonography-guided fine-needle aspiration biopsy caused dissemination. *J Gastroenterol Hepatol.* 2003;18:1323-1324.
20. Brandwein SL, Farrell JJ, Centeno BA, et al. Detection and tumor staging of malignancy in cystic, intraductal, and solid tumors of the pancreas by EUS. *Gastrointest Endosc.* 2001;53:722-727.
21. Hernandez LV, Mishra G, Forsmark C, et al. Role of endoscopic ultrasound (EUS) and EUS-guided fine needle aspiration in the diagnosis and treatment of cystic lesions of the pancreas. *Pancreas.* 2002;25:222-228.
22. Frossard JL, Amouyal P, Amouyal G, et al. Performance of endosonography-guided fine needle aspiration and biopsy in the diagnosis of pancreatic cystic lesions. *Am J Gastroenterol.* 2003;98:1516-1524.
23. Olson MT, Ali SZ. Cytotechnologist on-site evaluation of pancreas fine needle aspiration adequacy: comparison with cytopathologists and correlation with the final interpretation. *Acta Cytol.* 2012;56:340-346.
24. Maire F, Couvelard A, Hammel P, et al. Intraductal papillary mucinous tumors of the pancreas: the preoperative value of cytologic and histopathologic diagnosis. *Gastrointest Endosc.* 2003;58:701-706.
25. Lai R, Stanley MW, Bardales R, et al. Endoscopic ultrasound-guided pancreatic duct aspiration: diagnostic yield and safety. *Endoscopy.* 2002;34:715-720.
26. Hammel P, Voitot H, Vilgrain V, et al. Diagnostic value of CA 72-4 and carcinoembryonic antigen determination in the fluid of pancreatic cystic lesions. *Eur J Gastroenterol Hepatol.* 1998;10:345-348.
27. Rubin D, Warshaw AL, Southern JF, et al. Expression of CA 15.3 protein in the cyst contents distinguishes benign from malignant pancreatic mucinous cystic neoplasms. *Surgery.* 1994;115:52-55.
28. REFERENCE DELETED IN PROOFS.
29. Cizginer S, Turner BG, Bilge AR, et al. Cyst fluid carcinoembryonic antigen is an accurate diagnostic marker of pancreatic mucinous cysts. *Pancreas.* 2011;40:1024-1028.
30. van der Waaij LA, van Dullemen HM, Porte RJ. Cyst fluid analysis in the differential diagnosis of pancreatic cystic lesions: a pooled analysis. *Gastrointest Endosc.* 2005;62:383-389.
31. Hammel P, Levy P, Voitot H, et al. Preoperative cyst fluid analysis is useful for the differential diagnosis of cystic lesions of the pancreas. *Gastroenterology.* 1995;108:1230-1235.
32. Park WG, Mascarenhas R, Palaez-Luna M, et al. Diagnostic performance of cyst fluid carcinoembryonic antigen and amylase in histologically confirmed pancreatic cysts. *Pancreas.* 2011;40:42-45.
33. Al-Rashdan A, Schmidt CM, Al-Haddad M, et al. Fluid analysis prior to surgical resection of suspected mucinous pancreatic cysts. A single centre experience. *J Gastrointest Oncol.* 2011;2:208-214.
34. Yachida S, Jones S, Bozic I, et al. Distant metastasis occurs late during the genetic evolution of pancreatic cancer. *Nature.* 2010;467:1114-1117.
35. Jones S, Zhang X, Parsons DW, et al. Core signaling pathways in human pancreatic cancers revealed by global genomic analyses. *Science.* 2008;321:1801-1806.
36. Khalid A, Zahid M, Finkelstein SD, et al. Pancreatic cyst fluid DNA analysis in evaluating pancreatic cysts: a report of the PANDA study. *Gastrointest Endosc.* 2009;69:1095-1102.
37. Sreenarasimhaiah J, Lara LF, Jazrawi SF, et al. A comparative analysis of pancreas cyst fluid CEA and histology with DNA mutational analysis in the detection of mucin producing or malignant cysts. *JOP.* 2009;10:163-168.
38. Panarelli NC, Sela R, Schreiner AM, et al. Commercial molecular panels are of limited utility in the classification of pancreatic cystic lesions. *Am J Surg Pathol.* 2012;36:1434-1443.
39. Shen J, Brugge WR, Dimaio CJ, et al. Molecular analysis of pancreatic cyst fluid: a comparative analysis with current practice of diagnosis. *Cancer.* 2009;117:217-227.
40. Toll AD, Kowalski T, Loren D, et al. The added value of molecular testing in small pancreatic cysts. *JOP.* 2010;11:582-586.
41. Wu J, Jiao Y, Dal Molin M, et al. Whole-exome sequencing of neoplastic cysts of the pancreas reveals recurrent mutations in components of ubiquitin-dependent pathways. *Proc Natl Acad Sci U S A.* 2011;108:21188-21193.
42. Wu J, Matthaei H, Maitra A, et al. Recurrent GNAS mutations define an unexpected pathway for pancreatic cyst development. *Sci Transl Med.* 2011;3:92ra66.
43. Sakorafas GH, Smyrniotis V, Reid-Lombardo KM, et al. Primary pancreatic cystic neoplasms of the pancreas revisited. Part IV: rare cystic neoplasms. *Surg Oncol.* 2012;21:153-163.
44. Khashab MA, Shin EJ, Amateau S, et al. Tumor size and location correlate with behavior of pancreatic serous cystic neoplasms. *Am J Gastroenterol.* 2011;106:1521-1526.
45. Kimura W, Moriya T, Hanada K, et al. Multicenter study of serous cystic neoplasm of the Japan Pancreas Society. *Pancreas.* 2012;41:380-387.
46. Khalid A, Brugge W. ACG practice guidelines for the diagnosis and management of neoplastic pancreatic cysts. *Am J Gastroenterol.* 2007;102:2339-2349.
47. Malleo G, Bassi C, Rossini R, et al. Growth pattern of serous cystic neoplasms of the pancreas: observational study with long-term magnetic resonance surveillance and recommendations for treatment. *Gut.* 2012;61:746-751.
48. Yamao K, Yanagisawa A, Takahashi K, et al. Clinicopathological features and prognosis of mucinous cystic neoplasm with ovarian-type stroma: a multi-institutional study of the Japan Pancreas Society. *Pancreas.* 2011;40:67-71.
49. Reddy RP, Smyrk TC, Zapiach M, et al. Pancreatic mucinous cystic neoplasm defined by ovarian stroma: demographics, clinical features, and prevalence of cancer. *Clin Gastroenterol Hepatol.* 2004;2:1026-1031.

50. Crippa S, Salvia R, Warshaw AL, et al. Mucinous cystic neoplasm of the pancreas is not an aggressive entity: lessons from 163 resected patients. *Ann Surg.* 2008;247:571-579.

51. Tanaka M, Fernandez-Del Castillo C, Adsay V, et al. International consensus guidelines 2012 for the management of IPMN and MCN of the pancreas. *Pancreatology.* 2012;12:183-197.

52. Ohtsuka T, Kono H, Tanabe R, et al. Follow-up study after resection of intraductal papillary mucinous neoplasm of the pancreas; special references to the multifocal lesions and development of ductal carcinoma in the remnant pancreas. *Am J Surg.* 2012;204:44-48.

53. Mori Y, Ohtsuka T, Tsutsumi K, et al. Multifocal pancreatic ductal adenocarcinomas concomitant with intraductal papillary mucinous neoplasms of the pancreas detected by intraoperative pancreatic juice cytology. A case report. *JOP.* 2010;11:389-392.

54. Uehara H, Nakaizumi A, Ishikawa O, et al. Development of ductal carcinoma of the pancreas during follow-up of branch duct intraductal papillary mucinous neoplasm of the pancreas. *Gut.* 2008;57:1561-1565.

55. Kanno A, Satoh K, Hirota M, et al. Prediction of invasive carcinoma in branch type intraductal papillary mucinous neoplasms of the pancreas. *J Gastroenterol.* 2010;45:952-959.

56. He J, Cameron JL, Ahuja N, et al. Is it necessary to follow patients after resection of a benign pancreatic intraductal papillary mucinous neoplasm? *J Am Coll Surg.* 2013;216:657-665, discussion 665-667.

57. Ingkakul T, Sadakari Y, Ienaga J, et al. Predictors of the presence of concomitant invasive ductal carcinoma in intraductal papillary mucinous neoplasm of the pancreas. *Ann Surg.* 2010;251:70-75.

58. Furukawa T, Kloppel G, Volkan Adsay N, et al. Classification of types of intraductal papillary-mucinous neoplasm of the pancreas: a consensus study. *Virchows Arch.* 2005;447:794-799.

59. Maker AV, Katabi N, Gonen M, et al. Pancreatic cyst fluid and serum mucin levels predict dysplasia in intraductal papillary mucinous neoplasms of the pancreas. *Ann Surg Oncol.* 2011;18:199-206.

60. Tanaka M, Chari S, Adsay V, et al. International consensus guidelines for management of intraductal papillary mucinous neoplasms and mucinous cystic neoplasms of the pancreas. *Pancreatology.* 2006;6:17-32.

60a. Law JK, Ahmed A, Singh VK, et al. A systematic review of solid pseudopapillary neoplasms: Are these rare lesions? *Pancreas.* 2014;43:331-337.

61. Stoita A, Earls P, Williams D. Pancreatic solid pseudopapillary tumours—EUS FNA is the ideal tool for diagnosis. *ANZ J Surg.* 2010;80:615-618.

62. Song JS, Yoo CW, Kwon Y, et al. Endoscopic ultrasound-guided fine needle aspiration cytology diagnosis of solid pseudopapillary neoplasm: three case reports with review of literature. *Korean J Pathol.* 2012;46:399-406.

63. Salla C, Chatzipantelis P, Konstantinou P, et al. Endoscopic ultrasound-guided fine-needle aspiration cytology diagnosis of solid pseudopapillary tumor of the pancreas: a case report and literature review. *World J Gastroenterol.* 2007;13:5158-5163.

64. Nadler EP, Novikov A, Landzberg BR, et al. The use of endoscopic ultrasound in the diagnosis of solid pseudopapillary tumors of the pancreas in children. *J Pediatr Surg.* 2002;37:1370-1373.

65. Mergener K, Detweiler SE, Traverso LW. Solid pseudopapillary tumor of the pancreas: diagnosis by EUS-guided fine-needle aspiration. *Endoscopy.* 2003;35:1083-1084.

66. Master SS, Savides TJ. Diagnosis of solid-pseudopapillary neoplasm of the pancreas by EUS-guided FNA. *Gastrointest Endosc.* 2003;57:965-968.

67. Jhala N, Siegal GP, Jhala D. Large, clear cytoplasmic vacuolation: an under-recognized cytologic clue to distinguish solid pseudopapillary neoplasms of the pancreas from pancreatic endocrine neoplasms on fine-needle aspiration. *Cancer.* 2008;114:249-254.

68. Jani N, Dewitt J, Eloubeidi M, et al. Endoscopic ultrasound-guided fine-needle aspiration for diagnosis of solid pseudopapillary tumors of the pancreas: a multicenter experience. *Endoscopy.* 2008;40:200-203.

69. Cisco R, Jeffrey RB, Norton JA. Solid pseudopapillary tumor of the pancreas: an unexpected finding after minor abdominal trauma. *Dig Dis Sci.* 2010;55:240-241.

70. Chatzipantelis P, Salla C, Apostolou G, et al. Endoscopic ultrasound-guided fine needle aspiration cytology diagnosis of solid pseudopapillary tumor of the pancreas: a report of 3 cases. *Acta Cytol.* 2010;54:701-706.

71. Bardales RH, Centeno B, Mallery JS, et al. Endoscopic ultrasound-guided fine-needle aspiration cytology diagnosis of solid-pseudopapillary tumor of the pancreas: a rare neoplasm of elusive origin but characteristic cytomorphologic features. *Am J Clin Pathol.* 2004;121:654-662.

72. Konda VJ, Aslanian HR, Wallace MB, et al. First assessment of needle-based confocal laser endomicroscopy during EUS-FNA procedures of the pancreas (with videos). *Gastrointest Endosc.* 2011;74:1049-1060.

73. Iftimia N, Cizginer S, Deshpande V, et al. Differentiation of pancreatic cysts with optical coherence tomography (OCT) imaging: an ex vivo pilot study. *Biomed Opt Express.* 2011;2:2372-2382.

74. Kanda M, Knight S, Topazian MD, et al. Mutant GNAS detected in duodenal collections of secretin-stimulated pancreatic juice indicates the presence or emergence of pancreatic cysts. *Gut.* 2012.

75. Gan SI, Thompson CC, Lauwers GY, et al. Ethanol lavage of pancreatic cystic lesions: initial pilot study. *Gastrointest Endosc.* 2005;61:746-752.

76. Oh HC, Seo DW, Lee TY, et al. New treatment for cystic tumors of the pancreas: EUS-guided ethanol lavage with paclitaxel injection. *Gastrointest Endosc.* 2008;67:636-642.

77. Oh HC, Seo DW, Kim SC, et al. Septated cystic tumors of the pancreas: is it possible to treat them by endoscopic ultrasonography-guided intervention? *Scand J Gastroenterol.* 2009;44:242-247.

78. DeWitt J, McGreevy K, Schmidt CM, et al. EUS-guided ethanol versus saline solution lavage for pancreatic cysts: a randomized, double-blind study. *Gastrointest Endosc.* 2009;70:710-723.

79. Oh HC, Seo DW, Song TJ, et al. Endoscopic ultrasonography-guided ethanol lavage with paclitaxel injection treats patients with pancreatic cysts. *Gastroenterology.* 2011;140:172-179.

80. DiMaio CJ, DeWitt JM, Brugge WR. Ablation of pancreatic cystic lesions: the use of multiple endoscopic ultrasound-guided ethanol lavage sessions. *Pancreas.* 2011;40:664-668.

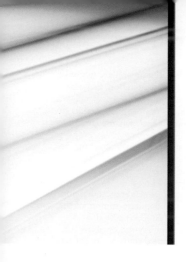

17

EUS in Bile Duct, Gallbladder, and Ampullary Lesions

Mohammad Al-Haddad

Key Points

- In patients with low to moderate clinical probability of CBD stones, EUS is recommended before ERCP is performed.
- In patients with acute pancreatitis of unknown origin or right upper quadrant pain with normal transabdominal ultrasound, EUS should be considered.
- In patients with a CBD stricture of unknown origin, EUS should be performed and, if inconclusive, ERCP should follow with tissue sampling with or without IDUS.
- Gallbladder polyps larger than 5 mm in size may be investigated with EUS to determine their malignant potential and to direct their subsequent therapeutic approach.
- Ampullary tumors can be staged with EUS and IDUS. EUS is better to differentiate between early (adenoma, T1) and advanced (T2-4) tumors. IDUS may help to stage early tumors.

General Examination Checklist for Biliary Stones and Tumors and Ampullary Lesions

Extrahepatic ducts (dilatation, stones)
Intrahepatic ducts (dilation)
Left and right liver lobes
Gallbladder
Ampulla (including IDUS in the case of T1 ampullary lesions)
Pancreatic main and accessory duct
Lymph nodes
Ascites
Portal hypertension

EUS and Biliary Stones

Bile Duct Stones

Endoscopic retrograde cholangiopancreatography (ERCP) has long been considered the best diagnostic method for common bile duct (CBD) stones. Moreover, ERCP allows stone removal during the same endoscopic session when combined with endoscopic sphincterotomy (ES). Nevertheless, it remains an invasive procedure and carries a substantial risk of complications,[1–3] although when performed by experienced endoscopists, the complication and mortality rates can be reduced to under 5% and 0.1%, respectively.[4] Furthermore, because it can be difficult to differentiate small stones from aerobilia, a substantial proportion of ERCP procedures are

completed with ES in order to confirm the diagnosis of choledocholithiasis. ES has a complication rate of 5% to 10%,[5–8] with a current mortality rate of less than 1%.[5–10] Long-term complications, such as stenosis and nonobstructive cholangitis, occur in approximately 10% of patients[11–13] because of permanent loss of biliary sphincter function.[14]

An accurate diagnostic tool associated with lower morbidity and mortality rates would reserve ERCP for patients with confirmed CBD stones. Transabdominal ultrasonography (TUS) is a noninvasive imaging modality, practically risk-free and widely available. Patients presenting with clinical and/or laboratory suspicion of CBD stones should undergo TUS as an initial diagnostic evaluation. However, although TUS is very sensitive and specific for cholelithiasis,[15] its sensitivity for the diagnosis of choledocholithiasis remains limited,[16,17] even in heavily calcified CBD stones. The location and orientation of the bile duct, along with adjacent duodenal air, make imaging of the distal bile duct difficult. Abdominal fat attenuates ultrasound waves, making this technique less effective in obese patients.

In the past decade, other imaging modalities such as multidetector computed tomography (CT), endoscopic ultrasonography (EUS), and magnetic resonance cholangiopancreatography (MRCP) have been effectively employed for the diagnosis of CBD stones, avoiding the need for the more invasive cholangiography (during ERCP or intraoperatively). The sensitivity, specificity, and accuracy of helical CT range from 85% to 88%, 88% to 97%, and 86% to 94%, respectively.[18,19] Nevertheless, the sensitivity of CT for detecting

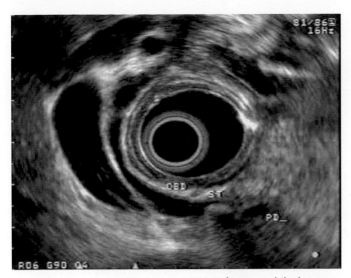

FIGURE 17-1 Linear EUS image (7.5 MHz) of common bile duct stone in a patient presenting with right upper quadrant pain and elevated transaminases.

Video 17-1. Interrogation of the head of the pancreas, distal bile duct, and pancreatic duct using a radial echoendoscope in a patient presenting with right upper quadrant pain and elevated transaminases. A free-floating nonshadowing echogenic structure, suggestive of a noncalcified stone, is noted in the common bile duct.

stones less than 5 mm in size remains significantly lower than those larger than 5 mm.[20] In one comparative study with MRCP and EUS, helical CT was inferior to both modalities,[21] although multiplanar reconstructions with multidetector CT can improve its specificity.[22,23] Therefore EUS and MRCP remain the most accurate minimally invasive methods for diagnosing CBD stones.

The Performance of EUS and MRCP for the Diagnosis of Choledocholithiasis

EUS provides excellent sonographic visualization of the extrahepatic biliary tree. Bile duct stones are shown as echo-dense structures (Figures 17-1 and 17-2) within the ampulla or CBD, sometimes freely moving within the duct, with or without acoustic shadowing or inflammatory thickening of the bile duct wall (Video 17-1). The accuracy of EUS was found to be higher than that of ERCP for the detection of small CBD stones[24] (Figure 17-3), with significantly reduced invasiveness[25–27] and a lower technical failure rate.[26,28] The specificity of EUS in ruling out the presence of CBD stones

was 98%[29] in some series. Additionally, EUS detects bile duct sludge as well as microlithiasis (Figure 17-4), often missed by the other imaging techniques.[30]

MRCP is a noninvasive, radiation-free imaging modality and is more accurate than CT for the diagnosis of choledocholithiasis.[21,31–41] The disadvantages of this technique include the limited spatial resolution, the difficulty of diagnosing CBD stones in the periampullary region, lack of availability in some areas, need for operator's experience to interpret findings, and high cost.[42] Moreover, MRCP is contraindicated in patients with metallic hardware such as pacemakers or cerebral aneurysm clips. Claustrophobic patients, estimated to represent 4% of the population,[43] often cannot complete the examination. EUS offers higher spatial resolution than MRCP (0.1 versus 1 to 1.5 mm), and its sensitivity for detecting choledocholithiasis does not vary with the stone size such as MRCP.[44] Thus it is not surprising that stones missed by MRCP were always smaller than 10 mm[45,46] and that the sensitivity of MRCP decreased to approximately 65% for diagnosing stones smaller than 5 mm.[21,44,45] Nevertheless, improvements in imaging may in the future permit the detection of smaller calculi, as shown in a recent series.[47]

To compare the performance of each technique, some parameters have to be considered. The first consideration is the delay between the performance of the technique being evaluated and the "gold standard" examination. Spontaneous stone migration between the two examinations increases with time and can lead to false-positive results. In a study comparing EUS and ERCP, when both were performed sequentially on every patient, stone migration was found to have occurred in 21% of patients within 1 month.[48] Ideally, in comparative studies the gold standard examination should be performed immediately or shortly after the evaluated technique. Second, the perfect gold standard is a matter of debate. ERCP and intraoperative cholangiography are the reference techniques most commonly chosen. Nevertheless, it is well known that opacification alone is not sufficient to exclude CBD stones because its sensitivity is only around 90%. The best reference standard comes from the association of ERCP, ES, and instrumental exploration of the CBD (with a Dormia basket or balloon). However, because of associated morbidity and mortality, this approach is not pursued in patients with low or moderate risk of CBD stones. Another approach in these patients would be to perform ERCP, ES, and bile duct exploration when a stone is found and to follow the patient when a stone has been excluded. Because some patients with CBD stones missed by this approach remain symptom-free for a

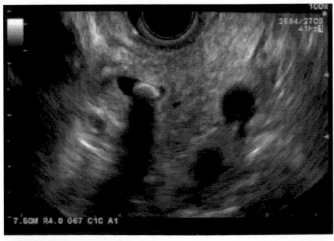

FIGURE 17-2 Linear EUS image (7.5 MHz) of a shadowing 5-mm common bile duct stone.

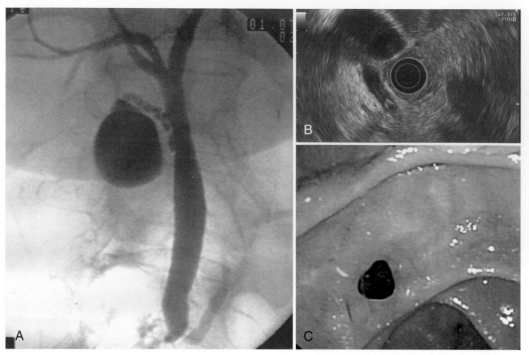

FIGURE 17-3 **A,** Fluoroscopy image of a CBD without any filling defects at ERCP, but identified on EUS (radial echoendoscope, 6 MHz) (**B**) and confirmed by biliary sphincterotomy and after balloon sweeping of the common bile duct (**C**).

long time, follow-up must be sufficiently long enough for firm conclusions to be drawn. In series in which patients were followed for up to 1 year, no stone was detected after 6 months of follow-up.[24,49]

The body of literature evaluating the respective performances of EUS and MRCP can therefore be classified into three groups (Tables 17-1 and 17-2) based on the level of proof, from the most to the least significant:

Level 1: Technique compared with the gold standard (ERCP, ES, and CBD instrumental exploration) with a very short interval between the two examinations.[50-53]

Level 2: Technique compared with ERCP and ES if a stone is found and with clinical and laboratory follow-up of at least 6 months if no stone is found.*

Level 3: Technique compared with cholangiography (ERCP or intraoperative).[21,28,61-75]

The diagnostic performance of EUS has been evaluated in two meta-analyses covering 3532 and 2673 patients.[76,77] The pooled sensitivity and specificity of EUS were 89% to 94% and 94% to 95%, respectively. The evidence for the use of MRCP for the diagnosis of CBD stones has been examined in a systematic review of 10 studies where MRCP achieved a high sensitivity (range 80% to 100%) and specificity (range 83% to 98%).[78] According to comparative studies, EUS was found to be either superior[47,48] or equivalent[2,47,61,68,69] to MRCP for the diagnosis of choledocholithiasis. One meta-analysis[79] and one systematic review[80] comparing EUS and MRCP for depicting CBD stones showed a high diagnostic performance for both modalities. Although no statistically significant differences were found between the two modalities, a trend toward higher sensitivity and specificity for EUS (93% and 88% to 96%) compared to MRCP (83% to 85% and 89% to 93%) was evident. This was especially obvious in the case of small stones causing acute biliary pancreatitis. Nevertheless, the choice between these two techniques should depend on others factors such as resource availability, operator experience, and cost.

Endosonographic Tools

In most EUS literature, EUS radial echoendoscopes were used for assessment of choledocholithiasis. Nevertheless, the

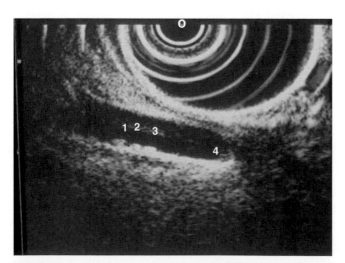

FIGURE 17-4 Radial EUS image of common bile duct microlithiasis (four small stones seen). *(Figure courtesy of Dr Mohamad Eloubeidi.)*

*24,25,47,49,54–60

TABLE 17-1

PERFORMANCE OF EUS IN THE DIAGNOSIS OF COMMON BILE DUCT STONES

Reference (Year)	Level of Evidence[a]	Number of Patients	Frequency of CBD Stones (%)	EUS Sensitivity (%)	Specificity (%)	PPV (%)	NPV (%)	Accuracy (%)
Aubertin et al[50] (1996)	1	50	24	96	96	92	100	98
Prat et al[53] (1996)	1	119	66	93	97	98	88	95
Kohut et al[51] (2002)	1	134	68	93	93	98	87	94
Meroni et al[52] (2004)	1	47	15	71	90	55	95	—
Dancygier et al[56] (1994)	2	31	39	96	50	100	—	98
Norton et al[59] (1997)	2	50	48	86	94	95	89	92
Burtin et al[54] (1997)	2	68	49	97	98	100	96	98
Canto et al[25] (1998)	2	64	30	84	98	94	93	94
Chak et al[115] (1999)	2	31	36	88	98	100	95	97
Liu et al[29] (2000)	2	139	35	98	98	100	96	99
Prat et al[60] (2001)	2	123	27	100	100	100	100	100
Berdah et al[49] (2001)	2	68	20	96	97	93	100	98
Buscarini et al[55] (2003)	2	463	52	98	99	99	98	97
Kohut et al[83] (2003)	2	55	9	75	99	100	98	98
Aubé et al[47] (2005)	2	45	34	94	97	94	97	96
Ney et al[58] (2005)	2	68	32	96	99	100	97	98
Amouyal et al[62] (1994)	3	62	36	97	100	94	97	96
Shim et al[71] (1995)	3	132	21	89	100	100	97	98
Palazzo et al[28] (1995)	3	422	36	95	98	—	—	96
Sugiyama et al[73] (1997)	3	142	36	97	99	100	95	98
Montariol et al[69] (1998)	3	215	19	85	93	75	96	92
De Ledinghen et al[64] (1999)	3	32	31	100	95	91	100	97
Lachter et al[67] (2000)	3	50	66	96	75	89	93	94
Materne et al[68] (2000)	3	50	26	97	88	94	93	94
Scheiman et al[70] (2001)	3	28	18	80	95	80	96	—
Ainsworth et al[61] (2004)	3	163	33	90	99	98	94	93
Kondo et al[21] (2005)	3	30	86	98	50	92	100	93
Dittrick et al[65] (2005)	3	30	37	100	84	56	100	—

[a]Level 1: technique compared with endoscopic retrograde cholangiopancreatography (ERCP) + systematic endoscopic sphincterotomy (ES) with a very short interval between the technique and ERCP; Level 2: technique compared with ERCP + ES if positive, and clinical and biological follow-up of at least 6 months if negative; Level 3: technique compared with ERC or with intraoperative cholangiography.
CBD, common bile duct; EUS, endoscopic ultrasound; NPV, negative predictive value; PPV, positive predictive value.

accuracy of linear EUS appeared to be comparable to that of the radial examination, as indicated in some series[51,67,81–83] comparing linear EUS with ERCP plus ES, or choledochotomy with choledochoscopy (see Table 17-1).

The use of extraductal catheter probe EUS (EDUS) has also been evaluated in two studies.[81,84] In the earlier published prospective study, EDUS with a radial scanning catheter probe was performed before ERCP and ES in patients with suspected CBD stones or other obstructive pathologies of the distal CBD.[84] EDUS detected 33 of 34 bile duct stones. In eight patients, the stones were missed on ERCP but seen after ES. More recently, the same group conducted another prospective trial to compare the diagnostic potential of EDUS with that of conventional EUS,[81] where EDUS was found to be nearly as accurate as linear array EUS.

Intraductal ultrasonography (IDUS) has also been proposed recently for this indication (Figure 17- 5). In a prospective study of patients with suspected CBD stones who underwent ERCP, 20-MHz IDUS was performed in those with equivocal cholangiograms or cholangiographic evidence of stones.[85] Interestingly, no stones were found in 36% of patients with a positive finding on ERCP. This, according to the

authors, was partly due to the existence of aerobilia. In 35% of patients with a negative ERCP, sludge or stones were found on IDUS and were confirmed on ES. Another study demonstrated that the addition of IDUS to confirm complete stone clearance after ES decreased the recurrence rate of CBD stones (13.2% in the non-IDUS group compared to 3.4% in the IDUS group).[86]

The sensitivity of MRCP, ERCP, and IDUS for the diagnosis of choledocholithiasis was 80%, 90%, and 95%, respectively, in a prospective trial, which also demonstrated that the accuracy of IDUS plus ERCP was superior to that of ERCP alone.[87] IDUS could be particularly helpful in non-opaque stones, as recently demonstrated in a study including patients with various calcium density CBD stones,[88] where IDUS identified all 148 patients with duct stones (100%) as opposed to ERCP, which missed three stones in the same group of patients. However, IDUS cannot be proposed as a routine procedure because of the morbidity associated with ERCP. It can be utilized prior to ES in patients in whom CBD stones have been found on EUS or MRCP but not on ERCP or following ES to confirm complete stone clearance.

TABLE 17-2

PERFORMANCE OF MAGNETIC RESONANCE CHOLANGIOPANCREATOGRAPHY IN THE DIAGNOSIS OF COMMON BILE DUCT STONES

Reference (year)	Level of Evidence[a]	Number of Patients	Magnetic Resonance Cholangiopancreatography				
			Sensitivity (%)	Specificity (%)	PPV (%)	NPV (%)	Accuracy (%)
Gautier et al[57] (2004)	2	99	96	99	—	—	—
Aubé et al[47] (2005)	2	45	88	97	93	93	—
Mofidi et al[32] (2008)	2	49	100	96	—	—	—
Topal et al[33] (2003)	2	315	95	100	100	98	—
Scaffidi et al[34] (2009)	2	120	88	72	87	72	83
De Ledinghen et al[64] (1999)	3	32	100	73	62	100	82
Cervi et al[63] (2000)	3	60	100	94	—	—	—
Demartines et al[75] (2000)	3	70	100	96	93	100	—
Stiris et al[72] (2000)	3	50	88	94	97	81	—
Materne et al[68] (2000)	3	50	91	94	88	95	92
Scheiman et al[70] (2001)	3	28	40	96	66	88	—
Kim et al[66] (2002)	3	121	95	95	—	—	95
Taylor et al[74] (2002)	3	146	98	89	84	99	—
Griffin et al[36] (2003)	3	115	84	96	91	93	92
Ainsworth et al[61] (2004)	3	163	87	97	95	93	—
Kondo et al[21] (2005)	3	30	88	75	96	50	86
Ausch et al[35] (2005)	3	773	94	98	80	99	—
Hallal et al[38] (2005)	3	29	100	91	50	100	92
Makary et al[96] (2005)	3	64	94	98	94	98	—
Moon et al[39] (2005)	3	32	80	83	89	71	81
De Waele et al[37] (2007)	3	104	83	98	91	95	94
Norero et al[41] (2008)	3	125	97	74	89	90	90
Richard et al[40] (2013)	3	70	27	83	36	77	69

[a]Level 1: technique compared with endoscopic retrograde cholangiopancreatography (ERCP) + systematic endoscopic sphincterotomy (ES) with a very short interval between the technique and ERCP; Level 2: technique compared with ERCP + ES if positive, and clinical and biological follow-up of at least 6 months if negative; Level 3: technique compared with ERC or with intraoperative cholangiography.
NPV, negative predictive value; PPV, positive predictive value.

The Use of EUS, MRCP, and ERCP in the Management of Choledocholithiasis

The use of noninvasive imaging modalities resulted in a considerable reduction in the number of inappropriate ERCP with bile duct instrumentation.[24,26,55,89,90] One meta-analysis comparing an EUS-guided ERCP strategy with an ERCP-only strategy found that the use of EUS significantly reduced the risk of overall complications (relative risk 0.35) by safely avoiding ERCP in 67.1% of patients.[90] Whether or not an EUS or MRCP would be necessary prior to ERCP depends on the pretest probability of having a stone in the CBD. Patients suspected of having choledocholithiasis on clinical and laboratory criteria and/or ultrasound (US) can be grouped into risk groups ranging from low to high.[91,92] The definition of each risk category has not been very accurately characterized in the literature[91,93,94] due to the variability of criteria used. When considering the published studies, the proportion of high-risk patients who actually have CBD stones was less than 80% (66% to 78%),[25,53,55,95] whereas fewer than 40% of patients classified as being at intermediate (also called moderate) risk had choledocholithiasis (19% to 44%).* Most experts agree that ERCP could be performed as a first-line approach in patients at high risk of CBD stones,[24,25,28] although it may be impossible to completely avoid unnecessary ERCP procedures altogether.[97]

EUS as a first-line approach in patients in the high-risk category has already found some support either to exclude a stone or to evaluate other causes of biliary symptoms.[31,55] Moreover, EUS confirming CBD stones would justify the use of aggressive techniques, such as precut papillotomy, if needed. However, there is still no general agreement in regard

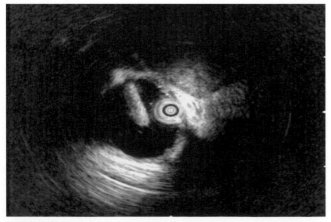

FIGURE 17-5 Two-dimensional intraductal ultrasound showing a shadowing common bile duct stone.

---

*25,28,49,53,62,71,73,96

to the routine utilization of EUS in such cases.[98] Practically, the best approach is probably to perform EUS followed by ERCP (with or without ES) when a stone is found during the same endoscopic session.[99,100]

Intermediate-risk patients include those who present with symptoms compatible with biliary origin, along with liver test abnormalities or dilated CBD on TUS. The general consensus is to consider EUS (or MRCP) as the first-line diagnostic approach (after TUS).[26,89,90,101,102] This approach was evaluated in the context of laparoscopic cholecystectomy.[49] First-line ERCP was performed in patients considered to be at high risk based on preoperative criteria, and EUS was performed before laparoscopic cholecystectomy in intermediate-risk patients. Choledocholithiases were found in 19% of the intermediate-risk patients and 78% of the high-risk patients. This EUS-based approach was efficient and optimized the surgical management of gallstones. After a mean follow-up of 32 months, no retained stones were found in this series of 300 patients.

For low-risk patients, who typically have no biliary symptoms or liver test abnormalities and have no CBD dilatation on TUS, no further examination is necessary. We suggest an algorithm to investigate patients with suspected choledocholithiasis based on their risk stratification (Figure 17-6).

The utilization of EUS as a first-line strategy was associated with potential advantages in cost-effectiveness studies. In a prospective study of 485 patients suspected of having CBD stones where EUS was always performed regardless of the risk classification, the mean cost for patients managed by the EUS-based strategy was significantly lower than that for patients who had ERCP.[55] In another study, the EUS-guided ERCP strategy resulted in a 14% reduction in ERCP procedures and was associated with significant cost savings.[103] Other studies

have found that EUS was the most cost-effective strategy in the intermediate-risk group, whereas in patients with a probability of CBD stones above 50% (high-risk group), the more cost-effective approach was to perform ERCP first.[25,61,97,104] In patients with acute biliary pancreatitis, an economic evaluation concluded that an EUS-based strategy was associated with lower costs, a reduction in the number of procedures, and fewer complications. This was especially obvious in patients with severe acute pancreatitis.[105] Finally, a randomized study comparing EUS and ERCP during the same endoscopic session versus EUS and ERCP in two separate sessions for the management of choledocholithiasis[100] showed that the average procedure time and days of hospitalization were significantly reduced in the first group, resulting in significant reductions in total costs. It is important to note that cost estimation in the literature can be difficult to assess from one country to another because of variability in health care systems and resources. In addition, cost assessment is also influenced by operator expertise, which is crucial not only for the accuracy of EUS but also for the performance and complications rate of ERCP and the subsequent need for repeated explorations.

In summary, EUS is the ideal alternative to cholangiography for the evaluation of choledocholithiasis, selecting only those patients with confirmed CBD stones for ERCP. MRCP can be utilized as an alternative when there are contraindications to sedation or when EUS is not available. ERCP should be avoided if biliary EUS is normal,[24,26,89,90] unless symptoms persist or recur during follow-up. Ideally, EUS and ERCP should be combined in a single endoscopic session whenever possible to reduce risks of repeated sedation and to minimize costs. When this approach is not feasible, high-risk patients could be managed with ERCP at first.

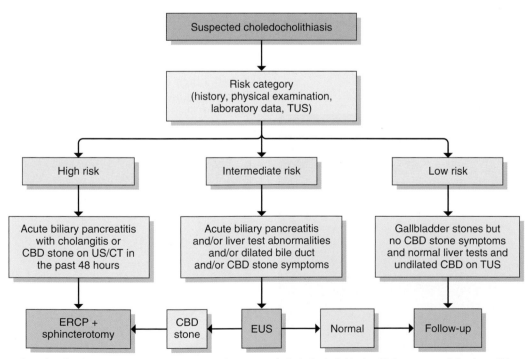

FIGURE 17-6 An algorithm for the management of patients with suspected choledocholithiasis. CBD, common bile duct; CT, computed tomography; ERCP, endoscopic retrograde cholangiopancreatography; US, ultrasonography.

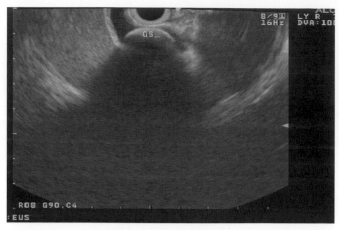

FIGURE 17-7 Linear EUS image (7.5 MHz) of a solitary shadowing gallstone incidentally noted during assessment of an esophageal subepithelial lesion.

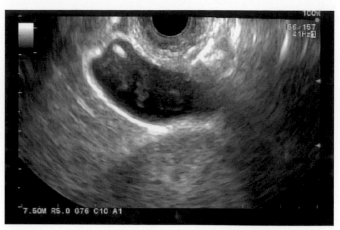

FIGURE 17-9 Linear EUS image (7.5 MHz) of a moderate amount of sludge adjacent to a small gallstone in an asymptomatic patient.

Gallstones

TUS is an excellent modality for the diagnosis of cholelithiasis, with a sensitivity and specificity of 97% and 95%, respectively, according to one meta-analysis.[106] Sensitivity is lower for small stones with a diameter of 3 mm or less and in obese patients with thick abdominal walls. The use of bile crystal analysis is justified when there is discordance in the clinical picture such as negative US findings but highly suggestive symptoms.[107] Because of its value in diagnosing small CBD stones, EUS has also been evaluated for detecting cholelithiasis (Figures 17-7 and 17-8). A study by Dill and colleagues[108] showed that EUS was as accurate as biliary crystal analysis for the diagnosis of microlithiasis (Figures 17-9 and 17-10) and failed in only one occasion in a group of 58 patients with biliary-type pain and negative TUS findings. The utility of EUS in the detection of cholelithiasis in patients with biliary pain and normal US has since been supported by several other studies showing EUS as an effective modality that can influence the management of these patients.[109–111] For example, Thorboll and colleagues[111] studied patients with a normal

TUS but with suspected gallstones based on clinical grounds and detected cholelithiasis in 18 of 35 patients (51.4%).

Idiopathic acute pancreatitis (IAP) can be the result of biliary sludge or microlithiasis undetected by other imaging techniques. Although the reported incidence of occult gallstones in IAP varies (ranging from 10% to 73%),[112–114] this remains the most common cause of pancreatitis in patients with an intact gallbladder. In one study, gallstones were found by EUS in 14 of 18 patients with negative findings on TUS.[29] Another study by Chak and colleagues[115] demonstrated that EUS and TUS had sensitivities of 91% and 50%, respectively, with corresponding accuracies of 97% and 83%, respectively. In a larger series[30] of 168 patients with IAP, EUS identified gallbladder sludge or very small stones in 40% of patients, with or without associated CBD stones that were missed by other examinations. Overall, EUS was able to detect a cause for acute pancreatitis in 80% of patients. In the study by Yusoff and colleagues, EUS established a presumptive diagnosis in 31% of 201 patients with a single episode of IAP.[116] The most frequent cause of pancreatitis in patients with a gallbladder was chronic pancreatitis or biliary sludge. A systematic review evaluating the role of EUS in idiopathic pancreatitis showed a high diagnostic yield, especially in patients with a single idiopathic episode and in patients with recurrent episodes and gallbladder in situ.[117] Moreover, a recent study

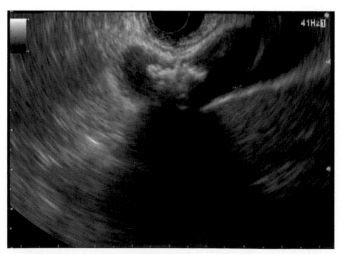

FIGURE 17-8 Linear EUS image (7.5 MHz) of multiple heavily calcified gallbladder stones.

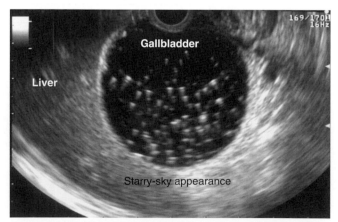

FIGURE 17-10 Radial EUS image (6 MHz) of extensive sludge in the gallbladder (starry-sky appearance).

concluded that EUS was the most cost-effective initial test in the evaluation of IAP when compared with other strategies, including ERCP with manometry, bile aspiration, and laparoscopic cholecystectomy.[118] Therefore an EUS-based strategy appears to be the best approach to evaluate patients with IAP because of the high diagnostic accuracy of EUS, not only for gallbladder sludge and stones but also for pancreatic diseases, and its minimally invasive nature. In patients with multiple unexplained attacks, particularly in postcholecystectomy cases, ERCP and sphincter of Oddi manometry should be considered after negative EUS results.

Summary

EUS is the most effective method for confirming the presence or absence of CBD stones. Its utility in avoiding unnecessary ERCP has been validated in patients at low or moderate risk of CBD stones. MRCP can probably be used as an alternative to EUS if available and there are no contraindications. EUS remains the preferred diagnostic test in the setting of acute pancreatitis, where biliary stones can be very small and can be missed on MRCP. For patients at high risk of CBD stones, ERCP with or without ES (in case CBD stones were found on cholangiography) can be considered as the first-line approach; however, EUS, if available and able to be performed during the same endoscopic session with ERCP, would be optimal. EUS is now a well-established modality after TUS for the diagnosis of gallstones and sludge in patients with unexplained right hypochondrial pain and also in those with an acute pancreatitis of unknown origin.

Diagnostic Checklist

CBD or gallstone
- Hyperechoic mobile structure with or without acoustic shadowing

Associated signs
- Dilation of extrahepatic ducts and/or cystic duct
- Thickening of the gallbladder and/or bile duct wall
- Thickening of the ampulla
- Pericholecystic fluid

EUS in Bile Duct Strictures

Benign and malignant bile duct strictures remain a diagnostic challenge for the gastroenterologist. Although TUS and CT can reliably demonstrate dilated bile ducts, they allow assessment of the cause in only two-thirds of cases.[17,119] Apart from contiguous tumor invasion or metastasis, MRCP appears to be no better than ERCP in the diagnosis of malignancy in this setting.[120] However, MRCP could be superior in investigating the anatomic extent of the lesion compared to ERCP because it displays the biliary tree proximal to the obstruction.[121] ERCP is highly accurate for the confirmation of obstructive jaundice, but little additional information could be obtained for tumor staging as only indirect tumor signs such as stenosis, suprastenotic dilation, or both can be visualized, and the tumor itself is generally not well seen.

Intraductal tissue sampling is commonly used at the time of ERCP. Brushing has a low sensitivity for the diagnosis of bile duct tumors of 27% to 56%,[122–126] because of their

desmoplastic nature or submucosal spread of the tumor, and is often negative for extrinsic tumors (pancreatic cancer, gallbladder cancer, metastatic lymph nodes). New ancillary cytology-based techniques have been recently developed to improve the sensitivity of routine cytology. Such techniques include fluorescent in situ hybridization (FISH) analysis that detects chromosomal polysomy using fluorescent probes and digital image analysis (DIA) technique to assess for the presence of aneuploidy.[127,128] FISH appears to be a promising technology that has been shown to increase the sensitivity of brush cytology from 21% to 58% in one recent study[129] and requires only a small amount of tissue.

Additional means of tissue sampling include direct forceps biopsies during ERCP, which has a higher sensitivity than brush cytology alone, with sensitivity ranging from 44% to 89% in cholangiocarcinoma and 33% to 71% in pancreatic cancer.[130–134] Nevertheless, this technique is limited by its low negative predictive value (NPV). This has led to the development of new methods to abrade the tumor surface in order to improve cytologic yield. For example, the combination of stricture dilation, endoscopic needle aspiration, and biliary brush cytology has been shown to improve the diagnostic yield in malignant strictures compared with brushings alone.[135] Nevertheless, these results have not been confirmed by others.[136] Currently, bile duct biopsy under direct cholangioscopy[137,138] presents a very promising method of biliary sampling using the new single operator cholangioscopy system, with a sensitivity up to 93% based on direct biopsies.[139–142] However, cholangioscopy remains an invasive procedure, carries a complication rate of 7%,[143] and is not widely available in all centers. Therefore biliary strictures often remain a diagnostic dilemma even after extensive invasive and noninvasive imaging procedures have been performed.[144,145]

The Performance of EUS and IDUS in Biliary Strictures

EUS has proved to be a useful tool in assessing biliary obstruction because it readily enables visualization of the entire CBD. Therefore it can be helpful in the differential diagnosis of bile duct strictures and neoplasia and local tumor staging[56,146–148] (Figures 17-11 and 17-12). In a meta-analysis of nine studies including a total of 555 patients, EUS had an estimated sensitivity of 78% and a specificity of 84% in detecting malignant biliary strictures.[76] The ability to acquire tissue by EUS-guided fine-needle aspiration (FNA) significantly improves the diagnostic yield when evaluating biliary strictures and is associated with a minimal risk of complications. Because the distal common bile duct is located immediately under the echoendoscope transducer when examined from the duodenal bulb, EUS performs extremely well for evaluating distal biliary strictures (Video 17.2). EUS FNA is highly accurate in diagnosing malignancy in distal biliary strictures, particularly in patients with masses within the pancreatic head.[149–157] In this setting, the overall EUS FNA sensitivity and specificity rates range from 81% to 91% and from 71% to 100%, respectively.* A meta-analysis of nine studies that included 284 patients who underwent EUS FNA of biliary strictures and gallbladder

---

*149,151,155,156,158,159

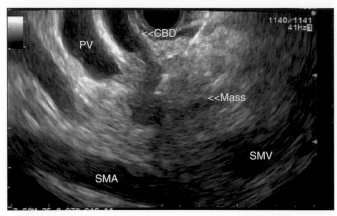

FIGURE 17-11 Linear EUS image (7.5 MHz) of a periampullary mass lesion originating from the distal common bile duct (CBD). The patient presented with painless jaundice. Superior mesenteric artery (SMA) and vein (SMV) appear free of tumor encasement, which abuts the portal vein (PV). Cholangiocarcinoma was confirmed on fine-needle aspiration of this mass.

masses showed a pooled sensitivity and specificity of 84% and 100%, respectively.[160] Nevertheless, the reported accuracies are lower for cholangiocarcinomas, mainly due to the inclusion of the hilar cholangiocarcinomas (Klatskin tumors) and the difficulty visualizing and sampling such tumors via EUS due to distance from the probe. Moreover, proximal biliary lesions tend to often be small and diffusely infiltrating, unlike distal biliary strictures that frequently present as focal solid masses. Cytologic diagnosis is an important adjunct to EUS and helps direct patient management and avoid unnecessary surgery. The sensitivity of EUS FNA is reported to be 45% to 100% for all biliary strictures whereas its sensitivity for proximal biliary strictures ranges from 25% to 89%* (Table 17-3). These figures might be an overestimation of the real performance of EUS FNA in hilar strictures because most of the studies included a mixture of proximal and distal strictures. Limited experience with a newly developed forward-viewing linear echoendoscope (GF-UCT160J-AL5, Olympus Medical Center Valley, PA, USA) suggests improved imaging of hilar strictures and easier EUS FNA technique.[172]

---

*159,161–165,157,163,166–171

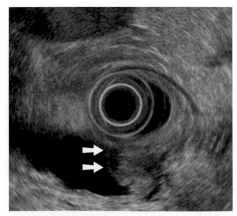

FIGURE 17-12 Radial EUS image (5 MHz) of a soft tissue mass (*arrows*) in the lumen of the common bile duct causing upstream obstruction. This was consistent with infiltrative cholangiocarcinoma.

Video 17-2. Interrogation of the bile duct using a linear echoendoscope in a patient presenting with obstructive jaundice. A solid distal bile duct mass is noted in association with loss of the characteristic layers of the bile duct wall in that location. A bile duct stent appears as a hyperechoic structure in the lumen of the bile duct. The bile duct wall upstream from the stricture appears thickened.

With the advent of high-frequency (20-MHz) mini-probes over a guidewire, IDUS has emerged as a feasible and promising imaging technique in the diagnosis of biliary strictures. Mini-probes can now be easily inserted through the papilla without the need for sphincterotomy in most cases.[173,174] IDUS provides an accurate image of the bile duct wall and surrounding tissue. Despite the limited depth of penetration, a precise image of an intraductal lesion is often possible, allowing assessment for invasion or compression of adjacent structures. IDUS is also faster and easier to learn than conventional EUS. It should be performed prior to drainage in order to avoid inflammatory artifacts and therefore is best performed by ERCP experts during the same procedure.[175] IDUS allows complete examination of bile duct strictures in 86% to 100% of cases,[135,174,176–180] generally without previous dilation. Most failures were due to tight strictures of the hilum or intrahepatic ducts that the guidewire could not traverse.[174,179] In Klatskin tumors, the examination is generally possible from the opposite side when the right or left hepatic duct stenosis cannot be traversed by the probe. The presence of a guidewire in the bile duct throughout the procedure does not usually interfere with US imaging (in case of artifact, the guidewire could be removed before IDUS). The recent generations of IDUS consist of an ultrasonic probe that is automatically moved for scanning within an external sheath and is capable of performing both linear and radial imaging simultaneously in real time with a single scanning operation. Three-dimensional images can also be generated automatically, and the time required for examination is reduced compared with two-dimensional IDUS. Although some authors[181] have suggested that three-dimensional IDUS can be more useful for evaluating the extent of cholangiocarcinoma, comparative studies between two- and three-dimensional systems would be necessary to assess other possible advantages of this technology.

As with EUS, three layers are seen in the bile duct wall. The first hyperechoic layer corresponds to the mucosa in addition to a border echo; the second hypoechoic layer is the smooth muscle fibers with fibroelastic tissue; and the third hyperechoic layer is the thin and loose connective tissue with a border echo.[182,183] The criteria for malignancy of a stricture are disruption of the normal three-layer sonographic pattern of the bile duct wall (outer echogenic, middle hypoechoic, inner echogenic) (Figures 17-13 and 17-14), a hypoechoic infiltrating lesion with irregular margins, heterogeneous echo-poor areas invading surrounding tissue, and continuation of

TABLE 17-3

OPERATING CHARACTERISTICS OF EUS FINE-NEEDLE ASPIRATION IN BILIARY STRICTURES

Reference (year)	Number of Strictures	Number of Strictures Confirmed Malignant[a]	Hilar Biliary Strictures	Overall Performance in All Strictures					Sensitivity in Hilar Strictures (%)
				Sensitivity (%)	Specificity (%)	PPV (%)	NPV (%)	Accuracy (%)	
Fritscher-Ravens et al[163] (2000)	10	10	10	80	—	100	—	—	80
Rösch et al[190] (2002)	43	26	3	79	62	76	66	—	—
Lee et al[159] (2004)	42	24	1	47	100	100	50	—	—
Eloubeidi et al[166] (2004)	28	21	15	86	100	100	57	88	67
Fritscher-Ravens et al[167] (2004)	44	32	44	89	100	100	67	91	89
Rösch et al[165] (2004)	50	28	11	75	100	100	58	70	25
Byrne et al[161] (2004)	35	11	3	45	100	100	—	—	—
Meara et al[164] (2006)	46	30	—	87	100	—	—	—	—
DeWitt et al[162] (2006)	24	23	24	77	100	100	29	79	77
Saifuku et al[171] (2010)	34	17	0	94	82	84	93	88	—
Mohamadnejad et al[157] (2011)	81	81	30	73	100	—	—	—	59
Ohshima et al[169] (2011)	22	18	2	100	100	100	100	100	—
Nayar et al[170] (2011)	32	24	32	52	100	100	54	68	52
Tummala et al[168] (2013)	342	248	—	92	—	—	81	92	—

[a]Based on surgical pathology, unequivocal cytology, or prolonged clinical follow-up.
NPV, negative predictive value; PPV, positive predictive value.

the main hypoechoic mass into adjacent structures. Findings considered diagnostic of a benign stricture (Figure 17-15) include preservation of the normal three-layer sonographic wall pattern, homogeneous echo patterns, smooth margins, hyperechogenic lesions, and the absence of a mass lesion. For lesions with intermediate echogenicity, asymmetric configuration suggests malignancy, whereas a symmetric one suggests a benign stricture; however, asymmetry has not been considered by all authors as a criterion for malignancy.[138,153,174,184] The accuracy of IDUS in differentiating benign from malignant strictures ranges from 76% to 92% in series of patients with various types of biliary strictures.* In 2002, Tamada and colleagues[185] proposed other IDUS criteria, including

*135,138,174,176,178,180,185

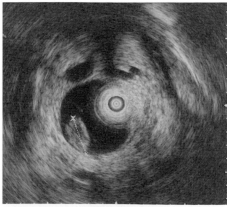

FIGURE 17-13 Two-dimensional intraductal ultrasonography image of a small solid mass *(white cross)* protruding in the lumen of the CBD consistent with early stage cholangiocarcinoma.

interruption of the bile duct wall that is considered specific for malignant stricture. Sessile tumors, even when they remain intraductal or extend outside the CBD wall, and tumor size greater than 10 mm are the other major criteria indicating malignancy. Echogenicity of the stricture, which is probably highly operator dependent, is no longer considered a factor predictive of malignancy. The vast majority of patients without the previously mentioned criteria and with negative samplings do not have a malignant lesion. The presence of two of the criteria, even with negative biopsies, is highly suspicious of malignancy. The absence of IDUS criteria of malignancy in addition to negative biopsies indicate a benign lesion with a 95% accuracy and 100% NPV.[185] History of choledocholithiasis or surgery of the biliary tract has been found to predict a benign lesion. Krishna and colleagues recently evaluated IDUS in 45 patients with biliary strictures with no mass lesion in CT or magnetic resonance imaging (MRI).[177] A wall thickness of ≤7 mm was a powerful parameter for excluding malignancy with 100% NPV in the absence of extrinsic compression. IDUS is very effective in confirming an extrinsic compression by a vascular structure or by a stone (Mirizzi's syndrome).[135,185,186] Biliary papillomatosis is also detected accurately by IDUS, whereas this pathology is frequently misdiagnosed with usual imaging techniques such as ERCP, EUS, or MRI. Biliary ducts with normal appearance alternating with areas covered by polypoid lesions protruding into the lumen establish the diagnosis.[187] In 30 patients with cholangiocarcinoma evaluated by IDUS, biliary papillomatosis was demonstrated in 3 (10%) and confirmed by biopsy or surgery.[186] When ERCP diagnosed a polypoid lesion inside the CBD, IDUS was the only test able to detect combined biliary papillomatosis inside the intrahepatic ducts (Figure 17-16). The clinical impact of this diagnosis can be important, because young patients with biliary papillomatosis without advanced cholangiocarcinoma should be treated with a Whipple

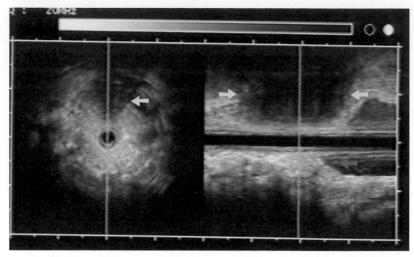

FIGURE 17-14 Three-dimensional intraductal ultrasonography showing biliary duct stenosis *(green arrows)* and pancreatic adenocarcinoma *(yellow arrows)*.

resection in combination with partial hepatectomy or liver transplantation.[187] In primary sclerosing cholangitis (PSC) presenting with dominant strictures, IDUS has been traditionally considered no more accurate than other imaging modalities in the diagnosis of cholangiocarcinoma (Figure 17-17).[188] However, recent studies show encouraging results.[128,189] In a prospective study,[189] 40 patients with PSC underwent ERCP with IDUS. The sensitivity, specificity, accuracy, positive predictive value (PPV), and NPV of IDUS for predicting malignancy were 87.5%, 91%, 90%, 70%, and 97%, respectively.

Practical Approach to Bile Duct Strictures

Because the performance of different diagnostic tests remains disappointing, the decision concerning the optimal use of the various imaging modalities is critical. In a prospective comparative study of 40 patients undergoing ERCP, MRCP, CT, and EUS for biliary strictures, the specificity improved when MRCP was combined with EUS.[190] Another prospective study of 142 patients with nonicteric cholestasis and common

hepatic duct dilatation of unclear etiology showed that a diagnostic algorithm with MRCP followed by EUS was highly sensitive and specific (90% and 98%, respectively) for the early diagnosis of extrahepatic bile duct carcinoma.[191]

The respective limitations and risks of EUS (with or without FNA) and ERCP with IDUS should also be considered prior to the assessment of any biliary stricture. If the stricture is localized at the level of the CBD, EUS should be proposed after noninvasive imaging modalities because of its excellent performance in distal biliary lesions and its ability to sample tissue. In patients with more proximal strictures, EUS and EUS FNA have several limitations, and ERCP-based tissue sampling should be considered as an alternative in addition to IDUS.[135,153,185] In view of its low NPV in proximal strictures, EUS FNA should be reserved for negative or nondiagnostic ERCP brush cytology results only if a high probability of malignancy exists. Nevertheless, some authors propose the systematic addition of EUS FNA to ERCP brushings to optimize the diagnostic yield.[192] With the increasing availability of peroral cholangioscopy, direct visualization and targeted biopsy of bile duct lesions should be performed whenever

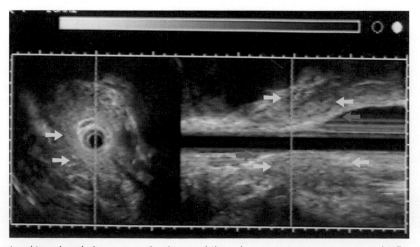

FIGURE 17-15 Three-dimensional intraductal ultrasonography showing biliary duct stenosis *(green arrows)* and inflammatory extrinsic compression following acute pancreatitis *(yellow arrows)*.

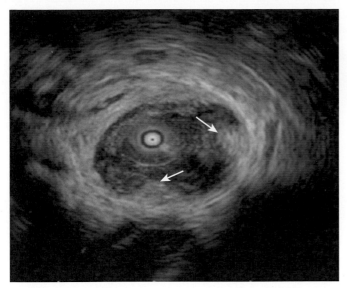

FIGURE 17-16 Two-dimensional intraductal ultrasonography image showing biliary papillomatosis with intrahepatic polypoid spread *(arrows)*.

possible. When compared with ERCP brush cytology, peroral cholangioscopy was 100% sensitive and 89% specific for biliary strictures and increased the diagnostic accuracy to more than 90% according to one study.[193] In a recent Japanese multicenter trial, the accuracy of endoscopic retrograde cholangiography (ERC) alone, ERC with cholangioscopy, and ERC with cholangioscopy and biopsy for the diagnosis of bile duct malignancy was 74%, 84%, and 93%, respectively.[142] More recently, Nguyen and colleagues reported on the utilization of EUS FNA before considering cholangioscopy in brushing-negative biliary strictures. The need for cholangioscopy was avoided in 60% of patients where EUS FNA provided tissue diagnosis, resulting in reduction of complications by 2.5% and in cost savings.[194] However, in patients with proximal biliary strictures, the performance of EUS FNA remains suboptimal. Siddiqui and colleagues demonstrated that cholangioscopy provided a definitive diagnosis in 77% of patients where ERCP-guided cytology brushing and EUS FNA were both inconclusive.[195] As the design, maneuverability, and optical resolution of cholangioscopes continue to improve,[196]

peroral cholangioscopy is emerging as an important adjunct to ERCP in the assessment of biliary strictures, particularly the proximal ones.

Visualizing and sampling biliary strictures during EUS can pose a challenge to the endosonographer. Bile duct lesions are best visualized and sampled from the duodenum. Distal lesions can sometimes be missed if the examination is only performed from the duodenal bulb. Therefore scope advancement to the second part of the duodenum followed by slow withdrawal through the duodenal sweep while maintaining full upward deflection is recommended to localize the lesion. During FNA, maintaining a close apposition of the echoendoscope to the duodenal wall is essential to help stabilize the scope and minimize the amount of tissue the needle has to traverse. This position creates an angulation in the tip of the scope, and therefore 25-G needles are recommended due to ease of advancement through the scope. Additionally, 25-G needles have been shown to be equivalent to 22-G needles in their diagnostic accuracy[197-199] and result in less bleeding during FNA, particularly when close to vascular structures such as the portal vein and hepatic artery.

In summary, we propose the following for the management of bile duct strictures (Figure 17-18):

- *For CBD strictures:* EUS plus FNA first, followed by ERCP with IDUS and brush cytology/cholangioscopy/forceps biopsy if needed.
- *For common hepatic duct and hilar strictures:* MRI plus ERCP with IDUS and brush cytology/forceps biopsy under fluoroscopy or cholangioscopy. EUS FNA can be considered when a strong clinical suspicion for malignancy persists after a negative ERCP-based workup.

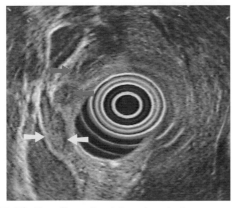

FIGURE 17-17 Two-dimensional intraductal ultrasonography image showing sclerosing cholangitis with thickened, irregular CBD *(green arrows)* and cystic wall *(yellow arrows)*.

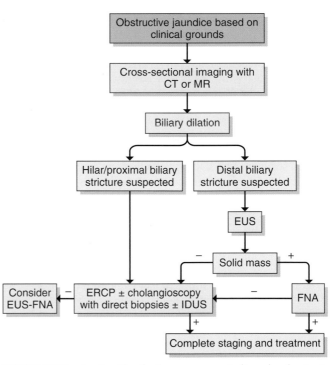

FIGURE 17-18 An algorithm for the management of jaundiced patients suspected to have cholangiocarcinoma. CT, computed tomography; ERCP, endoscopic retrograde cholangiopancreatography; FNA, fine-needle aspiration; IDUS, intraductal ultrasonography; MRI, magnetic resonance imaging.

Staging of Cholangiocarcinoma

When a bile duct carcinoma is diagnosed, the aim of the staging is primarily to determine candidacy for surgical resection, which offers the only practical chance of cure. Histologically, tumor invasion is limited to the mucosa or fibromuscular layer of the extrahepatic bile duct in early cancers, regardless of lymph node metastasis. Pathologically, bile duct carcinomas are generally staged according to the modified version of the TNM staging system: T1, where tumor is limited to the CBD wall; T2, tumor invasion beyond the CBD wall; and T3, tumor invasion of adjacent structures such as the pancreas, duodenum, and portal vein. From a cholangiographic standpoint, a common staging system describes the extent of tumor spread within the biliary tree according to the Bismuth classification.[200] Nevertheless, this system does not account for vascular or lymph node involvement and thus is limited in its ability to predict surgical resectability.

In a prospective study comparing EUS and IDUS in biliary strictures, the accuracy of IDUS in T staging (78%) was higher than that of EUS (54%).[153] EUS accuracy was inferior mainly in hilar or common hepatic duct strictures because of the limited field of examination. N-staging accuracy was comparable in both modalities, but other authors found that the depth of penetration of the standard 20-MHz catheter probe was not adequate for the evaluation of lymph nodes associated with advanced malignant strictures.[135] EUS and IDUS were limited in their ability to differentiate T1 from T2 bile duct cancers. In a large surgical series,[201] the sensitivity, specificity, and accuracy of IDUS for biliary strictures were 93%, 89%, and 91%, respectively. In the subgroup analysis of malignancy prediction, IDUS showed the best performance in cholangiocarcinoma (sensitivity of 98%) followed by pancreatic carcinoma (94%), gallbladder cancer (89%), and ampullary cancer (81%). The accuracy for discriminating T1 tumors was 84%, whereas for T2 and T3 malignancies it was 73% and 71%, respectively.[201]

From a practical perspective, the main question for the staging of biliary tumors is resectability, which relies on vascular, longitudinal, and tumor spread to adjacent organs such as the pancreas. Conventional cross-sectional imaging (e.g., MRI and CT) can be useful to identify non-resectable patients, such as those with a Bismuth type IV Klatskin tumors and those with metastatic disease. New generations of multidetector CT scanners and MRI provide high-resolution imaging to identify lateral spread of the tumor to vessels; however, the extent of longitudinal spread of tumors along the bile duct remains very difficult to assess. The accurate assessment of microscopic involvement of the bile duct wall remains challenging as well, resulting in understaging of the resection margins in some patients. Cholangiography and peroral choledochoscopy with biopsy are limited in determining the extent of longitudinal tumor spread and depth of spread.[202,203] To address this deficiency, Tamada and colleagues[204] initially evaluated IDUS in staging of cholangiocarcinoma and concluded that it has an accuracy of 72% for the assessment of longitudinal cancer extension to the hepatic side of the stricture using selected morphologic criteria (e.g., notching of the outer margins of the stricture). This accuracy was increased when asymmetric wall thickening was considered as a criterion of longitudinal tumor spread on both hepatic and duodenal sides, with an accuracy of 84% and 86%, respectively,

compared with cholangiography (47% and 43%, respectively).[179] In a later series by Inui and colleagues,[181] longitudinal spread was also diagnosed when irregular thickening of the bile duct was observed continuously and away from the main lesion. Overall accuracy of IDUS for assessing intraductal spreading was 85%. However, prior drainage of the biliary tract causes inflammatory thickening of the duct wall and limits the performance of IDUS.[175] Therefore IDUS must be carried out at the same time as the index ERCP or transhepatic drainage.

IDUS was also very accurate (100%) in defining portal vein and right hepatic artery involvement (Figure 17-19), which are the two most frequently involved vessels. Left and common hepatic arteries are more rarely involved and are not easily seen, as the area outside the hepatoduodenal ligament cannot be visualized with IDUS.[205,206] In the two most recent preoperative studies by Tamada and colleagues,[205,206] the accuracy of IDUS in detecting vascular involvement was significantly higher than angiography for both the portal vein (100% versus 50%) and the right hepatic artery (100% versus 33%). Invasion of the adjacent pancreatic parenchyma by a bile duct tumor should be determined presurgically, and in this case pancreaticoduodenectomy in combination with bile duct resection is recommended. IDUS was also superior to EUS in identifying slight invasion of the pancreatic parenchyma (accuracy 100% versus 78%),[175] but the therapeutic impact is probably small, because IDUS may understage intraductal infiltration.

Controlled series comparing the performance of each imaging modality (CT, MRCP, EUS, and IDUS) in staging of bile duct tumors are lacking. A clinical approach in patients with Klatskin tumors should be to start with MRI and MRCP. In patients with resectable tumors, ERCP plus IDUS should be the second step, carried out to assist in surgical planning. For bile duct tumors, EUS remains the most effective approach. ERCP plus IDUS could be utilized when the proximal part of the tumor cannot be seen with EUS or when there is suspicion of portal vein involvement. Finally, EUS and IDUS are useful tools in determining the nature of a biliary stenosis and for the staging of cholangiocarcinoma. As a result of their respective limitations (hilum imaging for EUS and the need for biliary access with IDUS), their use depends on the presence of local expertise, clinical presentation, and results of conventional imaging.

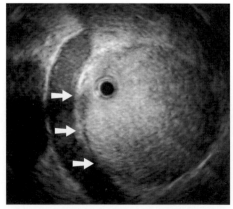

FIGURE 17-19   Two-dimensional intraductal ultrasonography obtained for staging of cholangiocarcinoma. It shows no infiltration of the right hepatic artery *(arrows)*.

Diagnostic Checklist

Cholangiocarcinoma
- Hypoechoic thickening of the wall with or without a mass
- Polypoid intraluminal tumor
- Involvement of vessels, pancreas, liver, ampulla, or duodenum
- Bile duct dilation
- Presence of adenopathy

Papillomatosis
- Polypoid intraluminal tumor alternating with normal bile duct wall

Mirizzi's syndrome
- Compression of CBD by intracystic stone
- Regular thickening of bile duct wall

Other benign stenoses
- Regular or symmetric thickening without wall disruption

EUS in Gallbladder Disease (Excluding Stones)

Gallbladder Polyps

The widespread use of US has led to the identification of an increasing number of polypoid lesions of the gallbladder. In fact, 4% to 7% of the healthy population has been reported to have polyps in the gallbladder.[207–209] Cholesterol, inflammatory polyps, and fibrous polyps have no malignant potential, and surgical intervention is not required as long as the patient is asymptomatic. In contrast, adenomatous polyps must be resected as the adenoma-carcinoma sequence is well characterized in the biliary epithelium of the gallbladder.[210] In a histologic review of a large series of 1605 sequential cholecystectomy specimens, the presence of histologic transition of adenoma into carcinoma was studied. All in situ carcinomas were associated with adenomatous components.[211] The same association was found in 19% of invasive carcinomas. Moreover, gallbladder carcinoma has one of the most dismal prognoses among malignancies of the digestive system, except at an early stage.

Laparoscopic cholecystectomy is a minimally invasive method for the removal of the gallbladder. However, the rate of procedure-related complications can be as high as 4%.[212,213] Moreover, postcholecystectomy syndrome can develop in up to 20% of patients after resection.[214,215] It is therefore important to establish criteria to select candidates for surgery among patients with gallbladder polyps. The incidental finding of a gallbladder polyp on TUS, CT, or MRI in an asymptomatic patient often leads to a clinical dilemma. The presence of a solitary lesion measuring greater than 10 mm in diameter and sessile appearance and hypoechogenicity on TUS are findings suggestive of a neoplastic polyp,[211,216] and cholecystectomy is recommended.[217,218] However, polyps smaller than 5 mm in diameter with echogenic and pedunculated appearance usually represent cholesterol and inflammatory polyps,[219] where only follow-up imaging is recommended. This approach, however, has been debated. In a study of 70 patients with polypoid lesions smaller than 2 cm, 35% of non-neoplastic polyps were more than 10 mm in diameter.[220] Moreover, it has been reported that as many as 30% of polyps

measuring 11 to 20 mm in diameter are cholesterol polyps.[221] Therefore offering cholecystectomy for gallbladder polyps larger than 10 mm will result in resection of otherwise benign polyps with low neoplastic potential. On the other hand, 19% to 29% of polyps between 5 and 10 mm in size were found to be adenomas in some studies.[216,219] Therefore a highly accurate diagnostic study is necessary to determine the best therapeutic approach. TUS is well suited as a first-line test because of its safety and availability; however, its sensitivity for diagnosing gallbladder polyps was only 50% in a recent large surgical series.[222] Owing to its high resolution, EUS is better positioned to provide more accurate imaging than TUS for gallbladder lesions.[216,219,223,224]

The gallbladder wall can readily be seen with EUS as a two-layered structure. The inner hypoechoic layer represents the mucosa, muscular layer, and subserosal fibrous layer. The outer hyperechoic layer represents the subserosal fat layer and serosa.[225,226] In some cases, a hyperechoic layer is demonstrated on the inner hypoechoic layer, which is mainly an interface echo. A gallbladder polyp is defined as a fixed echo structure protruding into the gallbladder lumen without acoustic shadowing on EUS. According to Azuma and colleagues,[223] EUS was superior to TUS in diagnosing the nature of gallbladder polyps: of 89 polyps smaller than 2 cm in size, 87% were correctly diagnosed by EUS, compared with only 52% by TUS. The sensitivity, specificity, PPV, and NPV of EUS in the diagnosis of carcinoma were 92%, 88%, 76%, and 97%, respectively.

Two series proposed a scoring system that relied on EUS findings in order to ascertain the risk of neoplasia.[219,220] In a retrospective analysis of EUS findings in 70 patients operated on for polypoid gallbladder lesions smaller than 20 mm, Sadamoto and colleagues[220] analyzed the morphologic characteristics of gallbladder polyps by multivariate stepwise logistic regression. The polypoid lesions confirmed by cholecystectomy were classified into two groups: neoplastic (adenomas and adenocarcinomas) and non-neoplastic (fibrous, inflammatory, and cholesterol polyps). The EUS variables studied were the maximum diameter and height/width ratio of the largest polyps, echo level, internal echo pattern, surface patterns, number and shape of polyps, presence of hyperechoic spots, and presence of gallstones. Internal echo pattern and size were positively associated with neoplasia whereas hyperechoic spots were negatively associated with neoplasia. All neoplastic polyps, including the smaller ones, were shown to have a relatively heterogeneous internal echo pattern on EUS. In contrast, large cholesterol polyps (more than 10 mm in diameter) had a homogeneous internal echo pattern. In this study, the sensitivity, specificity, and accuracy with an EUS-based scoring system developed from the above criteria were 78%, 83%, and 83%, respectively.[220] The hyperechoic spotting, which is specific for cholesterol polyps,[220,221] has been reported to represent a mass of foamy histiocytes containing cholesterol.[209,221] Nevertheless, in two cases of polypoid adenocarcinomas reported, hyperechoic spotting represented the accumulation of foamy cells underneath cancerous epithelium.[220] Another scoring system based on five EUS variables has been proposed to predict the malignancy of gallbladder polyps.[219] This system is based on layer structure, echo pattern, margin, stalk, and number of polyps. According to this study, size was the most significant predictor of neoplasia in polyps. All polyps with a diameter of 5 mm or less were non-neoplastic, whereas 94% of polyps larger than 15 mm were neoplastic. When the size of a gallbladder polyp exceeded 15 mm, the risk of neoplasia increased significantly compared with that of polyps measuring 5 to 10 mm or 10 to 15 mm in diameter. However, polyps of 5 to 10 mm and 10 to 15 mm in diameter showed no significant difference in risk of malignancy. For polyps measuring between 5 and 15 mm, the risk of neoplasia was significantly greater with a score of at least 6 than for those with a score of less than 6, with a sensitivity, specificity, and accuracy of 81%, 86%, and 84%, respectively. The authors concluded that use of the scoring system in patients with 5- to 15-mm gallbladder polyps could identify those patients at risk of neoplasia.

Despite the complexity of the EUS scoring systems discussed above, size remains a simple and strong factor, predicting neoplasia in gallbladder polyps. Although the presence of hypoechoic foci was the best individual predictive factor for neoplastic polyps in a more recent series,[227] polyps exceeding 15 mm in size were strongly associated with malignancy (OR of 22). In another study, EUS was always superior to TUS in accurately identifying neoplastic polyps of all sizes; however, EUS accuracy was only 44% among polyps smaller than 10 mm, in comparison to 89% for those greater than 10 mm.[228] Finally, the advent of EUS adjunct technologies has helped improve the ability of EUS to detect malignant gallbladder polyps. Choi and colleagues reported on the use of contrast-enhanced harmonic (CEH) EUS for this indication.[224] The presence of an irregular vessel pattern in malignant polyps resulted in an improved sensitivity and specificity of CEH EUS compared to conventional EUS (94% and 93% versus 90% and 91%, respectively). In another smaller series, Park and colleagues[229] found that CEH EUS also helped differentiate cholesterol polyps from gallbladder adenomas. In view of this performance, EUS can also be proposed as a surveillance tool for polyps not meeting resection criteria; however, longitudinal studies are lacking.

Considering the results of these studies, it appears that gallbladder polyps may be characterized more accurately with EUS than with TUS. Nevertheless, the results are inconclusive to make the choice between surgery and clinical follow-up, particularly in borderline-size polyps. EUS complements other relevant clinical data and cross-sectional imaging and is probably more useful in the management of high-risk surgical patients. A systematic surgical approach for gallbladder polyps more than 1 cm in size remains safe and widely practiced. It could be proposed to apply EUS for polyps that measure between 5 and 10 mm. In cases where EUS identifies suspicious features, surgery should be strongly considered. In other cases, EUS could serve as a reference tool for polyps that exhibit growth or changes in echo patterns and shape on TUS follow-up.[230,231] Nevertheless, more studies are needed to confirm the role of EUS for this indication.

Gallbladder Tumors

Preoperative differentiation of gallbladder adenomas from adenocarcinomas is unnecessary as adenomas have malignant potential,[211] and both lesions should be treated surgically. However, because of a significant difference between the open and laparoscopic cholecystectomy approaches, the preoperative diagnosis of cancer is important because of the increased risk of abdominal wall cancer recurrence after laparoscopic

cholecystectomy of carcinomas.[232,233] Recent advances in TUS and CT have made it possible to diagnose gallbladder carcinoma at an earlier stage. However, these modalities can stage only advanced lesions. Because EUS can be helpful in differentiating benign from malignant polyps, it can also help to guide the optimal surgical approach: laparoscopy for benign polyps or early cancer and open surgery for advanced cancer.[234]

Gallbladder cancer is staged according to the American Joint Committee on Cancer (AJCC) TNM Staging Classification System[235] (Table 17-4). The accuracy of EUS in gallbladder cancer staging depends on the criteria chosen. The integrity of the wall layers at the base of a gallbladder polyp remains the determinant criterion for deep invasion (Figure 17-20). Fujita and colleagues[225] classified the tumors into four groups based on depth of invasion in a retrospective EUS study with good interobserver correlation. Type A tumor was a pedunculated mass including a solid echo pattern with a fine nodular surface. Type B was a broad-based mass with an irregular surface and intact outer hyperechoic layer. In type C, the outer hyperechoic layer of the wall was irregular because of a mass echo, whereas in type D the entire layer structure was disrupted. After correlation of EUS and histopathology, the authors proposed that type A cancer on EUS be classified as Tis, because cancer was confined to the mucosa with no invasion of the surrounding epithelium. Type C cancer was found to invade the adipose layer of the subserosa; therefore it was staged preoperatively as T2. Type B cancer, on the other hand, can be either T1 or T2, because the depth of invasion varies from mucosa to the fibrous layer of the

---

TABLE 17-4

GALLBLADDER CANCER STAGED ACCORDING TO AJCC

Primary Tumor (T)

TX	Primary tumor cannot be assessed
T0	No evidence of primary tumor
Tis	Carcinoma in situ
T1	Tumor invades lamina propria or muscular layer
T1a	Tumor invades lamina propria
T1b	Tumor invades muscular layer
T2	Tumor invades perimuscular connective tissue; no extension beyond serosa or into liver
T3	Tumor perforates the serosa (visceral peritoneum) and/or directly invades the liver and/or one other adjacent organ or structure, such as the stomach, duodenum, colon, pancreas, omentum, or extrahepatic bile ducts
T4	Tumor invades main portal vein or hepatic artery or invades two or more extrahepatic organs or structures

Regional Lymph Nodes (N)

NX	Regional lymph nodes cannot be assessed
N0	No regional lymph node metastasis
N1	Metastases to nodes along the cystic duct, common bile duct, hepatic artery, and/or portal vein
N2	Metastases to periaortic, pericaval, superior mesenteric artery, and/or celiac artery lymph nodes

Distant Metastasis (M)

M0	No distant metastasis
M1	Distant metastasis

(From Edge S, Byrd DR, Compton CC, Fritz AG, Greene FL, Trotti A, eds. AJCC Cancer Staging Manual. 7th ed. New York, NY: Springer; 2010:215.)

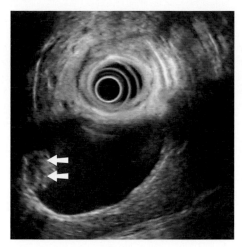

FIGURE 17-20 Radial EUS image of an adenomatous gallbladder polyp measuring 15 mm in diameter *(arrows)*.

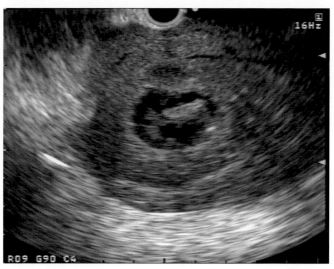

FIGURE 17-21 Linear EUS image (7.5 MHz) of a large gallbladder mass in a 55-year-old patient presenting with weight loss, right upper quadrant pain, and elevated liver enzymes. Substantial thickening of the gallbladder wall with complete loss of the wall layers, along with invasion of the adjacent liver parenchyma, were the basis of T3 staging in this case. The lumen of the gallbladder is restricted with sludge.

subserosa. This group is probably the most difficult to stage accurately, because diagnosing the depth of invasion is difficult when the outer hyperechoic layer is preserved.

In another retrospective study of 41 patients with gallbladder cancer,[236] a strong correlation between EUS and histopathologic tumor stage was demonstrated. EUS images were classified according to the shape of the tumor and the adjacent gallbladder wall structure: type A, pedunculated mass with preserved adjacent wall structure; type B, sessile and/or broad-based mass with a preserved outer hyperechoic layer of the gallbladder wall; type C, sessile and/or broad-based mass with a narrowed outer hyperechoic layer; and type D, sessile and/or broad-based mass with a disrupted outer hyperechoic layer. On histopathology, type A corresponded to Tis, type B to T1, type C to T2, and type D to T3-T4 stages with corresponding accuracies of 100%, 76%, 85%, and 93% for the four types, respectively. The best staging performance was for Tis and T3-T4 tumors.

FNA of gallbladder masses has been attempted and found to be accurate in diagnosing malignant tumors, with sensitivity ranging from 80% to 100%[164,237–241] (Table 17-5). The incidence of complications from direct puncture of the gallbladder appears to be low from the small published series, but biliary peritonitis and acute cholecystitis[240] have been reported following FNA of masses and during sampling of bile for crystals to evaluate for causes of acute pancreatitis.[242] To minimize this risk, 25-G needles should be utilized for this indication and the least number of passes performed.

From a management perspective, an extended cholecystectomy with systematic lymph node dissection and resection of the liver bed should be applied to all T3 (Figure 17-21) and

TABLE 17-5

PERFORMANCE CHARACTERISTICS OF EUS FINE-NEEDLE ASPIRATION FOR THE DIAGNOSIS OF GALLBLADDER MASSES

Reference (year)	Number of Patients	Sensitivity (%)	Specificity (%)	Complications	Comments
Kim et al[240] (2012)	13	84.6	100	Cholecystitis in one patient	Regional adenopathy sampled in 18 patients
Hijioka et al[237] (2012)	24	96	100	No complications	ERC had a diagnostic sensitivity of 47%
Hijioka et al[238] (2010)	15	89	100	No complications	Final diagnosis: xanthogranulomatous cholecystitis in five and adenocarcinoma in 10 FNA helped appropriately classify XGC in five of six suspected cases 22-G needles were used in all patients
Meara et al[164] (2006)	7	80	100	Not specified	22-G needles were used in all patients
Varadarajulu et al[241] (2005)	6	100	100	No complications	
Jacobson et al[239] (2003)	6	100	100	No complications	One case of XGC included Suspicious cytology was considered confirmatory 22-G needles were used in all patients

ERC, endoscopic retrograde cholangiography; EUS, endoscopic ultrasound; FNA, fine-needle aspiration; XGC, xanthogranulomatous cholecystitis.

T4 tumors, whereas laparoscopic cholecystectomy is likely sufficient for Tis tumors. The preoperative differentiation of T1 and T2 tumors is more difficult on EUS, and the appropriate surgical approach in this group of patients remains controversial.[243] When a hypoechoic area within the deeper part of the tumor was found on EUS, the differentiation between T1 and T2 tumors was possible and indicated subserosal invasion.[244] However, this finding is only valuable in polypoid gallbladder tumors.

In summary, the value of EUS FNA for the diagnosis and staging of gallbladder tumors remains questionable. This approach appears to be safe for obtaining samples from gallbladder masses for cytologic examination.[164,239,241] It could also be used for confirming lymph node involvement, because the existence of malignant lymph nodes indicates stage III disease irrespective of T staging (see Table 17.4). Nevertheless, because of the limited NPV of FNA, surgery should be pursued in all patients with suspicious gallbladder lesions despite a negative cytologic aspirate.

Because of the small and retrospective nature of EUS series in the staging of gallbladder cancer, the utility of EUS for the routine staging of this disease remains unclear. Nevertheless, EUS appears to be effective in the detection of early tumors and allows the appropriate classification of more advanced cases (T3, T4, and N1 disease), where open cholecystectomy with radical resection should be performed. In all other cases, open cholecystectomy should be undertaken with the extent of resection being pursued on a case-by-case basis.

Other Gallbladder Disorders Presenting with Wall Thickening

Localized or diffuse thickening of the gallbladder wall can be associated with a myriad of disorders (Table 17-6). When diffuse thickening and perivesicular fluid are present, differentiation of acute cholecystitis from other conditions such as ascites, portal hypertension, viral hepatitis, and hypoalbuminemia can be difficult.[245] Therefore it is important to rely on the clinical presentation and findings of other imaging studies in these cases.

Other conditions with diffuse or localized gallbladder wall thickening can be difficult to differentiate from neoplastic disease. Chronic cholecystitis is a common condition where gallstones are seen in association with a hyperechoic wall with a preserved layer structure. The wall is usually uniformly involved, but localized thickening is possible.[246] Adenomyomatosis of the gallbladder is generally considered a benign condition associated with diffuse thickening of its wall along with the presence of small cysts, which usually represent intramural diverticula (dilated Rokitansky-Aschoff sinuses). Ultrasonographically, wall layers are preserved despite a thickened wall, but the condition can sometimes be associated with hyperechoic echoes (comet-tail artifact).[216] According to the extent and site of involvement, adenomyomatosis can be classified into localized, generalized, and segmental types. The diagnosis is generally straightforward on TUS, and cancer mimicking adenomyomatosis is extremely rare.[247] Nevertheless, some cases can be difficult to diagnose, especially the localized type, and segmental adenomyomatosis has been linked to gallbladder carcinoma, especially in elderly patients.[248] Xanthogranulomatous cholecystitis (XGC) is an uncommon form of chronic inflammation of the gallbladder, the clinical presentation of which is similar to that of cholecystitis. In a large 15-year series of cholecystectomy, XGC was present in 1.46% of patients[249] and was associated with lithiasis in 85% of patients. XGC may simulate gallbladder cancer (see Table 17-6), and EUS can sometimes visualize hyperechoic nodules in the gallbladder wall, probably representing xanthogranulomas.[250]

Overall, the role of EUS in the diagnosis of gallbladder wall thickening remains poorly defined. Mizuguchi and colleagues[234] compared EUS, conventional US, CT, and MRI in the differential diagnosis of gallbladder wall thickening. The multiple-layer pattern was demonstrated more effectively by EUS than by other imaging modalities. Loss of multiple-layer patterns of the gallbladder wall demonstrated by EUS was the

---

TABLE 17-6

CHARACTERISTICS AND ETIOLOGIES OF GALLBLADDER WALL THICKENING ON EUS

	EUS Characteristics	
Disorder	**Thickening**	**Others Signs**
Acute cholecystitis	Localized or diffuse, layers preserved	Pericholecystic fluid
Chronic cholecystitis	High echogenicity	
Gallbladder carcinoma	Localized, layers inconsistently preserved	Polyp or mass
Adenomyomatosis	Localized or diffuse, layers preserved	Anechoic areas (cysts), hyperechoic echoes, comet-tail artifact
Xanthogranulomatous cholecystitis	Localized or diffuse, layers inconsistently preserved	Hyperechoic nodules in the gallbladder wall
Portal hypertension, viral hepatitis, ascites, or hypoalbuminemia	Diffuse, layers preserved	Extraluminal ascites
Extrahepatic portal venous obstruction	Localized, layers preserved	Varices inside the gallbladder wall
Primary sclerosing cholangitis	Diffuse, layers preserved	Irregular thickening
Diffuse papillomatosis	Localized or diffuse, layers inconsistently preserved	
Anomalous arrangement of the pancreatobiliary duct	Diffuse, layers preserved	Predominant thickening of the hypoechoic layer

EUS, endoscopic ultrasound.

most specific finding in diagnosing gallbladder cancer. It is nevertheless not pathognomonic, as this finding can also be seen in XGC.[250] In a recent series by Kim and colleagues, EUS characteristics were reviewed in 134 patients with gallbladder wall thickening including 11 patients with cancer who subsequently underwent cholecystectomy. Wall thickening >10 mm and hypoechoic internal echogenicity were associated with neoplastic wall thickening on multivariate analysis.[251] EUS can also help define gallbladder involvement in other less common conditions such as sclerosing cholangitis,[252] portal venous obstruction resulting in internal gallbladder varices,[253] and diffuse uniform wall thickenin in patients with anomalous arrangement of the pancreatobiliary ducts.[254,255] Finally, diffuse papillomatosis of the biliary tract may also involve the gallbladder presenting as wall thickening with a protruding mass[256] in association with bile duct polyps.

Summary

In conclusion, the utility of EUS for the diagnosis of gallbladder disease remains less defined than its role in bile duct tumors and stones. TUS, CT, or MRI are generally sufficient to determine the diagnosis and guide treatment. EUS could have a niche role in the preoperative assessment of patients with small gallbladder polyps, especially those 5 to 10 mm in size or those greater than 10 mm in poor operative candidates. It may also be helpful before surgery in patients with suspected gallbladder cancer or in those with large polyps suspected to be malignant. Finally, in cases of uncertainty on TUS, EUS could be useful in differentiating benign from malignant gallbladder lesions in the presence of diffuse wall thickening.

Ampullary Tumors

Tumors of the ampulla of Vater originate from the pancreaticobiliary-duodenal junction, guarded by the sphincter of Oddi. The pancreatic duct and common bile duct join in the ampulla of Vater and form a distal common channel in about 85% of individuals. The normal ampulla starts about 2 mm outside the duodenal wall and penetrates the muscularis propria somewhat more distally, forming an intraduodenal segment 9 to 25 mm in length.[257] A wide variety of tumors arise from the ampulla of Vater, including benign tubular and tubulovillous adenomas, carcinomas, and several rare other pathologic types, such as lipomas, fibromas, neurofibromas, leiomyomas, lymphangiomas, hemangiomas, and various neuroendocrine tumors. Adenomas can occur sporadically and in the setting of polyposis syndromes. They are considered premalignant, and the adenoma-carcinoma sequence has been assumed to be behind the pathogenesis of ampullary cancer.[258] Benign adenomas are increasingly detected during routine upper endoscopy performed for unrelated reasons and now represent an important proportion of endoscopically treated ampullary tumors.[259] Moreover, endoscopic surveillance programs are recommended for patients with familial adenomatosis polyposis (FAP) syndrome, where the major papilla is a common site of extracolonic adenomas or malignancy.[260] Tumors can also be found in symptomatic patients presenting with jaundice, abdominal pain, weight loss, pancreatitis, or anemia.

Carcinoma of the ampulla (papillary carcinoma) spreads by extension to contiguous organs and by invasion of lymphatic and/or blood vessels. Most ampullary cancers develop from the mucosa of the ampulla and infiltrate the sphincter of Oddi. They gradually invade the muscularis propria and the serosa of the duodenum and grow beyond the serosa toward the pancreas. Nevertheless, compared with pancreatic cancer, ampullary neoplasia carries a much better prognosis because of onset of symptoms at an earlier tumor stage.[261] Diagnosis of an ampullary tumor is not always easy endoscopically. Macroscopically, the tumors can be polypoid or ulcerative. Bile stasis often occurs and may contribute to gallstone formation. In fact, between 6% and 38% of patients with ampullary neoplasms also have coexistent choledocholithiasis.[262–266]

Confirming the diagnosis with pathology can also be difficult in ampullary cancers. Mucosal biopsies can be falsely negative because of intramural extension of the tumor in up to 38% of cases.[264,266–269] In these cases, ES is necessary to expose the endoampullary growth and allow adequate sampling of the tumor. In addition, the differential diagnosis between inflammatory changes and an adenoma with low-grade dysplasia can be difficult for the pathologist, and repeated biopsies may be necessary. Finally, standard forceps biopsies may not reliably represent the tumor: benign adenomas may harbor foci of carcinoma that may be either superficial or invasive, just as benign tissue elements may be found in ampullary carcinomas.[270] In fact, biopsies have been shown to underestimate the presence of adenocarcinoma in 19% to 30% of cases.[264,266–269]

In view of these limitations, the differential diagnosis between a normal ampulla, an inflamed one, or a real tumor can be difficult. EUS has been proposed to aid in the diagnosis of a suspected ampullary lesion when faced with a protruding ampulla without mucosal abnormalities. Will and colleagues[271] reported a series of 133 patients with a variety of ampullary and periampullary lesions found on duodenoscopy. The sensitivity and specificity of EUS in the detection of malignant lesions were 93% and 75%, respectively, using histopathology as the reference standard. This low specificity was also demonstrated by other series where the only specific signs confirming an ampullary mass were infiltration of the duodenal muscularis propria (Figure 17-22) or the main pancreatic duct (Video 17-3) or the presence of endoluminal growth in the CBD (Figure 17-23).[272,273] The other criteria including echogenicity (Figure 17-24), enlargement of the ampulla, and CBD

Video 17-3. Examination of the head of the pancreas along with the CBD and pancreatic duct using the radial echoendoscope in a patient with ampullary adenocarcinoma. The bile duct has been previously stented and appears decompressed. On the contrary, the pancreatic duct (PD) remains significantly dilated. The ampullary mass invades the duodenal wall and distal bile and pancreatic ducts.

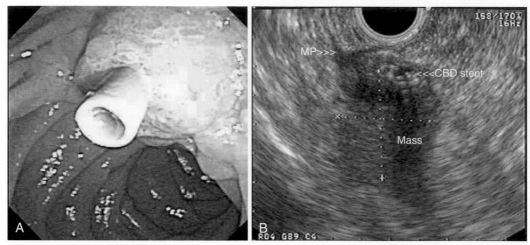

FIGURE 17-22 **A,** Endoscopic view of an ampullary mass in a patient who presented with painless jaundice. A plastic biliary stent was previously placed. **B,** Linear EUS image (7.5 MHz) of the same lesion. Tumor infiltration of the duodenal muscularis propria (MP) was strongly suspected. The patient was referred for pancreaticoduodenectomy. CBD, common bile duct.

or pancreatic duct dilation were not specific and were seen in non-neoplastic pathologies or even in normal ampullae. The detection sensitivity of an ampullary tumor remains high in symptomatic patients but is lower in asymptomatic ones. For example, it is not uncommon in patients with FAP syndrome to harbor ampullary tumors without EUS abnormalities. This emphasizes the fact that despite the high sensitivity of EUS for the diagnosis of ampullary tumors, its NPV remains limited, and sometimes only a mucosal biopsy can reliably confirm the diagnosis. In cases when mucosal biopsies are not conclusive because of intramural spread of the tumor, and to avoid the risks associated with ES to expose the tumor, FNA can be safely utilized as an alternative technique to confirm the diagnosis.[274,275] Therefore in patients with a suspicion of ampullary obstruction (based on clinical, biochemical, or imaging criteria) but with inconclusive biopsies and negative EUS, endoscopic sphincterotomy with repeated biopsies is needed. On the other hand, asymptomatic patients with a suspicion of an ampullary tumor on endoscopy but with

inconclusive biopsies and unremarkable EUS should undergo follow-up (Figure 17-25).

As in other luminal gastrointestinal malignancies, the aim of preoperative staging is to direct the patient to the most suitable therapeutic approach and to determine prognosis. Traditionally, pancreaticoduodenectomy has been the only potentially curative treatment for patients with benign ampullary tumors or early cancer.[276] Surgical ampullectomy was infrequently done, owing to its morbidity and the inability to rule out the presence of metastatic lymph nodes because of limited resection. In the last two decades, evolving endoscopic techniques for ampullectomy have made curative treatment of benign adenomas (Figure 17-26) or early cancers possible in 70% to 80% of patients.[277–282] Endoscopic ampullectomy has a lower morbidity rate (6% to 36%)[259,266,281,283–285] than local surgical excision[267,285]; nevertheless, careful selection is required to triage patients to the appropriate treatment approach. Despite its favorable outcomes, endoscopic ampullectomy is limited by its inability to assess for lymph node

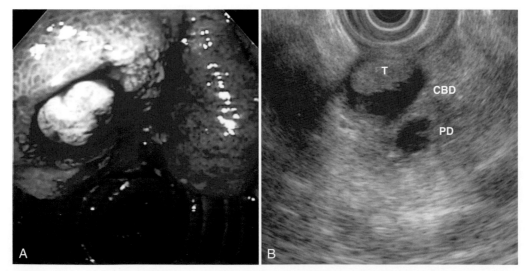

FIGURE 17-23 **A,** Endoscopic view of an ampullary cancer. **B,** Radial EUS image (6 MHz) of the mass. The tumor (T) is seen to invade the common bile duct (CBD), main pancreatic duct (PD), and duodenal wall.

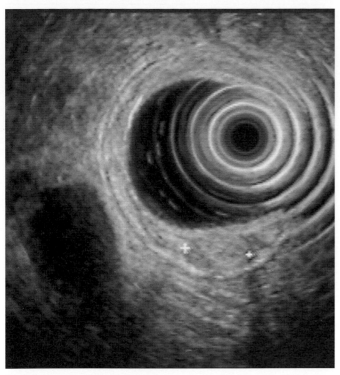

FIGURE 17-24 Radial EUS image (6 MHz) of a uT1 ampullary tumor (between the white cross signs).

metastasis, which is estimated to be present in up to 30% of patients with T1 disease.[286] Additionally, neoplastic tissue extending inside the pancreatic or bile ducts is inadequately removed using this approach. These limitations highlight the importance of pretreatment staging, not only to assess the resectability of the tumor but also to determine which tumors may be resected endoscopically versus surgically.

Ampullary tumors are staged according to the TNM classification[235] (Table 17-7). Nevertheless, this classification has limitations, because T1 encompasses early cancers invading the mucosa as well as those invading the duodenal

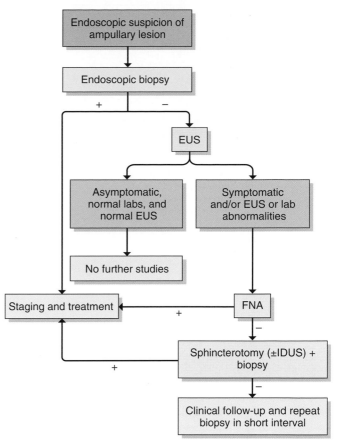

FIGURE 17-25 An algorithm for the management of patients with suspected ampullary lesions. *FNA,* fine-needle aspiration; *IDUS,* intraductal ultrasonography.

submucosa. An alternative but more selective staging system was developed to address those limitations, where T1 tumors are divided into d0 tumors limited to the sphincter of Oddi layer and d1 tumors that invade the duodenal submucosa. The biological behavior of d0 and d1 is significantly different

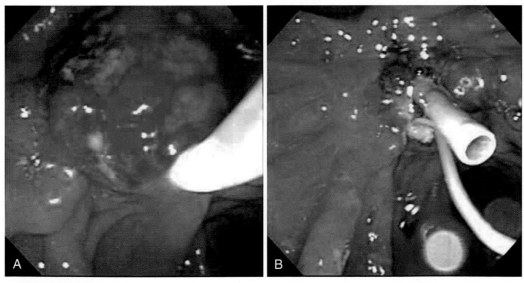

FIGURE 17-26 **A,** Endoscopic image of an ampullary adenoma confirmed by endoscopic mucosal biopsies. The patient was referred for endoscopic ampullectomy after EUS assessment. A snare is noted encircling the lesion. **B,** Endoscopic image of the adenoma after endoscopic resection is completed. Note the biliary stent *(blue)* and pancreatic stent *(orange).*

TABLE 17-7

TNM STAGING FOR AMPULLARY CARCINOMA

Primary Tumor (T)

TX   Primary tumor cannot be assessed
T0   No evidence of primary tumor
Tis Carcinoma in situ
T1   Tumor limited to the ampulla of Vater or sphincter of Oddi
T2   Tumor invades duodenal wall
T3   Tumor invades pancreas
T4   Tumor invades peripancreatic soft tissues or other adjacent organs or structures other than pancreas

Regional Lymph Nodes (N)

NX   Regional lymph nodes cannot be assessed
N0   No regional lymph node metastasis
N1   Regional lymph node metastasis

Distant Metastasis (M)

M0   No distant metastasis
M1   Distant metastasis

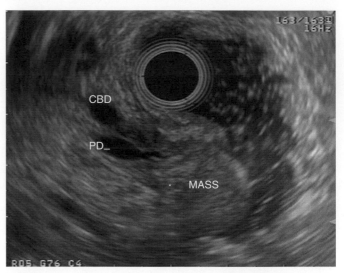

FIGURE 17-27 Radial EUS image (6 MHz) of a large ampullary mass infiltrating the duodenal wall and the head of the pancreas. CBD, common bile duct; PD, pancreatic duct.

in terms of the risk of lymph node metastasis,[286–289] which varies from 0% for d0 to 30% for d1 tumors.[290–292] The presence of metastatic lymph nodes correlates with the T stage for more advanced tumors: 55% for T2 and 78% for T3-T4 lesions.[292] Following this staging strictly makes d0 tumors the only true early cancer where endoscopic ampullectomy can be offered as the standard of care. Various imaging modalities, such as TUS, CT, angiography, ERCP, MRCP, and EUS, have been used to stage ampullary tumors and evaluate their resectability. These tumors often grow around the ampulla, far from the mesenteric and portal vessels, with rapid symptom development such as jaundice and pancreatitis. It is therefore rare to see a large tumor originating from the ampulla and invading the vessels. The resectability of those tumors is therefore easier to determine than for pancreatic and biliary adenocarcinomas. T staging is of ultimate importance as it determines prognosis and guides the choice of treatment (i.e., surgical versus endoscopic resection).

EUS remains the most reliable modality for local preoperative staging of ampullary lesions. In the earlier series, EUS was shown to be superior to CT, US, and angiography[146,273] for evaluation of T and N staging and to determine resectability, with 95% reported accuracy in assessing for portal venous

system involvement.[273] These results have been confirmed in recent studies comparing EUS (radial or linear) with conventional or helical CT for staging as well as for resectability.[293–299] In a series of 50 patients, EUS was more accurate for the T staging of ampullary neoplasms (78%) than CT (24%) or MRI (46%).[287] EUS understaging of true T3 lesions or overstaging of true T2 carcinomas accounted for most of the errors in the EUS T-stage assessment, probably due to desmoplastic peritumoral reaction, which cannot easily be differentiated from foci of invasive carcinoma.[288] Nevertheless, this differentiation is of little practical value because the same surgical treatment is recommended for T2 and T3 tumors (Figure 17-27). What is of more importance is the accuracy of EUS in determining whether or not endoscopic resection can be used with curative intent. The accuracy of EUS in confirming that the T stage is higher than T1 is around 90% (ranging from 78% to 94%; Table 17-8). Its ability to show an intraductal infiltration also seems to be good, although this has not yet been clearly evaluated in the literature. However, EUS is limited in its ability to differentiate infiltration of the duodenal submucosal layer because the sphincter of Oddi is not well recognized with the

TABLE 17-8

PERFORMANCE OF EUS IN THE STAGING OF AMPULLARY TUMORS

Reference (Year)	Number of Patients	Technique	Sensitivity (%)	Specificity (%)	PPV (%)	NPV (%)	Accuracy (%)
Mukai et al[146] (1992)	23	EUS	93	78	87	88	87
Tio et al[288] (1996)	32	EUS	100	60	93	100	94
Itoh et al[300] (1997)	40	IDUS	89	85	85	90	88
Menzel et al[301] (1999)	15	IDUS	100	80	91	100	93
Cannon et al[287] (1999)	50	EUS	88	100	100	80	90
Ito et al[296] (2007)	40	EUS/IDUS[a]	95	62	69	93	78
Artifon et al[293] (2009)	27	EUS	100	—	93	—	93
Chen et al[295] (2009)	31	EUS	96	57	89	80	88
Manta et al[303] (2010)	24	EUS	88	100	100	89	94
Wee et al[302] (2012)	79	EUS	69	88	66	88	—

EUS, endoscopic ultrasound; IDUS, intraductal ultrasound; NPV, negative predictive value; PPV, positive predictive value.
[a]IDUS was combined with EUS in all cases.

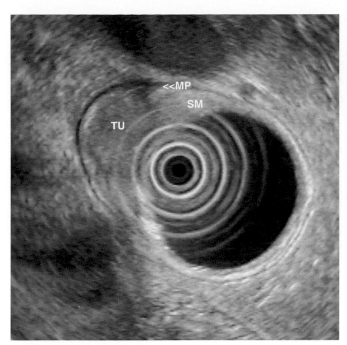

FIGURE 17-28 Radial EUS image (6 MHz) of a uT1sm ampullary tumor (TU) with disruption of the submucosa (SM). The muscularis propria (MP) is intact with no invasion.

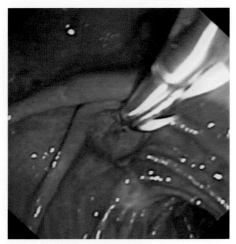

FIGURE 17-29 Endoscopic image of an intraductal ultrasonography probe being advanced over a guidewire for staging of ampullary tumor.

6- to 12-MHz EUS probes, even though the infiltration of the third hyperechoic layer of the duodenum sometimes enables the diagnosis of a d1 tumor (Figure 17-28). On the other hand, EUS also has low accuracy in the detection of lymph node metastases (53% to 87%), with an NPV of less than 75%.* In addition, MRI has been found to be not statistically superior to EUS for nodal staging,[164] whereas CT was less sensitive and specific.[293,295] EUS-guided FNA is highly accurate in sampling tissue from extraluminal lesions.[304] Use of this technique might increase the diagnostic accuracy of preoperative EUS, although the data to support this remain very limited.

EUS can therefore be considered to be highly accurate in predicting the unresectability of ampullary carcinoma and in determining the T stage. Nevertheless, EUS is limited by its inability to accurately demarcate the sphincter of Oddi, and its NPV for the presence of metastatic lymph nodes remains low. Therefore two complementary examinations (duodenoscopy and IDUS) may be useful. On duodenoscopy, ulceration above the roof of the ampulla, separated from the papilla by normal mucosa, indicates a lesion invading the duodenal submucosa and should be considered locally invasive.[305] To improve staging performance, IDUS has been proposed as a more accurate ultrasonographic imaging tool for the staging of ampullary neoplasms. Intraductal catheter probes (Figure 17-29) employ a higher frequency (20 MHz), resulting in enhanced resolution compared to the 7.5 or 12 MHz used for conventional EUS. However, the use of such probes has some restrictions: the ultrasonic probe should be inserted into the tumor via ERCP and the depth of penetration is limited because of the higher frequency, resulting in inadequate N staging.[301] However, IDUS is probably the only imaging

modality that can image the Oddi's muscle layer as a distinct layer.[300] The possibility of delineating the sphincter of Oddi and the duodenal submucosa allows superior T staging, particularly of early tumors that could be triaged to endoscopic therapy (Figure 17-30). In a series of 32 patients with cancer of the papilla of Vater, the accuracy of IDUS was 87.5%, and its sensitivity and specificity in assessing lymph node metastases were 66.7% and 91.3%, respectively.[300] The diagnostic accuracy for tumor dissemination was greatest for early tumors, with a rate of 100%, 92.3%, and 100% for d0, d1, and d2 lesions, respectively. IDUS was also very accurate in showing intraductal involvement, with 100% accuracy[300] (Figure 17-31).

Considering all three imaging modalities—duodenoscopy, EUS, and IDUS—a three-step approach could be applied to ascertain whether an ampullary tumor may be treated adequately by endoscopic ampullectomy:

1. *Duodenoscopy:* Large infiltrating tumors with ulcerations seen above the roof of the ampulla usually indicate submucosal infiltration; and pancreaticoduodenectomy should be considered in this case.
2. *EUS:* Any tumors staged above uT1 because of submucosal or muscularis propria invasion and all tumors with intraductal infiltration should be selected for pancreaticoduodenectomy.
3. *IDUS:* uT1 tumors confirmed to have no submucosal infiltration or intraductal spread should be considered for endoscopic ampullectomy with curative intent.

Because of the predisposition of ampullary tumors to recur after endoscopic ampullectomy (13%, range: 0% to 30%),* EUS is needed, in combination with endoscopy and biopsy, for the follow-up of patients with ampullary adenomas treated endoscopically, especially to detect intraductal recurrence. Lesions with high-grade dysplasia or adenocarcinoma, and those with incomplete endoscopic resection, are more likely to recur after endoscopic therapy.[259] Pancreaticoduodenec-

---

*146,273,282,287,288,293,295,297,300–303

*259,277–280,283,284,306–314

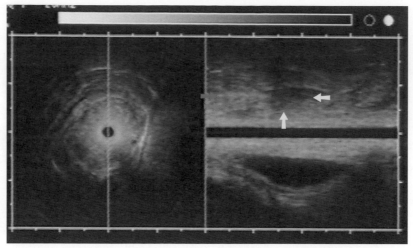

FIGURE 17-30 Three-dimensional intraductal ultrasonography showing a d1 ampullary tumor. *Yellow arrows*, tumor with disruption of the submucosa; *green arrow*, normal submucosa; *blue arrow*, sphincter of Oddi.

tomy should be considered in all surgically fit patients presenting with local recurrence.[259,315]

EUS and IDUS—if available—should be performed to stage ampullary tumors before any invasive treatment is pursued, particularly prior to diathermic biopsy, endoscopic sphincterotomy, or biliary stent insertion. Such interventions may compromise EUS interpretation by introducing air and creating artifacts. In one series, the presence of a transpapillary endobiliary stent resulted in a reduction of EUS T-stage accuracy from 84% to 72%,[287] which was most likely caused by the understaging of T2 and T3 carcinomas. Moreover, the bile duct wall thickness, measured by an intraductal ultrasonographic probe, was more than doubled in patients with an endobiliary drainage catheter in place for as little as 14 days[175] and could be interpreted as intraductal spread. Finally, economic studies assessing the value of pretherapeutic staging of ampullary tumors are scarce. Only one series has shown that use of EUS in the selection of patients for local resection may be a cost-effective approach in the management of ampullary tumors.[313]

Summary

EUS can be helpful in the diagnosis of ampullary tumors, especially lesions with intramural spread and negative mucosal biopsies. Its role in directing the management of ampullary cancer resides in its ability to accurately stage advanced tumors where surgical resection should be performed. For benign and early cancers of the ampulla, accurate staging could be achieved using a combination of endoscopic, EUS, IDUS, and cross-sectional imaging. In such cases, endoscopic resection appears to be adequate and provides good long-term results.

Diagnostic Checklist
Ampullary tumors
• Hypoechoic or hyperechoic thickening of the ampulla
• Polypoid intraductal tumor
• Involvement of vessels, pancreas, or duodenum
• Bile or pancreatic duct dilation
• Bile or pancreatic duct intraductal growth
• Presence of periduodenal adenopathy
Benign changes
• Hypoechoic or hyperechoic thickening of the ampulla
• Duodenal wall layers preserved
• No intraductal polypoid infiltration
• No bile or pancreatic duct dilation expected

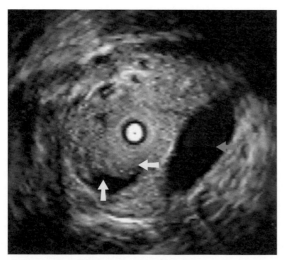

FIGURE 17-31 Two-dimensional intraductal ultrasonography showing an ampullary tumor. *Yellow arrows* demonstrate spread to the bile duct; *blue arrow* points to a normal pancreatic duct.

REFERENCES

1. Andriulli A, Loperfido S, Napolitano G, et al. Incidence rates of post-ERCP complications: a systematic survey of prospective studies. *Am J Gastroenterol.* 2007;102:1781-1788.
2. Davis WZ, Cotton PB, Arias R, et al. ERCP and sphincterotomy in the context of laparoscopic cholecystectomy: academic and community practice patterns and results. *Am J Gastroenterol.* 1997;92:597-601.
3. Loperfido S, Angelini G, Benedetti G, et al. Major early complications from diagnostic and therapeutic ERCP: a prospective multicenter study. *Gastrointest Endosc.* 1998;48:1-10.
4. Cotton PB, Garrow DA, Gallagher J, et al. Risk factors for complications after ERCP: a multivariate analysis of 11,497 procedures over 12 years. *Gastrointest Endosc.* 2009;70:80-88.

5. Barthet M, Lesavre N, Desjeux A, et al. Complications of endoscopic sphincterotomy: results from a single tertiary referral center. *Endoscopy.* 2002;34:991-997.

6. Cotton PB, Geenen JE, Sherman S, et al. Endoscopic sphincterotomy for stones by experts is safe, even in younger patients with normal ducts. *Ann Surg.* 1998;227:201-204.

7. Freeman ML, Nelson DB, Sherman S, et al. Complications of endoscopic biliary sphincterotomy. *N Engl J Med.* 1996;335:909-918.

8. Sherman S, Ruffolo TA, Hawes RH, et al. Complications of endoscopic sphincterotomy. A prospective series with emphasis on the increased risk associated with sphincter of Oddi dysfunction and nondilated bile ducts. *Gastroenterology.* 1991;101:1068-1075.

9. Lambert ME, Betts CD, Hill J, et al. Endoscopic sphincterotomy: the whole truth. *Br J Surg.* 1991;78:473-476.

10. Rabenstein T, Schneider HT, Nicklas M, et al. Impact of skill and experience of the endoscopist on the outcome of endoscopic sphincterotomy techniques. *Gastrointest Endosc.* 1999;50:628-636.

11. Folkers MT, Disario JA, Adler DG. Long-term complications of endoscopic biliary sphincterotomy for choledocholithiasis: a North-American perspective. *Am J Gastroenterol.* 2009;104:2868-2869.

12. Hawes RH, Cotton PB, Vallon AG. Follow-up 6 to 11 years after duodenoscopic sphincterotomy for stones in patients with prior cholecystectomy. *Gastroenterology.* 1990;98:1008-1012.

13. Sugiyama M, Atomi Y. Risk factors predictive of late complications after endoscopic sphincterotomy for bile duct stones: long-term (more than 10 years) follow-up study. *Am J Gastroenterol.* 2002;97:2763-2767.

14. Bergman JJ, van Berkel AM, Groen AK, et al. Biliary manometry, bacterial characteristics, bile composition, and histologic changes fifteen to seventeen years after endoscopic sphincterotomy. *Gastrointest Endosc.* 1997;45:400-405.

15. Vicary FR. Progress report. Ultrasound and gastroenterology. *Gut.* 1977;18:386-397.

16. Dong B, Chen M. Improved sonographic visualization of choledocholithiasis. *J Clin Ultrasound.* 1987;15:185-190.

17. Stott MA, Farrands PA, Guyer PB, et al. Ultrasound of the common bile duct in patients undergoing cholecystectomy. *J Clin Ultrasound.* 1991;19:73-76.

18. Neitlich JD, Topazian M, Smith RC, et al. Detection of choledocholithiasis: comparison of unenhanced helical CT and endoscopic retrograde cholangiopancreatography. *Radiology.* 1997;203:753-757.

19. Polkowski M, Palucki J, Regula J, et al. Helical computed tomographic cholangiography versus endosonography for suspected bile duct stones: a prospective blinded study in non-jaundiced patients. *Gut.* 1999;45:744-749.

20. Tseng CW, Chen CC, Chen TS, et al. Can computed tomography with coronal reconstruction improve the diagnosis of choledocholithiasis? *J Gastroenterol Hepatol.* 2008;23:1586-1589.

21. Kondo S, Isayama H, Akahane M, et al. Detection of common bile duct stones: comparison between endoscopic ultrasonography, magnetic resonance cholangiography, and helical-computed-tomographic cholangiography. *Eur J Radiol.* 2005;54:271-275.

22. Anderson SW, Rho E, Soto JA. Detection of biliary duct narrowing and choledocholithiasis: accuracy of portal venous phase multidetector CT. *Radiology.* 2008;247:418-427.

23. Okada M, Fukada J, Toya K, et al. The value of drip infusion cholangiography using multidetector-row helical CT in patients with choledocholithiasis. *Eur Radiol.* 2005;15:2140-2145.

24. Napoleon B, Dumortier J, Keriven-Souquet O, et al. Do normal findings at biliary endoscopic ultrasonography obviate the need for endoscopic retrograde cholangiography in patients with suspicion of common bile duct stone? A prospective follow-up study of 238 patients. *Endoscopy.* 2003;35:411-415.

25. Canto MI, Chak A, Stellato T, et al. Endoscopic ultrasonography versus cholangiography for the diagnosis of choledocholithiasis. *Gastrointest Endosc.* 1998;47:439-448.

26. Lee YT, Chan FK, Leung WK, et al. Comparison of EUS and ERCP in the investigation with suspected biliary obstruction caused by choledocholithiasis: a randomized study. *Gastrointest Endosc.* 2008;67:660-668.

27. Lightdale CJ. Indications, contraindications, and complications of endoscopic ultrasonography. *Gastrointest Endosc.* 1996;43:S15-S19.

28. Palazzo L, Girollet PP, Salmeron M, et al. Value of endoscopic ultrasonography in the diagnosis of common bile duct stones: comparison with surgical exploration and ERCP. *Gastrointest Endosc.* 1995;42:225-231.

29. Liu CL, Lo CM, Chan JK, et al. EUS for detection of occult cholelithiasis in patients with idiopathic pancreatitis. *Gastrointest Endosc.* 2000; 51:28-32.

30. Frossard JL, Sosa-Valencia L, Amouyal G, et al. Usefulness of endoscopic ultrasonography in patients with "idiopathic" acute pancreatitis. *Am J Med.* 2000;109:196-200.

31. Bret PM, Reinhold C. Magnetic resonance cholangiopancreatography. *Endoscopy.* 1997;29:472-486.

32. Mofidi R, Lee AC, Madhavan KK, et al. The selective use of magnetic resonance cholangiopancreatography in the imaging of the axial biliary tree in patients with acute gallstone pancreatitis. *Pancreatology.* 2008; 8:55-60.

33. Topal B, Van de Moortel M, Fieuws S, et al. The value of magnetic resonance cholangiopancreatography in predicting common bile duct stones in patients with gallstone disease. *Br J Surg.* 2003;90:42-47.

34. Scaffidi MG, Luigiano C, Consolo P, et al. Magnetic resonance cholangio-pancreatography versus endoscopic retrograde cholangio-pancreatography in the diagnosis of common bile duct stones: a prospective comparative study. *Minerva Med.* 2009;100:341-348.

35. Ausch C, Hochwarter G, Taher M, et al. Improving the safety of laparoscopic cholecystectomy: the routine use of preoperative magnetic resonance cholangiography. *Surg Endosc.* 2005;19:574-580.

36. Griffin N, Wastle ML, Dunn WK, et al. Magnetic resonance cholangiopancreatography versus endoscopic retrograde cholangiopancreatography in the diagnosis of choledocholithiasis. *Eur J Gastroenterol Hepatol.* 2003;15:809-813.

37. De Waele E, Op de Beeck B, De Waele B, et al. Magnetic resonance cholangiopancreatography in the preoperative assessment of patients with biliary pancreatitis. *Pancreatology.* 2007;7:347-351.

38. Hallal AH, Amortegui JD, Jeroukhimov IM, et al. Magnetic resonance cholangiopancreatography accurately detects common bile duct stones in resolving gallstone pancreatitis. *J Am Coll Surg.* 2005;200: 869-875.

39. Moon JH, Cho YD, Cha SW, et al. The detection of bile duct stones in suspected biliary pancreatitis: comparison of MRCP, ERCP, and intraductal US. *Am J Gastroenterol.* 2005;100:1051-1057.

40. Richard F, Boustany M, Britt LD. Accuracy of magnetic resonance cholangiopancreatography for diagnosing stones in the common bile duct in patients with abnormal intraoperative cholangiograms. *Am J Surg.* 2013;205:371-373.

41. Norero E, Norero B, Huete A, et al. [Accuracy of magnetic resonance cholangiopancreatography for the diagnosis of common bile duct stones]. *Rev Med Chil.* 2008;136:600-605.

42. MacEneaney P, Mitchell MT, McDermott R. Update on magnetic resonance cholangiopancreatography. *Gastroenterol Clin North Am.* 2002; 31:731-746.

43. Kay CL. Which test to replace diagnostic ERCP–MRCP or EUS? *Endoscopy.* 2003;35:426-428.

44. Savides TJ. EUS-guided ERCP for patients with intermediate probability for choledocholithiasis: is it time for all of us to start doing this? *Gastrointest Endosc.* 2008;67:669-672.

45. Mendler MH, Bouillet P, Sautereau D, et al. Value of MR cholangiography in the diagnosis of obstructive diseases of the biliary tree: a study of 58 cases. *Am J Gastroenterol.* 1998;93:2482-2490.

46. Zidi SH, Prat F, Le Guen O, et al. Use of magnetic resonance cholangiography in the diagnosis of choledocholithiasis: prospective comparison with a reference imaging method. *Gut.* 1999;44:118-122.

47. Aube C, Delorme B, Yzet T, et al. MR cholangiopancreatography versus endoscopic sonography in suspected common bile duct lithiasis: a prospective, comparative study. *AJR Am J Roentgenol.* 2005;184:55-62.

48. Frossard JL, Hadengue A, Amouyal G, et al. Choledocholithiasis: a prospective study of spontaneous common bile duct stone migration. *Gastrointest Endosc.* 2000;51:175-179.

49. Berdah SV, Orsoni P, Bege T, et al. Follow-up of selective endoscopic ultrasonography and/or endoscopic retrograde cholangiography prior to laparoscopic cholecystectomy: a prospective study of 300 patients. *Endoscopy.* 2001;33:216-220.

50. Aubertin JM, Levoir D, Bouillot JL, et al. Endoscopic ultrasonography immediately prior to laparoscopic cholecystectomy: a prospective evaluation. *Endoscopy.* 1996;28:667-673.

51. Kohut M, Nowakowska-Dulawa E, Marek T, et al. Accuracy of linear endoscopic ultrasonography in the evaluation of patients with suspected common bile duct stones. *Endoscopy.* 2002;34:299-303.

52. Meroni E, Bisagni P, Bona S, et al. Pre-operative endoscopic ultrasonography can optimise the management of patients undergoing laparoscopic cholecystectomy with abnormal liver function tests as the sole risk factor for choledocholithiasis: a prospective study. *Dig Liver Dis.* 2004;36:73-77.

53. Prat F, Amouyal G, Amouyal P, et al. Prospective controlled study of endoscopic ultrasonography and endoscopic retrograde cholangiography in patients with suspected common-bileduct lithiasis. *Lancet.* 1996;347:75-79.

54. Burtin P, Palazzo L, Canard JM, et al. Diagnostic strategies for extrahepatic cholestasis of indefinite origin: endoscopic ultrasonography or retrograde cholangiography? Results of a prospective study. *Endoscopy.* 1997;29:349-355.

55. Buscarini E, Tansini P, Vallisa D, et al. EUS for suspected choledocholithiasis: do benefits outweigh costs? A prospective, controlled study. *Gastrointest Endosc.* 2003;57:510-518.

56. Dancygier H, Nattermann C. The role of endoscopic ultrasonography in biliary tract disease: obstructive jaundice. *Endoscopy.* 1994;26:800-802.

57. Gautier G, Pilleul F, Crombe-Ternamian A, et al. Contribution of magnetic resonance cholangiopancreatography to the management of patients with suspected common bile duct stones. *Gastroenterol Clin Biol.* 2004;28:129-134.

58. Ney MV, Maluf-Filho F, Sakai P, et al. Echo-endoscopy versus endoscopic retrograde cholangiography for the diagnosis of choledocholithiasis: the influence of the size of the stone and diameter of the common bile duct. *Arq Gastroenterol.* 2005;42:239-243.

59. Norton SA, Alderson D. Prospective comparison of endoscopic ultrasonography and endoscopic retrograde cholangiopancreatography in the detection of bile duct stones. *Br J Surg.* 1997;84:1366-1369.

60. Prat F, Edery J, Meduri B, et al. Early EUS of the bile duct before endoscopic sphincterotomy for acute biliary pancreatitis. *Gastrointest Endosc.* 2001;54:724-729.

61. Ainsworth AP, Rafaelsen SR, Wamberg PA, et al. Cost-effectiveness of endoscopic ultrasonography, magnetic resonance cholangiopancreatography and endoscopic retrograde cholangiopancreatography in patients suspected of pancreaticobiliary disease. *Scand J Gastroenterol.* 2004;39:579-583.

62. Amouyal P, Amouyal G, Levy P, et al. Diagnosis of choledocholithiasis by endoscopic ultrasonography. *Gastroenterology.* 1994;106:1062-1067.

63. Cervi C, Aube C, Tuech JJ, et al. [Nuclear magnetic resonance cholangiography in biliary disease. Prospective study in 60 patients]. *Ann Chir.* 2000;125:428-434.

64. de Ledinghen V, Lecesne R, Raymond JM, et al. Diagnosis of choledocholithiasis: EUS or magnetic resonance cholangiography? A prospective controlled study. *Gastrointest Endosc.* 1999;49:26-31.

65. Dittrick G, Lamont JP, Kuhn JA, et al. Usefulness of endoscopic ultrasound in patients at high risk of choledocholithiasis. *Proc (Bayl Univ Med Cent).* 2005;18:211-213.

66. Kim JH, Kim MJ, Park SI, et al. MR cholangiography in symptomatic gallstones: diagnostic accuracy according to clinical risk group. *Radiology.* 2002;224:410-416.

67. Lachter J, Rubin A, Shiller M, et al. Linear EUS for bile duct stones. *Gastrointest Endosc.* 2000;51:51-54.

68. Materne R, Van Beers BE, Gigot JF, et al. Extrahepatic biliary obstruction: magnetic resonance imaging compared with endoscopic ultrasonography. *Endoscopy.* 2000;32:3-9.

69. Montariol T, Msika S, Charlier A, et al. Diagnosis of asymptomatic common bile duct stones: preoperative endoscopic ultrasonography versus intraoperative cholangiography—a multicenter, prospective controlled study. French Associations for Surgical Research. *Surgery.* 1998;124:6-13.

70. Scheiman JM, Carlos RC, Barnett JL, et al. Can endoscopic ultrasound or magnetic resonance cholangiopancreatography replace ERCP in patients with suspected biliary disease? A prospective trial and cost analysis. *Am J Gastroenterol.* 2001;96:2900-2904.

71. Shim CS, Joo JH, Park CW, et al. Effectiveness of endoscopic ultrasonography in the diagnosis of choledocholithiasis prior to laparoscopic cholecystectomy. *Endoscopy.* 1995;27:428-432.

72. Stiris MG, Tennoe B, Aadland E, et al. MR cholangiopancreaticography and endoscopic retrograde cholangiopancreaticography in patients with suspected common bile duct stones. *Acta Radiol.* 2000;41:269-272.

73. Sugiyama M, Atomi Y. Endoscopic ultrasonography for diagnosing choledocholithiasis: a prospective comparative study with ultrasonography and computed tomography. *Gastrointest Endosc.* 1997;45:143-146.

74. Taylor AC, Little AF, Hennessy OF, et al. Prospective assessment of magnetic resonance cholangiopancreatography for noninvasive imaging of the biliary tree. *Gastrointest Endosc.* 2002;55:17-22.

75. Demartines N, Eisner L, Schnabel K, et al. Evaluation of magnetic resonance cholangiography in the management of bile duct stones. *Arch Surg.* 2000;135:148-152.

76. Garrow D, Miller S, Sinha D, et al. Endoscopic ultrasound: a meta-analysis of test performance in suspected biliary obstruction. *Clin Gastroenterol Hepatol.* 2007;5:616-623.

77. Tse F, Liu L, Barkun AN, et al. EUS: a meta-analysis of test performance in suspected choledocholithiasis. *Gastrointest Endosc.* 2008;67:235-244.

78. Al Samaraee A, Khan U, Almashta Z, et al. Preoperative diagnosis of choledocholithiasis: the role of MRCP. *Br J Hosp Med (Lond).* 2009;70:339-343.

79. Ledro-Cano D. Suspected choledocholithiasis: endoscopic ultrasound or magnetic resonance cholangio-pancreatography? A systematic review. *Eur J Gastroenterol Hepatol.* 2007;19:1007-1011.

80. Verma D, Kapadia A, Eisen GM, et al. EUS vs MRCP for detection of choledocholithiasis. *Gastrointest Endosc.* 2006;64:248-254.

81. Wehrmann T, Martchenko K, Riphaus A. Catheter probe extraductal ultrasonography vs. conventional endoscopic ultrasonography for detection of bile duct stones. *Endoscopy.* 2009;41:133-137.

82. Katanuma A, Maguchi H, Osanai M, et al. The difference in the capability of delineation between convex and radial arrayed echoendoscope for pancreas and biliary tract; case reports from the standpoint of both convex and radial arrayed echoendoscope. *Dig Endosc.* 2011;23(suppl 1):2-8.

83. Kohut M, Nowak A, Nowakowska-Dulawa E, et al. Endosonography with linear array instead of endoscopic retrograde cholangiography as the diagnostic tool in patients with moderate suspicion of common bile duct stones. *World J Gastroenterol.* 2003;9:612-614.

84. Seifert H, Wehrmann T, Hilgers R, et al. Catheter probe extraductal EUS reliably detects distal common bile duct abnormalities. *Gastrointest Endosc.* 2004;60:61-67.

85. Catanzaro A, Pfau P, Isenberg GA, et al. Clinical utility of intraductal US for evaluation of choledocholithiasis. *Gastrointest Endosc.* 2003;57:648-652.

86. Tsuchiya S, Tsuyuguchi T, Sakai Y, et al. Clinical utility of intraductal US to decrease early recurrence rate of common bile duct stones after endoscopic papillotomy. *J Gastroenterol Hepatol.* 2008;23:1590-1595.

87. Sotoudehmanesh R, Kolahdoozan S, Asgari AA, et al. Role of endoscopic ultrasonography in prevention of unnecessary endoscopic retrograde cholangiopancreatography: a prospective study of 150 patients. *J Ultrasound Med.* 2007;26:455-460.

88. Lu J, Guo CY, Xu XF, et al. Efficacy of intraductal ultrasonography in the diagnosis of non-opaque choledocholith. *World J Gastroenterol.* 2012;18:275-278.

89. Karakan T, Cindoruk M, Alagozlu H, et al. EUS versus endoscopic retrograde cholangiography for patients with intermediate probability of bile duct stones: a prospective randomized trial. *Gastrointest Endosc.* 2009;69:244-252.

90. Petrov MS, Savides TJ. Systematic review of endoscopic ultrasonography versus endoscopic retrograde cholangiopancreatography for suspected choledocholithiasis. *Br J Surg.* 2009;96:967-974.

91. Cotton PB. Endoscopic retrograde cholangiopancreatography and laparoscopic cholecystectomy. *Am J Surg.* 1993;165:474-478.

92. Cotton PB, Baillie J, Pappas TN, et al. Laparoscopic cholecystectomy and the biliary endoscopist. *Gastrointest Endosc.* 1991;37:94-97.

93. O'Toole D, Palazzo L. Choledocholithiasis—a practical approach from the endosonographer. *Endoscopy.* 2006;38(suppl 1):S23-S29.

94. Sgouros SN, Bergele C. Endoscopic ultrasonography versus other diagnostic modalities in the diagnosis of choledocholithiasis. *Dig Dis Sci.* 2006;51:2280-2286.

95. Abboud PA, Malet PF, Berlin JA, et al. Predictors of common bile duct stones prior to cholecystectomy: a meta-analysis. *Gastrointest Endosc.* 1996;44:450-455.

96. Makary MA, Duncan MD, Harmon JW, et al. The role of magnetic resonance cholangiography in the management of patients with gallstone pancreatitis. *Ann Surg.* 2005;241:119-124.

97. Sahai AV, Mauldin PD, Marsi V, et al. Bile duct stones and laparoscopic cholecystectomy: a decision analysis to assess the roles of intraoperative

cholangiography, EUS, and ERCP. *Gastrointest Endosc.* 1999;49:334-343.

98. Das A, Chak A. Endoscopic ultrasonography. *Endoscopy.* 2004;36:17-22.

99. Benjaminov F, Stein A, Lichtman G, et al. Consecutive versus separate sessions of endoscopic ultrasound (EUS) and endoscopic retrograde cholangiopancreatography (ERCP) for symptomatic choledocholithiasis. *Surg Endosc.* 2013;27:2117-2121.

100. Fabbri C, Polifemo AM, Luigiano C, et al. Single session versus separate session endoscopic ultrasonography plus endoscopic retrograde cholangiography in patients with low to moderate risk for choledocholithiasis. *J Gastroenterol Hepatol.* 2009;24:1107-1112.

101. Polkowski M, Regula J, Tilszer A, et al. Endoscopic ultrasound versus endoscopic retrograde cholangiography for patients with intermediate probability of bile duct stones: a randomized trial comparing two management strategies. *Endoscopy.* 2007;39:296-303.

102. Kim KM, Lee JK, Bahng S, et al. Role of endoscopic ultrasonography in patients with intermediate probability of choledocholithiasis but a negative CT scan. *J Clin Gastroenterol.* 2013;47:449-456.

103. Alhayaf N, Lalor E, Bain V, et al. The clinical impact and cost implication of endoscopic ultrasound on use of endoscopic retrograde cholangiopancreatography in a Canadian university hospital. *Can J Gastroenterol.* 2008;22:138-142.

104. Arguedas MR, Dupont AW, Wilcox CM. Where do ERCP, endoscopic ultrasound, magnetic resonance cholangiopancreatography, and intraoperative cholangiography fit in the management of acute biliary pancreatitis? A decision analysis model. *Am J Gastroenterol.* 2001;96:2892-2899.

105. Romagnuolo J, Currie G. Noninvasive vs. selective invasive biliary imaging for acute biliary pancreatitis: an economic evaluation by using decision tree analysis. *Gastrointest Endosc.* 2005;61:86-97.

106. Shea JA, Berlin JA, Escarce JJ, et al. Revised estimates of diagnostic test sensitivity and specificity in suspected biliary tract disease. *Arch Intern Med.* 1994;154:2573-2581.

107. Ko CW, Sekijima JH, Lee SP. Biliary sludge. *Ann Intern Med.* 1999;130:301-311.

108. Dill JE, Hill S, Callis J, et al. Combined endoscopic ultrasound and stimulated biliary drainage in cholecystitis and microlithiasis—diagnoses and outcomes. *Endoscopy.* 1995;27:424-427.

109. Dahan P, Andant C, Levy P, et al. Prospective evaluation of endoscopic ultrasonography and microscopic examination of duodenal bile in the diagnosis of cholecystolithiasis in 45 patients with normal conventional ultrasonography. *Gut.* 1996;38:277-281.

110. Mirbagheri SA, Mohamadnejad M, Nasiri J, et al. Prospective evaluation of endoscopic ultrasonography in the diagnosis of biliary microlithiasis in patients with normal transabdominal ultrasonography. *J Gastrointest Surg.* 2005;9:961-964.

111. Thorboll J, Vilmann P, Jacobsen B, et al. Endoscopic ultrasonography in detection of cholelithiasis in patients with biliary pain and negative transabdominal ultrasonography. *Scand J Gastroenterol.* 2004;39:267-269.

112. Kaw M, Brodmerkel GJ Jr. ERCP, biliary crystal analysis, and sphincter of Oddi manometry in idiopathic recurrent pancreatitis. *Gastrointest Endosc.* 2002;55:157-162.

113. Lee SP, Hayashi A, Kim YS. Biliary sludge: curiosity or culprit? *Hepatology.* 1994;20:523-525.

114. Ros E, Navarro S, Bru C, et al. Occult microlithiasis in "idiopathic" acute pancreatitis: prevention of relapses by cholecystectomy or ursodeoxycholic acid therapy. *Gastroenterology.* 1991;101:1701-1709.

115. Chak A, Hawes RH, Cooper GS, et al. Prospective assessment of the utility of EUS in the evaluation of gallstone pancreatitis. *Gastrointest Endosc.* 1999;49:599-604.

116. Yusoff IF, Raymond G, Sahai AV. A prospective comparison of the yield of EUS in primary vs. recurrent idiopathic acute pancreatitis. *Gastrointest Endosc.* 2004;60:673-678.

117. Wilcox CM, Varadarajulu S, Eloubeidi M. Role of endoscopic evaluation in idiopathic pancreatitis: a systematic review. *Gastrointest Endosc.* 2006;63:1037-1045.

118. Wilcox CM, Kilgore M. Cost minimization analysis comparing diagnostic strategies in unexplained pancreatitis. *Pancreas.* 2009;38:117-121.

119. Lahde S. Helical CT in the examination of bile duct obstruction. *Acta Radiol.* 1996;37:660-664.

120. Park MS, Kim TK, Kim KW, et al. Differentiation of extrahepatic bile duct cholangiocarcinoma from benign stricture: findings at MRCP versus ERCP. *Radiology.* 2004;233:234-240.

121. Zidi SH, Prat F, Le Guen O, et al. Performance characteristics of magnetic resonance cholangiography in the staging of malignant hilar strictures. *Gut.* 2000;46:103-106.

122. Stewart CJ, Mills PR, Carter R, et al. Brush cytology in the assessment of pancreatico-biliary strictures: a review of 406 cases. *J Clin Pathol.* 2001;54:449-455.

123. Cote GA, Sherman S. Biliary stricture and negative cytology: what next? *Clin Gastroenterol Hepatol.* 2011;9:739-743.

124. Glasbrenner B, Ardan M, Boeck W, et al. Prospective evaluation of brush cytology of biliary strictures during endoscopic retrograde cholangiopancreatography. *Endoscopy.* 1999;31:712-717.

125. Kipp BR, Stadheim LM, Halling SA, et al. A comparison of routine cytology and fluorescence in situ hybridization for the detection of malignant bile duct strictures. *Am J Gastroenterol.* 2004;99:1675-1681.

126. Lee JG, Leung JW, Baillie J, et al. Benign, dysplastic, or malignant—making sense of endoscopic bile duct brush cytology: results in 149 consecutive patients. *Am J Gastroenterol.* 1995;90:722-726.

127. Fritcher EG, Kipp BR, Halling KC, et al. A multivariable model using advanced cytologic methods for the evaluation of indeterminate pancreatobiliary strictures. *Gastroenterology.* 2009;136:2180-2186.

128. Levy MJ, Baron TH, Clayton AC, et al. Prospective evaluation of advanced molecular markers and imaging techniques in patients with indeterminate bile duct strictures. *Am J Gastroenterol.* 2008;103:1263-1273.

129. Gonda TA, Glick MP, Sethi A, et al. Polysomy and p16 deletion by fluorescence in situ hybridization in the diagnosis of indeterminate biliary strictures. *Gastrointest Endosc.* 2012;75:74-79.

130. Ponchon T, Gagnon P, Berger F, et al. Value of endobiliary brush cytology and biopsies for the diagnosis of malignant bile duct stenosis: results of a prospective study. *Gastrointest Endosc.* 1995;42:565-572.

131. Schoefl R, Haefner M, Wrba F, et al. Forceps biopsy and brush cytology during endoscopic retrograde cholangiopancreatography for the diagnosis of biliary stenoses. *Scand J Gastroenterol.* 1997;32:363-368.

132. de Bellis M, Sherman S, Fogel EL, et al. Tissue sampling at ERCP in suspected malignant biliary strictures (Part 2). *Gastrointest Endosc.* 2002;56:720-730.

133. De Bellis M, Sherman S, Fogel EL, et al. Tissue sampling at ERCP in suspected malignant biliary strictures (Part 1). *Gastrointest Endosc.* 2002;56:552-561.

134. Higashizawa T, Tamada K, Tomiyama T, et al. Biliary guidewire facilitates bile duct biopsy and endoscopic drainage. *J Gastroenterol Hepatol.* 2002;17:332-336.

135. Farrell RJ, Jain AK, Brandwein SL, et al. The combination of stricture dilation, endoscopic needle aspiration, and biliary brushings significantly improves diagnostic yield from malignant bile duct strictures. *Gastrointest Endosc.* 2001;54:587-594.

136. de Bellis M, Fogel EL, Sherman S, et al. Influence of stricture dilation and repeat brushing on the cancer detection rate of brush cytology in the evaluation of malignant biliary obstruction. *Gastrointest Endosc.* 2003;58:176-182.

137. Tamada K, Kurihara K, Tomiyama T, et al. How many biopsies should be performed during percutaneous transhepatic cholangioscopy to diagnose biliary tract cancer? *Gastrointest Endosc.* 1999;50:653-658.

138. Tamada K, Ueno N, Tomiyama T, et al. Characterization of biliary strictures using intraductal ultrasonography: comparison with percutaneous cholangioscopic biopsy. *Gastrointest Endosc.* 1998;47:341-349.

139. Chen YK, Parsi MA, Binmoeller KF, et al. Single-operator cholangioscopy in patients requiring evaluation of bile duct disease or therapy of biliary stones (with videos). *Gastrointest Endosc.* 2011;74:805-814.

140. Chen YK, Pleskow DK. SpyGlass single-operator peroral cholangiopancreatoscopy system for the diagnosis and therapy of bile-duct disorders: a clinical feasibility study (with video). *Gastrointest Endosc.* 2007;65:832-841.

141. Draganov PV, Chauhan S, Wagh MS, et al. Diagnostic accuracy of conventional and cholangioscopy-guided sampling of indeterminate biliary lesions at the time of ERCP: a prospective, long-term follow-up study. *Gastrointest Endosc.* 2012;75:347-353.

142. Osanai M, Itoi T, Igarashi Y, et al. Peroral video cholangioscopy to evaluate indeterminate bile duct lesions and preoperative mucosal cancerous extension: a prospective multicenter study. *Endoscopy.* 2013.

143. Sethi A, Chen YK, Austin GL, et al. ERCP with cholangiopancreatoscopy may be associated with higher rates of complications than ERCP alone: a single-center experience. *Gastrointest Endosc.* 2011;73:251-256.

144. Devereaux CE, Binmoeller KF. Endoscopic retrograde cholangiopancreatography in the next millennium. *Gastrointest Endosc Clin N Am.* 2000;10:117-133, vii.
145. Fogel EL, Sherman S. How to improve the accuracy of diagnosis of malignant biliary strictures. *Endoscopy.* 1999;31:758-760.
146. Mukai H, Nakajima M, Yasuda K, et al. Evaluation of endoscopic ultrasonography in the pre-operative staging of carcinoma of the ampulla of Vater and common bile duct. *Gastrointest Endosc.* 1992;38:676-683.
147. Songur Y, Temucin G, Sahin B. Endoscopic ultrasonography in the evaluation of dilated common bile duct. *J Clin Gastroenterol.* 2001;33:302-305.
148. Tio TL, Cheng J, Wijers OB, et al. Endosonographic TNM staging of extrahepatic bile duct cancer: comparison with pathological staging. *Gastroenterology.* 1991;100:1351-1361.
149. Agarwal B, Abu-Hamda E, Molke KL, et al. Endoscopic ultrasound-guided fine needle aspiration and multidetector spiral CT in the diagnosis of pancreatic cancer. *Am J Gastroenterol.* 2004;99:844-850.
150. Gress F, Gottlieb K, Sherman S, et al. Endoscopic ultrasonography-guided fine-needle aspiration biopsy of suspected pancreatic cancer. *Ann Intern Med.* 2001;134:459-464.
151. Harewood GC, Wiersema MJ. Endosonography-guided fine needle aspiration biopsy in the evaluation of pancreatic masses. *Am J Gastroenterol.* 2002;97:1386-1391.
152. Hollerbach S, Klamann A, Topalidis T, et al. Endoscopic ultrasonography (EUS) and fine-needle aspiration (FNA) cytology for diagnosis of chronic pancreatitis. *Endoscopy.* 2001;33:824-831.
153. Menzel J, Poremba C, Dietl KH, et al. Preoperative diagnosis of bile duct strictures–comparison of intraductal ultrasonography with conventional endosonography. *Scand J Gastroenterol.* 2000;35:77-82.
154. Palazzo L, Roseau G, Gayet B, et al. Endoscopic ultrasonography in the diagnosis and staging of pancreatic adenocarcinoma. Results of a prospective study with comparison to ultrasonography and CT scan. *Endoscopy.* 1993;25:143-150.
155. Raut CP, Grau AM, Staerkel GA, et al. Diagnostic accuracy of endoscopic ultrasound-guided fine-needle aspiration in patients with presumed pancreatic cancer. *J Gastrointest Surg.* 2003;7:118-126, discussion 127-128.
156. Varadarajulu S, Tamhane A, Eloubeidi MA. Yield of EUS-guided FNA of pancreatic masses in the presence or the absence of chronic pancreatitis. *Gastrointest Endosc.* 2005;62:728-736, quiz 751, 753.
157. Mohamadnejad M, DeWitt JM, Sherman S, et al. Role of EUS for preoperative evaluation of cholangiocarcinoma: a large single-center experience. *Gastrointest Endosc.* 2011;73:71-78.
158. Horwhat JD, Paulson EK, McGrath K, et al. A randomized comparison of EUS-guided FNA versus CT or US-guided FNA for the evaluation of pancreatic mass lesions. *Gastrointest Endosc.* 2006;63:966-975.
159. Lee JH, Salem R, Aslanian H, et al. Endoscopic ultrasound and fine-needle aspiration of unexplained bile duct strictures. *Am J Gastroenterol.* 2004;99:1069-1073.
160. Wu LM, Jiang XX, Gu HY, et al. Endoscopic ultrasound-guided fine-needle aspiration biopsy in the evaluation of bile duct strictures and gallbladder masses: a systematic review and meta-analysis. *Eur J Gastroenterol Hepatol.* 2011;23:113-120.
161. Byrne MF, Gerke H, Mitchell RM, et al. Yield of endoscopic ultrasound-guided fine-needle aspiration of bile duct lesions. *Endoscopy.* 2004;36:715-719.
162. DeWitt J, Misra VL, Leblanc JK, et al. EUS-guided FNA of proximal biliary strictures after negative ERCP brush cytology results. *Gastrointest Endosc.* 2006;64:325-333.
163. Fritscher-Ravens A, Broering DC, Sriram PV, et al. EUS-guided fine-needle aspiration cytodiagnosis of hilar cholangiocarcinoma: a case series. *Gastrointest Endosc.* 2000;52:534-540.
164. Meara RS, Jhala D, Eloubeidi MA, et al. Endoscopic ultrasound-guided FNA biopsy of bile duct and gallbladder: analysis of 53 cases. *Cytopathology.* 2006;17:42-49.
165. Rosch T, Hofrichter K, Frimberger E, et al. ERCP or EUS for tissue diagnosis of biliary strictures? A prospective comparative study. *Gastrointest Endosc.* 2004;60:390-396.
166. Eloubeidi MA, Chen VK, Jhala NC, et al. Endoscopic ultrasound-guided fine needle aspiration biopsy of suspected cholangiocarcinoma. *Clin Gastroenterol Hepatol.* 2004;2:209-213.
167. Fritscher-Ravens A, Broering DC, Knoefel WT, et al. EUS-guided fine-needle aspiration of suspected hilar cholangiocarcinoma in potentially operable patients with negative brush cytology. *Am J Gastroenterol.* 2004;99:45-51.
168. Tummala P, Munigala S, Eloubeidi MA, et al. Patients with obstructive jaundice and biliary stricture +/- mass lesion on imaging: prevalence of malignancy and potential role of EUS-FNA. *J Clin Gastroenterol.* 2013;47:532-537.
169. Ohshima Y, Yasuda I, Kawakami H, et al. EUS-FNA for suspected malignant biliary strictures after negative endoscopic transpapillary brush cytology and forceps biopsy. *J Gastroenterol.* 2011;46:921-928.
170. Nayar MK, Manas DM, Wadehra V, et al. Role of EUS/EUS-guided FNA in the management of proximal biliary strictures. *Hepatogastroenterology.* 2011;58:1862-1865.
171. Saifuku Y, Yamagata M, Koike T, et al. Endoscopic ultrasonography can diagnose distal biliary strictures without a mass on computed tomography. *World J Gastroenterol.* 2010;16:237-244.
172. Larghi A, Lecca PG, Ardito F, et al. Evaluation of hilar biliary strictures by using a newly developed forward-viewing therapeutic echoendoscope: preliminary results of an ongoing experience. *Gastrointest Endosc.* 2009;69:356-360.
173. Farrell RJ, Agarwal B, Brandwein SL, et al. Intraductal US is a useful adjunct to ERCP for distinguishing malignant from benign biliary strictures. *Gastrointest Endosc.* 2002;56:681-687.
174. Vazquez-Sequeiros E, Baron TH, Clain JE, et al. Evaluation of indeterminate bile duct strictures by intraductal US. *Gastrointest Endosc.* 2002;56:372-379.
175. Tamada K, Tomiyama T, Ichiyama M, et al. Influence of biliary drainage catheter on bile duct wall thickness as measured by intraductal ultrasonography. *Gastrointest Endosc.* 1998;47:28-32.
176. Domagk D, Wessling J, Reimer P, et al. Endoscopic retrograde cholangiopancreatography, intraductal ultrasonography, and magnetic resonance cholangiopancreatography in bile duct strictures: a prospective comparison of imaging diagnostics with histopathological correlation. *Am J Gastroenterol.* 2004;99:1684-1689.
177. Krishna NB, Saripalli S, Safdar R, et al. Intraductal US in evaluation of biliary strictures without a mass lesion on CT scan or magnetic resonance imaging: significance of focal wall thickening and extrinsic compression at the stricture site. *Gastrointest Endosc.* 2007;66:90-96.
178. Stavropoulos S, Larghi A, Verna E, et al. Intraductal ultrasound for the evaluation of patients with biliary strictures and no abdominal mass on computed tomography. *Endoscopy.* 2005;37:715-721.
179. Tamada K, Nagai H, Yasuda Y, et al. Transpapillary intraductal US prior to biliary drainage in the assessment of longitudinal spread of extrahepatic bile duct carcinoma. *Gastrointest Endosc.* 2001;53:300-307.
180. Varadarajulu S, Eloubeidi MA, Wilcox CM. Prospective evaluation of indeterminate ERCP findings by intraductal ultrasound. *J Gastroenterol Hepatol.* 2007;22:2086-2092.
181. Inui K, Miyoshi H. Cholangiocarcinoma and intraductal sonography. *Gastrointest Endosc Clin N Am.* 2005;15:143-155, x.
182. Gress F, Chen YK, Sherman S, et al. Experience with a catheter-based ultrasound probe in the bile duct and pancreas. *Endoscopy.* 1995;27:178-184.
183. Kuroiwa M, Tsukamoto Y, Naitoh Y, et al. New technique using intraductal ultrasonography for the diagnosis of bile duct cancer. *J Ultrasound Med.* 1994;13:189-195.
184. Kuroiwa M, Goto H, Hirooka Y, et al. Intraductal ultrasonography for the diagnosis of proximal invasion in extrahepatic bile duct cancer. *J Gastroenterol Hepatol.* 1998;13:715-719.
185. Tamada K, Tomiyama T, Wada S, et al. Endoscopic transpapillary bile duct biopsy with the combination of intraductal ultrasonography in the diagnosis of biliary strictures. *Gut.* 2002;50:326-331.
186. Wehrmann T, Riphaus A, Martchenko K, et al. Intraductal ultrasonography in the diagnosis of Mirizzi syndrome. *Endoscopy.* 2006;38:717-722.
187. Dumortier J, Scoazec JY, Valette PJ, et al. Successful liver transplantation for diffuse biliary papillomatosis. *J Hepatol.* 2001;35:542-543.
188. Tamada K, Tomiyama T, Oohashi A, et al. Bile duct wall thickness measured by intraductal US in patients who have not undergone previous biliary drainage. *Gastrointest Endosc.* 1999;49:199-203.
189. Tischendorf JJ, Meier PN, Schneider A, et al. Transpapillary intraductal ultrasound in the evaluation of dominant bile duct stenoses in patients with primary sclerosing cholangitis. *Scand J Gastroenterol.* 2007;42:1011-1017.
190. Rosch T, Meining A, Fruhmorgen S, et al. A prospective comparison of the diagnostic accuracy of ERCP, MRCP, CT, and EUS in biliary strictures. *Gastrointest Endosc.* 2002;55:870-876.

191. Sai JK, Suyama M, Kubokawa Y, et al. Early detection of extrahepatic bile-duct carcinomas in the nonicteric stage by using MRCP followed by EUS. *Gastrointest Endosc.* 2009;70:29-36.
192. Mishra G, Conway JD. Endoscopic ultrasound in the evaluation of radiologic abnormalities of the liver and biliary tree. *Curr Gastroenterol Rep.* 2009;11:150-154.
193. Fukuda Y, Tsuyuguchi T, Sakai Y, et al. Diagnostic utility of peroral cholangioscopy for various bile-duct lesions. *Gastrointest Endosc.* 2005;62:374-382.
194. Nguyen NQ, Schoeman MN, Ruszkiewicz A. Clinical utility of EUS before cholangioscopy in the evaluation of difficult biliary strictures. *Gastrointest Endosc.* 2013;78(6):868-874.
195. Siddiqui AA, Mehendiratta V, Jackson W, et al. Identification of cholangiocarcinoma by using the Spyglass Spyscope system for peroral cholangioscopy and biopsy collection. *Clin Gastroenterol Hepatol.* 2012;10:466-471, quiz e48.
196. Itoi T, Reddy DN, Sofuni A, et al. Clinical evaluation of a prototype multi-bending peroral direct cholangioscope. *Dig Endosc.* 2013.
197. Siddiqui UD, Rossi F, Rosenthal LS, et al. EUS-guided FNA of solid pancreatic masses: a prospective, randomized trial comparing 22-gauge and 25-gauge needles. *Gastrointest Endosc.* 2009;70:1093-1097.
198. Lee JK, Lee KT, Choi ER, et al. A prospective, randomized trial comparing 25-gauge and 22-gauge needles for endoscopic ultrasound-guided fine needle aspiration of pancreatic masses. *Scand J Gastroenterol.* 2013;48:752-757.
199. Madhoun MF, Wani SB, Rastogi A, et al. The diagnostic accuracy of 22-gauge and 25-gauge needles in endoscopic ultrasound-guided fine needle aspiration of solid pancreatic lesions: a meta-analysis. *Endoscopy.* 2013;45:86-92.
200. Bismuth H, Castaing D, Traynor O. Resection or palliation: priority of surgery in the treatment of hilar cancer. *World J Surg.* 1988;12:39-47.
201. Meister T, Heinzow HS, Woestmeyer C, et al. Intraductal ultrasound substantiates diagnostics of bile duct strictures of uncertain etiology. *World J Gastroenterol.* 2013;19:874-881.
202. Nimura Y. Staging cholangiocarcinoma by cholangioscopy. *HPB (Oxford).* 2008;10:113-115.
203. Sato M, Inoue H, Ogawa S, et al. Limitations of percutaneous transhepatic cholangioscopy for the diagnosis of the intramural extension of bile duct carcinoma. *Endoscopy.* 1998;30:281-288.
204. Tamada K, Ueno N, Ichiyama M, et al. Assessment of pancreatic parenchymal invasion by bile duct cancer using intraductal ultrasonography. *Endoscopy.* 1996;28:492-496.
205. Tamada K, Ido K, Ueno N, et al. Assessment of hepatic artery invasion by bile duct cancer using intraductal ultrasonography. *Endoscopy.* 1995;27:579-583.
206. Tamada K, Ido K, Ueno N, et al. Assessment of portal vein invasion by bile duct cancer using intraductal ultrasonography. *Endoscopy.* 1995;27:573-578.
207. Chen CY, Lu CL, Chang FY, et al. Risk factors for gallbladder polyps in the Chinese population. *Am J Gastroenterol.* 1997;92:2066-2068.
208. Segawa K, Arisawa T, Niwa Y, et al. Prevalence of gallbladder polyps among apparently healthy Japanese: ultrasonographic study. *Am J Gastroenterol.* 1992;87:630-633.
209. Sugiyama M, Atomi Y, Kuroda A, et al. Large cholesterol polyps of the gallbladder: diagnosis by means of US and endoscopic US. *Radiology.* 1995;196:493-497.
210. Aldridge MC, Bismuth H. Gallbladder cancer: the polyp-cancer sequence. *Br J Surg.* 1990;77:363-364.
211. Kozuka S, Tsubone N, Yasui A, et al. Relation of adenoma to carcinoma in the gallbladder. *Cancer.* 1982;50:2226-2234.
212. Garcia-Olmo D, Vazquez P, Cifuentes J, et al. Postoperative gangrenous peritonitis after laparoscopic cholecystectomy: a new complication for a new technique. *Surg Laparosc Endosc.* 1996;6:224-225.
213. Zilberstein B, Cecconello I, Ramos AC, et al. Hemobilia as a complication of laparoscopic cholecystectomy. *Surg Laparosc Endosc.* 1994;4:301-303.
214. Black NA, Thompson E, Sanderson CF. Symptoms and health status before and six weeks after open cholecystectomy: a European cohort study. ECHSS Group. European Collaborative Health Services Study Group. *Gut.* 1994;35:1301-1305.
215. Desautels SG, Slivka A, Hutson WR, et al. Postcholecystectomy pain syndrome: pathophysiology of abdominal pain in sphincter of Oddi type III. *Gastroenterology.* 1999;116:900-905.

216. Sugiyama M, Atomi Y, Yamato T. Endoscopic ultrasonography for differential diagnosis of polypoid gall bladder lesions: analysis in surgical and follow up series. *Gut.* 2000;46:250-254.
217. Kubota K, Bandai Y, Noie T, et al. How should polypoid lesions of the gallbladder be treated in the era of laparoscopic cholecystectomy? *Surgery.* 1995;117:481-487.
218. Shinkai H, Kimura W, Muto T. Surgical indications for small polypoid lesions of the gallbladder. *Am J Surg.* 1998;175:114-117.
219. Choi WB, Lee SK, Kim MH, et al. A new strategy to predict the neoplastic polyps of the gallbladder based on a scoring system using EUS. *Gastrointest Endosc.* 2000;52:372-379.
220. Sadamoto Y, Oda S, Tanaka M, et al. A useful approach to the differential diagnosis of small polypoid lesions of the gallbladder, utilizing an endoscopic ultrasound scoring system. *Endoscopy.* 2002;34:959-965.
221. Sugiyama M, Xie XY, Atomi Y, et al. Differential diagnosis of small polypoid lesions of the gallbladder: the value of endoscopic ultrasonography. *Ann Surg.* 1999;229:498-504.
222. French DG, Allen PD, Ellsmere JC. The diagnostic accuracy of transabdominal ultrasonography needs to be considered when managing gallbladder polyps. *Surg Endosc.* 2013;27(11):4021-4025.
223. Azuma T, Yoshikawa T, Araida T, et al. Differential diagnosis of polypoid lesions of the gallbladder by endoscopic ultrasonography. *Am J Surg.* 2001;181:65-70.
224. Choi JH, Seo DW, Park DH, et al. Utility of contrast-enhanced harmonic EUS in the diagnosis of malignant gallbladder polyps (with videos). *Gastrointest Endosc.* 2013.
225. Fujita N, Noda Y, Kobayashi G, et al. Diagnosis of the depth of invasion of gallbladder carcinoma by EUS. *Gastrointest Endosc.* 1999;50:659-663.
226. Morita K, Nakazawa S, Naito Y, et al. [Endoscopic ultrasonography of the gallbladder compared with pathological findings]. *Nihon Shokakibyo Gakkai Zasshi.* 1986;83:86-95.
227. Cho JH, Park JY, Kim YJ, et al. Hypoechoic foci on EUS are simple and strong predictive factors for neoplastic gallbladder polyps. *Gastrointest Endosc.* 2009;69:1244-1250.
228. Cheon YK, Cho WY, Lee TH, et al. Endoscopic ultrasonography does not differentiate neoplastic from non-neoplastic small gallbladder polyps. *World J Gastroenterol.* 2009;15:2361-2366.
229. Park CH, Chung MJ, Oh TG, et al. Differential diagnosis between gallbladder adenomas and cholesterol polyps on contrast-enhanced harmonic endoscopic ultrasonography. *Surg Endosc.* 2013;27:1414-1421.
230. Chijiiwa K, Sumiyoshi K, Nakayama F. Impact of recent advances in hepatobiliary imaging techniques on the preoperative diagnosis of carcinoma of the gallbladder. *World J Surg.* 1991;15:322-327.
231. Kimura K, Fujita N, Noda Y, et al. Differential diagnosis of large-sized pedunculated polypoid lesions of the gallbladder by endoscopic ultrasonography: a prospective study. *J Gastroenterol.* 2001;36:619-622.
232. Nasiri S, Gafuri A, Karamnejad M, et al. Four port-site recurrences of gall bladder cancer after laparoscopic cholecystectomy. *ANZ J Surg.* 2009;79:75-76.
233. Hu JB, Sun XN, Xu J, et al. Port site and distant metastases of gallbladder cancer after laparoscopic cholecystectomy diagnosed by positron emission tomography. *World J Gastroenterol.* 2008;14:6428-6431.
234. Mizuguchi M, Kudo S, Fukahori T, et al. Endoscopic ultrasonography for demonstrating loss of multiple-layer pattern of the thickened gallbladder wall in the preoperative diagnosis of gallbladder cancer. *Eur Radiol.* 1997;7:1323-1327.
235. Edge SB, Byrd DR, Compton CC, et al., eds. *American Joint Committee on Cancer Staging Manual.* 7th ed. New York: Springer; 2010:211.
236. Sadamoto Y, Kubo H, Harada N, et al. Preoperative diagnosis and staging of gallbladder carcinoma by EUS. *Gastrointest Endosc.* 2003;58:536-541.
237. Hijioka S, Hara K, Mizuno N, et al. Diagnostic yield of endoscopic retrograde cholangiography and of EUS-guided fine needle aspiration sampling in gallbladder carcinomas. *J Hepatobiliary Pancreat Sci.* 2012;19:650-655.
238. Hijioka S, Mekky MA, Bhatia V, et al. Can EUS-guided FNA distinguish between gallbladder cancer and xanthogranulomatous cholecystitis? *Gastrointest Endosc.* 2010;72:622-627.
239. Jacobson BC, Pitman MB, Brugge WR. EUS-guided FNA for the diagnosis of gallbladder masses. *Gastrointest Endosc.* 2003;57:251-254.

240. Kim HJ, Lee SK, Jang JW, et al. Diagnostic role of endoscopic ultrasonography-guided fine needle aspiration of gallbladder lesions. *Hepatogastroenterology.* 2012;59:1691-1695.
241. Varadarajulu S, Eloubeidi MA. Endoscopic ultrasound-guided fine-needle aspiration in the evaluation of gallbladder masses. *Endoscopy.* 2005;37:751-754.
242. Jacobson BC, Waxman I, Parmar K, et al. Endoscopic ultrasound-guided gallbladder bile aspiration in idiopathic pancreatitis carries a significant risk of bile peritonitis. *Pancreatology.* 2002;2:26-29.
243. Downing SR, Cadogan KA, Ortega G, et al. Early-stage gallbladder cancer in the Surveillance, Epidemiology, and End Results database: effect of extended surgical resection. *Arch Surg.* 2011;146:734-738.
244. Fujimoto T, Kato Y, Kitamura T, et al. Case report: hypoechoic area as an ultrasound finding suggesting subserosal invasion in polypoid carcinoma of the gall bladder. *Br J Radiol.* 2001;74:455-457.
245. Kim MY, Baik SK, Choi YJ, et al. Endoscopic sonographic evaluation of the thickened gallbladder wall in patients with acute hepatitis. *J Clin Ultrasound.* 2003;31:245-249.
246. Sato M, Ishida H, Konno K, et al. Segmental chronic cholecystitis: sonographic findings and clinical manifestations. *Abdom Imaging.* 2002;27:43-46.
247. Ishizuka D, Shirai Y, Tsukada K, et al. Gallbladder cancer with intratumoral anechoic foci: a mimic of adenomyomatosis. *Hepatogastroenterology.* 1998;45:927-929.
248. Nabatame N, Shirai Y, Nishimura A, et al. High risk of gallbladder carcinoma in elderly patients with segmental adenomyomatosis of the gallbladder. *J Exp Clin Cancer Res.* 2004;23:593-598.
249. Guzman-Valdivia G. Xanthogranulomatous cholecystitis: 15 years' experience. *World J Surg.* 2004;28:254-257.
250. Muguruma N, Okamura S, Okahisa T, et al. Endoscopic sonography in the diagnosis of xanthogranulomatous cholecystitis. *J Clin Ultrasound.* 1999;27:347-350.
251. Kim HJ, Park JH, Park DI, et al. Clinical usefulness of endoscopic ultrasonography in the differential diagnosis of gallbladder wall thickening. *Dig Dis Sci.* 2012;57:508-515.
252. Eaton JE, Thackeray EW, Lindor KD. Likelihood of malignancy in gallbladder polyps and outcomes following cholecystectomy in primary sclerosing cholangitis. *Am J Gastroenterol.* 2012;107:431-439.
253. Palazzo L, Hochain P, Helmer C, et al. Biliary varices on endoscopic ultrasonography: clinical presentation and outcome. *Endoscopy.* 2000;32:520-524.
254. Tokiwa K, Iwai N. Early mucosal changes of the gallbladder in patients with anomalous arrangement of the pancreaticobiliary duct. *Gastroenterology.* 1996;110:1614-1618.
255. Tanno S, Obara T, Maguchi H, et al. Thickened inner hypoechoic layer of the gallbladder wall in the diagnosis of anomalous pancreaticobiliary ductal union with endosonography. *Gastrointest Endosc.* 1997;46:520-526.
256. Kawakatsu M, Vilgrain V, Zins M, et al. Radiologic features of papillary adenoma and papillomatosis of the biliary tract. *Abdom Imaging.* 1997;22:87-90.
257. Fockens P. The role of endoscopic ultrasonography in the biliary tract: ampullary tumors. *Endoscopy.* 1994;26:803-805.
258. Spigelman AD, Talbot IC, Penna C, et al. Evidence for adenoma-carcinoma sequence in the duodenum of patients with familial adenomatous polyposis. The Leeds Castle Polyposis Group (Upper Gastrointestinal Committee). *J Clin Pathol.* 1994;47:709-710.
259. Laleman W, Verreth A, Topal B, et al. Endoscopic resection of ampullary lesions: a single-center 8-year retrospective cohort study of 91 patients with long-term follow-up. *Surg Endosc.* 2013;27(10):3865-3876.
260. Burke CA, Beck GJ, Church JM, et al. The natural history of untreated duodenal and ampullary adenomas in patients with familial adenomatous polyposis followed in an endoscopic surveillance program. *Gastrointest Endosc.* 1999;49:358-364.
261. Sommerville CA, Limongelli P, Pai M, et al. Survival analysis after pancreatic resection for ampullary and pancreatic head carcinoma: an analysis of clinicopathological factors. *J Surg Oncol.* 2009;100:651-656.
262. Baczako K, Buchler M, Beger HG, et al. Morphogenesis and possible precursor lesions of invasive carcinoma of the papilla of Vater: epithelial dysplasia and adenoma. *Hum Pathol.* 1985;16:305-310.
263. Hayes DH, Bolton JS, Willis GW, et al. Carcinoma of the ampulla of Vater. *Ann Surg.* 1987;206:572-577.
264. Kimchi NA, Mindrul V, Broide E, et al. The contribution of endoscopy and biopsy to the diagnosis of periampullary tumors. *Endoscopy.* 1998;30:538-543.
265. Knox RA, Kingston RD. Carcinoma of the ampulla of Vater. *Br J Surg.* 1986;73:72-73.
266. Ponchon T, Berger F, Chavaillon A, et al. Contribution of endoscopy to diagnosis and treatment of tumors of the ampulla of Vater. *Cancer.* 1989;64:161-167.
267. Clary BM, Tyler DS, Dematos P, et al. Local ampullary resection with careful intraoperative frozen section evaluation for presumed benign ampullary neoplasms. *Surgery.* 2000;127:628-633.
268. Neoptolemos JP, Talbot IC, Carr-Locke DL, et al. Treatment and outcome in 52 consecutive cases of ampullary carcinoma. *Br J Surg.* 1987;74:957-961.
269. Yamaguchi K, Enjoji M, Kitamura K. Endoscopic biopsy has limited accuracy in diagnosis of ampullary tumors. *Gastrointest Endosc.* 1990;36:588-592.
270. Sivak MV. Clinical and endoscopic aspects of tumors of the ampulla of Vater. *Endoscopy.* 1988;20(suppl 1):211-217.
271. Will U, Bosseckert H, Meyer F. Correlation of endoscopic ultrasonography (EUS) for differential diagnostics between inflammatory and neoplastic lesions of the papilla of Vater and the peripapillary region with results of histologic investigation. *Ultraschall Med.* 2008;29:275-280.
272. Keriven O, Napoléon B, Souquet JC, et al. Patterns of the ampulla of Vater at endoscopic ultrasonography (abstract). *Gastrointest Endosc.* 1993;39:A290.
273. Rosch T, Braig C, Gain T, et al. Staging of pancreatic and ampullary carcinoma by endoscopic ultrasonography. Comparison with conventional sonography, computed tomography, and angiography. *Gastroenterology.* 1992;102:188-199.
274. Pang JC, Minter RM, Kwon RS, et al. The role of cytology in the preoperative assessment and management of patients with pancreaticobiliary tract neoplasms. *J Gastrointest Surg.* 2013;17:501-510.
275. Defrain C, Chang CY, Srikureja W, et al. Cytologic features and diagnostic pitfalls of primary ampullary tumors by endoscopic ultrasound-guided fine-needle aspiration biopsy. *Cancer.* 2005;105:289-297.
276. Brown KM, Tompkins AJ, Yong S, et al. Pancreaticoduodenectomy is curative in the majority of patients with node-negative ampullary cancer. *Arch Surg.* 2005;140:529-532, discussion 532-533.
277. Binmoeller KF, Boaventura S, Ramsperger K, et al. Endoscopic snare excision of benign adenomas of the papilla of Vater. *Gastrointest Endosc.* 1993;39:127-131.
278. Norton ID, Gostout CJ, Baron TH, et al. Safety and outcome of endoscopic snare excision of the major duodenal papilla. *Gastrointest Endosc.* 2002;56:239-243.
279. Saurin JC, Chavaillon A, Napoleon B, et al. Long-term follow-up of patients with endoscopic treatment of sporadic adenomas of the papilla of Vater. *Endoscopy.* 2003;35:402-406.
280. Zadorova Z, Dvofak M, Hajer J. Endoscopic therapy of benign tumors of the papilla of Vater. *Endoscopy.* 2001;33:345-347.
281. Patel R, Davitte J, Varadarajulu S, et al. Endoscopic resection of ampullary adenomas: complications and outcomes. *Dig Dis Sci.* 2011;56:3235-3240.
282. Roberts KJ, McCulloch N, Sutcliffe R, et al. Endoscopic ultrasound assessment of lesions of the ampulla of Vater is of particular value in low-grade dysplasia. *HPB (Oxford).* 2013;15:18-23.
283. Catalano MF, Linder JD, Chak A, et al. Endoscopic management of adenoma of the major duodenal papilla. *Gastrointest Endosc.* 2004;59:225-232.
284. Desilets DJ, Dy RM, Ku PM, et al. Endoscopic management of tumors of the major duodenal papilla: refined techniques to improve outcome and avoid complications. *Gastrointest Endosc.* 2001;54:202-208.
285. Ceppa EP, Burbridge RA, Rialon KL, et al. Endoscopic versus surgical ampullectomy: an algorithm to treat disease of the ampulla of Vater. *Ann Surg.* 2013;257:315-322.
286. Winter JM, Cameron JL, Olino K, et al. Clinicopathologic analysis of ampullary neoplasms in 450 patients: implications for surgical strategy and long-term prognosis. *J Gastrointest Surg.* 2010;14:379-387.
287. Cannon ME, Carpenter SL, Elta GH, et al. EUS compared with CT, magnetic resonance imaging, and angiography and the influence of biliary stenting on staging accuracy of ampullary neoplasms. *Gastrointest Endosc.* 1999;50:27-33.

288. Tio TL, Sie LH, Kallimanis G, et al. Staging of ampullary and pancreatic carcinoma: comparison between endosonography and surgery. *Gastrointest Endosc*. 1996;44:706-713.

289. Yoshida T, Matsumoto T, Shibata K, et al. Patterns of lymph node metastasis in carcinoma of the ampulla of Vater. *Hepatogastroenterology*. 2000;47:880-883.

290. Nakao A, Harada A, Nonami T, et al. Prognosis of cancer of the duodenal papilla of Vater in relation to clinicopathological tumor extension. *Hepatogastroenterology*. 1994;41:73-78.

291. Shirai Y, Tsukada K, Ohtani T, et al. Carcinoma of the ampulla of Vater: histopathologic analysis of tumor spread in Whipple pancreatoduodenectomy specimens. *World J Surg*. 1995;19:102-106, discussion 106-107.

292. Yamaguchi K, Enjoji M. Carcinoma of the ampulla of vater. A clinicopathologic study and pathologic staging of 109 cases of carcinoma and 5 cases of adenoma. *Cancer*. 1987;59:506-515.

293. Artifon EL, Couto D Jr, Sakai P, et al. Prospective evaluation of EUS versus CT scan for staging of ampullary cancer. *Gastrointest Endosc*. 2009;70:290-296.

294. Buscail L, Pages P, Berthelemy P, et al. Role of EUS in the management of pancreatic and ampullary carcinoma: a prospective study assessing resectability and prognosis. *Gastrointest Endosc*. 1999;50:34-40.

295. Chen CH, Yang CC, Yeh YH, et al. Reappraisal of endosonography of ampullary tumors: correlation with transabdominal sonography, CT, and MRI. *J Clin Ultrasound*. 2009;37:18-25.

296. Ito K, Fujita N, Noda Y, et al. Preoperative evaluation of ampullary neoplasm with EUS and transpapillary intraductal US: a prospective and histopathologically controlled study. *Gastrointest Endosc*. 2007;66:740-747.

297. Maluf-Filho F, Sakai P, Cunha JE, et al. Radial endoscopic ultrasound and spiral computed tomography in the diagnosis and staging of periampullary tumors. *Pancreatology*. 2004;4:122-128.

298. Midwinter MJ, Beveridge CJ, Wilsdon JB, et al. Correlation between spiral computed tomography, endoscopic ultrasonography and findings at operation in pancreatic and ampullary tumours. *Br J Surg*. 1999;86:189-193.

299. Rivadeneira DE, Pochapin M, Grobmyer SR, et al. Comparison of linear array endoscopic ultrasound and helical computed tomography for the staging of periampullary malignancies. *Ann Surg Oncol*. 2003;10:890-897.

300. Itoh A, Goto H, Naitoh Y, et al. Intraductal ultrasonography in diagnosing tumor extension of cancer of the papilla of Vater. *Gastrointest Endosc*. 1997;45:251-260.

301. Menzel J, Hoepffner N, Sulkowski U, et al. Polypoid tumors of the major duodenal papilla: preoperative staging with intraductal US, EUS, and CT—a prospective, histopathologically controlled study. *Gastrointest Endosc*. 1999;49:349-357.

302. Wee E, Lakhtakia S, Gupta R, et al. The diagnostic accuracy and strength of agreement between endoscopic ultrasound and histopathology in the staging of ampullary tumors. *Indian J Gastroenterol*. 2012;31:324-332.

303. Manta R, Conigliaro R, Castellani D, et al. Linear endoscopic ultrasonography vs magnetic resonance imaging in ampullary tumors. *World J Gastroenterol*. 2010;16:5592-5597.

304. Gress FG, Hawes RH, Savides TJ, et al. Endoscopic ultrasound-guided fine-needle aspiration biopsy using linear array and radial scanning endosonography. *Gastrointest Endosc*. 1997;45:243-250.

305. Napoleon B, Pialat J, Saurin JC, et al. [Adenomas and adenocarcinomas of the ampulla of Vater: endoscopic therapy]. *Gastroenterol Clin Biol*. 2004;28:385-392.

306. Cheng CL, Sherman S, Fogel EL, et al. Endoscopic snare papillectomy for tumors of the duodenal papillae. *Gastrointest Endosc*. 2004;60:757-764.

307. Han J, Lee SK, Park DH, et al. [Treatment outcome after endoscopic papillectomy of tumors of the major duodenal papilla]. *Korean J Gastroenterol*. 2005;46:110-119.

308. Irani S, Arai A, Ayub K, et al. Papillectomy for ampullary neoplasm: results of a single referral center over a 10-year period. *Gastrointest Endosc*. 2009;70:923-932.

309. Jung MK, Cho CM, Park SY, et al. Endoscopic resection of ampullary neoplasms: a single-center experience. *Surg Endosc*. 2009;23:2568-2574.

310. Katsinelos P, Paroutoglou G, Kountouras J, et al. Safety and long-term follow-up of endoscopic snare excision of ampullary adenomas. *Surg Endosc*. 2006;20:608-613.

311. Martin JA, Haber GB. Ampullary adenoma: clinical manifestations, diagnosis, and treatment. *Gastrointest Endosc Clin N Am*. 2003;13:649-669.

312. Moon JH, Cha SW, Cho YD, et al. Wire-guided endoscopic snare papillectomy for tumors of the major duodenal papilla. *Gastrointest Endosc*. 2005;61:461-466.

313. Vogt M, Jakobs R, Benz C, et al. Endoscopic therapy of adenomas of the papilla of Vater. A retrospective analysis with long-term follow-up. *Dig Liver Dis*. 2000;32:339-345.

314. Yamao T, Isomoto H, Kohno S, et al. Endoscopic snare papillectomy with biliary and pancreatic stent placement for tumors of the major duodenal papilla. *Surg Endosc*. 2010;24:119-124.

315. Boix J, Lorenzo-Zuniga V, Moreno de Vega V, et al. Endoscopic resection of ampullary tumors: 12-year review of 21 cases. *Surg Endosc*. 2009;23:45-49.

SECTION V

Anorectum

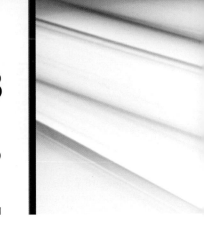

18

How to Perform Anorectal EUS

Paul Fockens • Steve Halligan • Robert H. Hawes • Shyam Varadarajulu

The Perianal Area

Examination of the perianal area is simplicity itself. No special patient preparation is required. The patient is told that any discomfort will be similar to having a finger in the anus and that the procedure will likely be less uncomfortable than digital rectal examination by a doctor. To the patient, the rigid probe is potentially a frightening piece of equipment, so it is worth mentioning that only the distal few centimeters will enter the anus (as opposed to rectal endosonography, in which insertion is obviously deeper). Some endosonographers place all patients in the left lateral position, whereas others prefer female patients to be in the prone position for examination. Placing women in the left lateral position can potentially distort anterior perineal anatomic features, with the result that the asymmetric images obtained will be difficult to interpret, especially with respect to perineal scarring.[1]

Appropriate equipment is essential for successful anal endoscopic ultrasonography (EUS). The standard (most commonly described in the literature) is the Bruel-Kjaer mechanical radial rigid probe. In the early days of EUS, when the principal instrument was the mechanical radial echoendoscope, examiners attempted to use this scope for anal EUS examination. However, the near-field imaging was poor, and the anal sphincters were often obscured by the ringdown artifact. Consequently, Olympus designed and marketed a rigid rectal probe compatible with its mechanical radial processor. However, with the introduction of electronic radial echoendoscopes, a flexible instrument is now available that can deliver high-quality images of anal anatomy and has rendered the dedicated rigid probe obsolete.

The rigid probe is prepared as necessary for the transducer being used. Some systems, for example, require the transducer head to be filled with degassed water to achieve acoustic coupling. This is accomplished by injection using a syringe through a side port. The probe must be maneuvered during filling so that all air is expelled through a pinhole located at the tip of the cone.

Whether or not water filling is required, the rigid probe tip is lubricated with ultrasound jelly and then is covered with a condom, which is itself lubricated to facilitate insertion. The probe is then inserted into the anus, and image acquisition is started by the operator. The probe is inserted so that its tip lies just in the distal rectum. The probe is then withdrawn gently to examine the anal sphincters. As for all ultrasound examinations, the clinical findings are generally based on the image displayed on the monitor screen in real time (with the exception of three-dimensional acquisition, in which case the examination in its entirety can be replayed later). However, still images are usually required, and it is convenient to obtain these at three levels: the proximal, middle, and distal anal canal. These three anatomic levels are imaged at standard magnification, and the examination is then repeated at a higher magnification so that six images are obtained, three at each magnification. The probe is oriented so that anterior (i.e., the 12-o'clock position) is uppermost and is then withdrawn. The examination is normally very quick, perhaps only a minute or so for the experienced operator who is familiar with normal and abnormal anatomy, especially when the sphincters are normal. The technique for imaging does not vary whether a rigid probe or an electronic radial flexible probe is used.

The Rectum

EUS of the rectum is mainly performed to examine suspicious rectal polyps or to stage rectal cancer. From country to country, huge differences exist in the use of EUS for this indication. Patients should be prepared with an enema or complete bowel preparation to evacuate all stool from the area to be investigated. For the start of the examination, the patient is usually placed in the left lateral position. The position may be changed during the examination. For noncircumferential masses or laterally spreading polyps, the patient should be positioned so that the mass or polyp is in the dependent position to allow easy submersion in water. This is also an easy way to determine which wall of the rectum is involved (anterior, posterior, left, or right). Sedation is not usually necessary because the rectosigmoid junction is not passed with the instrument.

The examination is usually begun with a therapeutic endoscope with a built-in washing function. This equipment allows inspection of the mass and provides an opportunity to clear any residual stool that could degrade imaging. It also allows filling of the rectum to indicate position of the patient that will optimize water filling.

There is no standard advice for the equipment to be used. For staging of tumors located very distally in the rectum, rigid radial scanning probes are often used. An alternative is a radial scanning echoendoscope, as used in the upper gastrointestinal tract. The advantage of echoendoscopes is that they can be advanced higher up into the rectum with help of the (oblique-viewing) optics. Linear echoendoscopes can also be used, with the advantage of enabling the examiner to perform EUS fine-needle aspiration (FNA) biopsy of extrarectal abnormalities such as lymph nodes or suspected tumor recurrences after

Video 18-1. Demonstrating the technique for endoscopic examination of the rectum using a radial echoendoscope.

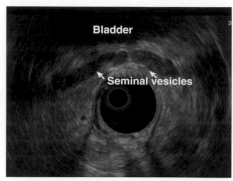

FIGURE 18-2   The anechoic structure at the 12-o'clock position represents the urinary bladder. In men, the echo-poor elongated structures seen below the urinary bladder represent the seminal vesicles.

surgery. The linear probes sometimes offer a further advantage because the tumor and mural layers can be followed in the same image. This sometimes makes it easier to determine the exact involvement of the deeper layers. Finally, mini-probes can be used in patients with superficial lesions. With 12-MHz mini-probes, a penetration depth of 2 cm is generally possible.

Using a balloon around the tip of the rigid probe or echoendoscope removes the air and allows for good acoustic coupling between probe and tumor. Filling of the rectum with water is sometimes helpful, especially in the case of smaller lesions that would otherwise be compressed with a balloon. Complete filling of the rectum with water is usually not possible and should not be attempted because it is much easier to change the patient's position. When the bowel has been prepared with an enema, care should be taken not to fill the colon extensively with water, because this may mobilize stool located in the proximal colon.

Usually, the instrument is positioned proximal to the tumor, the balloon is slowly inflated, and the lumen is filled with water (Video 18-1). From this position, the transducer should be positioned in the center of the colon to achieve perpendicular imaging of the rectal wall layers (Figure 18-1). One should then look for the perirectal anatomic features. The universal landmark is the urinary bladder. Once the bladder has been identified, the image should be mechanically rotated so the bladder is located at the 12-o'clock position (Figure 18-2). The instrument should be withdrawn slowly, with the

transducer kept in the middle of the colon. The left-right and up-down dials should be used to adjust the transducer to maintain its position in the middle of the colon. The examiner must *not* torque the instrument because this will cause tangential imaging and potentially lead to inaccurate assessment of the depth of tumor penetration. When withdrawing the probe in the male, the seminal vesicles will be seen as echo-poor, elongated structures at the 12-o'clock position (Figure 18-2). Further withdrawal will bring the prostate in view. The prostate is seen as a hypoechoic, bean-shaped structure at the 12-o'clock position (Figure 18-3). In female patients, withdrawal of the scope from the bladder first reveals the uterus (Figure 18-4A), which is a rounded, hypoechoic structure at the 12-o'clock position. Then the vagina is seen as an elongated oval, hypoechoic structure with a characteristic hyperechoic band in the center that represents air (Figure 18-4B). It is important to recognize perirectal structures because invasion into any of them represents T4 disease. In addition, one must distinguish these structures, especially the seminal vesicles, from lymph nodes.

Once the tumor is seen with EUS, the lesion is examined extensively, and all layers of the colon wall are followed underneath the tumor. Houston's valves and the rectosigmoid junction make it almost impossible to maintain a perpendicular view of the rectal wall at all times with a radial instrument scan. Adaptation of the plane of scanning with the controls of the echoendoscope is important to prevent overstaging by nonperpendicular imaging.

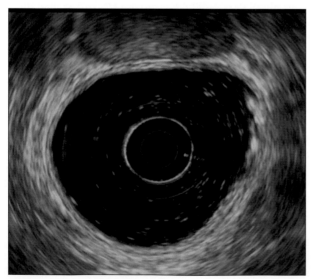

FIGURE 18-1   Rectal wall layers as imaged using a radial echoendoscope.

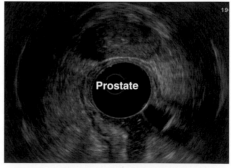

FIGURE 18-3   The prostate. On gradual withdrawal of the echoendoscope, a hypoechoic, bean-shaped structure is seen in men, which represents the prostate.

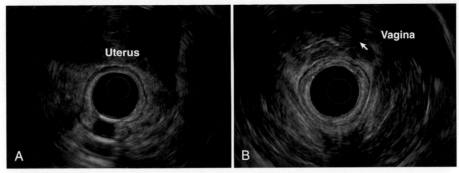

FIGURE 18-4 The uterus and vagina. In the female patient, withdrawal from the bladder first reveals the uterus (**A**), which is a rounded, hypoechoic structure at 12 o'clock, and then the vagina (**B**), which is seen as an elongated oval, hypoechoic structure with a characteristic hyperechoic band in the center that represents air.

After imaging of the tumor, the echoendoscope is advanced to the rectosigmoid junction to look for suspicious perirectal lymph nodes. Although it may be possible to advance the echoendoscope higher up, this maneuver is generally not advised. Images of the lesion and all other findings should be made; there are no standard positions at which images should be captured in every examination.

In cases of small mucosal or submucosal lesions of the rectum, the practitioner may find it easier to use a dual-channel endoscope and a mini-probe. This equipment allows simultaneous water instillation, endoscopic visualization of the lesion, and ultrasound imaging.

Transrectal EUS FNA is feasible and safe. Antibiotic administration is recommended before the needle is passed. Indications for transrectal EUS FNA include suspicious lymph nodes associated with known primary rectal cancer when the lymph nodes are not "protected" by the primary tumor (tumor lies between the transducer and the lymph node) and perirectal masses of unknown origin.

REFERENCES

1. Frudinger A, Bartram CI, Halligan S, et al. Examination techniques for endosonography of the anal canal. *Abdom Imaging.* 1998;23:301-303.

19

EUS in Rectal Cancer

Ferga C. Gleeson

Key Points

- The importance of nodal status guiding therapeutic decision making is increasingly recognized for rectal cancer.
- EUS FNA is recognized as being an essential component of locoregional clinical staging.
- Although EUS still has insufficient accuracy for T-staging, EUS FNA can accurately predict patients who have evidence of iliac vessel node disease by upstaging 7% of patients presenting for evaluation, in addition to establishing the presence of perirectal space nodal disease.
- Staging with EUS following neoadjuvant therapy should be approached with caution.
- The benefit of EUS FNA is in the postoperative surveillance period due to its ability to biopsy the extramural perirectal space to establish local disease recurrence.

An estimated 40,000 new cases of primary de novo rectal cancer occur per annum in the United States.[1] Based upon current data, the prognosis for such patients is directly related to several factors, with the most important being the extent of primary tumor invasion (T stage), the number of lymph nodes involved (N stage), involvement of the circumferential resection margin (CRM), and the presence of distant metastases (M stage). Contemporary staging and therapy are dependent upon presurgical diagnostic imaging modalities that include endoscopic ultrasonography (EUS), magnetic resonance imaging (MRI), or computed tomography (CT), which will influence the indication for neoadjuvant therapy and the decision-making process concerning the most appropriate surgical approach.

The diagnostic accuracy of lower gastrointestinal (GI) EUS assessments of rectal cancer staging has recently been questioned and criticized because clinical practice and current literature do not appear to support the early very positive literature reports. A German multicenter prospective quality assurance study ($n = 7000$ patients, from 2000 to 2008) compared radial EUS examination to surgical pathology T-stage biopsies, in the absence of neoadjuvant therapy.[2] The T-stage concordance was 65% but improved with increasing procedure volumes. The frequency of both understaging and overstaging was 18% and 17%, respectively. In addition, further scrutiny from a United States center revealed that EUS non–fine-needle aspiration (FNA) lymph node evaluation (from 1993 to 2007) did not reliably identify patients with nodal disease. The evidence to support this statement was based on a 29% lymph node morphology false-positive rate, and 23% of patients were understaged when using surgical pathology as the gold standard.[3] It is recognized that neither

studies included the important utility of EUS FNA with a view to enhanced disease staging and subsequent appropriate triage of care.

The objective of this chapter is to provide a comprehensive overview using practical up-to-date evidence to collectively enhance and consolidate our knowledge and skill mix. We discuss the incremental benefit of EUS and alternative imaging modalities for the assessment of primary de novo rectal cancer, evaluation following neoadjuvant therapy, and postoperative disease surveillance utility. The final section presents innovative interventions for lower gastrointestinal (GI) EUS.

Relevant Anorectal Anatomy and the AJCC 2010 Staging System for Rectal Cancer

Anorectal Anatomy

The rectum extends from the upper end of the anal canal to the rectosigmoid junction and is approximately 12 cm in length.[4] It is subdivided into proximal, middle, and distal thirds, depending upon the distance of the most distal aspect of the tumor from the anal verge. The surgical anal canal extends from the anorectal junction until the anal verge and measures between 2.5 and 4 cm in length.[5] The anatomic anal canal corresponds to the distal two thirds of the surgical anal canal and is separated from the proximal one third by the dentate line. Above the dentate line, the anal canal is lined with columnar epithelium, whereas it is lined with squamous epithelium distal to the dentate line. The anal transitional zone corresponds to an approximately 10-mm area between the columnar and squamous epithelial zones where the mucosa is of variable histology.[6]

The rectal wall is composed of mucosa, submucosa, and muscularis propria. The mucosa and submucosa complex appears as a three-layered wall structure on EUS. The mucosa is comprised of two wall layers: an inner hyperechoic layer (the interface between the mucosa and the ultrasound probe) and an outer hypoechoic wall layer. This is accompanied by the third wall layer, which is hyperechoic, representing the submucosa. The muscularis propria of the rectum, or fourth wall layer, is composed of an outer longitudinal and inner circular smooth muscle layer. The inner circular smooth muscle becomes thickened distally and continues as the internal anal sphincter. The outer longitudinal muscle fuses with fibers from the levator ani.[5] The outermost layer of the sphincter complex is formed by striated muscles: the levator ani and puborectalis muscles superiorly and the inferior part of the external anal sphincter inferiorly.

The rectum is surrounded by mesorectal fat containing lymph nodes, superior hemorrhoidal vessels, and fibrous tissue collectively known as the mesorectum. The mesorectum is continuous with the fat of the sigmoid mesocolon superiorly and is usually thicker along the posterior rectum in its intraperitoneal portion; on occasion it is absent anteriorly. It is bound circumferentially by the mesorectal fascia. This fascia extends inferiorly and coalesces with Denonvilliers' fascia in men, and anterior to it are the seminal vesicles and the prostate gland. Conversely, in women the anterior mesorectal fascia coalesces with rectovaginal fascia, anterior to which is the vagina. The mesorectal fascia forms an important barrier to the radial spread of upper and middle third rectal tumors and forms the plane of dissection used in total mesorectal excision (TME).

Nodal drainage of the rectum occurs initially to the perirectal lymph nodes within the mesorectum.[7] The majority of such nodes follow the rectal blood supply and are located superiorly and posteriorly. Common nodal spread is along the superior rectal artery into the apical mesorectum and the inferior mesenteric artery into the sigmoid mesocolon. The middle rectal artery arises from the internal iliac artery directly and the inferior rectal artery arises from the internal pudendal artery, which is a branch of the anterior division of the internal iliac artery. The inferior and middle rectal arteries anastomose at the anorectal junction and, although uncommon, distal rectal cancers can spread to the nodes along the internal pudendal and internal iliac arteries.

Rectal Cancer TNM Staging

The tumor-node-metastasis (TNM) system advocated by the American Joint Committee on Cancer (AJCC) and the International Union Against Cancer (UICC) have become the worldwide standard for staging colorectal cancer.[8,9] The TNM system classifies the extent of the tumor (T stage) by the depth of tumor invasion into and through the rectal wall. Nodal substations classified as regional lymph nodes for rectal cancer are perirectal, sigmoid mesenteric, inferior mesenteric, lateral sacral, presacral, sacral promontory, internal pudendal, internal iliac, superior rectal, middle rectal, and inferior rectal. Involvement of lymph nodes outside these groups, such as in the external or common iliac substations, is considered to be distant metastases (M stage) (Table 19-1).

TABLE 19-1

THE 2010 AMERICAN JOINT COMMITTEE ON CANCER (AJCC) STAGING SYSTEM FOR PRIMARY RECTAL CANCER

Primary Tumor (T)

TX	Primary tumor cannot be assessed
T0	No evidence of primary tumor
Tis	Carcinoma in situ: intraepithelial or invasion of lamina propria[a]
T1	Tumor invades submucosa
T2	Tumor invades muscularis propria
T3	Tumor invades through the muscularis propria into pericolorectal tissues
T4a	Tumor penetrates to the surface of the visceral peritoneum[b]
T4b	Tumor directly invades or is adherent to other organs or structures[b,c]

Regional Lymph Nodes (N)[d]

NX	Regional lymph nodes cannot be assessed
N0	No regional nodal metastasis
N1	Metastasis in 1-3 regional lymph nodes
N1a	Metastasis in one regional lymph node
N1b	Metastasis in 2-3 regional lymph nodes
N1c	Tumor deposit(s) in the subserosa, mesentery, or non-peritonealized pericolic or perirectal tissues without regional nodal metastasis
N2	Metastasis in 4 or more regional lymph nodes
N2a	Metastasis in 4-6 regional lymph nodes
N2b	Metastasis in 7 or more regional lymph nodes

Distant Metastasis (M)

M0	No distant metastasis
M1	Distant metastasis
M1a	Metastasis confined to one organ or site (i.e., liver, lung, ovary, non-regional node)
M1b	Metastases in more than one organ/site or the peritoneum

[a]Note: Tis include cancer cells confined within the glandular basement membrane (intraepithelial) or mucosal lamina propria (intramucosal) with no extension through the muscularis mucosa into the submucosa.

[b]Note: Direct invasion in T4 includes invasion of other organs or other segments of the colorectum as a result of direct extension through the serosa, as confirmed on microscopic examination (e.g., invasion of the sigmoid colon by a carcinoma of the cecum), for cancers in a retroperitoneal or subperitoneal location or direct invasion of other organs or structures by virtue of extension beyond the muscularis propria (i.e., respectively, a tumor on the posterior wall of the descending colon invading the left kidney or lateral abdominal wall or a mid or distal rectal cancer with invasion of prostate, seminal vesicles, cervix, or vagina).

[c]Note: Tumor that is adherent to other organs or structures, grossly, is classified xT4b. However, if no tumor is present in the adhesion, microscopically, the classification should be T1-4a depending on the anatomic depth of wall invasion. The V and L classifications should be used to identify the presence of absence of vascular or lymphatic invasion whereas the perineural (PN) site-specific factor should be used for perineural invasion.

[d]Note: A satellite peritumoral nodule in the pericolorectal adipose tissue of a primary carcinoma without histologic evidence of residual lymph node in the nodule may represent discontinuous spread, venous invasion with extravascular spread (V1/2), or a totally replaced lymph node (N1/2). Replaced nodes should be counted separately as positive nodes in the N category, whereas discontinuous spread or venous invasion should be classified and counted in the site-specific factor category tumor deposits (TD).

(From Edge S, Byrd DR, Compton CC, Fritz AG, Greene FL, Trotti A eds (2010). AJCC Cancer Staging Manual. 7th ed. New York, NY: Springer, pp 157).

Video 19-1. Demonstration of the technique for endosonographic examination of the rectum using a radial echoendoscope.

Video 19-2. Evaluation of rectal cancer, staged T3N1 by EUS.

Other tumor characteristics that are important to consider for imaging purposes include the proximal and distal tumor margins, extent of tumor annularity, presence of ulceration, anal sphincter complex invasion, and the relationship of the distal tumor margin to the middle valve of Houston. The valve of Houston is thought to be a surrogate marker for the anterior peritoneal reflection, and the location of a tumor proximal or distal to the anterior peritoneal reflection has important surgical planning implications.

Rectal EUS in the Setting of de Novo Rectal Cancer

The introduction of transrectal EUS has improved the ability to delineate the histologic layers of the rectal wall and as a result has improved treatment allocation by achieving a more accurate determination of the depth of tumor invasion (Video 19-1).[10–13] It has emerged as an important imaging modality for the pretreatment staging of rectal cancer, with superior T-staging accuracy compared to CT.[14–17] The technique of rectal EUS has been previously described (Chapter 18) and may be performed with either a radial or, more recently and frequently, a curvilinear echoendoscope.[18]

T-Staging Considerations

Rectal cancer usually appears as a hypoechoic lesion that disrupts the normal five-layer sonographic structure of the rectal wall. It is important to document where the distal border of the tumor is in relation to the seminal vesicles in males and the cervix in females in order to clarify the lesion location in relation to the anterior peritoneal reflection. This is then compared to the endoscopic estimate of the distal tumor border. In published studies, the accuracy of EUS T-staging ranges from 80% to 95% compared with 65% to 75% for CT and 75% to 85% for MRI[19–21] (Figure 19-1). With respect to T stage, one particular problem is the overstaging of T2 tumors due to the difficulty in differentiating peritumoral inflammation secondary to a desmoplastic reaction from tumor fibrosis[22] (Figure 19-2).

A T3 tumor must extend through the entire thickness of the muscularis propria into the perirectal fat, obliterating the sharp fat–muscle interface with features of pseudopodia (Video 19-2). It is thought that all T3 rectal tumors are not equal, with minimally invasive disease carrying a more favorable prognosis.[23] Therefore by discriminating minimally invasive from advanced T3 disease (invasion ≤2 mm or >3 mm beyond the muscularis propria), preoperative EUS may provide important prognostic information. However, the challenge is that overstaging is noted to be more common in minimally invasive T3 (50%) when compared to advanced T3 disease.[24] A maximum tumor thickness measured in a T3 cancer is also an independent prognostic factor for local and overall recurrence.[25] A maximum tumor thickness cutoff measurement ≥19 mm has been proposed to be useful when classifying patients preoperatively and to select patients for primary surgery or neoadjuvant therapy.

Conversely, understaging may be caused by a failure to detect microscopic cancer infiltration owing to the limits of EUS resolution. Resolution is improved by increasing ultrasound frequency but at the expense of a reduction in the depth of penetration, such that it may be impossible to visualize the leading edge of a tumor. This may limit the detection of invasion of adjacent organs. Important variables that influence the accuracy of tumor staging include operator experience and the location of the tumor within the rectum, with reduced accuracy for more distal tumors.[22,26–28]

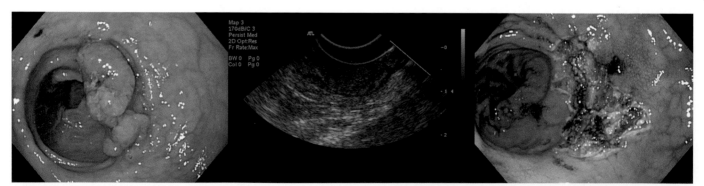

FIGURE 19-1 A superficial primary rectal cancer (T1N0) on the distal valve of Houston in an 84-year-old male, managed conservatively by a snare resection.

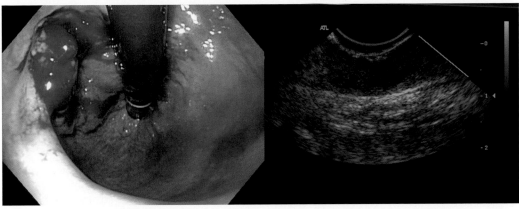

FIGURE 19-2 An ulcerated friable distal primary rectal cancer (T2N0) in a 62-year-old female who proceeded directly to an abdominoperineal resection. The tumor invaded the muscularis propria (hypoechoic fourth EUS layer) but did not penetrate through it (T3) or extend beyond the five echo layers into the surrounding perirectal tissue.

A meta-analysis of 42 studies (n = 5039 patients, from 1980 to 2008) that reviewed the EUS accuracy when differentiating T stages suggested that EUS sensitivity is greatest for advanced disease compared to early disease[29] (Table 19-2).

N-Staging Considerations

Conventional EUS nodal echo features that accurately predict nodal metastasis have been identified in patients with esophageal cancer.[30] These ultrasound features include lymph node short axis size, echogenicity, shape, and border. Features proposed to correlate with malignancy include an enlarged node (≥1 cm in short axis), hypoechoic appearance, round shape, and smooth border (Figure 19-3 and Table 19-3). However, these conventional EUS nodal criteria have proven inaccurate for staging many nonesophageal cancers.[30–32] No single criterion is predictive of malignancy in patients with lung, esophageal, and pancreatic cancer. If all four abnormal morphologic features are present, the accuracy for malignant invasion is 80%. However, all four features of malignant involvement are present in only 25% of malignant lymph nodes (Table 19-4).

Although EUS FNA is the most accurate modality for locoregional staging of cancer, the N-staging accuracy is only 70% to 75% and was recently reported to be as low as 42%.[33,34] It was previously assumed that EUS was incapable of detecting benign perirectal lymph nodes.[18] Therefore in patients with rectal cancer, visualization of lymph nodes was considered to be an accurate surrogate marker of nodal metastasis, thereby obviating the need for FNA. A meta-analysis (35

studies, n = 2732 patients, from 1966 to 2008) that reviewed the literature regarding N stage EUS accuracy suggested that the sensitivity and specificity of EUS is moderate and that further refinements in diagnostic criteria are needed to improve the diagnostic accuracy.[35] It is important to note that all of these studies were non-FNA, primarily radial EUS examinations.

Prior transrectal ultrasound studies identified a nodal size of ≥7 mm as an optimal size cutoff for predicting nodal metastases in rectal cancer, with an accuracy of 83% when compared with surgical pathology.[36] A dedicated FNA study based on a perception that metastatic locoregional nodes are only minimally different in morphologic appearance when compared to benign nodes noted that the number of conventional malignant echo features per lymph node did not accurately differentiate benign from malignant nodes, unless all four features were present.[37] The accuracy of conventional criteria to include short axis ≥10 mm, hypoechoic appearance, round shape, and smooth border for detecting malignant

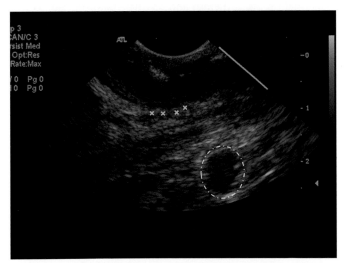

FIGURE 19-3 A T3N1 lesion in a 54-year-old male who proceeded to neoadjuvant therapy followed by surgery (++++ = tumor breaching through the fourth muscularis layer and making the lesion a T3 lesion). The highlighted node is perilesional and therefore not amenable to fine-needle aspiration. It has a hypoechoic appearance and short axis >5 mm but is oval in shape with an irregular border.

TABLE 19-2

EUS ACCURACY WHEN DIFFERENTIATING T STAGES SUGGESTS THAT EUS SENSITIVITY IS GREATEST FOR ADVANCED DISEASE RATHER THAN FOR EARLY DISEASE

T Stage	Sensitivity (%)	Specificity (%)
T1	87.8	98.3
T2	80.5	95.6
T3	96.4	90.6
T4	95.4	98.3

EUS MORPHOLOGIC FEATURES OF BENIGN AND MALIGNANT LYMPH NODES

EUS Features	Benign Features	Malignant Features
Echogenicity	Hyperechoic	Hypoechoic
Shape	Irregular	Round
Border	Irregular	Smooth
Size (short axis)	<10 mm	≥10 mm

lymphadenopathy was 61%, 65%, 51%, and 51%, respectively. A lymph node short-axis length ≥5 mm or hypoechoic appearance were the only conventional features predictive of malignant infiltration. An optimum short- and long-axis length of 6 mm and 9 mm yielded the best power distinction for malignancy. Using surgical histopathology specimens, Knight and colleagues assessed the performance characteristics for overall sensitivity, specificity, and positive and negative predictive values of FNA in the setting of primary or metastatic colorectal carcinoma, reflecting values of 89%, 79%, 89%, and 79%, respectively.[38]

The preoperative FNA identification of extramesenteric lymph node metastases upstages 7% of primary rectal cancers undergoing an EUS evaluation. For example, external iliac lymph node infiltration is outside the standard operative field for TME. This location, if recognized at EUS, may impact medical and surgical planning by altering the standard radiation fields or may alter surgical planning to extend the TME resection to include an extensive lymph node dissection.[39] Significant clinical, endoscopic, and sonographic features associated with such metastases include serum carcinoembryonic antigen (CEA) level, tumor length ≥4 cm, tumor annularity ≥50%, sessile morphology, and lymph node size.

The recent findings indicate that FNA should be used when verifying nodal status and when making critical decisions regarding the use of neoadjuvant therapy rather than relying on nodal appearance alone. Failure to use FNA risks stage-inappropriate therapy and, in turn, inappropriate patient outcomes. A note of caution is that luminal fluid cytology may be positive for malignancy in 48% of luminal cancers, including rectal cancer, but is not affected by performing FNA.[40] This translocated cell contamination in addition to endosonographer technique and cytologic misinterpretation are risk factors for false-positive EUS FNA cytology.[41]

EUS FNA of solid lesions in the lower GI tract is considered to be a low-risk procedure for infectious complications and does not warrant prophylactic administration of antibiotics for the prevention of bacterial endocarditis.[42] Until adverse event data become available, perirectal cystic structures should not be sampled, as abscess formation requiring percutaneous drainage has occurred despite the administration of prophylactic antibiotics.[43]

MRI Assessment versus EUS

The use of MRI for the local staging of rectal cancer, particularly with an endorectal coil technique, has been described.[44–46] It offers several theoretic advantages over EUS, as it reveals a larger field of view and permits the study of stenotic tumors.[26,47,48] Recently, the identification of the anterior peritoneal reflection, an important landmark to assist the surgical team, has been identified in 74% of patients.[49] A meta-analysis of 90 articles (from 1995 to 2002) compared the use of MRI, radial EUS without FNA, and CT for staging with histopathology correlation as the gold standard. The study came to the following conclusions: (1) for T1/T2 lesions, EUS and MRI had similar sensitivity but specificity was higher for EUS (86% vs 69%); and (2) for T3 tumors, the sensitivity of EUS was significantly higher than that of MRI or CT[50] (Figure 19-4). A more recent prospective study comparing radial EUS to MRI revealed that MRI was unable to visualize any T1 tumors, whereas EUS understaged all T4 tumors.[51] Furthermore, the presence of luminal stenosis and polypoid morphology was inversely associated with the accuracy of either EUS or MRI.

MRI may also be used to evaluate mesorectal nodal involvement, as lymph nodes are characterized by imaging features rather than by size criteria alone. The most reliable MRI criteria for lymph node metastasis are an irregular contour and inhomogeneous signal when correlated with histologic findings, and it may also identify nodal metastasis beyond the boundaries of the mesorectum.[52,53] Many studies have evaluated the prediction of lymph node involvement (Figure 19-5). A meta-analysis from 2004 revealed that the sensitivity and specificity of MRI were 66% and 76%, respectively, compared with 67% and 78% for radial EUS without FNA and 55% and 74% for CT.[46,50] In another meta-analysis there was similarly no significant difference in N-staging between MRI and EUS, although EUS had a slight advantage, mostly based upon specificity.[54]

PERFORMANCE CHARACTERISTICS RELATIVE TO THE NUMBER OF CONVENTIONAL EUS MALIGNANT NODAL FEATURES

	Two or More Features	Three or More Features	Four Features
Sensitivity (%)	77	68	23
Specificity (%)	29	52	100
PPV (%)	53	60	100
NPV (%)	55	61	55
Accuracy (%)	54	61	61

NPV, negative predictive value; PPV, positive predictive value.

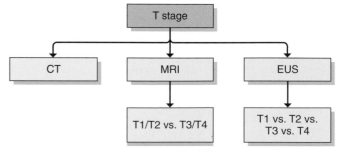

FIGURE 19-4 Imaging options to potentially assess T stage. CT, computed tomography; EUS, endoscopic ultrasonography; MRI, magnetic resonance imaging.

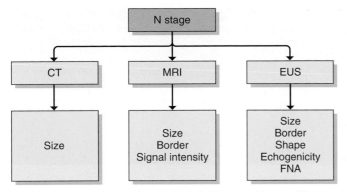

FIGURE 19-5 Imaging options to potentially assess N stage. CT, computed tomography; EUS, endoscopic ultrasonography; FNA, fine-needle aspiration; MRI, magnetic resonance imaging.

CT and Positron Emission Tomography (PET)-CT Evaluation versus EUS

Traditionally, the role of CT was to identify metastatic disease, as its resolution was considered to be inadequate to make a distinction between the various rectal wall layers.[55,56] More recently, however, multislice CT has been used for the assessment of mesorectal fascia involvement, especially when a lesion is located proximal to and including the mid-rectum; however, the accuracy of an involved margin in a distal rectal cancer is suboptimal.[57,58] The optimum CT lymph node size to predict nodal metastasis with the best negative predictive value was 7 mm.[59] However, an abdominal CT in addition to EUS is considered to be the most cost-effective staging strategy for nonmetastatic proximal rectal cancer, but this may change with increasing use of pelvic MRI.[60]

PET-CT provides additional information to conventional staging in primary rectal cancer and may be used selectively in more advanced stages and where indeterminate findings exist with conventional staging.[61] Contrast-enhanced PET-CT is superior to nonenhanced PET-CT for the precise definition of regional nodal status and is considered to enhance the staging/therapy in one-third of patients.[62,63] Some authorities suggest that the standardized uptake values $(SUV)_{max}$ following neoadjuvant therapy predicts downstaging and a complete pathologic response.[64,65] However, no EUS FNA versus PET-CT comparative study has been reported to date.

EUS Evaluation Following Neoadjuvant Therapy

Tumor response to neoadjuvant therapy is a strong predictor of disease-free survival. However, the accuracy of EUS for staging rectal cancer following such therapy is markedly decreased due to the effects of postradiation edema, inflammation, necrosis, and fibrosis.[66,67] EUS has not been extensively studied in this scenario, but it has been suggested that its routine use for staging purposes following such therapy should be discouraged.[68] The T-stage accuracy following neoadjuvant therapy is 50%.[69–74] As outcome is most accurately estimated by final pathologic stage; restaging tumors following such therapy is limited and clinical correlation is most

important to dictate operative and postoperative management modalities. However, the use of nonperitumoral lymph node FNA in this setting may establish the presence of residual nodal malignancy, which may offer useful information for further management decisions.

EUS for Recurrent Rectal Cancer Following Radical and Local Surgery

A positive CRM, serosal involvement, lymphovascular invasion, extramural venous invasion, and poor histologic differentiation are important independent predictive factors for the development of local recurrence (LR).[75] The combination of neoadjuvant therapy and total mesorectal excision has significantly reduced the incidence of LR (<10%), the incidence of which is greatest within the first 2 years following surgery.[76,77] Early detection of a recurrent local tumor may result in earlier treatment and improved survival. As LR often occurs in the extraluminal region, follow-up with forward-viewing endoscopy may fail to detect LR at a sufficiently early stage. EUS may not be able to visually distinguish recurrence from postoperative change due to fibrosis or inflammation, and images may be obscured by artifacts from surgically placed clips or sutures. However, FNA of the residual rectal wall or perirectal space (91% sensitivity, 93% specificity) may offer a diagnosis that is superior to clinical evaluation or EUS imaging alone. There is no clear strategy for early detection of local recurrence. Two prospective studies have demonstrated that EUS was superior to CT for local recurrence detection in rectal cancer.[78,79] The sensitivity of EUS was higher (100%) in both studies compared to CT (82% to 85%). EUS was also more sensitive than digital rectal examination, CT, and CEA levels to detect LR in asymptomatic patients.[80] The optimal interval for EUS surveillance following surgical intervention is unknown. However, performing EUS every 6 months for the first 2 years after low anterior resection may be a reasonable surveillance modality for recurrent rectal cancer.[81]

Local excision is an alternative management approach for early rectal cancers and for patients unfit for radical surgery. It is, however, associated with a high local recurrence rate. Mucosal scar biopsy and EUS FNA of either a lymph node or the deep rectal wall are methods to establish local recurrence.[82] In addition, EUS FNA with or without Tru-Cut biopsy (TCB) may be useful in the diagnostic evaluation of patients with extraluminal perirectal lesions to determine a therapeutic plan (Figure 19-6).[83]

Rectal implantation cysts occurring at an anastomotic site following a low anterior resection for rectal cancer need to be distinguished from locally recurrent rectal cancer. EUS may reveal cystic lesions at the anastomotic site with heterogeneous wall thickness, and FNA may reveal mucin containing some inflammatory cells in the absence of malignant cells.[84] EUS FNA and TCB are sensitive for the diagnosis of malignancy in pelvic masses but carry a 7% complication rate if cystic pelvic masses are sampled, and this should therefore be discouraged.[85,86]

EUS for Rectal Wall Metastases

Distant primary cancers, in general, rarely metastasize to the gastrointestinal wall. Such findings are estimated to be 1 of

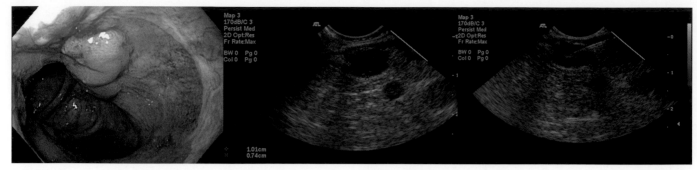

FIGURE 19-6 Post-transanal excision scar 18 months following local therapy. EUS detected an enlarged hypoechoic nonperilesional lymph node that was positive for malignancy.

3847 (0.03%) upper endoscopies and only 1 of 1871 (0.05%) colonoscopies.[87] The EUS appearance without FNA of secondary rectal linitis plastica is that of circumferential wall thickening affecting predominantly the submucosal and muscularis propria layers similar to that of primary gastric linitis plastica[88] (Figure 19-7). The role of FNA to aid the diagnosis secondary to prostate cancer has also been reported.[89] This appearance is in contrast to similar processes such as rectal endometriotic implants that are either hypoechoic or heterogeneous deposits involving the fourth and fifth layer with intact mucosal layers. It is also in contrast to local rectal cancer recurrence that is usually in an extraluminal location.[90,91] EUS FNA with or without TCB may confirm the diagnosis and identify the primary malignancy, which to date has included cancers originating from the bladder, breast, stomach, and cutaneous melanoma.[92]

Innovative Interventions for Lower GI EUS

EUS-guided drainage and stenting provides another option for the management of postoperative pelvic fluid collections.[93] EUS-guided drainage of abdominopelvic abscesses unrelated to diverticular disease may be another future therapeutic indication.[94] EUS fine-needle injection with ethanol for persistent malignant pelvic lymph nodes following therapy in nonsurgical candidates has also been reported, in addition to EUS-guided coil and glue placement for bleeding rectal varices.[95,96]

Conclusion

As the increasing importance of nodal status in therapeutic decision making is recognized for rectal cancer, EUS FNA has emerged as an essential component of locoregional clinical staging. Although EUS still has insufficient accuracy for T-staging, EUS FNA can accurately predict patients who have evidence of iliac vessel node disease by upstaging 7% of patients presenting for evaluation and establishing the presence of perirectal space nodal disease. Staging with EUS following neoadjuvant therapy should be approached with caution but overall may be of greater benefit in the postoperative surveillance period because of the possibility to biopsy the extramural perirectal space to establish local disease recurrence.

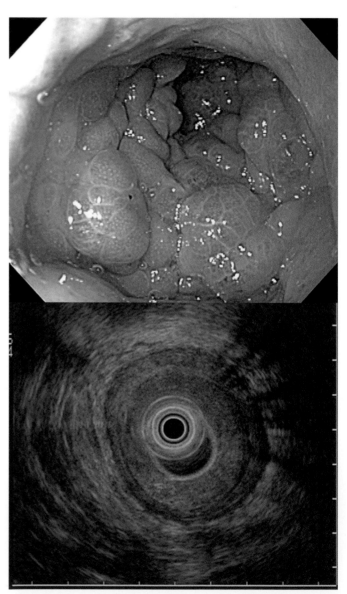

FIGURE 19-7 Circumferential cobblestone mucosal appearance with a corresponding hypoechoic wall thickness in a patient with a history of transitional cell cancer of the bladder, 2 years previously.

REFERENCES

1. http://www.cancer.gov/cancertopics/types/colon-and-rectal.
2. Marusch F, Ptok H, Sahm M, et al. Endorectal ultrasound in rectal carcinoma–do the literature results really correspond to the realities of routine clinical care? *Endoscopy*. 2011;43(5):425-431.
3. Shapiro R, Ali UA, Lavery IC, Kiran RP. Endorectal ultrasound does not reliably identify patients with uT3 rectal cancer who can avoid neo-adjuvant chemoradiotherapy. *Int J Colorectal Dis*. 2013;[Epub ahead of print].
4. Nelson H, Petrelli N, Carlin A, et al. Guidelines 2000 for colon and rectal cancer surgery. *J Natl Cancer Inst*. 2001;93:583-596.
5. Wexner SD, Jorge JMN. Anatomy and embryology of the anus, rectum, and colon. In: Corman ML, ed. *Colon and Rectal Surgery*. Philadelphia: Lippincott-Raven; 1998:1-26.
6. Kaiser AM, Ortega AE. Anorectal anatomy. *Surg Clin North Am*. 2002;82(6):1125-1138.
7. Canessa CE, Badia F, Fierro S, et al. Anatomic study of the lymph nodes of the mesorectum. *Dis Colon Rectum*. 2001;44:1333-1336.
8. Greene FL, Page DL, Fleming ID, et al., eds. *AJCC Cancer Staging Manual*. 7th ed. NewYork, NY: Springer; 2010.
9. Sobin LH, Wittekind C, eds. *TNM: Classification of Malignant Tumours*. 6th ed. NewYork, NY: Wiley-Liss; 2002.
10. Fedyaev EB, Volkova EA, Kuznetsova EE. Transrectal and transvaginal ultrasonography in the preoperative staging of rectal carcinoma. *Eur J Radiol*. 1995;20(1):35-38.
11. Dershaw DD, Enker WE, Cohen AM, Sigurdson ER. Transrectal ultrasonography of rectal carcinoma. *Cancer*. 1990;66(11):2336-2340.
12. Cohen JL, Grotz RL, Welch JP, Deckers PJ. Intrarectal sonography. A new technique for the assessment of rectal tumors. *Am Surg*. 1991;57(7):459-462.
13. Hawes RH. New staging techniques. Endoscopic ultrasound. *Cancer*. 1993;71(12 suppl):4207-4213.
14. Schwartz DA, Harewood GC, Wiersema MJ. EUS for rectal disease. *Gastrointest Endosc*. 2002;56(1):100-109.
15. Kwok H, Bissett IP, Hill GL. Preoperative staging of rectal cancer. *Int J Colorectal Dis*. 2000;15(1):9-20.
16. Rifkin MD, Ehrlich SM, Marks G. Staging of rectal carcinoma: prospective comparison of endorectal US and CT. *Radiology*. 1989;170(2):319-322.
17. Holdsworth PJ, Johnston D, Chalmers AG, et al. Endoluminal ultrasound and computed tomography in the staging of rectal cancer. *Br J Surg*. 1988;75(10):1019-1022.
18. Wiersema MJ, Harewood GC. Endoscopic ultrasound for rectal cancer. *Gastroenterol Clin North Am*. 2002;31:1093-1105.
19. Golfieri R, Giampalma E, Leo P, et al. Comparison of magnetic resonance (0, 5 T), computed tomography, and endorectal ultrasonography in the preoperative staging of neoplasms of the rectum-sigma. Correlation with surgical and anatomopathologic findings. *Radiol Med*. 1993;85(6):773-783.
20. Kim NK, Kim MJ, Yun SH, et al. Comparative study of transrectal ultrasonography, pelvic computerized tomography, and magnetic resonance imaging in preoperative staging of rectal cancer. *Dis Colon Rectum*. 1999;42(6):770-775.
21. Halefoglu AM, Yildirim S, Avlanmis O, et al. Endorectal ultrasonography versus phased-array magnetic resonance imaging for preoperative staging of rectal cancer. *World J Gastroenterol*. 2008;14(22):3504-3510.
22. Kauer WK, Prantl L, Dittler HJ, Siewert JR. The value of endosonographic rectal carcinoma staging in routine diagnostics: a 10-year analysis. *Surg Endosc*. 2004;18(7):1075-1078.
23. Harewood GC, Kumar KS, Clain JE, et al. Clinical implications of quantification of mesorectal tumor invasion by endoscopic ultrasound: all T3 rectal cancers are not equal. *Gastroenterol Hepatol*. 2004;19(7):750-755.
24. Jürgensen C, Teubner A, Habeck JO, et al. Staging of rectal cancer by EUS: depth of infiltration in T3 cancers is important. *Gastrointest Endosc*. 2011;73(2):325-328.
25. Esclapez P, Garcia-Granero E, Flor B, et al. Prognostic heterogeneity of endosonographic T3 rectal cancer. *Dis Colon Rectum*. 2009;52(4):685-691.
26. Orrom WJ, Wong WD, Rothenberger DA, et al. Endorectal ultrasound in the preoperative staging of rectal tumors. A learning experience. *Dis Colon Rectum*. 1990;33(8):654-659.
27. Solomon MJ, McLeod RS, Cohen EK, et al. Reliability and validity studies of endoluminal ultrasonography for anorectal disorders. *Dis Colon Rectum*. 1994;37(6):546-551.
28. Sailer M, Leppert R, Bussen D, et al. Influence of tumor position on accuracy of endorectal ultrasound staging. *Dis Colon Rectum*. 1997;40(10):1180-1186.
29. Puli SR, Bechtold ML, Reddy JB, et al. How good is endoscopic ultrasound in differentiating various T stages of rectal cancer? Meta-analysis and systematic review. *Ann Surg Oncol*. 2009;16(2):254-265.
30. Catalano MF, Sivak MV, Rice T, et al. Endosonographic features predictive of lymph node metastasis. *Gastrointest Endosc*. 1994;40:442-446.
31. Murata Y, Muroi M, Yoshida M, et al. Endoscopic ultrasonography in the diagnosis of esophageal carcinoma. *Surg Endosc*. 1987;1:11-16.
32. Tio TL, Coene PP, Luiken GJ, et al. Endosonography in the clinical staging of esophagogastric carcinoma. *Gastrointest Endosc*. 1990;36(suppl 2):S2-S10.
33. Rosen LS, Bilchik AJ, Beart RW Jr, et al. New approaches to assessing and treating early-stage colon and rectal cancer: summary statement from 2007 Santa Monica Conference. *Clin Cancer Res*. 2007;13:6853s-6856s.
34. Tsendsuren T, Jun SM, Mian XH. Usefulness of endoscopic ultrasonography in preoperative TNM staging of gastric cancer. *World J Gastroenterol*. 2006;12:43-47.
35. Puli SR, Reddy JB, Bechtold ML, et al. Accuracy of endoscopic ultrasound to diagnose nodal invasion by rectal cancers: a meta-analysis and systematic review. *Ann Surg Oncol*. 2009;16(5):1255-1265.
36. Heneghan JP, Salem RR, Lange RC, et al. Transrectal sonography in staging rectal carcinoma: the role of gray-scale, color-flow, and Doppler imaging analysis. *AJR Am J Roentgenol*. 1997;169:1247-1252.
37. Gleeson FC, Clain JE, Papachristou GI, et al. Prospective assessment of EUS criteria for lymphadenopathy associated with rectal cancer. *Gastrointest Endosc*. 2009;69(4):896-903.
38. Knight CS, Eloubeidi MA, Crowe R, et al. Utility of endoscopic ultrasound-guided fine-needle aspiration in the diagnosis and staging of colorectal carcinoma. *Diagn Cytopathol*. 2011;doi:10.1002/dc.21804; [Epub ahead of print].
39. Gleeson FC, Clain JE, Rajan E, et al. EUS-FNA assessment of extramesenteric lymph node status in primary rectal cancer. *Gastrointest Endosc*. 2011;74(4):897-905.
40. Levy MJ, Gleeson FC, Campion MB, et al. Prospective cytological assessment of gastrointestinal luminal fluid acquired during EUS: a potential source of false-positive FNA and needle tract seeding. *Am J Gastroenterol*. 2010;105(6):1311-1318.
41. Gleeson FC, Kipp BR, Caudill JL, et al. False positive endoscopic ultrasound fine needle aspiration cytology: incidence and risk factors. *Gut*. 2010;59(5):586-593.
42. Levy MJ, Norton ID, Clain JE, et al. Prospective study of bacteremia and complications With EUS FNA of rectal and perirectal lesions. *Clin Gastroenterol Hepatol*. 2007;5(6):684-689.
43. Mohamadnejad M, Al-Haddad MA, Sherman S, et al. Utility of EUS-guided biopsy of extramural pelvic masses. *Gastrointest Endosc*. 2012; 75(1):146-151.
44. Brown G, Richards CJ, Bourne MW, et al. Morphologic predictors of lymph node status in rectal cancer with use of high-spatial-resolution MR imaging with histopathologic comparison. *Radiology*. 2003;227:371-377.
45. Gualdi GF, Casciani E, Guadalaxara A, et al. Local staging of rectal cancer with transrectal ultrasound and endorectal magnetic resonance imaging: comparison with histologic findings. *Dis Colon Rectum*. 2000;43:338-345.
46. Bianchi P, Ceriani C, Palmisano A, et al. A prospective comparison of endorectal ultrasound and pelvic magnetic resonance in the preoperative staging of rectal cancer. *Ann Ital Chir*. 2006;77(1):41-46.
47. Hulsmans FJ, Tio TL, Fockens P, et al. Assessment of tumor infiltration depth in rectal cancer with transrectal sonography: caution is necessary. [see comment]. *Radiology*. 1994;190(3):715-720.
48. Hildebrandt U, Feifel G. Preoperative staging of rectal cancer by intrarectal ultrasound. *Dis Colon Rectum*. 1985;28(1):42-46.
49. Gollub MJ, Maas M, Weiser M, et al. Recognition of the anterior peritoneal reflection at rectal MRI. *AJR Am J Roentgenol*. 2013;200(1):97-101.
50. Bipat S, Glas AS, Slors FJ, et al. Rectal cancer: local staging and assessment of lymph node involvement with endoluminal US, CT, and MR imaging, a meta-analysis. *Radiology*. 2004;232:773-783.
51. Fernández-Esparrach G, Ayuso-Colella JR, Sendino O, et al. EUS and magnetic resonance imaging in the staging of rectal cancer: a prospective and comparative study. *Gastrointest Endosc*. 2011;74(2):347-354.
52. Brown G, Richards CJ, Bourne MW. Morphologic predictors of lymph node status in rectal cancer with use of high-spatial-resolution MR

imaging with histopathologic comparison. *Radiology.* 2003;227(2): 371-377.

53. Brown G, Kirkham A, Williams GT, et al. High-resolution MRI of the anatomy important in total mesorectal excision of the rectum. *AJR Am J Roentgenol.* 2004;182(2):431-439.

54. Lahaye MJ, Engelen SM, Kessels AG, et al. USPIO-enhanced MR imaging for nodal staging in patients with primary rectal cancer: predictive criteria. *Radiology.* 2008;246(3):804-811.

55. Heriot AG, Grundy A, Kumar D. Preoperative staging of rectal carcinoma. *Br J Surg.* 1999;86:17-28.

56. Kim NK, Kim MJ, Yun SH, et al. Comparative study of transrectal ultrasonography, pelvic computerized tomography, and magnetic resonance imaging in preoperative staging of rectal cancer. *Dis Colon Rectum.* 1999; 42:770-775.

57. Wolberink SV, Beets-Tan RG, de Haas-Kock DF, et al. Multislice CT as a primary screening tool for the prediction of an involved mesorectal fascia and distant metastases in primary rectal cancer: a multicenter study. *Dis Colon Rectum.* 2009;52(5):928-934.

58. Vliegen R, Dresen R, Beets G, et al. The accuracy of Multi-detector row CT for the assessment of tumor invasion of the mesorectal fascia in primary rectal cancer. *Abdom Imaging.* 2008;33(5):604-610.

59. Pomerri F, Maretto I, Pucciarelli S, et al. Prediction of rectal lymph node metastasis by pelvic computed tomography measurement. *Eur J Surg Oncol.* 2009;35(2):168-173.

60. Harewood GC, Wiersema MJ. Cost-effectiveness of endoscopic ultrasonography in the evaluation of proximal rectal cancer. *Am J Gastroenterol.* 2002;97(4):874-882.

61. Eglinton T, Luck A, Bartholomeusz D, et al. Positron-emission tomography/computed tomography (PET/CT) in the initial staging of primary rectal cancer. *Colorectal Dis.* 2010;12(7):667-673.

62. Davey K, Heriot AG, Mackay J, et al. The impact of 18-fluorodeoxyglucose positron emission tomography-computed tomography on the staging and management of primary rectal cancer. *Dis Colon Rectum.* 2008;51(7): 997-1003.

63. Tateishi U, Maeda T, Morimoto T, et al. Non-enhanced CT versus contrast-enhanced CT in integrated PET/CT studies for nodal staging of rectal cancer. *Eur J Nucl Mol Imaging.* 2007;34(10):1627-1634.

64. Kim JW, Kim HC, Park JW, et al. Predictive value of (18) FDG PET-CT for tumour response in patients with locally advanced rectal cancer treated by preoperative chemoradiotherapy. *Int J Colorectal Dis.* 2013;[Epub ahead of print].

65. Bampo C, Alessi A, Fantini S, et al. Is the standardized uptake value of FDG-PET/CT predictive of pathological complete response in locally advanced rectal cancer treated with capecitabine-based neoadjuvant chemoradiation? *Oncology.* 2013;84(4):191-199.

66. Siddiqui AA, Fayiga Y, Huerta S. The role of endoscopic ultrasound in the evaluation of rectal cancer. *Int Semin Surg Oncol.* 2006;3:36.

67. Williamson PR, Hellinger MD, Larach SW, Ferrara A. Endorectal ultrasound of T3 and T4 rectal cancers after preoperative chemoradiation. *Dis Colon Rectum.* 1996;39(1):45-49.

68. Marone P, de Bellis M, Avallone A, et al. Accuracy of endoscopic ultrasound in staging and restaging patients with locally advanced rectal cancer undergoing neoadjuvant chemoradiation. *Clin Res Hepatol Gastroenterol.* 2011;35(10):666-670.

69. Vanagunas A, Lin DE, Stryker SJ. Accuracy of endoscopic ultrasound for restaging rectal cancer following neoadjuvant chemoradiation therapy. *Am J Gastroenterol.* 2004;99(1):109-112.

70. Romagnuolo J, Parent J, Vuong T, et al. Predicting residual rectal adenocarcinoma in the surgical specimen after preoperative brachytherapy with endoscopic ultrasound. *Can J Gastroenterol.* 2004;18(7):435-440.

71. Rau B, Hunerbein M, Barth C, et al. Accuracy of endorectal ultrasound after preoperative radiochemotherapy in locally advanced rectal cancer. *Surg Endosc.* 1999;13:980-984.

72. Maor Y, Nadler M, Barshack I, et al. Endoscopic ultrasound staging of rectal cancer: diagnostic value before and following chemoradiation. *J Gastroenterol Hepatol.* 2006;21(2):454.

73. Napoleon B, Pujol B, Berger F, et al. Accuracy of endosonography in the staging of rectal cancer treated by radiotherapy. *Br J Surg.* 1991; 78:785-788.

74. Ramirez JM, Mortensen NJ, Takeuchi N, Humphreys MM. Endoluminal ultrasonography in the follow-up of patients with rectal cancer. *Br J Surg.* 1994;81:692-694.

75. Dresen RC, Peters EE, Rutten HJ, et al. Local recurrence in rectal cancer can be predicted by histopathological factors. *Eur J Surg Oncol.* 2009; 35(10):1071-1077.

76. Law WL, Chu KW. Anterior resection for rectal cancer with mesorectal excision: a prospective evaluation of 622 patients. *Ann Surg.* 2004;240(2):260-268.

77. Jörgren F, Johansson R, Damber L, Lindmark G. Risk factors of rectal cancer local recurrence: population-based survey and validation of the Swedish Rectal Cancer Registry. *Colorectal Dis.* 2010;12(10): 977-986.

78. Novell F, Pascual S, Viella P, Trias M. Endorectal ultrasonography in the follow-up of rectal cancer. Is it a better way to detect early local recurrence? *Int J Colorectal Dis.* 1997;12:78-81.

79. Lohnert M, Dohrmann P, Stoffregen C, Hamelmann H. [Value of endorectal sonography in the follow-up of patients treated surgically for rectum carcinoma]. *Zentralbl Chir.* 1991;116:461-464.

80. Mellgren A, Sirivongs P, Rothenberger DA, et al. Is local excision adequate therapy for early rectal cancer? *Dis Colon Rectum.* 2000;43: 1064-1071.

81. Rex DK, Kahi CJ, Levin B, et al. Guidelines for colonoscopy surveillance after cancer resection: a consensus update by the American Cancer Society and the US Multi-Society Task Force on Colorectal Cancer. *Gastroenterology.* 2006;130(6):1865-1871.

82. Gleeson FC, Larson DW, Dozois EJ, et al. Recurrence detection following transanal excision facilitated by EUS-FNA. *Hepatogastroenterology.* 2012;59(116):1102-1107.

83. Boo SJ, Byeon JS, Park do H, et al. EUS-guided fine needle aspiration and trucut needle biopsy for examination of rectal and perirectal lesions. *Scand J Gastroenterol.* 2011;46(12):1510-1518.

84. Honda K, Akahoshi K, Matsui N, et al. Role of EUS and EUS-guided FNA in the diagnosis of rectal implantation cyst at an anastomosis site after a previous low anterior resection for a rectal cancer without evidence of cancer recurrence. *Gastrointest Endosc.* 2008;68(4): 782-785.

85. Mohamadnejad M, Al-Haddad MA, Sherman S, et al. Utility of EUS-guided biopsy of extramural pelvic masses. *Gastrointest Endosc.* 2012;75(1):146-151.

86. Puri R, Eloubeidi MA, Sud R, et al. Endoscopic ultrasound-guided drainage of pelvic abscess without fluoroscopy guidance. *J Gastroenterol Hepatol.* 2010;25(8):1416-1419.

87. Wei SC, Su WC, Chang MC, et al. Incidence, endoscopic morphology and distribution of metastatic lesions in the gastrointestinal tract. *J Gastroenterol Hepatol.* 2007;22(6):827-831.

88. Dumontier I, Roseau G, Palazzo L, et al. Endoscopic ultrasonography in rectal linitis plastica. *Gastrointest Endosc.* 1997;46(6):532-536.

89. Bhutani MS. EUS and EUS-guided fine-needle aspiration for the diagnosis of rectal linitis plastica secondary to prostate carcinoma. *Gastrointest Endosc.* 1999;50(1):117-119.

90. Pishvaian AC, Ahlawat SK, Garvin D, Haddad NG. Role of EUS and EUS-guided FNA in the diagnosis of symptomatic rectosigmoid endometriosis. *Gastrointest Endosc.* 2006;63(2):331-335.

91. Mascagni D, Corbellini L, Urciuoli P, Di Matteo G. Endoluminal ultrasound for early detection of local recurrence of rectal cancer. *Br J Surg.* 1989;76(11):1176-1180.

92. Gleeson FC, Clain JE, Rajan E, et al. Secondary linitis plastica of the rectum: EUS features and tissue diagnosis (with video). *Gastrointest Endosc.* 2008;68(3):591-596.

93. Ulla-Rocha JL, Vilar-Cao Z, Sardina-Ferreiro R. EUS-guided drainage and stent placement for postoperative intra-abdominal and pelvic fluid collections in oncological surgery. *Therap Adv Gastroenterol.* 2012;5(2): 95-102.

94. Ramesh J, Bang JY, Trevino J, Varadarajulu S. Comparison of outcomes between EUS-guided trans-colonic and trans-rectal drainage of abdominopelvic abscesses. *J Gastroenterol Hepatol.* 2013;28(4):620-625.

95. DeWitt J, Mohamadnejad M. EUS-guided alcohol ablation of metastatic pelvic lymph nodes after endoscopic resection of polypoid rectal cancer: the need for long-term surveillance. *Gastrointest Endosc.* 2011;74(2): 446-447.

96. Weilert F, Shah JN, Marson FP, Binmoeller KF. EUS-guided coil and glue for bleeding rectal varix. *Gastrointest Endosc.* 2012;76(4):915-916.

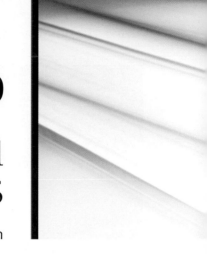

20

Evaluation of the Anal Sphincter by Anal EUS

Steve Halligan

Key Points

- AES is simple to perform and visualizes the anal sphincter complex, notably the external and internal anal sphincters.
- AES is able to image sphincter tears and defects.
- AES can also characterize sphincter morphology and determine muscular quality.
- AES is the single most important investigation in patients with anal incontinence.

First described in 1989,[1] anal endosonography (AES) was the first technique to visualize the anal sphincter complex with enough spatial resolution to resolve the individual components of the sphincter mechanism. Despite the advent of endoanal magnetic resonance imaging (MRI), AES remains the technique with the highest spatial resolution, and it is also quick and easy to perform. The introduction of AES precipitated a significant reappraisal of the causes of anal incontinence (and its treatment), which had hitherto been thought to be mainly the result of pelvic neuropathy.[2] When incontinent patients were studied with AES, it rapidly became clear that occult anal sphincter disruption was present in many cases. Patients with disrupted sphincters can be scheduled for surgical procedures that aim to restore integrity to the sphincter ring, whereas patients whose sphincters are intact, or whose muscles are thought to be of poor quality, can be directed toward conservative measures or alternative surgical approaches.

At present, AES has replaced physiologic testing as the pivotal examination in the clinical decision-making process for these patients. Although AES is probably used most often following obstetric injury, it has also facilitated the anatomic characterization of other causes of fecal incontinence. For example, with AES, the examiner can identify neurogenic incontinence by way of specific patterns of sphincter atrophy and can identify occult and unintended sphincter damage following anal surgical procedures.

Equipment and Examination Technique

Although it is possible to perform AES using an echoendoscope, the best results by far are obtained using a dedicated anal probe. The anus is a very superficial structure, and an echoendoscope is both cumbersome when compared with a probe designed specifically for the purpose and more expensive. AES first employed a 7.5-MHz transducer that had been designed initially for rectal cancer staging and prostatic imaging. The transducer was covered by a rubber balloon, it was inserted through the anus into the rectum, the balloon was inflated with degassed water, and the transducer was mechanically rotated to produce 360-degree images of the rectal wall. Professor Clive Bartram of St Mark's Hospital, London, realized that by simply replacing the soft rubber balloon with a rigid plastic cone, the rotating transducer could be safely withdrawn into the anus.[1] This maneuver was previously impossible because the balloon would be torn when compressed by the anus against the rotating metal transducer.

Modern probes encapsulate a fixed transducer within a permanent hard cover and are of higher frequency (Figure 20-1). Some also possess three-dimensional capacity, achieved either by withdrawing the probe during image acquisition (e.g., EUP-R54AW-19/33, Hitachi Medical Systems, Wellingborough, UK) or by incorporating a transducer that moves along the Z-axis of the probe, inside the exterior capsule, while the head is held stationary within the anal canal (e.g., 2052 transducer, BK Medical, Herlev, Denmark).

The examination is simple, easily tolerated by the patient, and very rapid when performed by an experienced operator. No special patient preparation is required. The patient is told that discomfort, if any, will be similar to having a small finger in the anus, and the procedure will likely be much less uncomfortable than digital rectal examination by a doctor. To the patient, the probe is potentially quite a frightening piece of equipment, so it is worth mentioning that only the distal few centimeters will enter the anus (as opposed to rectal endosonography, in which insertion is obviously deeper).

Men are examined in the left lateral patient position, but the prone patient position is preferable for examining women. Placing women in the left lateral position can occasionally

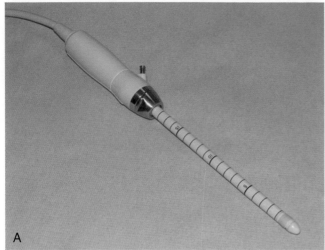

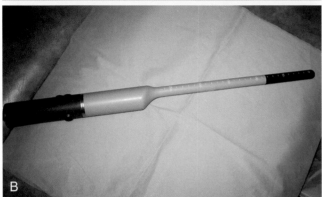

FIGURE 20-1 Probes for ultrasound examination of the anal sphincter complex. **A,** Hitachi EUP-R54AW-19/33 electronic radial probe. **B,** B and K medical 1846 probe. *(A, Courtesy of Hitachi Medical Systems, Wellingborough, UK; B, Courtesy of BK Medical, Herlev, Denmark.)*

distort anterior perineal anatomy and can induce an asymmetrical image, which makes it difficult to distinguish perineal scarring from normal anatomic features.[3] In the past, it was necessary to fill the transducer head with degassed water to achieve acoustic coupling, accomplished by injection using a syringe through a side port and then maneuvering the probe so that all air was expelled through a pinhole located at the tip of the cone. However, most modern probes merely require the tip to be lubricated with ultrasound jelly and then covered with a condom, which is itself lubricated to facilitate insertion. The probe is then inserted into the anus, and image acquisition is commenced. The aim is to insert the probe so that the transducer lies just in the distal rectum. The probe is then withdrawn gently and slowly to examine the anal sphincters.

As for all ultrasound examinations, clinical findings are generally based on the image displayed on the monitor screen in real time (with the exception of three-dimensional acquisition, in which case the examination in its entirety can be replayed later). However, still images are usually required for archival purposes, and it is convenient to obtain these still images at three levels: the proximal, middle, and distal anal canal (see later discussion). These three anatomic levels are imaged at standard magnification, and the examination is then repeated at a higher magnification, for a total of six images, three at each magnification. The probe is oriented so

that anterior (i.e., the 12-o'clock position) is uppermost. The examination is normally very quick, perhaps only a minute or so for the experienced operator who is familiar with normal and abnormal anatomy, and especially if the sphincters are normal.

Anal Sphincter Anatomy

Clearly, a sound understanding of basic anal anatomy is a prerequisite for accurate interpretation of endosonographic findings. There are two anal sphincters: the external anal sphincter (EAS) is composed of striated muscle, whereas the internal anal sphincter (IAS) is smooth muscle. These form two cylindrical layers, with the IAS innermost (Figure 20-2).

The EAS arises from the striated muscles of the pelvic floor and is composed of three cylindrical bundles lying on top of one another (deep, superficial, and subcutaneous) that are difficult to distinguish in practice. The deep portion is fused with the puborectalis (or pubococcygeus) muscle, which itself merges with the levator plate of the pelvic floor. The EAS extends approximately 1 cm distal to the IAS, where it forms the subcutaneous part of the EAS muscle. Anteriorly, the EAS is closely related to several surrounding structures, such as the superficial transverse muscle of the perineum and the perineal body. Posteriorly, it is continuous with the anococcygeal ligament, a structure that is often more prominent in men and should not be mistaken for a posterior sphincter defect. The EAS is much shorter anteriorly in women than in men, and this feature should not be confused with a sphincter defect.

The IAS is the distal termination and condensation of the circular smooth muscle of the gut tube. It extends from the anorectal junction to approximately 1 to 1.5 cm below the dentate line (see Figure 20-2). The longitudinal muscle of the gut tube also terminates in the anal canal, but it is less obvious than the IAS. The longitudinal muscle interdigitates between the EAS and the IAS and terminates in the subcutaneous EAS and subcutaneous anus. Its exact sphincteric action, if any, is much less clear than that of the EAS and IAS, and it is thought that its main purpose is to brace the anus and thus prevent anal eversion during defecation.[4] Lying between the EAS and the longitudinal muscle is a potential plane, the intersphincteric space, which may contain fat. The components of the anal sphincter are surrounded by the ischioanal space (often referred to as the ischiorectal fossa), which contains fat predominantly.

Directly anterior to the anal sphincter is the central perineal tendon or perineal body. In men, this lies posterior to the bulbospongiosus and corpus cavernosum and their related muscles, whereas in women, it lies within the anovaginal septum. Many structures insert fibers into the perineal body, such as the EAS, the deep and superficial transverse muscles of the perineum, the bulbocavernous muscle, and the puborectalis muscle. These structures should not be confused with sphincter defects. For example, normal variants of anal sphincter anatomy have been identified, such as differing relationships between the superficial transverse perineal muscle and the EAS.[5]

The distal anal canal is lined with stratified squamous epithelium, richly supplied by sensory receptors. These receptors are most concentrated at the dentate line, which demarcates the junction with proximal columnar epithelium. The

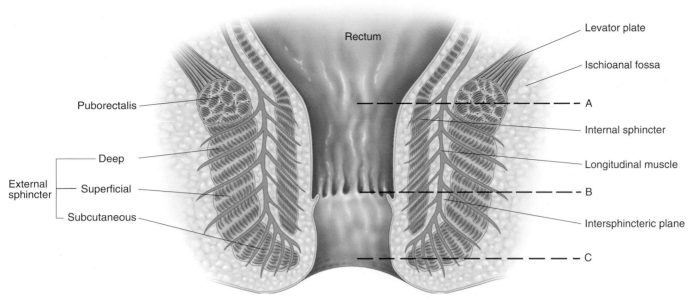

FIGURE 20-2 Coronal diagrammatic representation of important anal canal structures. The scan levels indicated correspond to Figure 20-3.

anal subepithelial tissues are relatively thick, and this lining and its underlining vascular spaces—the anal cushions—also play a role in maintaining continence.

Normal Endosonographic Findings

Because the anus and surrounding sphincter muscles are cylindrical, a 360-degree field of view is optimal, and the axial plane is also the most relevant surgically when considering sphincter defects. As stated earlier, it is convenient to obtain baseline images at three levels: the proximal, middle, and distal anal canal.

The proximal anal canal is primarily identified by the puborectalis and transverse perineal muscles (Figure 20-3A). The puborectalis slings around the anorectal junction and can be distinguished from the EAS, with which it blends imperceptibly, because its anterior ends splay outward as they travel toward their fusion with the pubic arch (see Figure 20-3A). The IAS is visible as a continuous hyperechoic ring and is generally the easiest structure to differentiate from other adjacent anal canal components because it is normally very hyporeflective. The subepithelial tissues, EAS, and longitudinal muscle all normally show varying degrees of hyperreflectivity, and their margins can often be difficult to define precisely, although direct comparisons with endoanal MRI have helped tremendously.[6] Increases in transducer frequency that improve spatial resolution have also helped to clarify the sonographic anatomy,[7] as has three-dimensional imaging.[8]

Sultan and colleagues[9] carefully imaged cadaveric specimens following sequential histologic dissection of anal layers and thereby validated the sonographic appearances. These investigators found that the echogenicity of normal muscle changed as its orientation was altered with respect to the transducer. Thus, normal variant striated muscle slips may appear hypoechoic, depending on their orientation to the transducer, and should not be confused with sphincter tears or scars.

If the probe is withdrawn just a centimeter or so from the proximal anal canal position, the anterior ends of the puborectalis muscle will converge anteriorly as they segue imperceptibly into the EAS. The midanal canal is thus defined where the EAS forms a complete ring anteriorly (see Figure 20-3B). The IAS is also normally thickest and best seen at this location. At this level, the intersphincteric plane and longitudinal muscle may be resolved as two distinct layers, with the longitudinal muscle forming distinct bundles of smooth muscle fibers.

Withdrawing the probe slightly more will move the field of view into the subcutaneous EAS (see Figure 20-3C). This structure is below the termination of the IAS, so it is either not visualized or only partially visualized if its termination is irregular (a common normal variant). It is usually impossible to visualize the longitudinal muscle reliably at this level because it has thinned out as it interdigitates into the EAS, and it is mainly composed of fibroelastic tissue rather than the smooth muscle found more proximally.

Correct interpretation of AES is possible only if the operator has a firm grasp of the normal sonographic anatomy described earlier. Disorder is defined by either muscular discontinuity (i.e., from sphincter tears or lacerations, secondary to a variety of causes) or abnormal muscular quality (which is usually caused by neuromuscular atrophy or degeneration). To appreciate muscular quality correctly, it is important to realize that normal sonographic appearances are contingent on both age and sex. Frudinger and colleagues[7] examined 150 nulliparous women with high-frequency AES to define normal age-related differences in sphincter morphology and found a highly significant positive correlation between IAS thickness and increasing age. In contrast, EAS thickness showed a highly significant negative correlation with increasing age.[7] Some evidence also suggested that the reflectivity of the IAS increased with age. No significant correlation was noted between age and thickness of subepithelial tissues, the longitudinal muscle, or the puborectalis muscle.[7]

On average, the IAS measures 2- to 3-mm thick (measured at either the 3-o'clock or 9-o'clock position in the midanal canal) in normal adults, but a thin IAS has more significance in an older person with symptoms (see later sections). In

Anterior

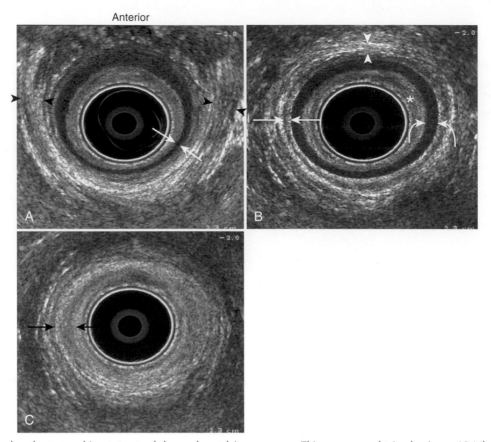

FIGURE 20-3   Normal endosonographic anatomy of the anal canal in a woman. This scan was obtained using a 10-Mhz 360-degree probe. **A,** Proximal anal canal level. At this level, the anterior ends of puborectalis muscle are well seen bilaterally *(between arrowheads)* as the muscle fibers course forward toward the pubis. The hyporeflective internal anal sphincter is also clearly seen *(between arrows)*. **B,** Midanal canal level. At this level, the external sphincter (superficial part) forms a complete ring around the anal canal, notably anteriorly *(between arrowheads)*. The internal sphincter is also at its thickest *(between curved arrows)*. The intersphincteric plane and longitudinal muscle *(between arrows)* lie between the external and internal sphincters. The subepithelial tissues *(asterisk)* lie medial to the internal sphincter. **C,** Distal anal canal level. At this level, the predominant muscle is the subcutaneous external sphincter *(between arrows)* because the scan plane is caudal to the termination of the internal sphincter.

addition, although the IAS can be measured easily because it contrasts with adjacent structures, other muscles may be more difficult to measure and are subject to greater interobserver variation. Gold and colleagues[10] measured anal canal structures in 51 consecutive referrals. These investigators found that although intraobserver agreement was superior to interobserver agreement, the 95% limits of agreement for EAS measurements spanned 5 mm, whereas those for the IAS spanned 1.5 mm.[10] More important from a diagnostic viewpoint, interobserver agreement for diagnosis of sphincter disruption and IAS echogenicity was very good ($\kappa = 0.80$ and 0.74, respectively).[10]

Clear sonographic differences exist between men and women with respect to the dimensions of anal canal structures and their sonographic appearances. Most importantly, the anterior complete ring of the EAS is shorter in women. This difference has been widely appreciated for some time, and Williams and colleagues[8] used three-dimensional AES to show that the craniocaudal length of the EAS was approximately 17 mm in women, as opposed to 30 mm in men. A short anterior canal in a woman should not be misinterpreted as a sphincter defect. In addition the various muscular components in men have a generally more striated appearance (Figure 20-4).

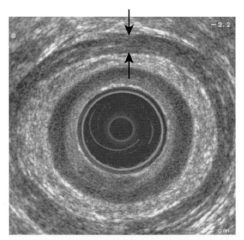

FIGURE 20-4   Anal endosonography at the midanal canal in an asymptomatic man. Note the generally more striated appearance when compared with Figure 20-3. The external sphincter *(between arrows)*, in particular, is relatively hyporeflective.

Anal Sphincter Function

Most clinical referrals for AES are in response to patients' complaining of anal incontinence, either to gas alone or to both gas and feces. It is therefore important to have some basic understanding of normal anal sphincter function.

The anal sphincter is the most complex sphincter in the human body. Continence is maintained by a multifaceted interrelationship between anal and pelvic floor musculature, integrating somatic and autonomic nervous pathways, the effects of which must be temporarily overcome during the act of defecation. The IAS is innervated by sympathetic presacral nerve fibers and is not under conscious control. It is primarily responsible for closing the anal canal at rest, at which time it is in a state of continuous involuntary contraction. Despite being striated muscle, the puborectalis and EAS also display some resting tone and can contract rapidly without conscious control in response to any sudden increase in intra-abdominal pressure to prevent anal incontinence. The EAS is innervated by the pudendal nerves (S2, S3, and S4).

Defecation is initiated by colonic smooth muscle contractions, which are provoked by waking and eating. These contractions propel stool from the sigmoid colon into the normally empty rectum and stimulate rectal sensory nerves that produce an urge to defecate. These nerves are also able to determine the nature of rectal content (i.e., solid, liquid, or gas). The sensation of a full rectum and the ability to discriminate among gaseous, liquid, and solid content are important components of continence, in addition to sphincter integrity. Sensation is retained after rectal excision, a finding suggesting that some sensory receptors reside in the pelvic floor itself.[11] Rectal filling causes reflex IAS relaxation (the rectoanal inhibitory reflex), rectal contraction, and contraction of the puborectalis and the EAS, both of which are heavily modulated by conscious control. Stool within the anal canal contacts sensory receptors concentrated at the dentate line and greatly intensifies the urge to defecate, which is resisted by vigorous striated muscle contraction until circumstances for defecation are appropriate. When this is so, pelvic floor relaxation and increased intra-abdominal pressure create a positive pressure gradient from rectum to anus to allow evacuation.

The normal function and contribution of the EAS and IAS to anal continence can be used to predict which muscles are abnormal in incontinent patients. For example, IAS abnormality generally results in passive incontinence (i.e., the patient is unaware that leakage is about to occur), whereas EAS abnormality is more frequently manifest as urge incontinence (i.e., the patient is unable consciously to defer defecation).[12]

Anorectal Physiologic Testing

Before the advent of AES, sphincter integrity and function were determined by anorectal physiologic testing, which tests nervous integrity, conduction, and muscular performance. Few physiologic tests are absolutely diagnostic, and most need to be considered together with symptoms, clinical findings, and imaging. However, these tests provide valuable complementary information and continue to be requested in combination with AES. Because of this, endosonographers working in this field need to be aware of these tests. Normal values vary among laboratories.

Manometry

Because digital assessment is unreliable, manometry is used to determine rectal and anal pressures. Systems vary in complexity, from simple balloons connected to a pressure transducer to perfused multichannel catheters capable of measuring pressure at several sites simultaneously, and even ambulatory systems that record over 24 hours or more. The pressure recorded rises when a rectal catheter is withdrawn into the anus, and it falls again when it reaches the anal margin. This zone defines the functional anal canal length (as opposed to anatomic length, which is usually shorter). The high-pressure zone generated at the anus is frequently diminished in incontinent patients. A static anal catheter can measure resting anal canal pressure, and it predominantly reflects IAS function. In general, reduced resting pressure points to IAS disease. In contrast, the squeeze pressure is the incremental rise over resting pressure elicited when the patient is asked to contract the anus voluntarily, and it reflects EAS function. This pressure is frequently reduced when incontinence is the result of EAS laceration, as occurs with obstetric injury. Dual-sphincter disease is implicated when both resting and squeeze pressures are abnormal, and neither finding is absolutely specific in an individual patient.

Pudendal Nerve Latency

The pudendal nerve terminal motor latency can be determined from the time taken for a digitally delivered pudendal nerve stimulus to elicit anal sphincter contraction. This is achieved by using a disposable glove with a stimulating electrode at the fingertip coupled with a pressure sensor at its base.[13] The nerve is stimulated near the ischial spine and has both sensory and motor components. Slow conduction is thought to be predominantly the result of stretch-induced injury. This may follow childbirth[2,14] or chronic straining,[15] and it can even be transiently demonstrated in physiologically normal individuals if they are asked to strain excessively. The clinical relevance of pudendal neuropathy remains unclear, especially because the degree of neuropathy, pelvic floor descent, and anal sensation should be directly related, but studies cannot demonstrate this.[16] Nevertheless, patients with abnormal latencies but intact sphincters usually have their incontinence attributed to neuropathic sphincter degeneration, and sphincter repair is less successful if underlying neuropathy is present.[17]

Electromyography

A needle electrode inserted into the EAS can determine both its activity and its muscular quality. Sphincter denervation is followed by reinnervation by neighboring healthy axons, which can be quantified electromyographically because the recorded action potentials become polyphasic. Until the advent of AES, electromyography was the only reliable way to diagnose sphincter tears preoperatively; the needle was inserted into the suspected defect, which was confirmed if no muscular potentials could be recorded subsequently (also possible if the needle tip missed the normal muscle because of incorrect placement—easily done when insertion is blind!). Needle passes were then made circumferentially around the anus until normal potentials were encountered, thus mapping the sphincter defect. Electromyography is painful because local anesthetic interferes with recording. Fortunately, AES is superior for detecting sphincter defects when the two modalities are compared directly.[18]

Sonographic Findings in Anal Incontinence

As mentioned earlier, most clinical referrals for AES are in response to patients' complaints of anal incontinence. Anal incontinence may have a variety of causes, many of which relate to the integrity and quality of the sphincter mechanism. AES has assumed a central role in the diagnostic workup for assessment of this problem because AES reliably identifies those patients who have a sphincter tear, selects individuals likely to benefit from surgery that aims to restore integrity to the sphincter ring, and prevents unnecessary surgery in other patients. Physical examination cannot reliably detect anal sphincter defects, and although anal canal pressures can help to determine whether sphincter function is normal, they cannot indicate whether the cause is loss of sphincter integrity or neuropathy.

Anal incontinence is common, especially in women, and its prevalence increases with age. Two percent of the general population older than 45 years have anal incontinence,[19] and the prevalence rises to 7% of persons more than 65 years old.[20] In retirement homes or hospitals, approximately one-third of individuals have anal incontinence.[19] Prevalence is also likely to be higher because of underreporting. Anal incontinence has considerable economic impact. A 1988 study estimated that more than $400 million annually was spent on incontinence appliances in the United States alone, and anal incontinence was the second most common cause of placement in a nursing home.[21] Several clinical grading systems for anal incontinence have been developed.

Obstetric Injury

Childbirth is a common cause of anal incontinence, either directly, from anal sphincter laceration, or indirectly, from damage to sphincter innervation. Until the advent of AES, it was assumed that neuropathy resulting from damage to sphincter innervation was the primary cause of obstetric-related incontinence because impaired pudendal nerve conduction can be demonstrated after vaginal delivery, presumably from stretch-induced injury.[2] Anal sphincter laceration was thought to be a relatively rare event because it could be identified clinically in only 1 of 200 vaginal deliveries.[22] However, AES revealed that anal sphincter tears were far more common than initially assumed. An early study of 11 women with a diagnosis of neurogenic fecal incontinence revealed that 4 had also sustained unsuspected anal sphincter tears.[23] A further study of 62 women whose incontinence was related to childbirth found EAS tears in 56 (90%).[24]

In a landmark study, Sultan and colleagues[25] used AES to study 202 consecutive unselected women before and after vaginal delivery and found anal sphincter tears in 28 of 79 of primiparous subjects (35%) and in 21 of 48 of multiparous subjects (44%). Furthermore, endosonographic evidence of sphincter laceration was associated with symptoms of anal incontinence 6 weeks following delivery and correlated with

evidence of physiologic impairment, namely reduced anal resting and squeeze pressures. No primiparous woman had a sphincter defect before childbirth, and no subject undergoing cesarean section developed a new defect. These findings confirmed that sphincter injury was caused by vaginal delivery, especially forceps extraction. Moreover, the study confirmed that clinical examination of the perineum immediately after vaginal delivery misses most sphincter tears.

Anal incontinence may occur immediately after delivery if trauma is substantial, but many women present later in life, presumably because the cumulative effects of multiple deliveries, progressive neuropathy, aging, and menopause overcome their compensatory mechanisms. Many women are also too embarrassed to complain, or they or their doctors believe that the condition is incurable. The accuracy of endosonography has been validated both histologically[9] and intraoperatively,[18] and it approaches 95%.[23,26,27] For example, a study of 44 patients found that all 23 EAS defects and 21 of 22 IAS defects visualized on preoperative AES were subsequently confirmed surgically.[26]

Sphincters are cylindrical structures, and discontinuity is diagnostic of a sphincter tear. A break in the hypoechoic IAS ring indicates an IAS defect, whereas EAS defects are defined by discontinuity of the more heterogeneous EAS, located peripheral to the intersphincteric plane and the longitudinal muscle. Obstetric injury is practically always anterior, because this is where the vagina lies. Because the EAS and IAS are in very close proximity, it is usual for obstetric injury to involve both sphincters. Isolated EAS injury is relatively uncommon, and isolated IAS injury is rarely the result of obstetric injury alone.

In severe disruptions, the entire sphincter mechanism is completely absent anteriorly, with a cloacal defect between the vagina and anal canal (Figure 20-5). However, it is usual for a primary repair of some sort to have been performed immediately after childbirth to close the perineum to a variable degree. The competence with which these repairs are performed varies enormously. Scar tissue forms between the sphincter ends and creates a sonographic defect (Figures 20-6 to 20-8). It is unclear how symptoms relate to the sonographic extent of the injury. For example, a study of 330 women

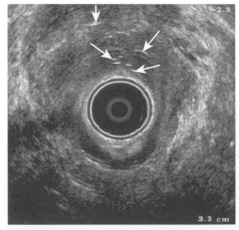

FIGURE 20-5 Obstetric injury. Anterior cloacal defect in a woman following vaginal delivery of a 5-kg baby. Note there is no external or internal sphincter anteriorly, and air within the defect *(arrows)* extends right to the probe surface.

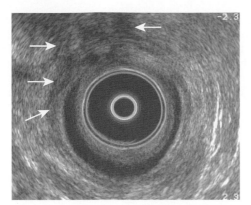

FIGURE 20-6 Typical anterior obstetric injury affecting both the external and internal anal sphincters. This 29-year-old woman was completely asymptomatic and was examined as part of a research study. The primary repair following delivery has opposed the external sphincter to some degree, but a sonographic defect remains *(arrows)*.

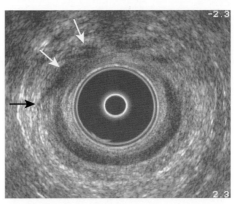

FIGURE 20-8 Typical anterior obstetric injury affecting both the external and internal anal sphincters. This 55-year-old woman had symptoms of anal incontinence that developed several years after vaginal delivery. Although it would be easy to ascribe this deterioration to progressive neuropathy, endosonography clearly reveals a sonographic defect centered on the right anterior quadrant *(arrows)*.

found that although women with an EAS tear had lower basal squeeze pressures than those without a tear, beyond this no consistent relationship was seen between the morphology of the tear (in terms of both its longitudinal and circumferential extent) and either symptoms or impaired anal pressures.[28] Patients may first present several years after the initial injury (see Figure 20-8), and some patients with large defects may be entirely asymptomatic initially (see Figure 20-6). Supporting this finding, a prospective study found that some women with clear evidence of sphincter disruption on AES were entirely asymptomatic following delivery,[29] and a study of 124 consecutive women with late-onset anal incontinence after vaginal delivery found that 71% had sonographic sphincter defects that were believed to be the cause of symptoms despite the temporal separation between childbirth and symptoms.[30]

It also seems that perineal tears that do not involve the sphincter muscles directly are much less likely to be associated with immediate symptoms (Figure 20-9). A prospective study of 55 nulliparous women that used three-dimensional AES found postpartum trauma in 29%. However, those women whose damage was limited to the puboanalis or transverse perineal muscles did not have symptoms, and no association with reduced anal pressures was noted.[31] It is also possible that anal canal morphology may change postpartum without any direct tearing of the perineum or sphincters. In particular, both two-dimensional and three-dimensional studies found that the anterior EAS may shorten following vaginal delivery but without any sonographic evidence of a tear (i.e., stretching of the sphincter during delivery changes its shape permanently but without frank tearing).[32,33] At the other extreme, AES may be used to examine women who have an anovaginal fistula following delivery because gas within the fistula is highly reflective and allows delineation of the tract and its relationship with the sphincter mechanism (Figure 20-10).

Perineal and sphincter trauma following vaginal delivery is generally repaired immediately afterward, usually using local anesthesia unless a significant disruption has been detected clinically. This sphincter surgery is known as a primary repair, and considerable attention has been focused on the sonographic assessment of such repairs. It is clear that many

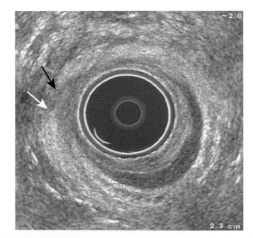

FIGURE 20-7 Typical anterior obstetric injury affecting both the external and internal sphincters. The sphincters have been reasonably well approximated *(arrows)* by primary repair, but the patient complained of anal incontinence immediately following childbirth.

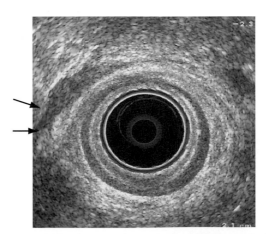

FIGURE 20-9 Perineal scar. Endosonography following vaginal delivery reveals a right anterior quadrant perineal scar *(arrows)* in this asymptomatic woman.

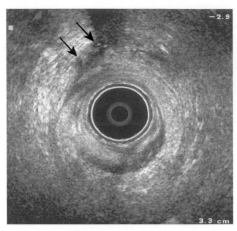

FIGURE 20-10 Anterior anovaginal fistula *(arrows)* in a woman following prolonged vaginal delivery.

women suffer symptoms of anal incontinence following primary repair, despite recognition of the tear and attempted repair. A study of 156 such women found that 40% of respondents were anally incontinent and that this was associated with a persistent sphincter defect on AES.[34] Another study found that 44 of 56 (79%) women who had undergone primary sphincter repair for a clinically recognized EAS tear following vaginal delivery had persistent sphincter defects on AES and were more symptomatic than those whose repair showed no sonographic defect.[35] These findings were confirmed by other workers.[36]

Primary sphincter repair aims to restore integrity to the sphincter ring but seems unable to achieve this objective in a significant proportion of cases (Figure 20-11). This may be because the perineum is very edematous and bruised immediately following vaginal delivery, factors that may conspire against successful repair. A study of 48 women 2 to 7 days following primary repair found that 90% had sonographic defects. Many of these defects were confined to the proximal anal canal, a finding suggesting that the initial repair had been incomplete.[37] The investigators concluded that inadequate repair was caused by surgical inexperience, rather than by the extent of sphincter damage, because junior doctors or midwives had undertaken many of the procedures.

If symptoms remain following primary repair and there is clear sonographic evidence of a persistent sphincter defect, patients then may be offered formal sphincter repair. An increasingly common option is to perform an anterior overlap repair, in which the disrupted EAS ends are mobilized, overlapped (thus tightening the anal canal), and then sutured together. Symptoms improve in approximately 85% of women immediately afterward, but this improvement is not sustained, and the percentage drops to approximately 50% at 5 years.[38] The cause of this deterioration is unclear, but concomitant progressive neuropathy is implicated, possibly resulting from pudendal damage or perhaps sphincter denervation and ischemia during the surgical procedure. However, repeated attempts at secondary sphincter repair are possible and can improve symptoms, even after many previous attempts, and delayed sphincter repair is also possible, with good symptomatic outcome.[39,40]

Endosonography has also assumed a role in the assessment of such secondary repairs. For example, the sonographic integrity of the repair correlates with symptoms and improved physiologic status.[41] Endosonography following a good anterior sphincter repair reveals sphincter ends that are well overlapped (Figure 20-12), whereas poor repairs are detected by persistent sphincter defects (Figure 20-13). Only the EAS is repaired, because attempts at IAS repair have not proved worthwhile. Residual IAS defects in the presence of a good EAS repair may underpin persistent symptoms, especially those of passive incontinence.

Endosonography has also been used to identify those women most at risk of obstetric injury. For example, some investigators have suggested that AES should be used routinely following vaginal delivery to identify those women with clinically occult sphincter tears whose sphincter may be at further risk from subsequent deliveries,[42] which is known to increase the risk of cumulative damage.[43,44] Endosonography has also been used to determine which routinely collected obstetric information best indicates the likelihood of associated sphincter disruption.

A study of 159 women found no correlation between sonographic tears and head circumference, baby weight, episiotomy, or the duration of active pushing.[45] However, forceps delivery was strongly associated with sphincter tears,[45] an association recognized by other workers.[25,46] Other

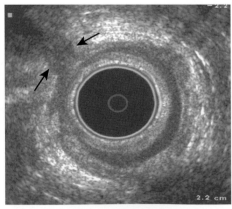

FIGURE 20-11 Anal endosonography following primary repair of a clinically recognized third-degree tear following vaginal delivery. A persistent external sphincter defect is visible *(arrows)*.

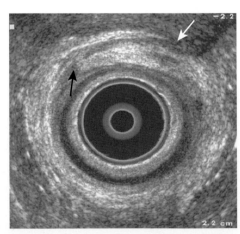

FIGURE 20-12 Good sonographic appearances following anterior overlapping sphincter repair. The external sphincter ends are well overlapped *(between arrows)*, and there is no residual defect.

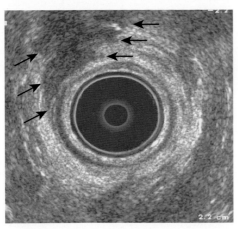

FIGURE 20-13 Poor sonographic appearance in a woman who remained symptomatic following a formal sphincter repair. A large persistent defect is visible *(arrows)*.

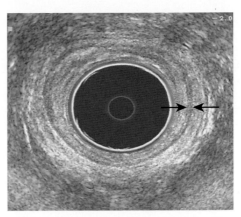

FIGURE 20-14 Anal endosonography in a 69-year-old woman with passive anal incontinence. The internal sphincter *(between arrows)* is intact but barely visible and measured 0.7 mm at its thickest. The findings suggest idiopathic degeneration of the internal anal sphincter.

investigators were able to identify a link between sphincter tears and a second stage of labor prolonged by epidural anesthesia, which increased the risk of disruption by an odds ratio of 2:1.[46] Where access to AES is limited, it may be possible to identify women who harbor sphincter tears by administering a simple incontinence questionnaire following delivery. Frudinger and colleagues[29] found that such an approach was able to identify 60% of women who sustained EAS tears following vaginal delivery.

AES revolutionized the management of women who sustain sphincter damage following vaginal delivery, but it is fair to say that some controversy persists regarding the exact incidence of EAS tears. For example, although the landmark study by Sultan and colleagues[25] found an incidence of 35% in primiparous women, Varma and colleagues[47] suggested that the true incidence was closer to 9%, and other investigators suggested 17%.[48] In an attempt to resolve this uncertainty, a meta-analysis of 717 vaginal deliveries found a 27% incidence of sphincter defects in nulliparous women, and 30% of these were symptomatic. The investigators concluded that the probability that postpartum anal incontinence was caused by sphincter disruption was closer to 80%.[49]

Idiopathic Internal Anal Sphincter Degeneration and External Anal Sphincter Atrophy

Not all anal incontinence is caused by sphincter disruption. Many incontinent patients have intact sphincters, but the functional quality of their sphincter muscle is impaired by neuromuscular degeneration. Vaizey and colleagues[50] reported 52 patients with anal incontinence who had an intact EAS and IAS on endosonography but whose IAS was thinned and hyperreflective. Resting pressures, reflecting IAS function, were significantly lowered in this group, but squeeze pressures and pudendal nerve latencies were normal. The investigators concluded that discrete and isolated primary degeneration of the IAS was likely responsible for anal incontinence in these patients. Because the IAS normally thickens with age,[7] IAS thinning is relatively easy to diagnose, and the diagnosis should be considered in any older patient

whose IAS measures 1 mm or less in thickness (Figure 20-14). A rare cause of isolated IAS thinning is systemic sclerosis (scleroderma).[51]

The EAS may also degenerate, a process termed *atrophy*. This phenomenon was first recognized using endoanal MRI because the striated fibers of the EAS contrast strongly against ischioanal fat, and it is therefore easier to appreciate muscular bulk than on AES.[52] Although the mechanisms are unclear, one possibility being long-standing pudendal neuropathy, EAS atrophy is important because it adversely affects the outcome of sphincter repair. Briel and colleagues[52] found that surgical procedures for concomitant EAS defects in this group were unsuccessful because the functional quality of the EAS was compromised by atrophy. Using both endoanal MRI and AES, Williams and colleagues[53] were able to define the sonographic features of EAS atrophy and found that the EAS in these patients was patchy and poorly defined. In particular, the lateral edge of the EAS was indistinct, and the muscle was thinner than normal.[53] IAS degeneration and EAS atrophy may be combined in the same patient, and these are probably the sonographic features of what has long been termed *neurogenic* fecal incontinence (Figure 20-15). Indeed, atrophy

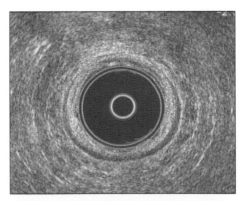

FIGURE 20-15 Anal endosonography in a 50-year-old woman complaining of anal incontinence. Both sphincters are intact but are very poorly seen. The lateral margins of the external anal sphincter (EAS) are indistinct, suggesting EAS atrophy, and the internal anal sphincter is very thin, suggesting degeneration.

of both sphincters and concomitant tears can be found in the same patient.

Although endoanal MRI is likely superior to AES for diagnosis of EAS atrophy, investigators found that both modalities are equivalent for diagnosis of sphincter tears. AES is particularly adept at the diagnosis of IAS degeneration because this muscle is normally well visualized during endosonography and is thinned in these patients, whereas it is normally thicker in older people, an observation that facilitates a distinction between normal and abnormal.[54] EAS atrophy is more difficult to diagnose reliably with AES, not only because the sphincter is difficult to define but also because the normal EAS tends to thin with age.[7]

Iatrogenic Sphincter Injury and Anal Trauma

Unfortunately, iatrogenic damage is a relatively common cause of anal incontinence. A study of 50 patients following a variety of anal surgical procedures found subsequent sphincter defects in 46%.[55] Although some procedures purposely seek to divide the sphincter mechanism, most obviously IAS sphincterotomy, other procedures should not normally cause sphincter damage. An association between unintentional sphincter division and hemorrhoidectomy is now well recognized (Figure 20-16). A study of 16 patients undergoing hemorrhoidectomy found subsequent sphincter defects in 50%.[56] Quadrantic IAS division is relatively common in symptomatic patients, but occasionally the incision is sufficiently deep to lacerate the longitudinal muscle and the EAS as well.

The IAS may also be damaged in patients who have undergone procedures that require anal dilatation. In these cases, the appearances tend to be those of generalized IAS fragmentation around the circumference (Figure 20-17). Anal stretch (the Lord procedure) for anal fissure is a common cause of such disruption, as is manual rectal evacuation for intractable constipation if it is not carefully performed.[57] Transanal stapling instruments, such as those used for low anterior resection, may also unintentionally incorporate the IAS in their firing path and result in IAS defects and subsequent passive incontinence.[58,59] Whereas the IAS is purposefully divided during lateral sphincterotomy, the intent is usually to divide the muscle for only the most caudal one-third of its

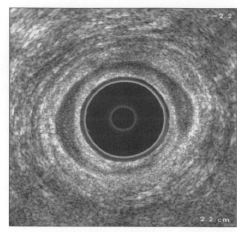

FIGURE 20-17 Internal anal sphincter fragmentation. Endosonography reveals internal sphincter fragmentation in this woman who had anal dilatation for an anal fissure and who now complains of anal incontinence.

length. However, prospective sonographic studies of IAS morphology following this procedure revealed that division is often more extensive than actually intended, notably in women, probably because their anatomic anal canal is shorter than in men.[60] Such studies have increased physician awareness of overextensive IAS division, and operators are probably now more cautious than they were before the advent of AES. The result is that sonographic studies have revealed that some patients whose anal fissure persisted after sphincterotomy may not actually have had any muscle divided during the procedure.[61]

A current role is also emerging for AES in the treatment of anal incontinence, although this work is largely preliminary. For example, AES is necessary to monitor injection of bulking material, such as silicone, into the anal sphincter that may possibly treat incontinence.[62,63] More recent work has used AES to deliver autologous myoblasts into EAS defects, with the hope that the engineered cells will integrate into their surroundings and restore functionality to the damaged striated muscle.[64]

Sonographic Findings in Other Anal Disorders

Although the main role for AES is in patients with anal incontinence, AES has other useful applications. The most prominent of these is probably for imaging fistula-in-ano. Surgeons operating on these patients need to know the relationship of the fistula tract to the anal sphincter mechanism because treatment usually involves cutting down onto the fistula and laying it open so that infection can drain and heal subsequently. This practically always necessitates a degree of unavoidable sphincter division, the extent of which may be predicted by AES.

Early attempts to use AES for preoperative assessment of fistula-in-ano were relatively disappointing, and assessment was no better than that achieved by digital examination by an experienced colorectal surgeon.[65] However, more recent studies using 10-MHz AES were more optimistic. A study of 108 fistulas in 104 patients found that AES correctly classified the primary fistula tract in 81% of cases, as opposed to 61%

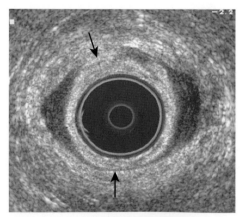

FIGURE 20-16 Endosonography in a man who became incontinent following hemorrhoidectomy. The scan reveals extensive internal sphincter division, with large anterior and posterior defects *(arrows)*.

for digital examination by an experienced surgeon.[66] Endosonography was particularly accurate in predicting the site of the internal enteric opening in the anal canal; the prediction was correct in 91% of cases.[66] The reason is that the internal opening is inevitably close to the transducer surface and is therefore visualized with high spatial resolution. However, AES has specific disadvantages in several areas. For example, insufficient penetration beyond the EAS, especially with high-frequency transducers, limits the ability to resolve tracts and abscesses that are remote from the anal canal. Unfortunately, these lesions are especially common in patients with recurrent disease.[67] Moreover, AES cannot reliably distinguish infection from fibrosis, given that both appear hypoechoic on ultrasound. This inability causes particular difficulties in patients with recurrent disease because active tracts and fibrotic scars are frequently combined. Attempts have been made to clarify the course of patent tracts by injecting hydrogen peroxide or ultrasound contrast agents into the external opening during examination.[68]

Another disadvantage of AES is the inability to image in the surgically important (for fistulas) coronal plane, so it may be very difficult to distinguish supralevator from infralevator extensions. Some investigators have attempted to overcome this disadvantage by employing three-dimensional acquisition[69,70] (Figure 20-18), but this technique remains relatively experimental. However, there is little doubt that MRI is a superior technique overall, and therefore the major role of AES in fistula disease is probably to assess the degree of sphincter disruption in those patients who become anally incontinent. AES also has a particular role in those patients who may have a small intersphincteric abscess that could be difficult to resolve using standard body or phased array surface coil MRI (Figure 20-19).

Endosonography has revealed sphincter abnormalities in patients who are severely constipated, although the significance of these abnormalities remains largely uncertain. For example, patients with solitary rectal ulcer syndrome are known to have an abnormally thickened IAS (Figure 20-20),[71] and this finding has been correlated with the presence of

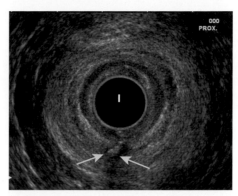

FIGURE 20-19 Endosonography clearly reveals a posterior intersphincteric abscess *(arrows)* in this patient with anal pain. The digital rectal examination had been normal.

high-grade prolapse of rectal mucosa.[72] IAS hypertrophy has also been demonstrated by AES in children with intractable constipation.[73] A study of 144 constipated children found that this finding correlated with duration and severity of symptoms, size of megarectum, and amplitude of rectal contraction.[74] The investigators suggested that IAS thickening was caused by hypertrophy as a result of chronic stimulation owing to the presence of feces in the rectum.[74] Endosonography may also be useful when it is necessary to determine the correct anatomic position of the neoanus with respect to any residual musculature in children with imperforate anus and, unlike MRI, can be easily performed perioperatively.[75,76]

Endosonography may also be used to stage anal tumors locally because it can determine the depth of penetration into surrounding tissues (Figure 20-21).[77] However, some investigators have found the technique less useful for detecting local recurrence because all 14 recurrences in a series of 82 patients were detected by visual inspection and digital examination alone.[78]

Recent Developments

The last few years have seen a rash of publications describing results from three-dimensional imaging, for example, describing the longitudinal extent of internal sphincter division

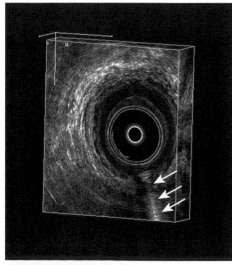

FIGURE 20-18 Three-dimensional anal endosonography following hydrogen peroxide injection through the external opening of a fistula-in-ano. Echogenic gas is present within an intersphincteric tract *(arrows)*.

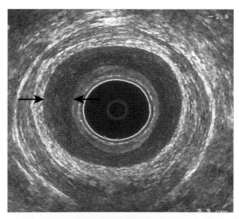

FIGURE 20-20 Male patient with solitary rectal ulcer syndrome. The internal sphincter *(between arrows)* measured 7.5 mm, far greater than normal.

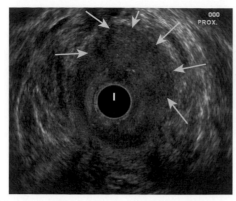

FIGURE 20-21 Anal squamous tumor. Endosonography in a man with a primary anal squamous tumor reveals a large left anterior quadrant mass *(arrows)* that has breached the anal sphincter complex to reach the surrounding tissues.

following sphincterotomy for anal fissure.[79] Although very useful as a research tool, the author believes that three-dimensional acquisition is not substantially superior to standard two-dimensional imaging when the latter is used by experienced practitioners; the author uses only two-dimensional imaging for his clinical work. The major advantage of three-dimensional imaging would seem to be a practical one—because a volume of data is acquired that encompasses the whole anal canal, the entire examination can be retrieved and reviewed subsequently, whereas only selected "slices" are available in two dimensions.

Transperineal ultrasound has also attracted significant attention recently. Although often cited as "less invasive, more user-friendly, more accessible, and more patient-acceptable,"[80] the author would argue that there is no substantial difference between rubbing an ultrasound probe over a patient's perineum versus inserting a small-diameter probe a couple of centimeters into his or her anus. However, the ability to use a standard ultrasound probe is a distinct advantage if the technique is accurate. Transperineal ultrasound is performed with the patient supine and the hips flexed, with the probe placed directly on the perineum. Clearly, the anatomic display is very different from that obtained by endoanal imaging. An alternative approach is to image the "undisturbed" anal sphincter via transvaginal ultrasound. There are few comparative studies of these various modalities, but a recent review of available literature concluded that, for anal sphincter defects, AES was likely to be the most accurate diagnostic test.[80]

REFERENCES

1. Law PJ, Bartram CI. Anal endosonography: technique and normal anatomy. *Gastrointest Radiol.* 1989;14:349-353.
2. Snooks SJ, Setchell M, Swash M, Henry MM. Injury to the innervation of the pelvic floor sphincter musculature in childbirth. *Lancet.* 1984;2:546-550.
3. Frudinger A, Bartram CI, Halligan S, Kamm M. Examination techniques for endosonography of the anal canal. *Abdom Imaging.* 1998;23:301-303.
4. Lunniss PJ, Phillips RK. Anatomy and function of the anal longitudinal muscle. *Br J Surg.* 1992;79:882-884.
5. Stoker J, Rociu E, Zwamborn AW, et al. Endoluminal MR imaging of the rectum and anus: technique, applications, and pitfalls. *Radiographics.* 1999;19:383-398.
6. Williams AB, Bartram CI, Halligan S, et al. Endosonographic anatomy of the normal anal canal compared with endocoil magnetic resonance imaging. *Dis Colon Rectum.* 2002;45:176-183.
7. Frudinger A, Halligan S, Bartram CI, et al. Female anal sphincter: age-related differences in asymptomatic volunteers with high-frequency endoanal US. *Radiology.* 2002;224:417-423.
8. Williams AB, Bartram CI, Halligan S, et al. Multiplanar anal endosonography: normal anal canal anatomy. *Colorectal Dis.* 2001;3:169-174.
9. Sultan AH, Nicholls RJ, Kamm MA, et al. Anal endosonography and correlation with in vitro and in vivo anatomy. *Br J Surg.* 1993;80:508-511.
10. Gold DM, Halligan S, Kmiot WA, Bartram CI. Intraobserver and interobserver agreement in anal endosonography. *Br J Surg.* 1999;86:371-375.
11. Lane RH, Parks AG. Function of the anal sphincters following colo-anal anastomosis. *Br J Surg.* 1977;64:596-599.
12. Engel AG, Kamm MA. Relationship of symptoms in faecal incontinence to specific sphincter abnormalities. *Int J Colorectal Dis.* 1995;10:152-155.
13. Rogers J, Henry MM, Misiewicz JJ. Disposable pudendal nerve stimulator: evaluation of the standard instrument and new device. *Gut.* 1988;29:1131-1133.
14. Kiff ES, Swash M. Slowed conduction in the pudendal nerves in idiopathic (neurogenic) faecal incontinence. *Br J Surg.* 1984;71:614-616.
15. Parks AG, Porter NH, Hardcastle JD. The syndrome of the descending perineum. *Proc R Soc Med.* 1966;59:477-482.
16. Jorge JMN, Wexner SD, Ehrenpreis ED, et al. Does perineal descent correlate with pudendal neuropathy? *Dis Colon Rectum.* 1993;36:475-483.
17. Gilliand R, Altomare DF, Moreira H, et al. Pudendal neuropathy is predictive of failure following anterior overlapping sphincteroplasty. *Dis Colon Rectum.* 1998;41:1516-1522.
18. Sultan AH, Kamm MA, Talbot IC, et al. Anal endosonography for identifying external sphincter defects confirmed histologically. *Br J Surg.* 1994;81:463-465.
19. Denis P, Bercoff E, Bizien MF. Etude de la prevalence di l'incontinence anale chez l'adulte. *Gastroenterol Clin Biol.* 1992;16:344-350.
20. Talley NJ, O'Keefe EA, Zinsmeister AR, Melton JL. Prevalence of gastrointestinal symptoms in the elderly: a population based study. *Gastroenterology.* 1992;102:895-901.
21. Lahr CJ. Evaluation and treatment of incontinence. *Pract Gastroenterol.* 1988;12:27-35.
22. Sultan AH, Kamm MA, Hudson CN, Bartram CI. Third degree obstetric tears: risk factors and outcome of primary repair. *BMJ.* 1994;308:887-891.
23. Law PJ, Kamm MA, Bartram CI. Anal endosonography in the investigation of faecal incontinence. *Br J Surg.* 1991;78:312-314.
24. Burnett SJD, Spence-Jones C, Speakman CTM, et al. Unsuspected sphincter damage following childbirth revealed by anal endosonography. *Br J Radiol.* 1991;64:225-227.
25. Sultan AH, Kamm MA, Hudson CN, et al. Anal sphincter disruption during vaginal delivery. *N Engl J Med.* 1993;329:1905-1911.
26. Deen KI, Kumar D, Williams JG, et al. Anal sphincter defects: correlation between endoanal ultrasound and surgery. *Ann Surg.* 1993;218:201-205.
27. Sentovich SM, Wong WD, Blatchford GJ. Accuracy and reliability of transanal ultrasound for anterior anal sphincter injury. *Dis Colon Rectum.* 1998;41:1000-1004.
28. Voyvodic F, Rieger NA, Skinner S, et al. Endosonographic imaging of anal sphincter injury: does the size of the tear correlate with the degree of dysfunction? *Dis Colon Rectum.* 2003;46:735-741.
29. Frudinger A, Halligan S, Bartram CI, et al. Assessment of the predictive value of a bowel symptom questionnaire in identifying perianal and anal sphincter trauma after vaginal delivery. *Dis Colon Rectum.* 2003;46:742-747.
30. Oberwalder M, Dinnewitzer A, Baig MK, et al. The association between late-onset fecal incontinence and obstetric anal sphincter defects. *Arch Surg.* 2004;139:429-432.
31. Williams AB, Bartram CI, Halligan S, et al. Anal sphincter damage after vaginal delivery using three-dimensional endosonography. *Obstet Gynaecol.* 2001;97:770-775.
32. Frudinger A, Halligan S, Bartram CI, et al. Changes in anal anatomy following vaginal delivery revealed by anal endosonography. *Br J Obstet Gynaecol.* 1999;106:233-237.
33. Williams AB, Bartram CI, Halligan S, et al. Alteration of anal sphincter morphology following vaginal delivery revealed by multiplanar anal endosonography. *BJOG.* 2002;109:942-946.

34. Poen AC, Felt-Bersma RJ, Strijers RL, et al. Third-degree obstetric perineal tear: long-term clinical and functional results after primary repair. *Br J Surg.* 1998;85:1433-1438.

35. Davis K, Kumar D, Stanton SL, et al. Symptoms and anal sphincter morphology following primary repair of third-degree tears. *Br J Surg.* 2003;90:1573-1579.

36. Savoye-Collet C, Savoye G, Koning E, et al. Endosonography in the evaluation of anal function after primary repair of a third-degree obstetric tear. *Scand J Gastroenterol.* 2003;38:1149-1153.

37. Starck M, Bohe M, Valentin L. Results of endosonographic imaging of the anal sphincter 2-7 days after primary repair of third- or fourth-degree obstetric sphincter tears. *Ultrasound Obstet Gynecol.* 2003;22:609-615.

38. Malouf AJ, Norton CS, Engel AF, et al. Long-term results of overlapping anterior anal-sphincter repair for obstetric trauma. *Lancet.* 2000;355:260-265.

39. Pinedo G, Vaizey CJ, Nicholls RJ, et al. Results of repeat anal sphincter repair. *Br J Surg.* 1999;86:66-69.

40. Giordano P, Renzi A, Efron J, et al. Previous sphincter repair does not affect the outcome of repeat repair. *Dis Colon Rectum.* 2002;45:635-640.

41. Felt-Bersma RJ, Cuesta MA, Koorevaar M. Anal sphincter repair improves anorectal function and endosonographic image: a prospective clinical study. *Dis Colon Rectum.* 1996;39:878-885.

42. Faltin DL, Boulvain M, Irion O, et al. Diagnosis of anal sphincter tears by postpartum endosonography to predict fecal incontinence. *Obstet Gynecol.* 2000;95:643-647.

43. Fines M, Donnelly V, Behan M, et al. Effect of second vaginal delivery on anorectal physiology and faecal continence: a prospective study. *Lancet.* 1999;354:983-986.

44. Faltin DL, Sangalli MR, Roche B, et al. Does a second delivery increase the risk of anal incontinence? *BJOG.* 2001;108:684-688.

45. Varma A, Gunn J, Lindow SW, Duthie GS. Do routinely measured delivery variables predict anal sphincter outcome? *Dis Colon Rectum.* 1999;42:1261-1264.

46. Donnelly V, Fynes M, Campbell D, et al. Obstetric events leading to anal sphincter damage. *Obstet Gynecol.* 1998;92:955-961.

47. Varma A, Gunn J, Gardiner A, et al. Obstetric anal sphincter injury: prospective evaluation of incidence. *Dis Colon Rectum.* 1999;42:1537-1543.

48. Abramowitz L, Sobhani I, Ganansia R, et al. Are sphincter defects the cause of anal incontinence after vaginal delivery? Results of a prospective study. *Dis Colon Rectum.* 2000;43:590-596, discussion 596–598.

49. Oberwalder M, Connor J, Wexner SD. Meta-analysis to determine the incidence of obstetric anal sphincter damage. *Br J Surg.* 2003;90:1333-1337.

50. Vaizey CJ, Kamm MA, Bartram CI. Primary degeneration of the internal anal sphincter as a cause of passive faecal incontinence. *Lancet.* 1997;349:612-615.

51. Engel AF, Kamm MA, Talbot IC. Progressive systemic sclerosis of the internal anal sphincter leading to passive faecal incontinence. *Gut.* 1994;35:857-859.

52. Briel JW, Stoker J, Rociu E, et al. External anal sphincter atrophy on endoanal magnetic resonance imaging adversely affects continence after sphincteroplasty. *Br J Surg.* 1999;86:1322-1327.

53. Williams AB, Bartram CI, Modhwadia D, et al. Endocoil magnetic resonance imaging quantification of external anal sphincter atrophy. *Br J Surg.* 2001;88:853-859.

54. Malouf AJ, Williams AB, Halligan S, et al. Prospective assessment of accuracy of endoanal MR imaging and endosonography in patients with fecal incontinence. *AJR Am J Roentgenol.* 2000;175:741-745.

55. Felt-Bersma RJ, van Baren R, Koorevaar M, et al. Unsuspected sphincter defects shown by anal endosonography after anorectal surgery: a prospective study. *Dis Colon Rectum.* 1995;38:249-253.

56. Abbasakoor F, Nelson M, Beynon J, et al. Anal endosonography in patients with anorectal symptoms after haemorrhoidectomy. *Br J Surg.* 1998;85:1522-1524.

57. Gattuso JM, Kamm MA, Halligan SM, Bartram CI. The anal sphincter in idiopathic megarectum: effects of manual disimpaction under general anesthetic. *Dis Colon Rectum.* 1996;39:435-439.

58. Ho YH, Tsang C, Tang CL, et al. Anal sphincter injuries from stapling instruments introduced transanally: randomized, controlled study with endoanal ultrasound and anorectal manometry. *Dis Colon Rectum.* 2000;43:169-173.

59. Farouk R, Duthie GS, Lee PW, Monson JR. Endosonographic evidence of injury to the internal anal sphincter after low anterior resection: long-term follow-up. *Dis Colon Rectum.* 1998;41:888-891.

60. Sultan AH, Kamm MA, Nicholls RJ, Bartram CI. Prospective study of the extent of internal anal sphincter division during lateral sphincterotomy. *Dis Colon Rectum.* 1994;37:1031-1033.

61. Garcia-Granero E, Sanahuja A, Garcia-Armengol J, et al. Anal endosonographic evaluation after closed lateral subcutaneous sphincterotomy. *Dis Colon Rectum.* 1998;41:598-601.

62. Tjandra JJ, Lim JF, Hiscock R, Rajendra P. Injectable silicone biomaterial for fecal incontinence caused by internal anal sphincter dysfunction is effective. *Dis Colon Rectum.* 2004;47:2138-2146.

63. Maeda Y, Vaizey CJ, Kamm MA. Long-term results of perianal silicone injection for faecal incontinence. *Colorectal Dis.* 2007;9:357-361.

64. Frudinger A, Kölle D, Schwaiger W, et al. Muscle-derived cell injection to treat anal incontinence due to obstetric trauma: pilot study with 1 year follow-up. *Gut.* 2010;59:55-61.

65. Choen S, Burnett S, Bartram CI, Nicholls RJ. Comparison between anal endosonography and digital examination in the evaluation of anal fistulae. *Br J Surg.* 1991;78:445-447.

66. Buchanan GN, Halligan S, Bartram CI, et al. Clinical examination, endosonography, and magnetic resonance imaging for preoperative assessment of fistula-in-ano: comparison to an outcome based reference standard. *Radiology.* 2004;233:674-681.

67. Buchanan G, Halligan S, Williams A, et al. Effect of MRI on clinical outcome of recurrent fistula-in-ano. *Lancet.* 2002;360:1661-1662.

68. Kruskal JB, Kane RA, Morrin MM. Peroxide-enhanced anal endosonography: technique, image interpretation, and clinical applications. *Radiographics.* 2001;21:173-189.

69. Buchanan GN, Bartram CI, Williams AB, et al. Value of hydrogen peroxide enhancement of three-dimensional endoanal ultrasound in fistula-in-ano. *Dis Colon Rectum.* 2005;48:141-147.

70. West RL, Zimmerman DD, Dwarkasing S, et al. Prospective comparison of hydrogen peroxide-enhanced three-dimensional endoanal ultrasonography and endoanal magnetic resonance imaging of perianal fistulas. *Dis Colon Rectum.* 2003;46:1407-1415.

71. Halligan S, Sultan A, Rottenberg G, Bartram CI. Endosonography of the anal sphincters in solitary rectal ulcer syndrome. *Int J Colorectal Dis.* 1995;10:79-82.

72. Marshall M, Halligan S, Fotheringham T, et al. Predictive value of internal anal sphincter thickness for diagnosis of rectal intussusception in patients with solitary rectal ulcer syndrome. *Br J Surg.* 2002;89:1281-1285.

73. Hosie GP, Spitz L. Idiopathic constipation in childhood is associated with thickening of the internal anal sphincter. *J Pediatr Surg.* 1997;32:1041-1043, discussion 1043-1044.

74. Keshtgar AS, Ward HC, Clayden GS, Sanei A. Thickening of the internal anal sphincter in idiopathic constipation in children. *Pediatr Surg Int.* 2004;20:817-823.

75. Jones NM, Humphreys MS, Goodman TR, et al. The value of anal endosonography compared with magnetic resonance imaging following the repair of anorectal malformations. *Pediatr Radiol.* 2003;33:183-185.

76. Yamataka A, Yoshida R, Kobayashi H, et al. Intraoperative endosonography enhances laparoscopy-assisted colon pull-through for high imperforate anus. *J Pediatr Surg.* 2002;37:1657-1660.

77. Tarantino D, Bernstein MA. Endoanal ultrasound in the staging and management of squamous-cell carcinoma of the anal canal: potential implications of a new ultrasound staging system. *Dis Colon Rectum.* 2002;45:16-22.

78. Lund JA, Sundstrom SH, Haaverstad R, et al. Endoanal ultrasound is of little value in follow-up of anal carcinomas. *Dis Colon Rectum.* 2004;47:839-842.

79. Murad-Regadas SM, Fernandes GO, Regadas FS, et al. How much of the internal sphincter may be divided during lateral sphincterotomy for chronic anal fissure in women? Morphologic and functional evaluation after sphincterotomy. *Dis Colon Rectum.* 2013;56:645-651.

80. Abdool Z, Sultan AH, Thakar R. Ultrasound imaging of the anal sphincter complex: a review. *Br J Radiol.* 2012;85:865-875.

SECTION VI

EUS-Guided Tissue Acquisition

21

How to Perform EUS-Guided Fine-Needle Aspiration

Anand V. Sahai • Sarto C. Paquin

Key Points

- Because movement of the needle is easier when the echoendoscope is straight, the endosonographer should try to achieve a position in which up-down and left-right tip angulation is minimal and no elevator is required.
- Before insertion of a needle, the needle pathway should be scanned using color Doppler mode.
- Excessive force should never be used to pass the needle sheath past an acute bend in the endoscope tip.
- The needle is kept in the visual plane at all times during EUS FNA.
- During aspiration of cysts without a mass component, the endosonographer should fully aspirate all fluid, make only one pass, use antibiotics, and not try to perform aspiration cytology from the cyst wall.

Fine-needle aspiration (FNA) provides some of the most clinically powerful information that endoscopic ultrasound (EUS) has to offer—pathological confirmation of the presence (or absence) of malignancy and/or metastasis to secondary sites ("histologic staging"). Like any procedure, proficiency requires adequate experience, but EUS FNA is not a universally difficult technique to master. Some cases are more technically demanding than others. Sampling a 5-mm pancreatic nodule buried deep in the uncinate process is certainly more challenging than sampling a 4-cm subcarinal lymph node. Interestingly, some of the easiest cases provide information that can have a tremendous impact on patient management (e.g., prevention of surgery by documentation of mediastinal node involvement in a patient with non–small-cell lung cancer).

EUS FNA can be broken down into a series of steps. Proper execution of each step will make EUS FNA easier and probably increase the yield for malignancy. Experts have varying opinions of the best way to perform EUS FNA; however, objective data are constantly emerging to help clarify which procedural variables improve results and which have no clear impact.

This chapter will provide a detailed description of a generic EUS FNA technique that can be applied to the great majority of lesions, to obtain specimens for cytologic analysis, and/or to prepare a cell block. Special consideration will also be given to issues that provide particular challenges.

Cytological specimens are adequate for diagnostic purposes in most cases. They can be used to confirm or exclude epithelial malignancies, allow for immunochemical staining (e.g., to diagnose neuroendocrine tumors and small cell lung cancer, to look for specific tumor receptors, etc.), and permit flow cytometry, which can help diagnose or exclude monoclonal lymphoid processes. Cytological specimens may also be sufficient to identify granulomas, which may help diagnose diseases such as sarcoidosis. However, in some cases, true histologic specimens may be required, and core specimens should be sought using larger gauge needles. The techniques required to obtain a "core" biopsy specimen for true histologic analysis are addressed in Chapter 22.

Indications and Contraindications

Indications for EUS FNA for tissue acquisition have broadened over time. Tissue sampling is performed most often to confirm suspected cancer,[1] although it may also be useful in benign conditions such as diagnosing sarcoidosis or infections (e.g., tuberculosis or fungal disease). Box 21-1 summarizes the common sites for performing EUS FNA.

Contraindications to EUS FNA are limited. Before performing EUS FNA, the endosonographer must be certain that there is a reasonable chance that tissue sampling will be clinically useful.

As a general rule, FNA should be avoided in patients with significant coagulopathy (INR > 1.5, platelets < 100,000, recent use of thienopyridines [e.g., clopidogrel], etc.).[2] However, the use of aspirin or nonsteroidal anti-inflammatory drugs is not a problem. Patients receiving anticoagulant therapy (e.g., warfarin or dabigatran) should discontinue their

| BOX 21-1 | Common Sites for Performing EUS FNA |

Pancreas
Bile duct
Digestive wall lesions[a]
    Suspicious wall thickening
    Subepithelial lesions
Adrenal glands
Liver
Retroperitoneal masses
Lymph nodes
Posterior mediastinum
    Suspicious lymph nodes
    Pulmonary masses[b]

[a]Digestive wall lesions include the esophagus, stomach, duodenum, and rectum.
[b]Pulmonary masses must abut the posterior mediastinum to be visualized under EUS.

medication prior to the procedure (3 to 5 days for warfarin, 48 hours for dabigatran). If the patient is at high risk for thromboembolic events, bridge therapy with low molecular weight heparin should be considered. Patients receiving antiplatelet therapy such as clopidogrel should also withhold them for 7 to 10 days prior to the procedure if they carry a low thromboembolic risk.

Some high-risk patients may not safely discontinue their treatment. In these situations, where the risk of stopping anticoagulation is potentially greater than the risk of FNA-induced bleeding (e.g., FNA of a large mediastinal node in a patient anticoagulated for massive pulmonary embolus), it may be reasonable to attempt EUS FNA without stopping anticoagulants, while using a small-gauge (25-G) needle and minimizing the number of passes (e.g., with on-site cytology).

Finally, certain anatomical challenges may also contraindicate EUS FNA, such as a large vessel or duct interposing itself between the targeted lesion and the ultrasound probe. Lymph nodes may not be accessible if the primary mass is preventing direct node sampling, carrying the risk of false-positive results. Box 21-2 provides an overview to EUS FNA contraindications.

| BOX 21-2 | Contraindications for Performing EUS FNA |

Contraindication for endoscopic examination
    Cardiac or respiratory instability
    Suspected perforated viscus
    Nonfasting patient or undecompressed upper
        gastrointestinal obstruction
Coagulation disorder
    Anticoagulants
    Antiplatelet therapy[a]
Inaccessible lesion
    Lesion not visualized
    Large vessel or duct interposition
    Metastatic lesion with primary mass interposition
EUS FNA results will not alter subsequent management

[a]Aspirin or nonsteroidal anti-inflammatory drug use is not contraindicated.

Steps for EUS FNA

1. Verify the indication.
2. Localize the lesion and position the echoendoscope.
3. Choose the correct needle.
4. Insert the EUS FNA needle into the echoendoscope.
5. Position the lesion in the needle path.
6. Puncture the lesion and move the needle within the lesion.
7. Withdraw the needle and process the aspirate.
8. Prepare the needle for subsequent passes.
9. Evolving trends in EUS FNA:
    a. use of the stylet
    b. use of suction
10. FNA particularities according to site:
    a. esophagus
    b. stomach
    c. duodenal bulb
    d. duodenal sweep (D2)

Verify the Indication

Before performing EUS FNA, the indication should be clear and the endoscopy suite and team adequately prepared. Like any test, EUS FNA does not need to "change management" to be useful. However, before considering EUS FNA in a given patient, it should be clear that the information obtained has a reasonable chance of being clinically useful (to those managing the patient and/or to the patient). If the endosonographer is not in charge of the patient's management, his or her opinion as to the value of the information need not affect the decision to perform EUS FNA, unless there is compelling evidence that the risks of the procedure will likely far outweigh the possible benefits. If there is any doubt, these issues should be addressed with the referring physician before the procedure (or even *during* the procedure) if necessary.

EUS FNA should be avoided if it will clearly not influence management or treatment, if there is a risk of tumor seeding that could worsen clinical outcomes, or if there is an excessive risk of puncture-related complications (e.g., bleeding, infection, or trauma to surrounding structures).

When faced with the possibility of performing FNA on multiple sites, one should focus on the lesion likely to provide the most relevant information first. For instance, in the setting of a pancreatic head mass with suspicious liver nodules, FNA of the liver lesions may provide a positive cytologic diagnosis *and* confirm that the patient is not a surgical candidate.

Localize the Lesion and Position the Echoendoscope

Whenever possible, the echoendoscope should be straight. This makes needle movement easier and reduces the risks of damage to the accessory channel during insertion of the needle into the scope.

In our experience, most pancreatic lesions (including pancreatic head/uncinate lesions) can also be sampled with the scope in a straight position. To do so, the scope should be passed into the second duodenum and then withdrawn into a "short" position. By withdrawing the scope toward the duodenal bulb, most pancreatic head lesions can be accessed and punctured. However, when withdrawn sufficiently, this position will become unstable and the scope may slip into the stomach. Lesions near the pancreatic genu are often difficult to biopsy with this withdrawal technique, because they often become visible just at the moment that the position becomes unstable.

For these lesions (and any other lesions that cannot be accessed with the scope in a straight position), it is necessary to assume a "long" position, with the scope in the bulb or prepyloric region. This position will also provide a mechanical advantage when trying to puncture indurated lesions in the pancreatic head region.

Choose the Correct Needle

At the time of this writing, there are three needle sizes available for EUS FNA that can be used to obtain material for cytology: 19 G, 22 G, and 25 G. These needle sizes are also available in models featuring a beveled side-hole near the tip, which may help scrape more material into the needle.

There is increasing evidence that smaller needles offer at least similar results in diagnostic yield compared to larger needles and are also easier to manipulate.[3-8] Large-diameter needles tend to be harder to maneuver (particularly the 19-G needle), are more traumatic, and may provide bloodier samples—which may actually reduce their effectiveness when compared to smaller-diameter needles. Traditionally, 22-G needles were used for solid lesions, mainly because it was the first size that was commercially available. However, 25-G needles eventually came to market, and some hypothesized that a 25-G needle would be better (easier to penetrate hard lesions, more maneuverable, provide less bloody aspirates), particularly for challenging pancreatic head lesions.[7,9-12] The first retrospective comparisons of the 22-G and 25-G needles showed the 25-G needle to be more sensitive for cancer in pancreatic masses,[9,10] but subsequent prospective studies failed to show statistically significant advantages.[7,11] However, a recent meta-analysis showed that for pancreatic masses the sensitivity of the 22-G needle is clearly inferior to that of the 25-G needle (85% [95% CI: 82% to 88%] vs 93% [95% CI: 91% to 96%], $p = 0.0003$).[8] Given that the 25-G needle is more flexible, and hence easier to manipulate, it appears reasonable to favor the 25-G needle for all cases of solid-lesion EUS-guided FNA when the objective is to obtain material for cytology.

A detailed review of the value (if any) of adding the beveled side-hole near the tip of the needle is beyond the scope of this chapter. The only published prospective, comparative study showed no advantage for the beveled side-hole for the purpose of obtaining cytology specimens.[13] Further comparative trials are required before any firm conclusions can be drawn.

Insert the EUS FNA Needle into the Echoendoscope

Whether or not the needle system is inserted into the biopsy channel before or after the echoendoscope is in position for FNA is a matter of personal preference. However, it should be noted that, once the echoendoscope is in position, it might be difficult or impossible to pass the needle system completely into position if the echoendoscope is not sufficiently straight. In this situation, the sheath may become stuck in the bending portion of the instrument near the tip. One should *never* use excessive force to push the sheath past an excessive bend at this location because the needle sheath may perforate the inner sheath of the biopsy channel. Instead, the echoendoscope should be withdrawn into a straight configuration before attempting to re-insert the needle system completely.

For lesions to be accessed from the second duodenum, the needle should be inserted into the scope only *after* the scope has been placed into the second duodenum. In other words, the duodenal sweep should not be negotiated with the needle and/or sheath protruding from the biopsy channel, because there is a risk of duodenal laceration during this maneuver. The scope should be positioned in a "short-scope" fashion prior to attempting needle insertion.

The rubber cap covering the operating channel must be removed prior to inserting the needle system. Once the needle is fully inserted into the echoendoscope, the base of the needle should be Luer-locked to the operating channel (Figure 21-1).

In some cases, a lesion that is clearly visible before the needle deployment may become difficult to see once the needle assembly is in place. The needle/sheath may produce an artifact or may slightly reduce complete coupling between the ultrasound probe and the gut wall, producing an air artifact. Slight repositioning of the echoendoscope, application of suction, or reinsertion of the needle assembly may help correct the problem.

Position the Lesion in the Needle Path

Optimal positioning of the echoendoscope with respect to the lesion should make EUS FNA easier, safer, and more effective. The needle sheath should be adjusted so that it protrudes just beyond the elevator. Most commercially available needles are manufactured with a sheath length adjuster. This device is located near the bottom of the needle shaft and allows the endosonographer to determine the proper length of sheath to exit the echoendoscope into the gut lumen (see Figure 21-1). In order to minimize ultrasound artifacts caused by the shaft and to maximize elevator deflection capabilities, the needle

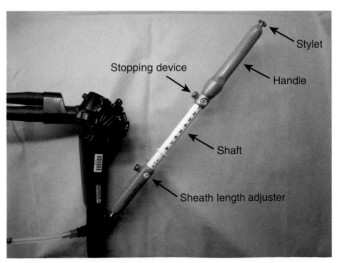

FIGURE 21-1   The needle system is firmly Luer-locked to the operating channel of the echoendoscope.

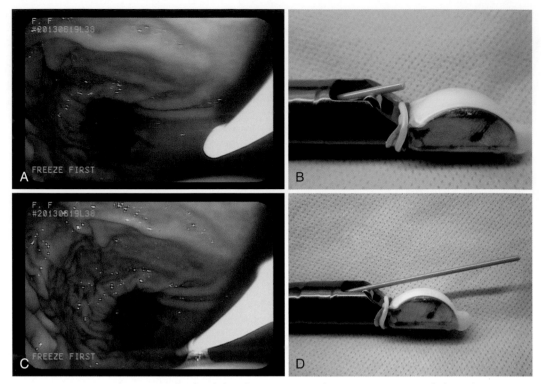

FIGURE 21-2 Adjusting needle sheath length. **A,B,** Correct distance. **C,D,** Excessively long distance.

sheath should be kept at a short distance from the operating channel exit. However, to avoid traumatizing the inner lining of the operating channel during needle deployment, one must be certain that the needle sheath terminates outside the operating channel (Figure 21-2).

After needle sheath adjustment is performed, the screw must be tightly wound to avoid inadvertently advancing the sheath during needle thrusting, which could result in gut wall trauma. Needle sheath adjustment is usually performed when the needle is first used and rarely requires further manipulation during the subsequent passes.

Once the lesion is identified, it should be positioned as much as possible within the natural path of the needle (i.e., the path taken by the needle when no elevator is applied) (Figure 21-3). This varies depending on the instrument used. If this is not possible, it should be positioned within the range of deflection offered by the elevator (Figure 21-4). The

elevator can be used to *increase* the angle formed between the echoendoscope shaft and the needle. It cannot *reduce* this angle (Figure 21-5). Once adequate elevator adjustment is attained, it is best to lock the up-down control so that the thumb can then be used to move the elevator if needed.

A stopping device locks the needle inside the sheath, avoiding accidental injury or scope trauma during manipulation and insertion of the needle into the echoendoscope. Prior to puncturing the lesion, the stopping device must be unscrewed to allow needle deployment. The stopping device can be set so as to limit the maximum distance that the needle can travel (Figure 21-6). This can be helpful in situations where inserting the needle beyond the limits of the target lesion would be dangerous (e.g., the target lies directly over a vascular structure). Once the target lesion is in position on the screen, the caliper function can be used to measure the distance between the ultrasound probe and the desired

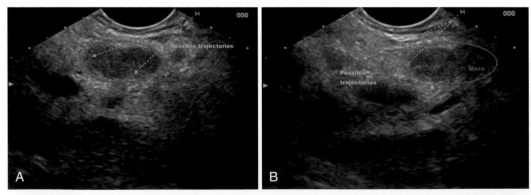

FIGURE 21-3 Correct positioning of a peri-gastric lymph node prior to FNA. **A,** The lesion is within the natural path of the needle and elevator path. **B,** Incorrect positioning.

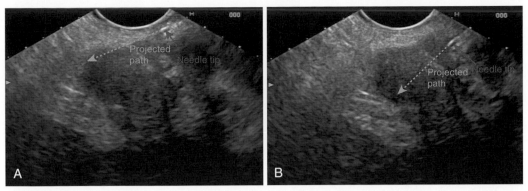

FIGURE 21-4 Using the elevator to provide adequate needle trajectory. **A,** The needle is in its natural state with the elevator in neutral position, resulting in inadequate positioning. **B,** Elevator use deflects the needle trajectory into a correct path.

area to sample. The stopping device can then be set to this distance.

To ensure maximum control, the fixed component of the needle handle should be grasped between the palm and the last two or three fingers of the right hand. The movable portion should be held between the thumb and index finger. This allows fine or vigorous needle movements to be performed, but with control. Any method that does not allow such control should be avoided (Figure 21-7).

As discussed earlier, movement of the FNA needle is easier if it is straight. Any bend in the needle induced by excessively tipping up and/or torquing the echoendoscope, or by applying pressure with the elevator, will increase resistance during needle deployment, and may cause the needle to bend in an axis that will make it disappear from the ultrasound field of view. This situation is encountered most often when the EUS probe is placed in the duodenal bulb or the second duodenum.

In order to minimize risks of puncturing other vital structures, one should try to limit the distance the needle must travel to reach the target. Undrained, obstructed ducts should not be punctured because this may provoke cholangitis or pancreatitis.

Should a structure such as a bile duct or blood vessel be punctured, it is logical to assume that the risk of leakage is lower if the needle enters perpendicular to the vessel/duct as opposed to passing tangentially and causing a linear laceration. Therefore contact with all vessels should be avoided, but particularly when passing the needle laterally to a vessel.

Scanning the FNA path with power Doppler prior to needle insertion is a good way to exclude any unsuspected significant blood vessels in the targeted path.

Puncture the Lesion and Move the Needle within the Lesion

Once the needle assembly and lesion are in adequate position, tissue sampling may begin. The needle should always be seen under real-time ultrasound guidance during tissue sampling to avoid traumatizing other structures. The goal is to insert the needle into the lesion, making repetitive back-and-forth thrusting movements into the lesion to shear off cells and collect them within the needle lumen. This requires that the needle be kept in the ultrasound-imaging plane and that thrusting movements be deliberate, always keeping an eye on the distal tip of the needle. Care should be taken to ensure that the needle does not exit the confines of the lesion during sampling. This will avoid contamination of the specimen with unwanted surrounding tissues.

Once the lesion is ready for puncture, sweeping the projected needle path with power Doppler to detect blood vessels can be performed. Before beginning to advance the needle, firm upward tip deflection should be applied using the up-down dial. This tends to bring the lesion closer to the echoendoscope and to reduce the tendency of the needle to push the ultrasound probe away from the gut wall, which can reduce the ultrasound image quality by allowing air to seep in between the probe and the gut wall. It also provides a

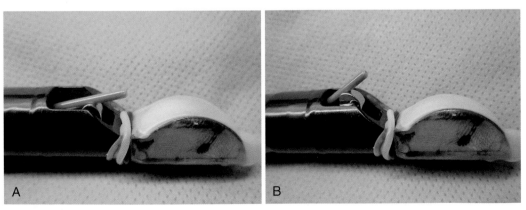

FIGURE 21-5 Elevator range of movement. **A,** No elevator use. **B,** Maximal deflection of elevator.

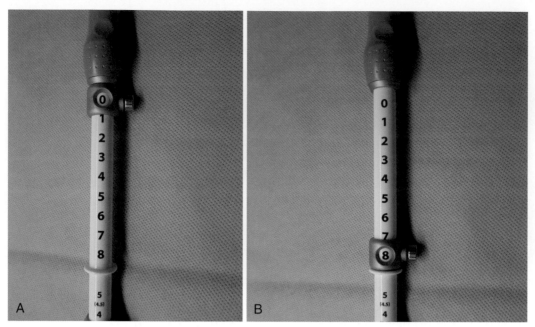

FIGURE 21-6   Stopper adjustment. **A,** Stopper on. **B,** Stopper off.

mechanical advantage when trying to puncture an indurated lesion. Firm upward tip deflection also increases tension on the gut wall, thereby facilitating the puncture of mobile and thick walls such as the stomach body.

The needle should first be advanced approximately 1 cm out of the sheath, just enough to localize the tip in the ultrasound field. Once the tip has been identified, the elevator can

be used to adjust the needle trajectory if needed. The needle can then be advanced into the lesion under ultrasound guidance.

If, for some reason, the needle tip can no longer be seen once the lesion has been punctured, all forward movement of the needle should be stopped. Continuing to advance the needle in the hope that the tip will become visible is a mistake

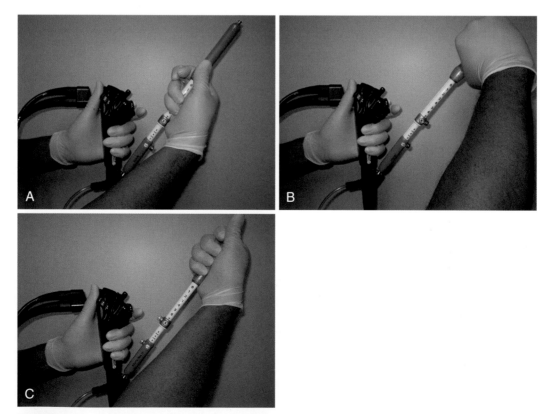

FIGURE 21-7   Holding the needle. **A,** Correct positioning. **B,** Incorrect method. **C,** Another incorrect method.

Video 21-1. Video demonstrating the fanning technique of FNA.

Video 21-2. Video demonstrating the multiple pass technique of FNA.

and can result in inadvertent puncture of structures deep or lateral to the target lesion. Instead, the first reflex should be to slowly withdraw the needle. This will help localize the tip without risking puncture of deep structures. If this is ineffective, slow left and right movement of the shoulders can help bring the needle into the ultrasound-imaging plane.

If both these techniques fail, the needle should be withdrawn completely from the lesion into the sheath. If it is possible that the scope position could have caused the needle to bend, the needle assembly should be removed from the echoendoscope and the needle straightened if needed (see later in the chapter). The puncture can then be attempted again. This situation may be frequently encountered when the scope is torqued, especially in the duodenal bulb or sweep.

Once the needle is in the lesion and the tip clearly seen, the needle is moved back and forth several times within the lesion, with adequate force to produce cell shearing. Should needle thrusting reduce visibility by separating the transducer from the gut wall, slight forward pressure applied to the echoendoscope shaft will push the probe back against the wall. Constant gut lumen suctioning with the echoendoscope during needle deployment can also reduce any air seepage risk between the probe and gut wall.

If the elevator deflection tip was used to adjust the needle angle, it may be helpful to return the elevator to the relaxed position once the needle is inside the lesion. This will allow the needle to move more freely.

Sampling Different Areas of the Same Lesion: "Fanning" or "Multiple Pass" Techniques

In order to gather as much material as possible, several areas within the lesion should be sampled before processing it on the slide.[14]

To sample different areas of the same lesion during the same pass, a "fanning" technique may be possible if the lesion is sufficiently soft (Video 21-1). Fanning is obtained by manipulation of the elevator and/or up-down tip deflection to guide the needle into different regions of the target lesion or to orient the needle into the long axis of an oval or oblong lesion—without withdrawing the needle from the lesion.[15]

However, if the lesion is too hard, adequate fanning may be impossible. In this case, the "multiple pass" technique may be used (Video 21-2). This involves sampling widely through the lesion many times, before removing the needle from the scope. The needle is moved through the entire diameter of the lesion for 5 to 10 strokes, and then the needle is withdrawn from the lesion and moved to a different region of the lesion. Approximately five regions per lesion are sampled before processing the sample. The multi-pass technique differs from the "fanning" technique in that the latter involves trying to sample different regions without removing the needle completely from the lesion[16] (Figure 21-8).

Withdraw the Needle and Process the Aspirate

After completing a pass, the needle should be completely withdrawn into the sheath. The locking device should be returned to its original upmost position and secured with the screw. In order to confirm complete needle withdrawal, the "0" numeral should be clearly seen within the locking device (see Figure 21-6A)

To avoid clotting in the needle, the aspirate should be expressed from the needle as quickly as possible. The authors expel all samples onto a glass slide using a 10-mL air-filled syringe. The sample is then smeared using a second slide. This

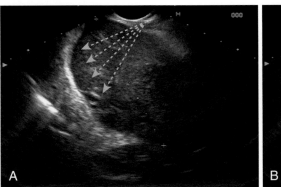
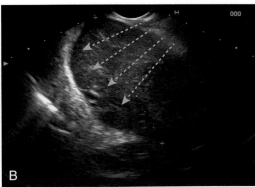

FIGURE 21-8 FNA sampling of multiple sites. **A,** The fanning technique. **B,** The multiple pass technique.

produces two slides per pass. If a cell block is required, a different sample is expelled with an air-filled syringe into a receptacle containing 20 mL of 50% alcohol.

If the needle is blocked, the aspirate can be forced out by inserting the stylet. Once the clot has been expressed onto a slide or container, the syringe should be used to express any remaining material from the needle.

Prepare the Needle for Subsequent Passes

The same needle can be used for several passes and need not be changed unless it malfunctions or the needle tip becomes too dull. If previous aspirates were bloody, it may be helpful to rinse the lumen with normal saline before the next pass.

If the needle is bent, it must be straightened; otherwise it will deflect out of the ultrasound beam on subsequent passes. To straighten the needle, push it completely out of the sheath, then use your fingers to straighten it manually (Figure 21-9). An alcohol swab can then be used to clean the outer surface of the needle.

If a cytologist is available, passes should be performed until he or she makes a diagnosis or determines that adequate material is obtained. If not, the available data suggest that approximately three to five passes should be sufficient to obtain a diagnosis (if cancer is indeed present).[17–21] There is no absolute limit to the number of passes that can be performed with the same needle. However, it should be changed if it malfunctions or it becomes too difficult to re-insert the stylet.

Evolving Trends in EUS FNA

Use of the Stylet

All commercially available EUS FNA systems include a removable stylet. It was believed that the stylet helps prevent clogging of the needle by gut wall tissue, which could limit the ability to aspirate cells from the target lesion. This is a logical assumption, but there are no data clearly demonstrating that the use of a stylet increases the yield of EUS FNA. Manipulation of the stylet increases the time and energy required to perform EUS FNA, increases the risks of needle stick injury, and likely increases the costs of EUS FNA needle systems. In some circumstances, the stylet may actually make EUS FNA impossible. For example, it may be impossible to advance or

to remove the stylet once the target has been punctured. This tends to occur only if the echoendoscope is bent (particularly when sampling from the bulb or duodenal sweep) and a large (19-G) needle is being used.

Three randomized trials and several retrospective series are now available comparing the results of EUS FNA with and without the stylet. There is universal agreement that the stylet adds no value to EUS FNA.[22–24] EUS FNA without the stylet is also technically much simpler and faster because the stylet withdrawal and reinsertion maneuvers are eliminated. Therefore it is currently recommended to *not* use the stylet for EUS FNA. However, the stylet may be used to expel the aspirate or to unblock the needle if necesary. The stylet may also be useful in certain select indications, such as preventing a mucosal plug when aspirating cyst fluid or delivering fiducial markers in solid lesions. Theoretically, it may also be helpful if a large amount of normal tissue (>2 to 3 cm) must be traversed before reaching the target lesion (e.g., a deep-seated liver mass); however, this remains speculative.

Use of Suction

There is conflicting evidence in the literature concerning the use of suction to obtain adequate material. While some experts recommend the use of suction, others state that it may actually hinder adequate cytologic analysis by causing aspirates to become diluted with blood. Two randomized trials showed that using suction when performing FNA of lymph nodes and pancreatic masses did not improve the diagnostic yield of the FNA.[19,25] It may be reasonable to initially perform FNA without suction. However, if in-room cytologic analysis of aspirates shows inadequate cellularity, it may be helpful to apply 5 to 10 mL of suction for a few seconds immediately before withdrawing the needle from the lesion or to use continuous suction (however, this remains unproven).

Traditionally, suction is applied with an empty syringe. More recently, methods involving application of suction using a water-filled syringe ("wet technique" or "liquid stylet") or slow withdrawal of the stylet ("slow pull" technique) have gained some notoriety. However, there are currently no published comparative data to support their use.

FNA Particularities According to Site

The site in the gut from which EUS FNA is performed may make the technique easier or more difficult. The following

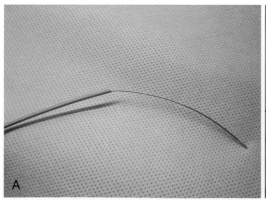
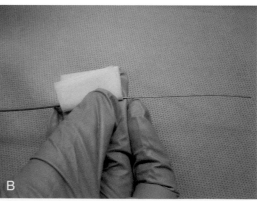

FIGURE 21-9 Straightening the needle. **A,** Bent needle. **B,** Straightening the needle.

describes common pitfalls and solutions based on the EUS FNA site.

Esophagus

This region is commonly the easiest area from which to perform EUS FNA. Most lesions accessed through this site are mediastinal lymph nodes or masses. The echoendoscope is virtually always in a straight position, and the tubular anatomy of the esophagus will naturally prevent the scope from bending.

Stomach

The stomach probably has the thickest wall of all the sites from which EUS FNA is commonly performed. It is also very compliant, meaning that it will tend to recoil during needle advancement. This can make traversing the gastric wall difficult and targeting perigastric lesions problematic, particularly if they are small and/or mobile (e.g., gastrohepatic ligament lymph nodes). If this problem arises, it may be helpful to divide the EUS FNA maneuver into two stages. First, focus on traversing the gastric wall. To facilitate wall puncture, collapse the stomach by sucking out the air. The wall will be more stable if the echoendoscope is withdrawn into position (from the antrum), rather than if it is pushed into position from the region of the gastroesophageal junction. A strong tip up maneuver will also help hold the echoendoscope close to the wall. Successful gastric puncture may require an unusually quick, strong, yet controlled jab. If present, the safety stopper on the needle may be used to prevent inadvertently advancing the needle too far. Once the needle has successfully been passed through the gastric wall into the perigastric space, attention should be focused on the second stage—puncturing the target lesion.

Duodenal Bulb

When positioning the echoendoscope in the duodenal bulb, it naturally assumes a "long-scope" position. Whereas this position may offer a mechanical advantage to more forcefully puncture an indurated lesion, the bending in the scope may render needle insertion into the scope difficult. To avoid this situation, the needle should be inserted into the scope while it is still in the stomach antrum. Once the needle is loaded in the scope, the pylorus should be intubated and the needle repositioned in the bulb.

Accessing hilar lesions from the bulb usually requires a large amount of counterclockwise torquing. When excessive torquing is applied, this will create a bend in the needle. As the needle is deployed out of the sheath, it may deflect out of the ultrasound plane and may not be visible. Removing the needle from the scope and correcting any bend should be attempted at this point. If the problem recurs, the needle should be deployed a few millimeters out of the sheath into the gut lumen when facing the lesion. Gentle *counterclockwise* rotation will usually make the needle tip appear. The amount of left rotation needed to identify the needle should be checked, and the needle should be withdrawn back into its sheath. The sheath should be repositioned at the level of the lesion and the rotated away from the lesion by torquing *clockwise*. The needle should be deployed for a few millimeters and counter-rotated *counterclockwise*. If a sufficient amount of "extra" rotation was applied, the needle should be in front of the lesion. Ideally, the needle should be visualized at *all times*

during FNA. It should be remembered that it may be easier to access hilar lesions from the stomach because the echoendoscope will be in a straight configuration, and little torque is needed.

Duodenal Sweep (D2)

Similar difficulties can be encountered when performing FNA from the duodenal sweep. Needle scope insertion can be problematic. To avoid this, the scope should be withdrawn completely into a "short-scope" position while remaining in the sweep. This should remove any bend in the scope and make initial needle insertion easy. One may still encounter some resistance a few centimeters before being able to Luer-lock the needle. Any locks applied to the dials of the echoendoscope should be removed, and a large amount of tip deflection should be generated down using the up-down dial. This should remove any resistance to scope needle insertion. Once properly Luer-locked to the scope shaft, the shaft can be repositioned as necessary into the duodenal sweep. The authors find that this technique can enable needle insertion of any caliber, including the 19-G needle in most situations.

Needle bending can also occur in this location based on the amount of torquing needed to visualize the lesion. The same technique described for duodenal bulb lesions can be applied.

Special Issues
Sampling of Multiple Lesions

When there are several potential biopsy sites or lesions in an individual patient (e.g., pancreatic mass, celiac node, liver lesion, and mediastinal node), sampling should be performed starting with the lesion that, if positive, will confirm the most advanced stage. If the first lesion is negative, the lesion offering the next highest stage should be sampled. If a metastatic lesion is confirmed, the primary lesion need not necessarily be biopsied, unless there is a compelling reason to do so. If the above sequence of biopsy sites is employed (i.e., from distant lesions toward the primary lesion), then several lesions can be sampled using a single EUS FNA needle. If not, a new needle should be used for each lesion, to avoid the risk of creating false-positive results and/or seeding distant sites.

EUS FNA of Cystic Lesions

Cystic lesions may be punctured for cyst fluid analysis, sampling of the cyst wall, and/or treatment. The primary concerns relate to the risk of infection and bleeding. Bleeding is alarming but rarely serious, because it is usually contained by the cyst cavity. Infections, however, can lead to serious morbidity and mortality. Therefore, perhaps more than with other lesions, cysts should not be punctured unless it is clear that the information obtained will likely be useful to someone. Prophylactic antibiotics are indicated prior to FNA of a cystic lesion.[26]

Unless there is clear evidence of a mass component, it is the authors' opinion that sampling of the wall is rarely productive and only increases the risk of bleeding. Likewise, cyst fluid cytology is almost always negative. Therefore, for cysts *without* a significant mass component, the primary goal should be to aspirate sufficient fluid to perform tumor marker analysis. Conversely, if there is a significant mass component, it is reasonable to perform EUS FNA of the mass alone and avoid the risks of cyst puncture. Biochemistry laboratory personnel should be consulted to determine the minimum quantity of cyst fluid that will be required to perform the desired analyses.

For larger diameter lesions (>1 to 2 cm), the authors prefer using a 19-G needle instead of a smaller gauge needle to allow for more rapid and complete cyst fluid aspiration (especially if the fluid is viscous). As indicated earlier, use of the stylet is reasonable in this setting to avoid clogging the needle with a mucosal plug that will hinder aspiration. Once the needle is in the cyst cavity, the stylet can be withdrawn and suction may begin. A *new* needle should always be used to puncture a cyst and, if possible, only one pass should be performed. If more than one pass is required, a new needle should be used.

Many experts believe that the risk of infection is lower if the cyst is drained completely, so this is probably a reasonable goal. However, in the case of a multiloculated cyst, it may be safer to focus on draining only a single, superficial loculation—one that appears to contain sufficient fluid for marker analysis.

Once the cyst has been punctured, an attempt should be made to place the tip in the center of the cavity before aspirating the cyst. During aspiration and as the cyst collapses, the needle should be repositioned as necessary to stay away from the wall or any debris that may clog the needle lumen. If the needle clogs before the cyst has collapsed completely, one may halt suction and try to reposition the needle gently, *without removing it from the cyst.* When the cyst is almost completely collapsed, drainage frequently stops, and it often becomes difficult to locate the needle tip. Attempts to reposition the needle to get "every last drop" should be avoided because this may lead to bleeding. Once adequate fluid has been obtained for analysis, the remaining fluid can be drained by repeatedly filling a syringe or by connecting the aspiration port of the needle to wall suction. After cyst drainage, the cyst should be observed for a short time to look for early recurrence or bleeding.

Mobile Lesions

Lesions that are not fixed, such as retroperitoneal nodes, can be difficult to puncture because they tend to bounce off the needle tip. This situation may be compounded if the lesion is not directly adjacent to the gut wall or is small, or if there is excessive respiratory movement. To effectively puncture these lesions, it may be helpful first to focus on traversing the gut wall with the needle. Once the needle tip is in the extraluminal space, one can then focus on puncturing the lesion.

To puncture the lesion, the needle tip should be advanced so that it is abutting the lesion wall. Coordination with respiratory movement may be required. To enter the lesion, a rapid single thrust should be used to stab the lesion effectively. It may be necessary to actually pass the needle completely through the lesion. If this occurs, the lesion will be immobilized and the needle tip can then be slowly withdrawn until it is within the confines of the lesion.

Indurated Lesions

Occasionally, it may be difficult to penetrate a lesion because it is indurated. If a lesion is difficult to penetrate one must first verify that the needle is functioning correctly. The needle tip may have become dull, for example due to multiple previous passes, or may not be exiting the sheath effectively.

If the needle is functioning properly, the lesion can be punctured by using more forceful stabbing maneuvers. However, this should be a last resort because it is difficult to stab forcefully *and* to simultaneously control the depth of penetration. Instead, firm upward tip deflection should be applied, the needle tip should be placed against the leading edge of the lesion, and firm, progressively increasing pressure should be applied to the needle. If this fails, it may be helpful to apply force by actually advancing the echoendoscope (assuming that the echoendoscope is in a position that ensures that pressure can be applied in the same axis as the needle).

Tumor Seeding

Although very rare, tumor seeding has been described with EUS FNA.[27-32] In the presence of a potentially resectable malignant lesion, EUS FNA should be reconsidered if the biopsy tract will not be included in the surgical specimen (e.g., FNA through the gastric wall in the case of a pancreatic body lesion). Instead, if at all possible, an attempt should be made to perform biopsies through a part of the gut wall that will be removed should the patient go to surgery (e.g., lesions of the pancreatic genu should be biopsied through the duodenum if possible).

To avoid seeding extraluminal sites, such as nodes, EUS FNA should never be performed through an area of the gut wall that is overtly or possibly infiltrated by malignancy or dysplasia.

Conclusion

EUS FNA is a powerful clinical tool. It can be technically challenging but is often straightforward if the lesion can be located, is sufficiently large, and can be brought into the needle path with the echoendoscope in a fairly straight position. Many additions to the basic EUS FNA technique have been described, but none appear to clearly improve the yield other than: (1) moving the needle effectively; (2) sampling many different areas of the lesion; and (3) using a smaller (25-G) needle. The stylet should not be used, because all the data show that it does not improve results but increases procedural complexity. There is also no clear evidence that suction of any type or newer needle designs improve outcomes. Quality comparative trials will be required before modifications to the basic FNA technique that have been described in this chapter can be recommended.

REFERENCES

1. Dumonceau JM, Polkowski M, Larghi A, et al. Indications, results, and clinical impact of endoscopic ultrasound (EUS)-guided sampling in gastroenterology: European Society of Gastrointestinal Endoscopy (ESGE) Clinical Guideline. *Endoscopy*. 2011;43:1-16.
2. ASGE Standards of Practice Committee, Anderson MA, Ben-Menachem T, et al. Management of antithrombotic agents for endoscopic procedures. *Gastrointest Endosc*. 2009;70(6):1060-1070.
3. Lee JK, Lee KT, Choi ER, et al. A prospective, randomized trial comparing 25-gauge and 22-gauge needles for endoscopic ultrasound-guided fine needle aspiration of pancreatic masses. *Scand J Gastroenterol*. 2013;48(6):752-757.
4. Affolter KE, Schmidt RL, Matynia AP, et al. Needle size has only a limited effect on outcomes in EUS-guided fine needle aspiration: a systematic review and meta-analysis. *Dig Dis Sci*. 2013;58(4):1026-1034.

5. Camellini L, Carlinfante G, Azzolini F, et al. A randomized clinical trial comparing 22G and 25G needles in endoscopic ultrasound-guided fine-needle aspiration of solid lesions. *Endoscopy*. 2011;43:709-715.

6. Fabbri C, Polifemo AM, Luigiano C, et al. Endoscopic ultrasound-guided fine needle aspiration with 22- and 25-gauge needles in solid pancreatic masses: a prospective comparative study with randomisation of needle sequence. *Dig Liver Dis*. 2011;43:647-652.

7. Siddiqui UD, Rossi F, Rosenthal LS, et al. EUS-guided FNA of solid pancreatic masses: A prospective, randomized trial comparing 22-gauge and 25-gauge needles. *Gastrointest Endosc*. 2009;70:1093-1097.

8. Madhoun MF, Wani SB, Rastogi A, et al. The diagnostic accuracy of 22-gauge and 25-gauge needles in endoscopic ultrasound-guided fine needle aspiration of solid pancreatic lesions: A meta-analysis. *Endoscopy*. 2013;45:86-92.

9. Yusuf TE, Ho S, Pavey DA, et al. Retrospective analysis of the utility of endoscopic ultrasound-guided fine-needle aspiration (EUS-FNA) in pancreatic masses, using a 22-gauge or 25-gauge needle system: a multicenter experience. *Endoscopy*. 2009;41(5):445-448.

10. Nguyen TT, Lee CE, Whang CS, et al. A comparison of the diagnostic yield and specimen adequacy between 22 and 25 gauge needles for endoscopic ultrasound guided fine-needle aspiration (EUS-FNA) of solid pancreatic lesions (SPL): is bigger better? *Gastrointest Endosc*. 2008; 67(5):AB100.

11. Lee JH, Stewart J, Ross WA, et al. Blinded prospective comparison of the performance of 22-gauge and 25-gauge needles in endoscopic ultrasound-guided fine needle aspiration of the pancreas and peri-pancreatic lesions. *Dig Dis Sci*. 2009;54(10):2274-2281.

12. Paquin SC, Gariepy G, Sahai AV. A Prospective, randomized, controlled trial of EUS-FNA with and without a stylet: no stylet is better. *Gastrointest Endosc*. 2007;65(5):AB198.

13. Bang JY, Hebert-Magee S, Trevino J, et al. Randomized trial comparing the 22-gauge aspiration and 22-gauge biopsy needles for EUS-guided sampling of solid pancreatic mass lesions. *Gastrointest Endosc*. 2012; 76(2):321-327.

14. Varadarajulu S, Fockens P, Hawes RH. Best practices in endoscopic ultrasound-guided fine-needle aspiration. *Clin Gastroenterol Hepatol*. 2012;10(7):697-703.

15. Bang JY, Magee SH, Ramesh J, et al. Randomized trial comparing fanning with standard technique for endoscopic ultrasound-guided fine-needle aspiration of solid pancreatic mass lesions. *Endoscopy*. 2013;45(6): 445-450.

16. Wyse JM, Paquin SC, Joseph L, et al. EUS-FNA without the stylet: the yield is comparable to that with the stylet and sampling of multiple sites during the same pass may improve sample quality and yield. *Gastrointest Endosc*. 2009;69(5):AB330-AB331.

17. Rong L, Kida M, Yamauchi H, et al. Factors affecting the diagnostic accuracy of endoscopic ultrasonography-guided fine-needle aspiration (EUS-FNA) for upper gastrointestinal submucosal or extraluminal solid mass lesions. *Dig Endosc*. 2012;24(5):358-363.

18. Suzuki R, Irisawa A, Bhutani MS, et al. Prospective evaluation of the optimal number of 25-gauge needle passes for endoscopic ultrasound-guided fine-needle aspiration biopsy of solid pancreatic lesions in the absence of an onsite cytopathologist. *Dig Endosc*. 2012;24(6):452-456.

19. Wallace MB, Kennedy T, Durkalski V, et al. Randomized controlled trial of EUS-guided fine needle aspiration techniques for the detection of malignant lymphadenopathy. *Gastrointest Endosc*. 2001;54(4):441-447.

20. LeBlanc JK, Ciaccia D, Al-Assi MT, et al. Optimal number of EUS-guided fine needle passes needed to obtain a correct diagnosis. *Gastrointest Endosc*. 2004;59(4):475-481.

21. Savides TJ. Tricks for improving EUS-FNA accuracy and maximizing cellular yield. *Gastrointest Endosc*. 2009;69(suppl 2):S130-S133.

22. Sahai AV, Paquin SC, Gariépy G. A prospective comparison of endoscopic ultrasound-guided fine needle aspiration results obtained in the same lesion, with and without the needle stylet. *Endoscopy*. 2010;42: 900-903.

23. Rastogi A, Wani S, Gupta N, et al. A prospective, single-blind, randomized, controlled trial of EUS-guided FNA with and without a stylet. *Gastrointest Endosc*. 2011;74:58-64.

24. Wani S, Gupta N, Gaddam S, et al. A comparative study of endoscopic ultrasound guided fine needle aspiration with and without a stylet. *Dig Dis Sci*. 2011;56:2409-2414.

25. Puri R, Vilmann P, Săftoiu A, et al. Randomized controlled trial of endoscopic ultrasound-guided fine-needle sampling with or without suction for better cytological diagnosis. *Scand J Gastroenterol*. 2009;44(4): 499-504.

26. ASGE Guideline. Antibiotic prophylaxis for GI endoscopy. *Gastrointest Endosc*. 2008;67:791-798.

27. Hirooka Y, Goto H, Itoh A, et al. Case of intraductal papillary mucinous tumor in which endosonography-guided fine-needle aspiration biopsy caused dissemination (letter). *J Gastroenterol Hepatol*. 2003;18: 1323-1324.

28. Shah JN, Fraker D, Guerry D, et al. Melanoma seeding of an EUS-guided fine needle track. *Gastrointest Endosc*. 2004;59:923-924.

29. Paquin SC, Gariépy G, Lepanto L, et al. A first report of tumor seeding because of EUS-guided FNA of a pancreatic adenocarcinoma. *Gastrointest Endosc*. 2005;61(4):610-611.

30. Doi S, Yasuda I, Iwashita T, et al. Needle tract implantation on the esophageal wall after EUS-guided FNA of metastatic mediastinal lymphadenopathy. *Gastrointest Endosc*. 2008;67(6):988-990.

31. Chong A, Venugopal K, Segarajasingam D, et al. Tumor seeding after EUS-guided FNA of pancreatic tail neoplasia. *Gastrointest Endosc*. 2011;74(4):933-935.

32. Katanuma A, Maguchi H, Hashigo S, et al. Tumor seeding after endoscopic ultrasound-guided fine-needle aspiration of cancer in the body of the pancreas. *Endoscopy*. 2012;44(suppl 2 UCTN):E160-E161.

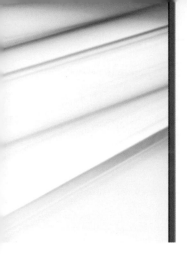

22

How to Perform EUS-Guided Fine-Needle Biopsy

Nikola Panić • Alberto Larghi

Key Points

- Although EUS FNA is very accurate, it cannot fully characterize certain neoplasms, and lack of cytology expertise may result in a limited perceived utility of EUS.
- EUS TCB does not offer any clear advantage as compared to EUS FNA and is technically very demanding with a low transduodenal yield.
- Standard 19-G and 22-G FNA needles with or without high negative pressure have proven to be reliable in obtaining high-quality histologic samples for various indications. Because most data are from single-center experiences, multicenter studies to demonstrate reproducibility of the results are warranted.
- The novel 19-G and 22-G ProCore needles have demonstrated a high yield and reproducibility in obtaining histologic samples in multicenter studies, whereas the 25-G ProCore appears unsuitable for histology.
- EUS FNB is expected to refine differential diagnostic capabilities, favor widespread EUS utilization, and enable targeted therapies and monitoring of treatment response.

Since its initial description in 1992,[1] endoscopic ultrasound-guided fine-needle aspiration (EUS FNA) has become an increasingly important tool to achieve a definitive diagnosis and proper staging of lesions of the gastrointestinal (GI) tract and of adjacent organs.[2] The diagnostic accuracy of EUS FNA ranges from 60% to 90% depending on the site of investigation,[3] and it is particularly low for neoplasms such as stromal tumors, lymphomas, and well-differentiated adenocarcinomas that are difficult to diagnose by cytology alone.[4-6] In addition, the accuracy of EUS FNA relies on the assessment of the adequacy of the collected specimens by an on-site cytopathologist,[7-9] which requires a high degree of expertise and is not available in many centers.[10] This has created a barrier to the dissemination of EUS in the community and in many countries limits the overall utility of EUS because the lack of cytology expertise results in low diagnostic accuracy.[11,12]

The procurement of a specimen for histologic examination may overcome this main limitation of EUS FNA. A tissue core biopsy with preserved architecture is critical to diagnose and fully characterize certain neoplasms, such as lymphomas and GI stromal tumors. Moreover, tissue specimens for histologic examination also provide the opportunity to: (1) easily immunostain the tissue, further increasing differential diagnostic capabilities; (2) reach a specific diagnosis for benign diseases not always obtainable with a cytologic sample, thus sparing patients from more invasive and risky sampling procedures or costly and unnecessary follow-up examinations; and (3) potentially perform tissue profiling and/or cell culture needed

to guide targeted therapies for individualized treatment of patients with cancer of the GI tract.[13-15]

The ability to obtain fragments of tissue for histologic examination with FNA needles of various diameters was tested,[16-18] and a Tru-Cut biopsy needle dedicated for EUS-guided fine-needle biopsy (EUS FNB), the Quick-Core needle, was developed. However, the technique had no meaningful advantages over EUS FNA.[19-22] More recently, a new technique called EUS fine-needle tissue acquisition (EUS FNTA) using standard 22-G and 19-G needles has been developed and evaluated in a few studies.[23-25] New needles, the ProCore needles, have been specifically designed to obtain histologic samples. These needles are now being tested in clinical practice.[26-29] These new techniques and needles, coupled with refinements in specimen processing, should change the practice of EUS from cytology to histology, thereby facilitating the expansion of EUS utilization throughout the world.

This chapter will present the techniques developed so far to perform EUS FNB, their clinical results and limitations, and their future perspective.

EUS-Guided Tru-Cut Biopsy (EUS TCB)

Background

Large-caliber cutting needles to acquire tissue core biopsy specimens for histologic examination have been used via the percutaneous (under conventional ultrasound [US] or computed tomography [CT] guidance), intraluminal (transanal, transrectal, transvaginal, transjugular), and surgical (laparoscopic, open) routes.[30–32] Based on these experiences, it seemed reasonable to translate this technology to develop a needle able to perform Tru-Cut biopsy under EUS guidance. In 2002, the first case report using the Quick-Core needle (Cook Medical Inc., Bloomington, IN, US), a 19-G needle capable of collecting an 18-mm tissue specimen sufficient for histologic examination, was published.[33] The study was conducted in swine models, reporting the safety and feasibility of EUS TCB using the Quick-Core needle that enabled histologic sampling from the liver, spleen, left kidney, and body of the pancreas through a transgastric approach.[33] A few months later, the same group reported the results of the first study in humans, where 19 patients with intestinal and extraintestinal lesions were evaluated.[22] Patients underwent both EUS TCB and EUS FNA. Overall, EUS TCB was found to be more accurate than EUS FNA (85% versus 60%), with a significantly reduced number of needle passes for establishing diagnosis (mean 2 versus 3.3, respectively; $p < 0.05$). No complications were encountered.

Since then a number of studies have examined the feasibility and safety of EUS TCB, as well as comparing its performance with other EUS-guided sampling techniques.[19–22,34–51]

Design and Technique

The EUS TCB device has a spring-loaded mechanism built into the handle of the needle, making automated acquisition of biopsy specimens possible (Figure 22-1). The handle also contains a screw-stop lock that allows advancement up to 8 cm and an adjustment wheel, which rotates the device to orient into the proper position. The nonhandle portion consists of an outer catheter sheath, an internal 19-G cutting sheath, an 18-mm-long specimen tray, and a 5-mm-long stylet tip (Figure 22-2). Before insertion in the working channel of the echoendoscope, the needle should be prepared in the "firing position" by retraction of the handle that causes withdrawal of both the cutting sheath and the specimen tray (Figure 22-3). The needle is then advanced until the tip is nearly flush with the catheter sheath (Figure 22-4). After this preparation, the device is introduced in the working channel of the echoendoscope and screwed securely into the biopsy channel Luer-lock adapter. In order to improve sampling collection, the device needs to be oriented by rotating the needle so that the 19-G marker on the handle is aligned with the model number on the echoendoscope. In this position, the specimen tray directly faces the transducer. Once the target lesion has been placed in the proper position, the needle is

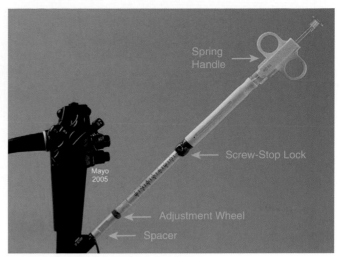

FIGURE 22-1 Tru-Cut needle affixed to a linear echoendoscope demarcating the individual components of the handle portion of the device, including the following: spring-loaded mechanism built into the handle, which permits automated collection of a biopsy specimen; a "screw-stop lock," which when unlocked allows advancement of the needle up to 8 cm and protects against inadvertent advancement; an "adjustment wheel," which rotates the device into the proper orientation; and a "spacer," which may be used, depending on the length of the linear echoendoscope by the manufacturer. *(Adapted with permission from Levy MJ, Wiersema MJ. EUS-guided Trucut biopsy. Gastrointest Endosc. 2005;62:417-426.)*

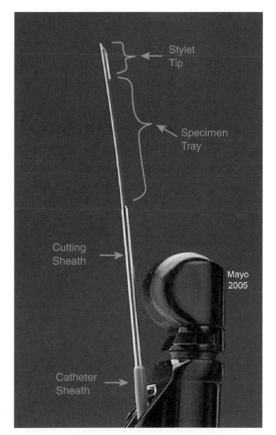

FIGURE 22-2 Nonhandle portion of the Tru-Cut needle demonstrating the following: outer "catheter sheath," an internal 19-G "cutting sheath" that shaves off the tissue specimen; an 18-mm-long "specimen tray," which contains the tissue core; and a 5-mm-long "stylet tip." *(Adapted with permission from Levy MJ, Wiersema MJ. EUS-guided Trucut biopsy. Gastrointest Endosc. 2005;62:417-426.)*

Video 22-1. Technique of EUS-guided Tru-Cut biopsy.

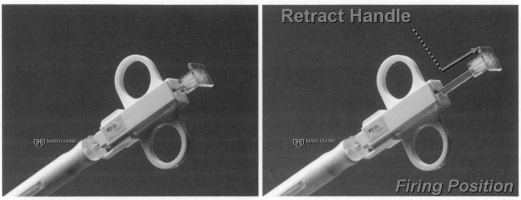

FIGURE 22-3 Tru-Cut needle handle, which uses a spring-loaded firing mechanism for activating the cutting sheath. Retraction of the handle readies the device in the "firing" position. *(Adapted with permission from Levy MJ, Wiersema MJ. EUS-guided Trucut biopsy. Gastrointest Endosc. 2005;62:417-426.)*

advanced under real-time EUS guidance with all controls of the endoscope, including the elevator, released. The spring handle is then pressed forward, resulting in the advancement of the specimen tray into the target lesion that is done under continuous EUS monitoring. After at least 30 seconds, further pressure is applied on the spring handle that fires the device and obtains a biopsy specimen. Once the procedure is completed, the screw-stop is locked and the needle removed from the echoendoscope.

Results

Table 22-1 summarizes the results of the published studies that have evaluated the performance of EUS TCB in patients with various indications. Following the initial study by Levy and colleagues[22] who evaluated a small group of patients with

intestinal and extraintestinal lesions and reported that transgastric EUS TCB was more accurate and required fewer passes than transgastric FNA, Larghi and colleagues[34] reported their experience in a cohort of patients with pancreatic solid masses. They were able to collect pancreatic tissue samples in 74% of the patients, with a diagnostic accuracy of 87%. Interestingly, they showed a high rate of failures (40%) when the procedure was performed through the duodenum, thus reflecting the difficulty in using the device with the scope in a bent position. Similar failure rates for transduodenal puncture of pancreatic masses have been reported by Itoi and colleagues,[35] and Sakamoto and colleagues reported a lower failure rate of 17%.[40]

Subsequently, various studies have been published, most of which involved small patient populations and will not be reviewed in detail in this chapter (see Table 22-1). Three studies, including a meaningful number of patients, are

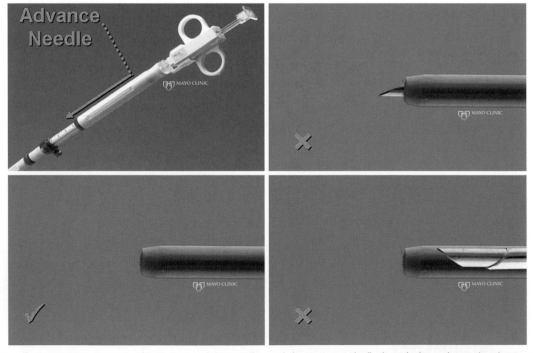

FIGURE 22-4 Needle preparation requires advancement of the needle until the tip is nearly flush with the catheter sheath. Overadvancement of the needle tip exposes the sharp stylet tip, risking damage to the echoendoscope accessory channel. Failure to advance the needle tip far enough may result in inadvertent puncture of catheter and echoendoscope. *(Adapted with permission from Levy MJ, Wiersema MJ. EUS-guided Trucut biopsy. Gastrointest Endosc. 2005;62:417-426.)*

TABLE 22-1

STUDIES EVALUATING THE PERFORMANCE OF THE QUICK-CORE NEEDLE FOR EUS-GUIDED TRU-CUT BIOPSY (EUS TCB)

Author (year)	No. of Patients	Patient Population	EUS TCB Yield (%)	EUS TCB Accuracy (%)	EUS FNA Accuracy (%)	Yield of Transduodenal Biopsy
Levy et al[22] (2003)	19	Intestinal and extraintestinal lesions	NA	85	60	NA
Larghi et al[34] (2004)	23	Pancreatic masses	74	61	NA	40
Varadarajulu et al[19] (2004)	18	Abdominal and mediastinal lesions	89	78	89	NR
Itoi et al[35] (2005)	16	Pancreatic masses	69	NR	NA	40
Storch et al[36] (2006)	41	Abdominal and mediastinal lesions	NR	76	76	NA
Wittmann et al[37] (2006)	96	Abdominal and mediastinal lesions	88	73	77	NR
Aithal et al[38] (2007)[a]	167	Abdominal and extra-abdominal masses	89	89	82	NR
Saftoiu et al[39] (2007)	30	Abdominal and mediastinal lesions	89	68	73	NA
Sakamoto et al[40] (2008)[b]	24	Pancreatic masses	50	54	92	17
Shah et al[20] (2008)	51	Pancreatic masses	86	52	89	NR
Storch et al[41] (2008)	48	Lymph nodes, lung masses, esophageal wall masses	94	79	79	NA
Berger et al[42] (2009)	70	Mediastinal lesions	94	90	93	NA
DeWitt et al[43] (2009)	21	Suspected hepatic parenchymal disease	100	90	NA	NA
Mizuno et al[44] (2009)	14	Suspected autoimmune pancreatitis	100	76	88	NR
Polkowski et al[45] (2009)	49	Gastric subepithelial lesions	63	89	NA	NA
Thomas et al[21] (2009)	247	Masses in pancreas, esophagogastric wall and extrapancreatic lesions	87	75	NA	NR[c]
Wahnschaffe et al[46] (2009)	24	Abdominal and extra-abdominal lesions	83	95	NA	NA
DeWitt et al[47] (2010)	38	Suspected upper gastrointestinal or rectal gastrointestinal mesenchymal tumors	97	79	76	NA
Ribeiro et al[48] (2010)	24	Suspected lymphomas	100	73[d]	0[d]	NA
Lee et al[49] (2011)	65	Gastric subepithelial lesions	57	NP	NP	NA
Mohamadneja et al[50] (2011)	6	Extramural pelvic masses	83	80	NR	NA
Cho[51] (2013)	27	Mediastinal lesions	NR	67	78	NA

FNA, fine-needle aspiration; NA, not applicable; NR, not reported.

[a]Patients with lesions that needed a transduodenal approach were included only when the lesion could be approached with the scope in a relatively straight position.

[b]FNA accuracy using 25-G needle.

[c]Site of biopsy (stomach versus duodenum versus esophagus) was identified as predictor of positive diagnostic yield.

[d]Accuracy for diagnosis and subclassification of lymphomas.

available that evaluated the use of both EUS TCB and EUS FNA with different sampling strategies.[37,38,42] Wittmann and colleagues[37] evaluated 159 patients with a variety of solid lesions (83 pancreatic, 76 nonpancreatic) who underwent EUS FNA alone (maximum four passes) in cases of lesions less than 2 cm in diameter and EUS FNA followed by EUS TCB (maximum three passes) for lesions with a diameter greater than 2 cm. A trend toward an increased number of adequate samples with the combination of both techniques versus EUS FNA alone was found ($p = 0.056$), which was statistically significant if only nonpancreatic sites were considered ($p = 0.044$). No major complications for EUS TCB were reported. The overall accuracy for FNA, TCB, and FNA

plus TCB was 77%, 73%, and 91%, respectively. The combination of both sampling modalities versus EUS FNA alone resulted in a significant improvement in accuracy ($p = 0.008$), which was mainly due to the additional value of EUS TCB in sampling nonpancreatic sites (EUS FNA alone was 78%, EUS TCB alone 83%, and EUS FNA/TCB 95%, $p = 0.006$). These findings prompted the authors to conclude that the combination of EUS FNA/TCB can improve adequacy of sampling and diagnostic accuracy for lesions greater than 2 cm compared with either technique alone.[37]

Subsequently, Aithal and colleagues[38] compared the efficacy of a strategy of "dual sampling" (performing both FNA and TCB in 95 patients) with a strategy of "sequential sampling" (performing FNA only when TCB samples were macroscopically inadequate in 72 patients) in 167 patients with solid lesions. In 86% of the cases the sampling procedure was performed through the esophagus or the stomach. The results of the dual sampling strategy revealed that the combined accuracy of EUS FNA and EUS TCB was significantly higher than that of FNA alone (92.6% versus 82.1%, $p = 0.048$), but not that of TCB alone (92.6% versus 89.5%, $p = 0.61$). Using the sequential sampling strategy, an accurate diagnosis was achieved in 92% of the patients, a rate very similar to the 93% observed with the dual sampling strategy, suggesting that the former strategy could save the use of an additional needle, and thereby costs, in a substantial proportion of patients.[38] Of note, one patient with mediastinal tuberculosis developed a cold abscess after EUS TCB.

Finally, Berger and colleagues[42] in a retrospective study evaluated the performance of EUS FNA followed by EUS TCB in 70 consecutive patients with mediastinal lesions. The diagnostic accuracy of EUS FNA, EUS TCB, and both procedures combined did not differ significantly (93%, 90%, and 98%, respectively). No complications were observed. Interestingly, in 15 of the 20 patients with cytologic specimens demonstrating malignancy, the diagnosis could be further specified with histologic analysis (tumor origin in 8, clear-cut lymphoma diagnosis in 4, and specification of tumor characteristics in 3). Despite these latter findings, the authors suggested that clinicians should limit the use of EUS TCB to specific cases in which EUS FNA was inconclusive.[42]

The study that has assessed the performance of EUS TCB in the largest patient population did not, however, involve a comparison with EUS FNA.[21] Of the 247 patients evaluated, 113 had pancreatic masses, 34 esophagogastric wall thickening, and 100 extrapancreatic lesions. A median of three needle passes per patient was done, and in 14 of the 247 patients (6%) a technical failure occurred that in 57% of the cases was related to transduodenal puncture. The overall diagnostic accuracy was 75%, with a 2% complication rate. Independent predictors for a positive diagnostic yield included the number of passes greater than 2 ($p = 0.05$) and the route of biopsy (stomach versus duodenum, $p = 0.001$; stomach versus esophagus, $p = 0.041$).[21]

Taking into consideration all the published studies, no clear advantage for EUS TCB over EUS FNA has been demonstrated (see Table 22-1), even in patients with suspected lymphomas or subepithelial lesions that are considered a class IIa indication for the use of EUS TCB.[40] In addition, the Tru-Cut needle is very difficult to handle, and the technique is less intuitive than EUS FNA and is associated with an increased risk for complications. For these reasons, this technically demanding needle has failed to reach widespread use outside of tertiary care centers but is considered as the primer to future developments in EUS FNB.

EUS-Guided Fine-Needle Biopsy Using a Standard 22-G Needle
Background

In 2000, Voss and colleagues,[18] in an attempt to overcome some of the limitations of EUS FNA, described their experience in obtaining tissue specimens from pancreatic masses

Video 22-2. Technique of EUS-guided fine-needle tissue acquisition using a standard 22-G needle.

using a standard 22-G FNA needle in association with high negative suction pressure by using a 30-mL syringe. They were able to gather tissue core specimens in 81% of the patients, with a diagnostic accuracy of 74.4%. Subsequently, other groups reported their experience in using a standard 22-G FNA needle with or without high negative suction pressure to obtain samples for histologic evaluation.[23,52-55] In particular, Larghi and colleagues[23] used the Alliance II inflation system to obtain a high steady and continuous negative suction. They named their procedure EUS-guided FNTA to distinguish it from standard EUS FNA.

Design and Technique

The EUS FNTA technique with high negative pressure[23] is performed using the Alliance II inflation system (Boston Scientific Corp., Natick, MA, US) (Figure 22-5), which is attached to a standard 22-G FNA needle. Once the needle is advanced in the target lesion under real-time EUS imaging, the stylet is withdrawn and the Alliance II system is attached to the proximal end of the needle. The Alliance II system is then turned into the suction mode and a high negative continuous suctioning pressure corresponding to 35 mL of the 60-mL syringe, a value arbitrarily chosen, is applied. The lock of the

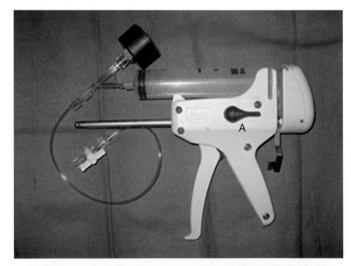

FIGURE 22-5 The Alliance II system used to perform EUS-guided fine-needle tissue acquisition. This system was attached to the proximal end of a standard FNA needle and after turning it into the suction mode (*A*) was used to apply steady and high negative continuous suctioning at 35 mL of the 60-mL syringe. *(From Larghi A, Noffsinger A, Dye CE, et al. EUS-guided fine-needle tissue acquisition by using high negative pressure suction for the evaluation of solid masses: a pilot study. Gastrointest Endosc. 2005;62:768-774.)*

syringe is then opened to apply steady and continuously high negative suction pressure during the back-and-forth movements of the needle inside the target lesion.

Results

Results of studies evaluating the possibility of acquiring a tissue biopsy sample for histologic examination using a standard 22-G needle are summarized in Table 22-2.[13,18,52–55] Variable yield and diagnostic accuracy have been found in the different studies, the reason for which may be related to the different technique used and how the samples were handled. The group from Clichy, France, first reported the use of a standard 22-G needle to acquire tissue sample for histologic examination allowing analysis of tissue structure with serial section and the possibility to perform better immunostaining to increase diagnostic accuracy.[18] To theoretically increase the possibility of acquiring a tissue sample they utilized high negative suction pressure by using a 30-mL syringe in a large cohort of patients with pancreatic solid lesions. Overall, the procedure was feasible in 90 of the 99 patients (90.9%), with the obtainment of material that could be analyzed for histology in 73 patients (81% of the patients in whom the procedure was feasible and 73.7% of the entire cohort), which was diagnostic in 67 patients (74.4% of the patients in whom the procedure was feasible and 67.7% of the entire cohort). Minor bleeding occurred in 5% of all cases that were managed conservatively. Interestingly, diagnostic accuracy was significantly better for adenocarcinomas than for neuroendocrine tumors (81% versus 47%, $p < 0.02$), whereas tumor size did not influence the results. This promising report was not followed by any other confirmatory or negative study until 5 years later by Larghi and colleagues,[23] using a similar amount of negative suction pressure steadily applied through the use of the Alliance II inflation system in patients with solid masses. They included 27 patients with pancreatic, mediastinal, left adrenal, liver, gallbladder, and gastric wall masses. All patients first underwent EUS FNA with a total of five passes performed. Using the same 22-G FNA needle an extra pass was done with the technique described above, and in all but one patient a tissue specimen for histologic examination was procured with no complications. EUS FNA and EUS FNTA reached the same diagnostic accuracy of 76.9% (in some patients with negative results using both procedures, a definitive diagnosis was not reached, and results were considered false negative), prompting the authors to speculate that EUS FNTA could have the potential for better performance if done as the starting sampling technique.[23] This inference, however, was partially disproved by the only other study that further investigated the role of this technique,[53] which involved mainly patients with enlarged lymph nodes that represented 61% of the entire patient population studied. The content of the needle after EUS FNTA was placed directly into formalin for histologic examination. Tissue core biopsy specimens were found in only 27.8% of the 36 patients evaluated. On the other hand, diagnostic accuracy was found to be 77.8%, a result very similar to the one described by Larghi and colleagues,[23] thus implying that a sample for at least cytologic evaluation was obtained.

Without using high negative suction pressure, Iglesias-Garcia and colleagues[52] assessed the value of an extra pass performed using the same 22-G needle utilized for two previous FNA passes in obtaining tissue core specimens in 62 patients with pancreatic masses. Histologic samples were adequate in 83.9% of the cases, with a 6.5 ± 5.3-mm mean length of the retrieved core specimen. Overall, correct diagnosis from the samples collected at the third needle pass was 88.7%, meaning that a few samples had some cells that were sufficient to reach a cytologic diagnosis but not to render a histologic core for evaluation. In a subsequent study, Möller and colleagues[54] further investigated the capability of collecting tissue samples from 192 patients with pancreatic masses using a 22-G needle without high negative suction pressure. The material, which was retrieved by reinserting the stylet in the needle, was first visually evaluated for the presence of core specimens that were subsequently carefully harvested by syringe suction and placed in formalin. The remaining liquid material was placed in saline solution or smeared onto glass slides for cytologic analysis. Using this technique, adequate samples for histologic evaluation were found in 85.9% of patients with only one or two passes performed. In these cases an adequate cytologic specimen was also available in 93.2% of the cases. Overall diagnostic accuracy was 71.4% for histologic and 77.6% for cytologic samples, with an overall 87.5% accuracy when both histologic and cytologic results were combined.[54] Finally, Noda and colleagues[55] performed a

TABLE 22-2

STUDIES EVALUATING THE POSSIBILITY OF ACQUIRING A TISSUE BIOPSY SAMPLE FOR HISTOLOGIC EXAMINATION USING A STANDARD 22-G NEEDLE

Author (year)	No. of Patients	Patient Population	Yield of Core Tissue (%)	Diagnostic Accuracy (%)
Voss et al[18] (2000)[a]	99	Pancreatic masses	81	68
Larghi et al[23] (2005)[b,c]	27	Solid masses	96	76.9
Iglesias-Garcia et al[52] (2007)	62	Pancreatic masses	83.9	88.7
Gerke et al[53] (2009)[b]	120	Solid masses and lymph nodes	27.8	77.8[d]
Möller et al[54] (2009)	192	Pancreatic masses	86.5	71.4
Noda et al[55] (2010)	32	Solid masses and lymph nodes	NA	93.9

NA, not applicable.
[a]Using high negative suction pressure with a 30-mL syringe.
[b]Using high negative suction pressure obtained using the Alliance II inflation system.
[c]Results obtained with a single needle pass for tissue acquisition was performed at the end of a standard FNA.
[d]Diagnostic accuracy calculated based on both histologic and cytologic specimens.

similar study on 33 patients where one half of the pancreatic mass sample was evaluated by cytologic methods and the other half by the cell block histologic method. Reading of the cell block was diagnostic in 25 of the 33 patients (75.8%) and in 31 of the 33 (93.9%) after immunostaining was performed.

EUS Fine-Needle Biopsy Using a Standard 19-G Needle
Background

Between 2005 and 2006, two Japanese investigators first reported their experiences in using a standard 19-G needle to procure core biopsy specimens for histologic examination in patients with solid pancreatic masses and with mediastinal and/or intra-abdominal lymphadenopathy of unknown origin.[35,56] They reported an overall diagnostic accuracy of 68.8% and 98%, respectively. This discrepancy in the overall reported accuracy was due to the high rate of failure (five of eight patients, 62.5%) of the sampling procedure when performed through the duodenum as required for patients with pancreatic head and uncinate process masses.[35] However, the impressively high capability (88%) to correctly subtype lymphomas in patients with lymphadenopathy of unknown origin reported in the study by Yasuda and colleagues[56] clearly showed that tissue specimens acquired with a standard 19-G needle could have a very important role in establishing a definitive diagnosis in selected patient populations.

Inspired by these promising results and in an attempt to overcome the limitation of the use of a standard 19-G needle through the duodenum, the authors modified the technique described by Itoi[35] and by Yasuda[56] by removing the stylet before insertion of the needle into the working channel of the EUS scope in order to increase needle flexibility and improve its performance.[24] This technique, which the authors continued to name EUS FNTA to distinguish it from EUS FNA, has been tested in different patient populations and in some specific cases in which it was thought that a histologic sample could be more useful than a cytologic aspirate to reach a definitive diagnosis.[24,25,57–59]

EUS Fine-Needle Tissue Acquisition Technique

The EUS FNTA technique is performed using a disposable standard 19-G needle. The needle is prepared before insertion into the working channel of the echoendoscope by removing the stylet and attaching to its proximal end a 10-mL syringe

Video 22-3. Technique of EUS-guided fine-needle tissue acquisition using a standard 19-G needle.

already preloaded with 10 mL of negative pressure. The needle is then advanced under EUS guidance a few millimeters inside the target lesion. After opening the lock of the syringe to apply negative pressure, two or three back-and-forth motions inside the lesion using the fanning technique[60] are made, which together account for one needle pass. The needle is removed after closing the lock of the syringe and the collected specimens are placed directly in formalin by flushing the needle with saline and sent for histologic examination.

Results

Table 22-3 summarizes the results of all studies in which a standard 19-G needle has been used to gather samples for histologic analysis, independent of the technique utilized.[24,25,35,56,61–67] As shown in the Table 22-3, apart from the study by Itoi and colleagues[35] in which a high technical failure rate was observed when the procedure was performed through the duodenum, the overall technical success and yield in all the published studies were above 90%. Moreover, overall diagnostic accuracy was also found to be above 90%, with the only exception of the study by Iwashita and colleagues,[63] in which patients with a pancreatic mass suspicious for autoimmune pancreatitis were evaluated. In the latter study, despite specimens for histologic analysis being obtained in 93% of the patients, a definitive histologic diagnosis of autoimmune pancreatitis (AIP) based on lymphoplasmacytic infiltration around pancreatic ducts, obliterative phlebitis, and/or positive IgG4 immunostaining could be achieved in only 43% of the cases. In the remaining 50% of patients with available tissue for histologic analysis, specific histologic findings of AIP could not be established and a diagnosis of idiopathic chronic pancreatitis was made.[63] This low diagnostic yield can be attributed to the patchy distribution of the specific histologic changes of AIP,[68] thus rendering the amount of tissue obtained with EUS-guided biopsy insufficient to establish a definitive diagnosis. On the other hand, in all patients with available tissue, a malignant etiology could be excluded, which is extremely important in order to safely start empirical therapy for AIP with steroids.[63]

After the first publication in 2006,[56] the Japanese group from Gifu University Hospital published its subsequent experiences in patients with mediastinal lymphadenopathy and a clinical presentation suggestive of sarcoidosis[61] and in a larger cohort of patients with mediastinal and/or abdominal lesions suspicious for lymphoma.[66] Both studies demonstrated the value of using a standard 19-G needle to: (1) confirm the clinical suspicion of sarcoidosis;[61] and (2) to establish a diagnosis of lymphoma with subclassification in a very high percentage of patients, thus sparing them from more invasive diagnostic procedures.[66] These results suggest that the 19-G needle should be used as the sampling procedure of choice in these patient populations.

In the authors' first experience using the modified EUS FNTA technique, besides patients with lymphadenopathy of unknown origin they also evaluated patients with subepithelial lesions, esophagogastric wall thickening, and with pancreatic body or tail solid lesions after a negative FNA, in whom we deemed histologic samples to be more appropriate than cytologic aspirates.[18] Overall, in the cohort of 120 patients consecutively enrolled, the procedure was technically successful in all but one patient without any complications, with a

TABLE 22-3

STUDIES EVALUATING THE POSSIBILITY OF ACQUIRING A TISSUE BIOPSY SAMPLE FOR HISTOLOGIC EXAMINATION USING A STANDARD 19-GAUGE NEEDLE

Author (year)	No. of Patients	Patient Population	Technical Success (%)	Yield (%)	Diagnostic Accuracy (%)
Itoi et al[35] (2005)[a]	16	Pancreatic masses	81	68.8	68.8
Yasuda et al[56] (2006)	104	Mediastinal and/or abdominal lymphadenopathy	100	100	98.1; 88% accuracy in subclassification of lymphoma
Iwashita et al[61] (2008)	41	Mediastinal lymphadenopathy suspicious for sarcoidosis	100	95.1	95.1
Larghi et al[24] (2011)[b,c]	120	Heterogeneous patient population	99.2	96.7	93.2
Eckardt et al[62] (2012)	46	Gastric subepithelial lesions	71.7	59	52
Iwashita et al[63] (2012)	44	Pancreatic masses suggestive of autoimmune pancreatitis	100	93	43.2
Larghi et al[25] (2012)[c]	30	Pancreatic masses suspicious for nonfunctional neuroendocrine neoplasia	100	93.3	93.3
Stavropoulos et al[64] (2012)[d]	31	Patients with abnormal liver tests undergoing EUS to rule out biliary obstruction	100	91	91
Varadarajulu et al[65] (2012)	38	Pancreatic masses/subepithelial lesions	100	94.7	94.7
Yasuda et al[66] (2012)	152	Mediastinal and/or abdominal lesions suspicious for lymphoma	97	97	93.4; 95% accuracy in subclassification of lymphoma (142 patients)
Gor et al[67] (2013)	10	Patients with abnormal liver tests	100	100	100
Larghi et al[57] (2013)[c,e]	121	Gastrointestinal subepithelial lesions	99.2	93.4	93.4

[a]All failures occurred when sampling was performed from the duodenum.
[b]Consecutive patients with subepithelial lesions, esophagogastric wall thickening, mediastinal and abdominal masses/lymphadenopathy of unknown origin, pancreatic body or tail lesions after a negative FNA were included in the study.
[c]The EUS FNTA technique was used.
[d]Adequate specimen defined as a length of 15 mm with the presence of at least six portal tracts.
[e]All procedures were performed using the forward-viewing EUS scope.

diagnostic yield of 96.7% and a diagnostic accuracy of 93.2%. Remarkably, not only specimens gathered with the EUS FNTA could be of help to establish a diagnosis of malignancy, but also a definitive diagnosis of benign disease was established in 20 patients who were spared more invasive diagnostic procedures and unnecessary follow-up examinations.[24]

Representative cases of benign and malignant diagnoses are shown in Figure 22-6. In this first experience, it was decided not to enroll patients with pancreatic head/uncinate masses after a negative FNA because of the fear that the presence of a stent usually placed after EUS FNA could interfere with the procedure.[24] Subsequently, a second study was performed in patients with pancreatic lesions suspicious for nonfunctional neuroendocrine neoplasia (NF-NEN).[25] In these patients, ki-67 proliferation index determination was perfomred that can be better determined on tissue biopsy specimens and has an important prognostic value on management decisions.[25] Thirty consecutive patients with a pancreatic mass with a mean diameter of 16.9 ± 6.1 mm were enrolled. The lesions were located throughout the pancreas, including the pancreatic head and uncinate process (eight patients, representing 27% of the cohort) that could be approached only from the duodenum. The procedure was technically successful in all cases, and in 28 of 30 patients a specimen for histologic examination was retrieved and confirmed the suspicious diagnosis of NF-NEN. Moreover, in 26 patients (92.9% of those with an available specimen and 86.6% of the entire cohort),

ki-67 determination could be performed (Figure 22-7). Comparison with the ki-67 determination on surgical specimens, which represent the gold standard, was feasible in 12 patients and showed an agreement in 10 cases when a cutoff of >2% to define G2 tumors was applied. Conversely when a cutoff of 5% was used, which is suggested to be more useful than the 2% value to stratify prognosis of patients with pancreatic NF-NEN,[69,70] an agreement was found in all patients.[25] These results indicate that preoperative ki-67 determination on EUS FNTA specimens may be used for the discussion with a patient regarding the available therapeutic options.

Two other patient populations in which the use of a standard 19-G needle has been evaluated are patients with abnormal liver tests of unclear etiology referred for EUS to exclude biliary obstruction and those with subepithelial lesions.[57,62,64,67] In the first patient population, after an unrevealing EUS, Stavropoulos and colleagues[64] investigated the value of EUS-guided liver biopsy performed in the same session using a standard 19-G needle. An adequate specimen was defined as a specimen that was at least 15 mm in length and with at least six complete portal tracts. Among the 22 patients evaluated, a specimen with these characteristics could be retrieved in 20 of them (91%), and was diagnostic in all cases. Importantly, there were no procedural complications, including five higher risk patients with relative coagulopathy (platelets <100,000/μL, INR > 1.3). These results have been replicated by Gor and colleagues[67] in a case series of 10 patients in whom

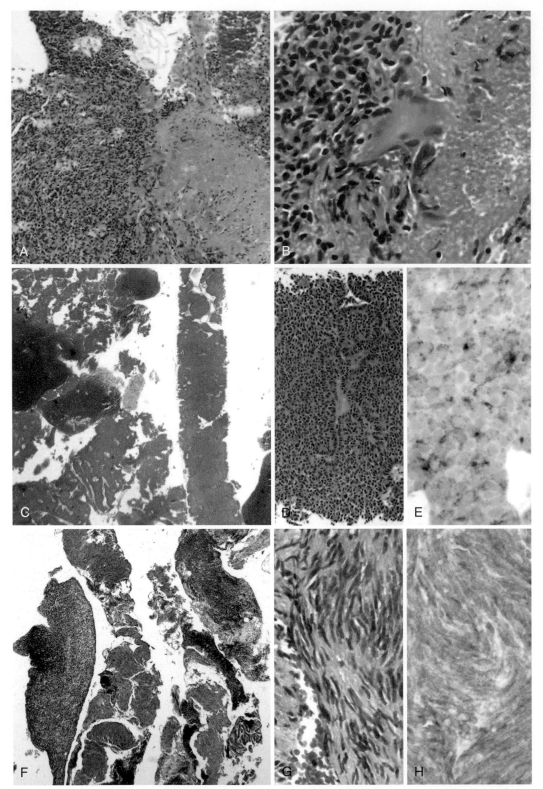

FIGURE 22-6 Representative cases of specimens obtained by EUS FNTA. **A, B,** Mediastinal lymph node: **A,** abundant tissue fragments, **B,** at higher magnification showing caseous material (left part of the micrograph) and polynucleated giant cells consistent with a tubercular granuloma, as also later confirmed by PCR methods; H&E. **C-E,** Body-tail of the pancreas: **C, D,** multiple large tissue fragments of a well-differentiated, nonfunctioning, neuroendocrine tumor, with a typical trabecular structure, low-grade histology void of necrosis and mitotic figures (**D**) and chromogranin A expression at immunohistochemistry (**E**); **C, D,** H&E; **E,** immunoperoxidase. **F-H,** Perigastric lesion: **F,** abundant, large fragments of neoplastic tissue with solid structure, in absence of necrosis, composed of regular, fused cell with mild atypia (**G**) intensely immunoreactive for c-Kit and consistent with gastrointestinal stromal tumor (GIST); **F, G,** H&E, **H,** immunoperoxidase. H&E, hematoxylin and eosin; PCR, polymerase chain reaction. *(Larghi A, Verna EC, Ricci R, et al. EUS-guided fine-needle tissue acquisition by using a 19-G needle in a selected patient population: a prospective study.* Gastrointest Endosc. *2011;74:504-510.)*

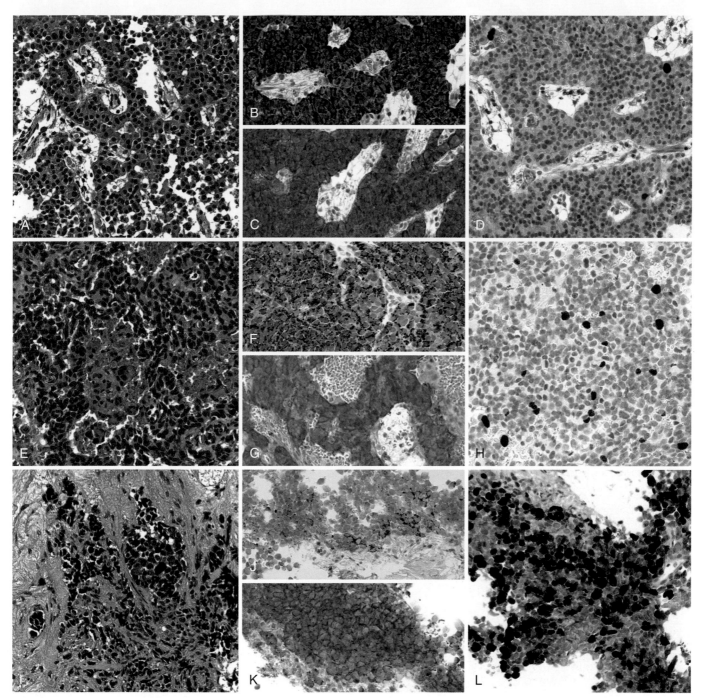

FIGURE 22-7 Examples of grading for neuroendocrine neoplasms in EUS FNTA samples. **A-D,** Grade 1 PNET showing trabecular histology, mild atypia (**A**), intense immunoreactivity for chromogranin A (**B**) and synaptophysin (**C**), and rare cells with nuclear labeling for ki-67 (**D**). **E-H,** Grade 2 PNET showing large trabecular structure, moderate cell atypia (**E**), intense immunoreactivity for chromogranin A (**F**) and synaptophysin (**G**), and discrete cells with nuclear labeling for ki-67 (**H**). **I-L,** High-grade, G3, p-NEC fragmented sample showing abundant desmoplasia and solid islets of cells with severe atypia and scarce cytoplasm (**I**), focal and often faint immunoreactivity for chromogranin A (**J**), intense and diffuse immunoreactivity for synaptophysin (**K**), and diffuse nuclear labeling for ki-67 (**L**). **A, E, I,** hematoxylin and eosin; **B-D, F-H,** and **J-L,** immunoperoxidase. PNET, pancreatic neuroendocrine tumor. pNEC, xxxxxxx. *(Larghi A, Capurso G, Carnuccio A, et al. Ki-67 grading of nonfunctioning pancreatic neuroendocrine tumors on histologic samples obtained by EUS-guided fine-needle tissue acquisition: a prospective study. Gastrointest Endosc. 2012;76:570-577.)* *p-NEC,* high-grade pancreatic neuroendocrine carcinoma; *p-NET,* low-grade to intermediate-grade pancreatic neuroendocrine tumor.

EUS FNB using the standard 19-G needle provided diagnostic core specimens in all patients, a mean length of 14.4 mm, and contained a mean of 9.2 complete portal tracts per sample. In patients with subepithelial lesions, two studies have reached opposite conclusions reporting a diagnostic accuracy of 52%[62] versus 93.4%.[57] The reason for this discrepancy is unclear. It was speculated that in the study[57] the employment of the EUS

FNTA technique with removal of the stylet before the procedure, which renders the needle more flexible and easy to operate, coupled with the utilization of the forward-viewing therapeutic linear echoendoscope that seems to ensure easier deployment of a 19-G needle,[71–73] could account for the better results reported. Interestingly, with the specimens collected (representative cases are shown in Figure 22-8) the authors

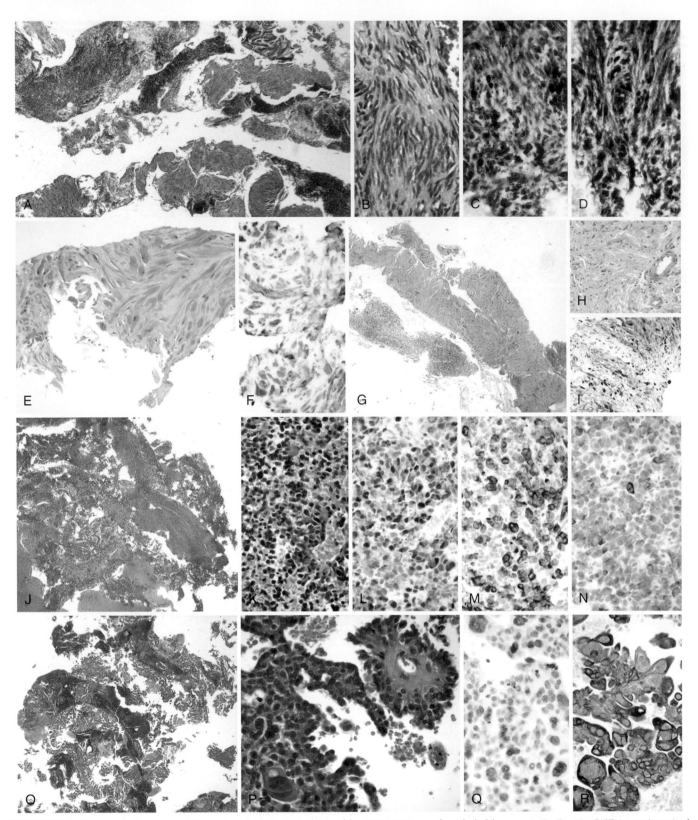

FIGURE 22-8 Representative cases of tissue type and amount obtained by EUS FNTA in subepithelial lesions. **A-D,** Gastric GIST (gastrointestinal stromal tumor): abundant tissue fragments (**A**) at higher magnification showing a spindle cell neoplasm (**B**) whose strong and diffuse immune positivity for CD117 (**C**) and DOG1 (**D**) unequivocally qualified as a GIST (**A** and **B,** H&E; **C,** CD117 IHC; **D,** DOG1 IHC; original magnification: **A,** ×20; **B, C,** and **D,** ×400). **E, F,** Esophageal leiomyoma. The abundance of the available fragments allowed us not only to detect the presence of spindle cells with abundant eosinophilic cytoplasm with bland nuclei and no mitotic activity, but also allowed us to appreciate their arrangement in intersecting fascicles (**E**); these findings, together with an intense desmin reactivity (**F**) in the absence of staining with CD117 and DOG1 (not shown) led to a straight-forward diagnosis of leiomyoma (**E,** H&E; **F,** desmin IHC; original magnification: **E,** ×200; **F,** ×400). **G-I,** Gastric schwannoma: the bioptic specimen showed a spindle cell neoplasm (**G, H**); the preservation of architectural details such as the presence of hyaline thickening of vessel walls (**H**) and the diffuse S-100 positivity (**I**) in the absence of CD117 and DOG1 staining (not shown) were diagnostic for a schwannoma (**G, H,** H&E; **I,** S-100 IHC; original magnification: **G,** ×40; **H, I** ×400). **J-N,** Gastric metastasis of melanoma: the bioptic sample was composed of fragments of highly cellular neoplasm composed of atypical epithelioid cells (**J, K**) intensely and diffusely positive for S-100 (**L**), HMB-45 (**M**), and Melan-A (**N**), typical features of melanoma (**J, K,** H&E; **L,** S-100 IHC; **M, H,** MB-45 IHC; **N,** Melan-A IHC; original magnification: **J,** ×40; **K, L, M, N** ×400). **O-R,** Gastric metastasis of ovarian serous papillary carcinoma: the bioptic fragments showed a neoplasm composed of epithelioid cells with marked atypia arranged in papillae (**O, P**), with nuclear WT1 immunoreactivity (**Q**) and intense staining for cytokeratin 7 (**R**) (**O, P,** H&E; **Q,** WT1 IHC; **R,** cytokeratin 7 IHC; original magnification: **O,** ×20; **P, Q, R,** ×400). H&E, hematoxylin and eosin; IHC, immunohistochemistry. *(Larghi A, Fuccio L, Chiarello G et al. Fine-needle tissue acquisition from subepithelial lesions using a forward-viewing linear echoendoscope. Endoscopy 2014;46:39-45.)*

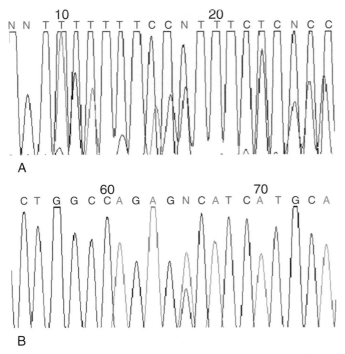

FIGURE 22-9 Mutational analyses performed on tissue core biopsy specimens obtained by EUS FNTA in two patients with a subepithelial lesion after histologic features were consistent with the diagnosis of gastrointestinal stromal tumor but with negative immunohistochemical studies. Partial nucleotide sequence of exon 11 of *KIT* gene showed a reading-frameshift mutation caused by a heterozygous deletion of six nucleotides (from position 1666 to 1671) (**A**). This determines a deletion of two amino acids (glutamine and tryptophan at position 556 and 557, respectively) (ΔQ556-W557). Partial nucleotide sequence of exon 18 of *PDGFRA* gene showed a heterozygous A→T change at base 2526 (**B**). This determines a substitution of an aspartic acid with a valine at position 842 (D842 V).

were able to perform genetic analysis for diagnostic purposes in three patients in whom immunohistochemical studies were negative despite histopathologic features that were suggestive of GIST (Figure 22-9). The capability of performing genotype profiling of GISTs is relevant beyond its diagnostic significance because it has a prognostic impact and allows optimizing chemotherapy for unresectable cases and for other selected cases where neoadjuvant therapy may be a useful option.[74,75]

Finally, Varadarajulu and colleagues[65] recently published their experience in using a newly developed flexible 19-G needle (Expect™ 19 Flex, Boston Scientific Corp., Natick, MA, US) made of nitinol, which is supposed to have a better performance for transduodenal puncture. They evaluated 32 patients with pancreatic head/uncinate masses or peripancreatic masses approached from the duodenum and 6 patients with subepithelial lesions in the stomach (5 patients) and in the rectum (1 patient). On-site cytopathology evaluation and cell block analysis were performed. The procedure was successful in all patients, and examination of cell block specimens revealed optimal histologic core tissue in 36 of 38 (93.7%) patients, which was diagnostic in all cases. Based on these results,[66] the same group proposed an algorithm in which, in centers where an on-site cytopathologist is not available, they recommended performance of EUS FNB instead of EUS FNA by using a standard 19-G needle for lesions approached from the esophagus, stomach, and rectum, and

to use the flex 19-G needle for transduodenal puncture.[76,77] To date, however, there is insufficient data to make this suggestion a standard procedure, and further experiences with EUS FNB using different needles and techniques are necessary before a definitive conclusion on the value of the proposed algorithm can be drawn.

All together, the results of the above-mentioned studies strongly suggest that standard 19-G needles are valuable in obtaining tissue core biopsy specimens. All these data, however, are from single-center studies by clinicians highly experienced in the use of standard 19-G needles; thus the reproducibility in other centers with less experience and in the community remains unknown. Future studies to answer these important questions are warranted.

EUS-Guided Fine-Needle Biopsy Using ProCore Needles

Background

Although the Quick-Core needle failed to reach widespread use due to technical difficulty associated with its utilization and the relative lack of advantages over standard FNA needles, the same manufacturer developed a new needle with a different design, the ProCore needle.[26] To meet all the needs and have a needle to cover for any different clinical scenarios and difficulty, three needle sizes have been developed, the 19-G, the 22-G, and the 25-G ProCore needles.

Design and Technique

All ProCore needles are 1.705 m long and made of stainless steel with a nitinol stylet. The stylet that runs through the cannula of the needle matches the bevel tip. There is a lateral opening of varying length depending on the needle size (Figure 22-10), which presents a reverse bevel to hook and cut the tissue entrapping it into the needle. This reverse bevel is located at a different distance from the tip of the needle depending on the needle size. Characteristics and differences between ProCore needles are shown in Table 22-4.

In the first published study,[26] which involved five European centers, each participating center used a different sampling technique. At univariate and multivariate analyses, the only variable associated with the obtainment of an optimal sample for histologic analysis and to make a correct final diagnosis was the intervention of an experienced pathologist to evaluate the sample. Site of puncture (duodenum versus other sites), use or not of the stylet, number of back-and-forth movements (three to four versus one), number of needle

Video 22-4. Technique of EUS-guided fine-needle biopsy using a ProCore needle.

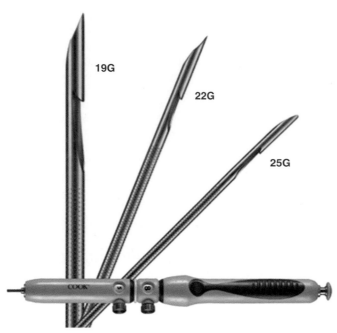

FIGURE 22-10 Novel 19-G, 22-G, and 25-G ProCore needles with reverse bevel technology for acquisition of tissue samples.

Video 22-5. Technique of EUS-guided fine-needle biopsy using the stylet-pull technique.

as compared to the suction method used in both the European ProCore studies.[26,27]

Results

The performance of the 19-G ProCore needle in the diagnosis of intraintestinal and extraintestinal lesions was evaluated in a multicenter study by Iglesias-Garcia and colleagues.[26] Among 109 patients with 114 heterogeneous lesions, EUS FNB using this newly developed biopsy needle was technically feasible in 112 cases (98.24%), with no complications. The only two technical failures occurred when the sampling procedure was performed through the duodenum, accounting for an overall success rate of 94.3% (33 of 35) for transduodenal sampling. In both patients, who respectively had an aortocaval lymph node and a pancreatic head tumor, failure was due to impossibility of removal of the stylet from the needle once inside the lesion. Overall, in all lesions in which the procedure was technically successful a sample suitable for pathological evaluation was obtained, which was adequate for histologic examination in 102 lesions (89.5%) and for cytologic evaluation in the remaining 10 cases (sample was processed as a cell block). Diagnostic accuracy was 86% for all lesions and 92.9% when only considering malignant lesions. Interestingly, the only factor that positively correlated with a significant increase in the potential of making a definitive histologic diagnosis was the involvement of an expert pathologist.[26]

A study evaluating the interobserver agreement in grading the quality of specimens obtained with the 19-G ProCore needle among five expert pathologists from the five participating centers was performed.[79] Overall, an excellent interobserver agreement in the assessment of the histologic material

passes (two to three versus one), and modality of sample retrieval (air, stylet, or saline solution) did not have any impact on tissue sample acquisition.[26] In a subsequent study from the same European group,[27] a standardized sample acquisition protocol was developed: (1) the needle is advanced into the target lesion under EUS guidance; (2) once inside the lesion, the stylet is removed and negative suction pressure is applied using a 10-mL syringe for 30 seconds; (3) three back-and-forth movements within the lesion are made; and (4) suction is then released by closing the lock of the syringe and the needle is finally removed. Tissue samples are recovered in formalin or CytoLyt by flushing the needle with saline.[27]

A different sampling technique, the slow pull technique, has been proposed for the tissue acquisition procedure performed using the 25-G ProCore needle.[29] With this technique, once the needle is inside the lesion, the negative suction pressure is obtained by slowly and continuously pulling out the stylet from the needle while 10 to 20 back-and-forth movements are performed (Video 22-5). Preliminary results[78] have reported this technique to result in a significantly higher yield

---

TABLE 22-4

MAIN CHARACTERISTICS OF THE DIFFERENT AVAILABLE PROCORE NEEDLES

	ECHO-HD-25-C	ECHO-HD-22-C	ECHO-HD-19-C
Needle outer diameter (mm)	0.56	0.71	1.07
Needle inner diameter (mm)	0.37	0.51	0.94
Needle length (m)	1.705	1.705	1.705
Needle bevel	Lancet	Lancet	Lancet
Stylet tip design	Lancet	Recessed Ball	Recessed Ball
Reverse bevel length (mm)	2	2	4
Distance of the needle tip from the reverse bevel (mm)	3	3.9	5
Sheath size	5.2 Fr	5.2 Fr	4.8 Fr
Needle material	Stainless steel	Stainless steel	Stainless steel
Stylet material	Nitinol	Nitinol	Nitinol

was found among the involved pathologists, and this was particularly high (91.2%) with regard to sample adequacy, with a Fleiss' κ that was 0.73 (95% CI 0.61 to 0.81).[79] Moreover, when the same samples were evaluated by nonexpert pathologists, the interobserver agreement substantially decreased (unpublished data), thus suggesting the paramount importance of a pathologist dedicated to reading EUS samples. It is the authors' opinion that efforts to establish pathology expertise by combining their educational activities with those of endosonographers should be strongly encouraged.

The same study group subsequently evaluated the performance of the 22-G ProCore needle in a cohort of 61 patients with pancreatic masses, in which 57.4% of the lesions were localized in the pancreatic head/uncinate, thus requiring a transduodenal approach.[27] Only one needle pass was performed using the protocol described above. In one patient with an uncinate process mass, the procedure failed because of the inability to extend the needle out of the working channel of the echoendoscope. In the remaining patients with a successful sampling procedure, tissue specimens for histologic examination were retrieved in 55 patients (90.2%), which in all but one patient (88.5%) were judged adequate to make a definitive diagnosis. All adequate specimens were found to be diagnostic, thus accounting for an overall accuracy of 88.5%. These very promising results prompted another group to design a randomized trial to compare the capability of this needle with that of a standard 22-G FNA needle in the obtainment of cytologic and histologic samples in 56 patients with pancreatic masses.[28] No significant difference in the median number of passes required for establishing on-site diagnosis, rates of diagnostic accuracy, or technical failure between the FNA and FNB needles were detected. Moreover, no significant difference between the two groups was found in the proportion of samples in which histologic core tissue was present (FNA 100% versus FNB 83.3%, $p = 0.26$).[28] On the other hand, histologic core of optimal quality was present in 66.7% of FNA specimens and 80% of FNB specimens ($p = 0.66$).[28] In a study with a similar design that included both pancreatic masses and other types of lesions (e.g., lymph nodes and intraintestinal and extraintestinal lesions), the 22-G ProCore needle required significantly fewer needle passes as compared with a standard 22-G FNA needle to achieve diagnostic adequacy.[80] Despite similar cytologic interpretability, diagnostic accuracy, and procured amount of cell block material between the two needles, this finding can result in less procedural time and cost savings.[80] Future multicenter studies in large patient populations with heterogeneous indications are needed to better clarify if the 22-G ProCore needle has any advantages over a standard 22-G FNA needle for the evaluation of solid lesions.

Interestingly, the performance of the 22-G ProCore needle has been recently evaluated in pancreatic cystic lesions.[81] Among 60 cysts punctured, adequate amount of fluid for carcinoembryonic antigen and amylase levels and for verification of k-*ras* mutation was obtained in 32 (53.3%) and in 24 (40%) of the aspirated cysts, respectively. Moreover, samples for cytohistologic diagnosis were retrieved in 65% of the cysts, with an adequacy that reached 94.4% and 100% for lesions with a solid component and with already malignant transformation, respectively.

Finally, Iwashita and colleagues[29] reported the first experience in using the 25-G ProCore needle for the evaluation of 50 consecutive patients with solid pancreatic masses. They applied the slow stylet-pull technique described above. After FNB, the obtained material was expressed onto a glass slide by reinsertion of the stylet, and any visible core was lifted off and placed in formalin. Smears for on-site cytopathologic evaluation were made from the residual material. The authors found an impressively high sensitivity (83%) for cytologic diagnosis on the first pass, which increased to 91% and 96% at the second and third passes, respectively. On the first pass, where the histologic analysis was performed on a per pass basis, they found a sensitivity of 63%. This value increased to 87% at the subsequent two to four passes. Interestingly, the presence of a histologic core was found in only 12% of the patients after the first needle pass and in 32% of the patients at the subsequent two to four passes. In the authors' opinion, these results indicate that the 25-G ProCore needle is a proficient needle to gather diagnostic cytologic specimens, probably even more efficient than a standard 25-G FNA needle, but cannot be used when a tissue core biopsy specimen is required to make the diagnosis.

Conclusions and Future Perspective

In the last decade, in an attempt to overcome some of the limitations of EUS FNA, alternative sampling techniques and dedicated needles to obtain core tissue biopsy specimens for histologic examination under EUS guidance have been developed and tested with different success. These efforts may lead to a shift in this field from cytology to histology, which is easier to interpret, thus potentially contributing to the widespread expansion of EUS utilization in the community and in countries where cytology expertise may be difficult to be developed. Moreover, in the era of individualized medicine, this shift will likely pave the road to targeted therapies and better approaches to the treatment of most GI malignancies, because tissue samples for histologic examination are more adequate than cytologic aspirates to perform predictive molecular markers or cell culture with chemosensitivity testing to guide individualized therapies. This will transform diagnostic EUS into a more therapeutic procedure that not only provides a diagnostic answer, but also offers the possibility to deliver the best treatment for individual patients. Based on these premises, current thought patterns need to be changed, and a search needs to be made for the right technique and/or the right needle that will give enough tissue to perform all studies necessary to reach the diagnosis and to allow for personalized treatment for individual patients. This needle should be able to meet the needs not only of experts, but also those of all individual endosonographers. The authors firmly believe that a close collaboration between endosonographers and pathologists is of paramount importance to succeed in this balanced effort to develop the right EUS FNB needle/technique to achieve the best possible clinical outcomes.

REFERENCES

1. Vilmann P, Jacobsen GK, Henriksen FW, et al. Endoscopic ultrasonography with guided fine needle aspiration biopsy in pancreatic disease. *Gastrointest Endosc.* 1992;38:172-173.
2. Dumonceau JM, Polkowski M, Larghi A, et al. European Society of Gastrointestinal Endoscopy. Indications, results, and clinical impact of endoscopic ultrasound (EUS)-guided sampling in gastroenterology:

European Society of Gastrointestinal Endoscopy (ESGE) Clinical Guideline. *Endoscopy*. 2011;43:897-912.

3. Dumonceau JM, Polkowski M, Larghi A, et al. Indications, results, and clinical impact of endoscopic ultrasound (EUS)-guided sampling in gastroenterology: European Society of Gastrointestinal Endoscopy (ESGE) Clinical Guideline. *Endoscopy*. 2011;43:897-912.

4. Erickson RA, Sayage-Rabie L, Beissner RS. Factors predicting the number of EUS-guided fine-needle passes for diagnosis of pancreatic malignancies. *Gastrointest Endosc*. 2000;51:184-190.

5. Turner MS, Goldsmith JD. Best practices in diagnostic immunohistochemistry: spindle cell neoplasms of the gastrointestinal tract. *Arch Pathol Lab Med*. 2009;133:1370-1374.

6. Garcia CF, Swerdlow SH. Best practices in contemporary diagnostic immunohistochemistry: panel approach to hematolymphoid proliferations. *Arch Pathol Lab Med*. 2009;133:756-765.

7. Hébert-Magee S, Bae S, Varadarajulu S, et al. The presence of a cytopathologist increases the diagnostic accuracy of endoscopic ultrasound-guided fine needle aspiration cytology for pancreatic adenocarcinoma: a meta-analysis. *Cytopathology*. 2013;24:159-171.

8. Iglesias-Garcia J, Dominguez-Munoz JE, Abdulkader I, et al. Influence of on-site cytopathology evaluation on the diagnostic accuracy of endoscopic ultrasound-guided fine needle aspiration (EUS-FNA) of solid pancreatic masses. *Am J Gastroenterol*. 2011;106:1705-1710.

9. Eloubeidi MA, Tamhane A, Jhala N, et al. Agreement between rapid onsite and final cytologic interpretations of EUS-guided FNA specimens: implications for the endosonographer and patient management. *Am J Gastroenterol*. 2006;101:2841-2847.

10. Jhala NC, Jhala DN, Chhieng DC, et al. Endoscopic ultrasound-guided fine-needle aspiration. A cytopathologist's perspective. *Am J Clin Pathol*. 2003;120:351-367.

11. Kalaitzakis E, Panos M, Sadik R, et al. Clinicians' attitudes towards endoscopic ultrasound: a survey of four European countries. *Scand J Gastroenterol*. 2009;44:100-107.

12. Larghi A, Eguia V, Hassan C, et al. Economic crisis: the right time to widen the utilization of endoscopic ultrasound. *Endoscopy*. 2014;46(1):80-81.

13. Braat H, Bruno M, Kuipers EJ, et al. Pancreatic cancer: promise for personalised medicine? *Cancer Lett*. 2012;318:1-8.

14. Wakatsuki T, Irisawa A, Terashima M, et al. ATP assay-guided chemosensitivity testing for gemcitabine with biopsy specimens obtained from unresectable pancreatic cancer using endoscopic ultrasonography-guided fine-needle aspiration. *Int J Clin Oncol*. 2011;16:387-394.

15. Brais RJ, Davies SE, O'Donovan M, et al. Direct histological processing of EUS biopsies enables rapid molecular biomarker analysis for interventional pancreatic cancer trials. *Pancreatology*. 2012;12:8-15.

16. Harada N, Kouzu T, Arima M, et al. Endoscopic ultrasound-guided histologic needle biopsy: preliminary results using a newly developed endoscopic ultrasound transducer. *Gastrointest Endosc*. 1996;44:327-330.

17. Binmoeller KF, Thul R, Rathod V, et al. Endoscopic ultrasound-guided, 18-gauge, fine needle aspiration biopsy of the pancreas using a 2.8 mm channel convex array echoendoscope. *Gastrointest Endosc*. 1998;47:121-127.

18. Voss M, Hammel P, Molas G, et al. Value of endoscopic ultrasound guided fine needle aspiration biopsy in the diagnosis of solid pancreatic masses. *Gut*. 2000;46:244-249.

19. Varadarajulu S, Fraig M, Schmulewitz N, et al. Comparison of EUS guided 19-gauge Trucut needle biopsy with EUS-guided fine-needle aspiration. *Endoscopy*. 2004;36:397-401.

20. Shah SM, Ribeiro A, Levi J, et al. EUS-guided fine needle aspiration with and without trucut biopsy of pancreatic masses. *JOP*. 2008;9:422-430.

21. Thomas T, Kaye PV, Ragunath K, et al. Efficacy, safety, and predictive factors for a positive yield of EUS-guided Trucut biopsy: a large tertiary referral center experience. *Am J Gastroenterol*. 2009;104:584-591.

22. Levy MJ, Jondal ML, Clain J, et al. Preliminary experience with an EUS guided trucut biopsy needle compared with EUS-guided FNA. *Gastrointest Endosc*. 2003;57:101-106.

23. Larghi A, Noffsinger A, Dye CE, et al. EUS-guided fine needle tissue acquisition by using high negative pressure suction for the evaluation of solid masses: a pilot study. *Gastrointest Endosc*. 2005;62:768-774.

24. Larghi A, Verna EC, Ricci R, et al. EUS-guided fine-needle tissue acquisition by using a 19-gauge needle in a selected patient population: a prospective study. *Gastrointest Endosc*. 2011;74:504-510.

25. Larghi A, Capurso G, Carnuccio A, et al. Ki-67 grading of nonfunctioning pancreatic neuroendocrine tumors on histologic samples obtained by EUS-guided fine-needle tissue acquisition: a prospective study. *Gastrointest Endosc*. 2012;76:570-577.

26. Iglesias-Garcia J, Poley JW, Larghi A, et al. Feasibility and yield of a new EUS histology needle: results from a multicenter, pooled, cohort study. *Gastrointest Endosc*. 2011;73:1189-1196.

27. Larghi A, Iglesias-Garcia J, Poley JW, et al. Feasibility and yield of a novel 22-gauge histology EUS needle in patients with pancreatic masses: a multicenter prospective cohort study. *Surg Endosc*. 2013;27:3733-3738.

28. Bang JY, Hebert-Magee S, Trevino J, et al. Randomized trial comparing the 22-gauge aspiration and 22-gauge biopsy needles for EUS-guided sampling of solid pancreatic mass lesions. *Gastrointest Endosc*. 2012;76:321-327.

29. Iwashita T, Nakai Y, Samarasena JB, et al. High single-pass diagnostic yield of a new 25-gauge core biopsy needle for EUS-guided FNA biopsy in solid pancreatic lesions. *Gastrointest Endosc*. 2013;7:909-915.

30. Hatada T, Ishii H, Ichii S, et al. Diagnostic value of ultrasound-guided fine-needle aspiration biopsy, core-needle biopsy, and evaluation of combined use in the diagnosis of breast lesions. *J Am Coll Surg*. 2000;190:299-303.

31. Rodriguez LV, Terris MK. Risks and complications of transrectal ultrasound guided prostate needle biopsy: a prospective study and review of the literature. *J Urol*. 1998;160:2115-2120.

32. Durup Scheel-Hincke J, Mortensen MB, Pless T, et al. Laparoscopic four-way ultrasound probe with histologic biopsy facility using a flexible tru-cut needle. *Surg Endosc*. 2000;14:867-869.

33. Wiersema MJ, Levy MJ, Harewood GC, et al. Initial experience with EUS-guided trucut needle biopsies of perigastric organs. *Gastrointest Endosc*. 2002;56:275-278.

34. Larghi A, Verna EC, Stavropoulos SN, et al. EUS-guided trucut needle biopsies in patients with solid pancreatic masses: a prospective study. *Gastrointest Endosc*. 2004;59:185-190.

35. Itoi T, Itokawa F, Sofuni A, et al. Puncture of solid pancreatic tumors guided by endoscopic ultrasonography: a pilot study series comparing Trucut and 19-gauge and 22-gauge aspiration needles. *Endoscopy*. 2005;37:362-366.

36. Storch I, Jorda M, Thurer R, et al. Advantage of EUS Trucut biopsy combined with fine-needle aspiration without immediate on-site cytopathologic examination. *Gastrointest Endosc*. 2006;64:505-511.

37. Wittmann J, Kocjan G, Sgouros SN, et al. Endoscopic ultrasound-guided tissue sampling by combined fine needle aspiration and trucut needle biopsy: a prospective study. *Cytopathology*. 2006;17:27-33.

38. Aithal GP, Anagnostopoulos GK, Tam W, et al. EUS-guided tissue sampling: comparison of "dual sampling" (Trucut biopsy plus FNA) with "sequential sampling" (Trucut biopsy and then FNA). *Endoscopy*. 2007;39:725-730.

39. Saftoiu A, Vilmann P, Guldhammer SB, et al. Endoscopic ultrasound (EUS)-guided Trucut biopsy adds significant information to EUS-guided fine-needle aspiration in selected patients: a prospective study. *Scand J Gastroenterol*. 2007;42:117-125.

40. Sakamoto H, Kitano M, Komaki T, et al. Prospective comparative study of the EUS guided 25-gauge FNA needle with the 19-gauge Trucut needle and 22-gauge FNA needle in patients with solid pancreatic masses. *J Gastroenterol Hepatol*. 2009;24:384-390.

41. Storch I, Shah M, Thurer R, et al. Endoscopic ultrasound-guided fine-needle aspiration and trucut biopsy in thoracic lesions: when tissue is the issue. *Surg Endosc*. 2008;22:86-90.

42. Berger LP, Scheffer RC, Weusten BL, et al. The additional value of EUS guided Tru-cut biopsy to EUS guided FNA in patients with mediastinal lesions. *Gastrointest Endosc*. 2009;69:1045-1051.

43. Dewitt J, McGreevy K, Cummings O, et al. Initial experience with EUS-guided Tru-cut biopsy of benign liver disease. *Gastrointest Endosc*. 2009;69:535-542.

44. Mizuno N, Bhatia V, Hosoda W, et al. Histological diagnosis of autoimmune pancreatitis using EUS-guided trucut biopsy: a comparison study with EUS-FNA. *J Gastroenterol*. 2009;44:742-750.

45. Polkowski M, Gerke W, Jarosz D, et al. Diagnostic yield and safety of endoscopic ultrasound-guided trucut biopsy in patients with gastric submucosal tumors: a prospective study. *Endoscopy*. 2009;41:329-334.

46. Wahnschaffe U, Ullrich R, Mayerle J, et al. EUS-guided Trucut needle biopsies as first-line diagnostic method for patients with intestinal or extraintestinal mass lesions. *Surg Endosc*. 2009;23:2351-2355.

47. DeWitt J, Emerson RE, Sherman S, et al. Endoscopic ultrasound-guided Trucut biopsy of gastrointestinal mesenchymal tumor. *Surg Endosc*. 2011;25:2192-2202.

48. Ribeiro A, Pereira D, Escalón MP, et al. EUS-guided biopsy for the diagnosis and classification of lymphoma. *Gastrointest Endosc.* 2010;71: 851-855.

49. Lee JH, Choi KD, Kim MY, et al. Clinical impact of EUS-guided Trucut biopsy results on decision making for patients with gastric subepithelial tumors ≥ 2 cm in diameter. *Gastrointest Endosc.* 2011;74:1010-1018.

50. Mohamadnejad M, Al-Haddad MA, Sherman S, et al. Utility of EUS-guided biopsy of extramural pelvic masses. *Gastrointest Endosc.* 2012;75:146-151.

51. Cho CM, Al-Haddad M, Leblanc JK, et al. Rescue endoscopic ultrasound (EUS)-guided Trucut biopsy following suboptimal EUS-guided fine needle aspiration for mediastinal Lesions. *Gut Liver.* 2013;7:150-156.

52. Iglesias-Garcia J, Dominguez-Munoz E, Lozano-Leon A, et al. Impact of endoscopic ultrasound-guided fine needle biopsy for diagnosis of pancreatic masses. *World J Gastroenterol.* 2007;13:289-293.

53. Gerke H, Rizk MK, Vanderheyden AD, et al. Randomized study comparing endoscopic ultrasound-guided Trucut biopsy and fine needle aspiration with high suction. *Cytopathology.* 2010;21:44-51.

54. Möller K, Papanikolaou IS, Toermer T, et al. EUS-guided FNA of solid pancreatic masses: high yield of 2 passes with combined histologic-cytologic analysis. *Gastrointest Endosc.* 2009;70:60-69.

55. Noda Y, Fujita N, Kobayashi G, et al. Diagnostic efficacy of the cellblock method in comparison with smear cytology of tissue samples obtained by endoscopic ultrasound-guided fine-needle aspiration. *J Gastroenterol.* 2010;45:868-875.

56. Yasuda I, Tsurumi H, Omar S, et al. Endoscopic ultrasound-guided fine needle aspiration biopsy for lymphadenopathy of unknown origin. *Endoscopy.* 2006;38:919-924.

57. Larghi A, Fuccio L, Chiarello G, et al. Fine-needle tissue acquisition from subepithelial lesions using a forward-viewing linear echoendoscope. *Endoscopy.* 2014;46:39-45.

58. Larghi A, Lococo F, Ricci R, et al. Pleural tuberculosis diagnosed by EUS-guided fine-needle tissue acquisition. *Gastrointest Endosc.* 2010;272: 1307-1309.

59. Larghi A, Lugli F, Sharma V, et al. Pancreatic metastases from a broncho-pulmonary carcinoid diagnosed by endoscopic ultrasonography-guided fine-needle tissue acquisition. *Pancreas.* 2012;41:502-504.

60. Bang JY, Magee SH, Ramesh J, et al. Randomized trial comparing fanning with standard technique for endoscopic ultrasound-guided fine-needle aspiration of solid pancreatic mass lesions. *Endoscopy.* 2013;45: 445-450.

61. Iwashita T, Yasuda I, Doi S, et al. The yield of endoscopic ultrasound-guided fine needle aspiration for histological diagnosis in patients suspected of stage I sarcoidosis. *Endoscopy.* 2008;40:400-405.

62. Eckardt AJ, Adler A, Gomes EM, et al. Endosonographic large-bore biopsy of gastric subepithelial tumors: a prospective multicenter study. *Eur J Gastroenterol Hepatol.* 2012;24:1135-1144.

63. Iwashita T, Yasuda I, Doi S, et al. Use of samples from endoscopic ultrasound-guided 19-gauge fine-needle aspiration in diagnosis of auto-immune pancreatitis. *Clin Gastroenterol Hepatol.* 2012;10:316-322.

64. Stavropoulos SN, Im GY, Jlayer Z, et al. High yield of same-session EUS-guided liver biopsy by 19-gauge FNA needle in patients undergoing EUS to exclude biliary obstruction. *Gastrointest Endosc.* 2012;75:310-318.

65. Varadarajulu S, Bang JY, Hebert-Magee S. Assessment of the technical performance of the flexible 19-gauge EUS-FNA needle. *Gastrointest Endosc.* 2012;76:336-343.

66. Yasuda I, Goto N, Tsurumi H, et al. Endoscopic ultrasound-guided fine needle aspiration biopsy for diagnosis of lymphoproliferative disorders: feasibility of immunohistological, flow cytometric, and cytogenetic assessments. *Am J Gastroenterol.* 2012;107:397-404.

67. Gor N, Salem SB, Jakate S, et al. Histological adequacy of EUS-guided liver biopsy when using a 19-gauge non-Tru-Cut FNA needle. *Gastrointest Endosc.* 2013;79:170-172.

68. Zamboni G, Lüttges J, Capelli P, et al. Histopathological features of diagnostic and clinical relevance in autoimmune pancreatitis: a study on 53 resection specimens and 9 biopsy specimens. *Virchows Arch.* 2004;445:552-563.

69. Scarpa A, Mantovani W, Capelli P, et al. Pancreatic endocrine tumors: improved TNM staging and histopathological grading permit a clinically efficient prognostic stratification of patients. *Mod Pathol.* 2010;23: 824-833.

70. Rindi G, Falconi M, Klersy C, et al. TNM staging of neoplasms of the endocrine pancreas: results from a large international cohort study. *J Natl Cancer Inst.* 2012;104:764-777.

71. Larghi A, Lecca PG, Ardito F, et al. Evaluation of hilar biliary strictures by using a newly developed forward-viewing therapeutic echoendoscope: preliminary results of an ongoing experience. *Gastrointest Endosc.* 2009;69:356-360.

72. Trevino JM, Varadarajulu S. Initial experience with the prototype forward-viewing echoendoscope for therapeutic interventions other than pancreatic pseudocyst drainage (with videos). *Gastrointest Endosc.* 2009;69:361-365.

73. Larghi A, Seerden TC, Galasso D, et al. EUS-guided therapeutic interventions for uncommon benign pancreaticobiliary disorders by using a newly developed forward-viewing echoendoscope (with videos). *Gastrointest Endosc.* 2010;72:213-215.

74. Corless CL, Barnett CM, Heinrich MC. Gastrointestinal stromal tumours: origin and molecular oncology. *Nat Rev Cancer.* 2011;11: 865-878.

75. Eisenberg BL, Smith KD. Adjuvant and neoadjuvant therapy for primary GIST. *Cancer Chemother Pharmacol.* 2011;67(suppl 1):S3-S8.

76. Itoi T, Tsuchiya T, Itokawa F, et al. Histological diagnosis by EUS-guided fine-needle aspiration biopsy in pancreatic solid masses without on-site cytopathologist: a single-center experience. *Dig Endosc.* 2011;23(suppl 1):34-38.

77. Bang JY, Ramesh J, Trevino J, et al. Objective assessment of an algorithmic approach to EUS-guided FNA and interventions. *Gastrointest Endosc.* 2013;77:739-744.

78. Iwashita T, Nakai Y, Samarasena JB, et al. Endoscopic ultrasound-guided fine needle aspiration and biopsy (EUS-FNAB) using a novel 25-gauge core biopsy needle: optimizing the yield of both cytology and histology. *Gastrointest Endosc.* 2012;75:AB183.

79. Petrone MC, Poley JW, Bonzini M, et al. Interobserver agreement among pathologists regarding core tissue specimens obtained with a new endoscopic ultrasound histology needle; a prospective multicentre study in 50 cases. *Histopathology.* 2013;62:602-608.

80. Witt BL, Adler DG, Hilden K, et al. A comparative needle study: EUS-FNA procedures using the HD ProCore(™) and EchoTip(®) 22-gauge needle types. *Diagn Cytopathol.* 2013;41:1069-1074.

81. Barresi L, Tarantino I, Traina M, et al. Endoscopic ultrasound-guided fine needle aspiration and biopsy using a 22-gauge needle with side fenestration in pancreatic cystic lesions. *Dig Liver Dis.* 2013;46:45-50.

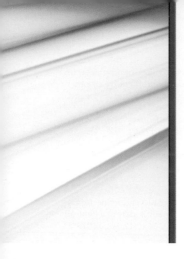

23

Cytology Primer for Endosonographers

Darshana Jhala • Nirag Jhala

Key Points

- Communication between the endosonographer and the cytopathologist is the key to a successful EUS FNA service.
- A cytopathology service should be involved early in the planning process for establishing an EUS-guided FNA service.
- Using an algorithmic approach to diagnosing a patient will facilitate a correct diagnosis.

Conceptual breakthroughs, based on developed theories, and discoveries in science bring accolades. Advances in the biotechnology field are signs of the dominance of creative imagination expressed through technology over abstract conceptual thinking. Despite such subtle differences in the concepts put forth, most clinicians involved in patient care agree that advances in the biomedical sciences have significantly broadened horizons and have redefined patient management.

The field of endoscopic ultrasonography (EUS)-guided fine-needle aspiration (FNA) should be viewed as no different. It could be said that the keystone events in the development of modern endosonography were the conceptualization and production of flexible endoscopes for human use in the late 1950s.[1] In the 1980s, ultrasound probes were attached to endoscopes, and Doppler imaging capability was introduced. These improvements allowed better visualization of lesions and an understanding of vascular flow. These powerful scopes could characterize lesions not only of the luminal gastrointestinal tract, but also of the gastrointestinal tract wall, the periluminal lymph nodes (intrathoracic and intra-abdominal), the pancreas, the liver (mostly the left side), the left kidney, the spleen, and the adrenal glands. The list continues to grow.[2–6] EUS imaging alone, however, may not be sufficient to differentiate neoplastic from non-neoplastic and a benign from malignant lesion.[7] Further advances in technology made since the early 1990s permit the performance of FNA under EUS guidance.[8,9] The ability to obtain cytologic material safely under real-time visualization makes this a powerful modality that offers an opportunity for prompt and accurate diagnosis and staging.

The outcome of the EUS FNA diagnosis depends on effective collaboration between the cytopathologist and endoscopist. The best results are achieved by those clinicians who really believe in cytology for their own patients and who work in close cooperation with cytologists. Thus, an understanding of relevant issues by both endosonographers and

cytopathologists involved in obtaining and interpreting cytologic specimens optimizes the diagnostic yield.[3,10] When such visions are synchronized, the diagnostic performance of EUS FNA far exceeds expectations.[11] As predicted earlier,[2] this technique has now become a standard of care at many institutions and continues to replace other modalities for tissue diagnoses, staging, and adequate management of patients.

The objective of this chapter is to help both endosonographers and cytopathologists to learn the technical aspects of cytology procedures and to understand the basic principles of interpretive cytopathology diagnosis. Thus, the chapter reviews pertinent technical aspects that may influence cytology interpretation and affect outcome. It also discusses the algorithmic approach and salient cytologic features of benign and malignant lesions commonly sampled by EUS FNA.

Technical Aspects of EUS That Improve Diagnostic Yield

Fundamental to the success of EUS FNA is the procurement of adequate cells to provide the most effective diagnosis. This requires careful planning and understanding of factors that can affect cellularity of the target lesion.

Preliminary Planning

Ideally, an interested pathologist should be involved in the development of the EUS FNA service from the earliest stages of the planning process. This includes such crucial factors as the location of the endosonography suite, the type of instrument and needle used, the personnel involved, the scheduling of FNA, the type of preparation, the transport medium, the need for immediate cytologic evaluation (ICE) for determination of adequacy and diagnosis, the need for performing ancillary studies, and the role of the procedure in the patient

TABLE 23-1

FACTORS TO CONSIDER IN PRELIMINARY PLANNING FOR CYTOLOGY SERVICES

Factor	Details
Type of biopsy	Needle core or cytology (fine needle)
Size of needle	25 G, 22 G, 19 G, or other
Fixation or processing for cores	Formalin, other
Type of preparation of cells for FNA	Direct smears, transport media (proprietary, culture media [RPMI-1640], formalin, other)
Type of smear	Air dried, alcohol fixed, or both
Personnel	GI suite staff, laboratory staff, training
Immediate cytologic assessment	Cytopathologist, cytotechnologist, advanced trainee, not performed
Database archives for cytology information	Diagnosis, number of passes, pathologist, type of smears prepared, cell block available, special studies

FNA, fine-needle aspiration; GI, gastrointestinal.

management algorithm (Table 23-1). Further planning should also involve ordering of supplies, stocking and provision of the FNA cart or cabinet, or maintenance of a permanent small space for supplies in the endoscopy suite area.

The type of tissue specimen preparation (direct smear, liquid-based cytologic preparation, cell block, core biopsy, or a combination) depends on institutional practice, staffing issues, and the physical distance between the pathologist and the endoscopy suite, in addition to the relative sensitivity, specificity, and diagnostic accuracy of the various choices. Developing adequate skills for accurate interpretation of EUS

samples not only depends on an experienced cytopathologist but may also require additional specific experience in interpreting these samples. Experience indicates that cytopathologists who are specifically interested in gastrointestinal diseases tend to be more effective in providing accurate diagnoses.[12]

For the pathologist and laboratory staff, a comprehensive understanding of their direct role in the EUS procedure and the patient care algorithm ensures appropriate support. Diagnostic strategies depend on whether the procedure is a screening test, a diagnostic test in a patient who may not undergo further diagnostic workup, or a test to procure material for performance of ancillary studies to enhance patient management decisions.

A further preliminary planning step is consideration of database archives of cytology and diagnostic data. In combination with the EUS characteristics of lesions and other clinical information, these data can provide valuable feedback regarding diagnostic accuracy, individual practitioner competency, utility of ICE, and other quality assurance measures.

Professional staff should be properly trained and should understand the limitations of their expertise and of the technique. In the United States, both the technical and the interpretive services in the cytology laboratory are regulated at state and federal levels by the provisions of the Clinical Laboratory Improvement Amendments of 1988 (CLIA 1988), the Laboratory Accreditation Program of the College of American Pathologists (CAP), and others. Such mandatory and voluntary standards ensure high-quality laboratories.

The following sections discuss technical factors that may improve diagnostic yield for EUS biopsy procedures, including needle type and size, suction or "capillary" aspiration, number of passes, and direction of passes. These factors are listed in Table 23-2.

Fine-Needle Aspirates

Fine-needle biopsies are used widely for EUS, computed tomography (CT), and other image-guided biopsy techniques,

TABLE 23-2

TECHNICAL ASPECTS THAT MAY POSITIVELY INFLUENCE DIAGNOSTIC YIELD

Technical Feature	Advantage	Disadvantage
Preliminary planning	Optimal laboratory support	None
Endoscopist skill	More likely to procure adequate specimen	None
Pathologist skill	Few if any false-positive or "atypical" diagnoses	None
Core biopsy	Histologic diagnosis	Possible more tissue injury
	Tissue for special stains	No capacity for on-site evaluation for adequacy
	Does not require on-site laboratory personnel for specimen processing or evaluation	
Aspiration biopsy	More cells	Few disadvantages
		Risk of inadequate sample for some lesions or sites
Smaller needle size	Less tissue injury	Relatively fewer cells
Suction	Retrieves more cells	Increases bleeding in tissue
		May compromise some cell features
More passes	More cells	Injury to tissue
Cytopathologist in room	Specimens adequate for diagnosis	Time and cost
Air-dried and alcohol-fixed smears	Complementary stains yield optimal nuclear and cytologic detail	Increased technical effort required
Cell block	Tissue available for special stains	Not a stand-alone preparation; best in combination with smears

as well as for percutaneous biopsies of palpable masses. The material contained within a fine needle is usually smeared onto slides, and the resulting monolayer of cells is fixed or dried and stained. Material obtained from a fine needle is generally dispersed as single and small groups of cells, rather than intact tissue cores. Because the preparation is not sectioned, the cells represented on an aspirate smear are intact, and they round up or splay out depending on how they are treated in further processing steps. The monolayer smear created from a fine-needle biopsy allows resolution of microarchitecture and of details of the nucleus and cytoplasm that is superior to many other modalities.

Choice of Needles

Fine-needle biopsies are defined as being performed with a 22-G or smaller needle. Varying sizes of EUS instruments and needles are available on the market, and the choice of needle may also influence cytology findings. The cutting edge of the needle plays a role in obtaining samples; for example, a beveled edge requires less force in comparison with circular edges. Similarly, needle sizes also have an impact on the procurement of tissue samples. In current practice, EUS needles range from 19 G to 25 G.[13–15] Contrary to intuitive thinking that larger size is always better for FNA samples, sometimes the smaller-bore needle provides better sampling.

Several prospective studies and meta-analysis of published literature have been attempted to determine the impact on cell yield and diagnostic performance of samples obtained by the various EUS FNA needle types.[14–18] Some of these investigators suggested that needle aspirates from 25-G needles provide less hypocellular or acellular and bloody specimens, have better diagnostic performance, and perhaps induce less tissue injury in comparison with samples from a 22-G needle.[14,15,19] Other investigators, however, could not independently confirm this finding and found either no or minimal difference between 22-G and 25-G needles with regard to the ability to render a diagnosis.[13,17,20]

FNA samples are also increasingly used for ancillary studies. In a study designed to determine the optimum needle size and number of passes to obtain material for RNA quantitation, the number of cells obtained from needles of varying sizes was counted. With 10 needle excursions into a tumor, 32,000 cells were obtained with a 25-G needle.[21] Although large numbers of cells are important for some tests, such as RNA extraction, it is generally accepted that diagnoses can be made on smears containing fewer than 100 cells. Investigators have suggested that a larger needle (e.g., 22 G) may be useful for lesions associated with less risk of complication or that require large numbers of cells for classification. Unraveling of underlying molecular targets that may affect diagnosis, prognosis, or therapeutic predictions are increasingly being characterized. This has resulted in increased utilization of small tissue samples in performance of molecular tests such as fluorescence in situ hybridization (FISH) analysis, pyrosequencing, and newer platforms to generate genetic profiles utilizing techniques such as next-generation sequencing.[22–24] As a unique technique, the authors have also de-stained Diff-Quik–stained smears and performed FISH analysis to detect specific chromosomal translocations in lymphomas to improve diagnostic performance.[25] This method has the clear advantage of making a morphologic determination and then using the same cells for detection of characteristic chromosomal translocations to clinch the diagnosis.

Given the tradeoff between more cells and more complications with larger fine needles, the choice of needle size should be based on the site and type of lesion to be aspirated. Indications for a smaller needle (e.g., 25 G) include patients with coagulopathy, organs in which leakage of fluid or air may occur, organs in which tissue trauma may increase complications (e.g., pancreas), and vascular organs or lesions. A smaller needle size decreases potential complications such as bleeding into the tissue and hemodilution or obscuring of the cytology sample by excessive blood. Smaller needles also cause less tissue damage and thus possibly less risk of pancreatitis.

Needle Core Biopsy versus Fine-Needle Aspiration

For numerous reasons some clinicians and pathologists believe that a tissue core yields unequivocally better diagnostic material. This belief perhaps stems from the concept that tissue cores will result in adequate samples with fewer needle passes, they do not involve on-site specimen assessment, they provide architecture, and ancillary studies can be performed on these samples.[11,26–28] It is also true that needle core biopsies (14 G to 19 G) have been used for a long time to obtain tissue samples. Sections made from these core biopsies are thin, 3- to 5-μm slices of the tissue that, when stained and viewed microscopically, show cells or portions of cells within their intact tissue stroma. Most histopathologists are very familiar with this method of tissue-based assessment.

Conversely, however, one should also be aware that analysis of tissue core may not always provide adequate diagnostic clues. Tru-Cut biopsy also induces greater tissue injury than a fine-needle biopsy and is considered more invasive. Such considerations should deter clinicians from using large-bore Tru-Cut needles routinely. It is also true that needle core biopsies can pose greater challenges for diagnosing well-differentiated carcinomas of the pancreas in comparison with FNA samples. In preliminary analyses, the success of FNA sampling using EUS guidance led to a sharp decline in performance of percutaneous needle core biopsies and CT-guided FNA. Such a change dramatically altered practice management decisions for pancreatic neoplasms.

A possible explanation for the failure of core needles to sample the lesion may be the attributes of the lesion itself, given that a larger needle may deflect from the surface of a firm or rubbery lesion. In addition, a Tru-Cut biopsy represents a single pass into the tissue and is not able to sample the lesion widely without further passes into the tissue. The use of larger needles increases the risk of bleeding and complications, although these risks remain very low. In addition, technical limitations of the currently available EUS-guided Tru-Cut biopsy equipment limit the anatomic regions that can be sampled for biopsy successfully.

Although studies of the pancreas show mixed results, the use of EUS-guided Tru-Cut biopsies showed significant promise in a review of lymphadenopathy. Tru-Cut biopsy is useful not only to establish the diagnosis of lymphoma but also to characterize cellular architecture, which is more important in disorders such as follicular center cell lymphomas. Tru-Cut biopsy also may be more useful in cases in which flow cytometry results can provide false-negative results, such as large B-cell lymphomas.[25] EUS-guided Tru-Cut biopsy may also be helpful in establishing the difficult diagnosis of Hodgkin lymphoma in which morphology is varied and often challenging to identify.

The decision to obtain cores instead of, or in addition to, aspirates rests on certain factors, including the available equipment and personnel, the training and expertise of the pathologists and staff, and the endoscopist's preference. Each type of biopsy has advantages and disadvantages that must be considered for individual lesions or patients. Overall, FNA is considered a more sensitive diagnostic method, and it can be complemented by core biopsy or cell block.

To Apply or Not to Apply Suction

For many fine-needle biopsies, suction is applied to the needle to attempt to increase cell yield. This is the origin of the term *fine-needle aspirate,* which is often used more generally for any fine-needle biopsy. The purpose of suction is not to draw cells into the needle, but rather to "hole" the tissue against the cutting edge of the needle. Suction should be turned off before the needle is withdrawn.

In another technique, the cells are obtained without applying suction. The lumen is filled with cells by the direct cutting action of the needle through the tissue or capillary action. A study of 670 superficial and deep lesions sampled by biopsy with a fine needle without suction showed that diagnostic material was obtained in more than 90% of the cases.[29] Specific to EUS FNA, a study by Wallace and colleagues[30] found no difference in suction versus no suction in terms of overall diagnostic yield for lymph nodes, but these investigators noted excess blood in the specimens to which suction was applied. Another study demonstrated that EUS-guided fine-needle sampling with suction increased the number of slides (17.8 ± 7.1 slides) needed to be prepared as compared with a significantly ($p < 0.0001$) reduced number of slides to be prepared for samples in which no suction was applied.[31]

In general, applying suction to the needle increases cellular yield but potentially increases artifact and blood, especially in vascular organs and lesions. Suction is commonly used because the increased cellular yield of specimens often outweighs the disadvantages. Some clinicians attempt up to three passes without suction and add further passes with suction if the cellular yield is low. While no suction improves analysis, the choice to use or not to use suction should be dictated by the type of lesion.[32]

When a large amount of blood is aspirated and the specimen clots, a less desirable but useful salvage of material is with gentle microdissection of the clot or fragment with a small scalpel blade or separate needle tip. The fragments are then lifted from the slide and are placed in formalin for subsequent cell block preparation. Forceful smearing of the clot to disperse the cells may cause significant crush artifact and may render the cells uninterruptible.

Number of Passes

A pass usually comprises 10 or more needle excursions or movements of the needle to-and-fro once the needle is within the lesion. The number of passes needed to obtain diagnostic material depends on multiple factors, including experience of the endosonographer, location of the lesion, type of lesion, cellularity of the lesion, and risk of complications. Many investigators suggest that after a certain number of passes, the procedure reaches a state of diminishing returns for obtaining diagnostic cellularity.

In our early analysis of more than 204 cases, diagnostic cellularity was obtained after five passes in more than 90% of cases. It also emerged in this study that the rate of diminishing returns was reached earlier for lymph nodes and later for the pancreas. For solid pancreatic lesions, adequate cellularity was achieved with fewer numbers of passes when the lesion was smaller (≤25 mm) compared with larger lesions.[33] This study also demonstrated that after five passes, lymph nodes offered little benefit in obtaining diagnostic cells. It was also evident that for lymph nodes, a mean of only three passes was needed for obtaining diagnostic cellularity. LeBlanc and colleagues determined that at least seven passes were needed in pancreatic lesions to obtain a sensitivity and specificity of 83% and 100%, respectively, although only five passes were needed in lymph node aspirates for a respective sensitivity and specificity of 77% and 100%.[34] In recent years, better technique and understanding has led to reduction in the number of passes needed to procure adequate diagnostic cellularity.

A well-known advantage of real-time image-guided biopsies, especially EUS, is the ability to direct the needle to a small point of interest. Selection of the exact site of biopsy may influence the cytologic yield. Biopsy of the necrotic center of a tumor may be nondiagnostic, whereas the edge may contain viable tumor cells. Conversely, biopsy of the edge of a pancreatic carcinoma may show only chronic pancreatitis, a common reactive change in the surrounding pancreatic tissue.

Depending on the anatomic site, directing the needle to specific portions of the lesion may be advantageous. Metastatic tumor in lymph nodes may be histologically more apparent in the subcapsular sinus, but in lymph node aspirates evaluated by EUS FNA, aspiration of the edge of the node did not increase the likelihood of a correct diagnosis. Nonetheless, because EUS allows visualization of the lesion, biopsy of a necrotic area can be avoided, and, as discussed later, on-site evaluation of the specimen can provide guidance to another location if the first site is necrotic.

A main advantage of the FNA technique is the wide sampling of a lesion by maneuvering the needle in different directions with each back-and-forth movement. Small redirections of the needle to make a fan shape will result in sampling of new areas of the lesion each time. Utilization of the fanning technique as described in Chapter 21 in comparison to the standard multiple pass technique to obtain cells helps reduce the number of passes and improves diagnostic cellularity rates.[35] Repeated needle excursions in the same direction, along the same needle tract, result in biopsy of the blood or fluid that can fill the area with blood.

Immediate Cytologic Evaluation

One way to ensure adequate material from an FNA procedure is the use of ICE (Video 23-1). The goal of ICE is to provide real-time feedback about the content and quality of the smears, to reduce the number of nondiagnostic or atypical biopsies, and to maximize the efficiency of the procedure. We as well as other investigators have demonstrated that ICE yields increased highly reliable preliminary diagnosis and will

Video 23-1. Video of on-site processing of specimen procured by EUS-guided FNA.

also help triage the specimen for performing ancillary studies.[36] Other investigators have demonstrated that specimen adequacy is more than 90% when a cytopathologist is present in the endoscopy suite for ICE.[33] Such high specimen adequacy rates drop when cytopathologists are not present in the endoscopy suite for ICE.[37] In a direct comparison of EUS FNA procedures performed by the same endoscopist at two institutions, with and without a pathologist present during the procedure, ICE was more likely to result in a definitive diagnosis and less likely to involve an inadequate specimen.[37] Most false-negative EUS results are caused by inadequate sampling, which may necessitate a second procedure. It is also true that the most effective way to reduce sampling error is ICE.

A retrospective analysis was conducted of changes noted after the transition from CT-guided FNA to EUS-guided FNA sampling from the pancreas. Cytopathologists were present to provide ICE in an endoscopy suite, whereas this practice was not in place for samples obtained under CT guidance. The results demonstrated that EUS FNA provided more definitive diagnoses and fewer unsatisfactory or equivocal diagnoses. The investigators were also able to procure additional samples for ancillary studies. Such efforts at other institutions have also seen greater than 90% specimen adequacy rates and reductions in equivocal diagnosis. When ICE is performed, selected air-dried slides are stained in the endoscopy suite or an adjacent room and are reviewed immediately by the pathologist, so that feedback can be given to the endoscopist regarding the adequacy of the pass. If diagnostic material is present, additional passes are not made, and the procedure is stopped. If the smears are nondiagnostic, further passes are made. If there are no cells or only necrosis, the needle can be redirected for the next pass, and the procedure can be continued until adequate material for diagnosis is obtained.

In addition to minimizing the number of passes needed to obtain diagnostic material, another advantage of ICE is the triage of specimens for special studies. Such a practice may allow procurement of samples for ancillary studies such as lymphoma workup or for cell block when the initial smears show a tumor that may need classification by immune histochemistry, in situ hybridization, or other studies for better patient management. Thus, obtaining additional directed passes is encouraged for making an adequate cell block.

Although ICE clearly improves diagnostic yield, this practice is variable throughout the world. The use of ICE is influenced by the physical location of the laboratory and gastrointestinal suite, personnel, and cost issues. Reluctance of a pathologist to attend EUS FNA procedures may relate to lack of time and inadequate reimbursement for the time investment required.

Unfortunately, however, lack of will on the part of consumers of these services has not helped to change the conventional stance on reimbursements in the United States. Instead, the reimbursement rates are increasingly becoming more cost prohibitive. All institutions and regions of any country are different, and they need to develop their own cost-effective strategies for the sake of providing optimal health care for their patients.

In an attempt to minimize the impact of the lack of ICE, different investigators, with variable success, have investigated alternatives. These alternatives include assessment of cellularity by visual inspection, performance of smears and evaluation by endosonography personnel, and the use of services of advanced cytotechnologists following adequate training[38,39] or advanced trainees in cytopathology. In this context, the use of dynamic telecytology for adequacy assessment was also investigated.[40–42]

Regardless of whether ICE is used or not, an adequate sample is the foundation of the diagnosis. The needle must be placed into the lesion, and the technical aspects of the sampling must be optimized to obtain cells for evaluation, and the smears must be free of crush, drying, staining, or other artifact and obscuring blood, inflammation, or necrosis.

Factors Associated with Improved Cytologic Preparation

The material from EUS-guided biopsy can be prepared in many different ways, each of which has advantages and disadvantages. Some preparations are complementary, and two or three types are often prepared from the same biopsy specimen. The following sections define preparation of air-dried and alcohol-fixed smears, cell block, and the stains used for highlighting various cell features.

Cytology Smears and Cell Block

A smear slide is the standard method of preparing cells obtained from a fine-needle biopsy for viewing. As in a blood smear, the biopsy material is dispersed or "smeared" onto a glass slide, stained, and viewed as individual cells. For EUS FNA, after the needle is removed from the endoscope, the tip is placed near the frosted end of a labeled slide, and a single small drop is expressed onto the slide by slowly advancing the stylet into the needle. Dropping the material from a distance, squirting, or spraying it onto the slide can result in drying of the specimen and unwanted artifact. A second slide is then drawn over the drop of material, to pull the material into a monolayer. The technique requires practice. If the smear is too thick, the cells are obscured by one another or by background cells; if too much pressure is applied, the cells are artificially disrupted from their normal microarchitecture or are lysed. Imperfect smears may reduce the diagnostic yield.

In contrast to smears, a cell block is a preparation in which the cells are placed into a liquid medium or fixative, transported to the laboratory, spun into a pellet, formalin fixed, paraffin embedded, and selected for standard hematoxylin and eosin (H&E) staining. This routine formalin fixation and paraffin embedding is not optimal for preserving cytologic detail. A cell block is often made from leftover material rinsed from the needle. Its value as an adjunct to diagnosis can improve if an additional directed pass is obtained at the end of the procedure. This technique is highly recommended, especially for lesions that may require special stains.

Air-Dried or Alcohol-Fixed Smears

Generally, smears prepared from FNA material are either air dried or alcohol fixed. Air-dried smears are stained rapidly (using a modified Romanowsky stain [e.g., Diff-Quik]) and are typically used for ICE. Some institutions use H&E or rapid Papanicolaou (Pap) stains for ICE.

Diff-Quik–stained, air-dried smear preparations highlight intracytoplasmic material and extracellular substances. Alcohol fixation causes cells to shrink and round up but it preserves nuclear features and is followed by Pap or H&E staining. The Pap stain highlights nuclear detail and chromatin quality, as well as demonstrating keratinization of squamous cells. The cytoplasm appears more transparent in Pap-stained slides. Slides can be fixed in preparation for a Pap stain by immersing or spraying them with alcohol. The Pap and Diff-Quik stains are complementary, and optimal cytologic detail is provided when both alcohol-fixed and air-dried smears are prepared from the FNA.

Transport Media and Liquid-Based Preparations

Samples are frequently collected in transport media for subsequent preparations. Although many media are available, Hank's balanced salt solution is preferred. This medium allows for preparation of cytospins and cell blocks, and should one require lymphoma consideration later, this medium can also be used for flow cytometric analysis. For consideration of any lymphoma workup, many institutions also collect their samples in RPMI 1640. This is also a useful medium to collect for cytogenetic analysis, as well as gene rearrangement studies.

Liquid-based cytology is increasingly being investigated. Currently, two methods have been approved by the Food and Drug Administration: ThinPrep (Cytyc Co, Marlborough, MA) and SurePath (TriPath Inc, Burlington, NC). There are slight differences between the two methods but both offer advantages of monolayer cell dispersion, elimination of obscuring mucus and blood, and consistent cell preparation without artifacts of preparation, as noted with smear preparations.

These techniques, however, increase the cost of preparation and cannot be used for ICE. Because the preparations may disaggregate cells (loss of architecture) and alter some cytologic details, they offer challenges to interpretation. Some of the proprietary liquid fixatives contain methanol, a coagulative fixative (rather than a protein cross-linking fixative such as formalin), which may lead to suboptimal fixation for immunohistochemistry. Liquid-based cytology preparations do not fare as well as direct smear preparations. However, liquid-based cytology offers a viable alternative when ICE is not a consideration. Samples from pancreas prepared using liquid-based cytology preparations demonstrated smaller cell clusters, smaller cell size in comparison with air-dried smears, better nuclear characteristics, and diminished or absent mucin. Furthermore, these samples could not be used at a later time for flow cytometry analysis. Such considerations

should be taken into account during selection of transport media and preparations. A detailed model of an optimized EUS FNA procedure is shown in Table 23-3.

Cytology Interpretation

Evaluation of the biopsy begins the moment material is expressed from the needle onto a slide or into a fixative. An adequate aspirate, or one that is likely to yield a diagnosis, is cellular, so that when placed on the slides and smeared out, a finely granular quality is apparent. In contrast, in a hypocellular or purely bloody smear, the thin sheen of material is smooth. When the material is placed in fixative, visible particulate matter or cloudiness is usually present. Mucus, pus, and necrosis may also be grossly apparent.

Adequacy

Once under the microscope, the smear is first assessed for adequacy. For an aspirate to be interpretable, it must be free of technical artifacts and must contain cells for evaluation. A global assessment of cellularity as a measure of adequacy, however, may be misleading in FNA, because the number of cells relates to the lesion. For example, aspiration of neuroendocrine tumors usually yields highly cellular smears, whereas aspiration of a gastrointestinal stromal tumor (GIST) may yield few cells but both may be equally adequate for diagnosis.

For diagnostic nongynecologic cytology specimens, a sample is adequate when it explains the clinical situation or target lesion. The aspirator must be certain that the lesion has been sampled, and the pathologist must be able to interpret the slides. The concept of the "triple test" is also applicable to EUS FNA. The clinical, imaging, and FNA findings should agree and correlate on whether the lesion is benign or malignant. Some lesions have characteristic morphologic features, and therefore a cell number criterion for such tumors is not a requirement.

Diagnostic Evaluation of the Slide

Whether on-site or in the laboratory, the cytotechnologist or pathologist begins the slide evaluation by assessing the cell types, cell arrangement, and cellular features on the smear. Central to a cytology diagnosis is the appearance of the nuclear and cytoplasmic features of individual cells; these are quite distinct, depending on the lesion sampled. No single feature is diagnostic of malignancy, but rather the composite picture of cell type, microarchitecture, and nuclear and cytoplasmic characteristics determines the diagnosis. It is useful to know the common pathologic diagnoses as well as the characteristic of the normal tissue in the region sampled (Table 23-4 and Figure 23-1).

As in histologic sections, order and aesthetics reign in cytologic preparations of benign tissue. The appearance and composition of a benign aspirate reflect the various cell populations in normal tissue. Epithelial cells are round to oval, have moderate to abundant cytoplasm, and are cohesive. Benign epithelial cells show evidence of differentiation. Squamous cells acquire keratin as they mature, whereas their nuclei become progressively smaller and darker (pyknotic). A benign superficial squamous cell exfoliated from the esophagus has a large, polyhedral shape, with a small, uniformly

TABLE 23-3

OPTIMIZED EUS FINE-NEEDLE ASPIRATION MODEL TECHNIQUE

Stage	Description
Preparation	When the procedure is scheduled, arrangements are made for the cytology technician and pathologist to be at the site. Clinical findings are discussed with the pathologist at the start of the procedure. The locations of the lesions or other details must be known, based on previous imaging studies. Conscious sedation is provided to the patient with intravenous meperidine and midazolam.
Needle preparation	The stylet is removed completely from a 22-G EUS FNA needle, and the needle is flushed with heparin. Air is then flushed through the needle to expel the excess heparin. The stylet is replaced, and the needle is ready for use. The needle may also be straightened manually between passes if necessary.
Radial EUS	A radial echoendoscope is first used for an overview of appropriate anatomic landmarks. The location of lesions is noted.
Linear array EUS FNA	The radial echoendoscope is replaced with a linear array echoendoscope. The scope is advanced to the distance at which the lesion of interest was identified with radial endosonography. The lesion is visualized, and color Doppler is used if there is concern about intervening blood vessels. The EUS FNA needle is inserted and fastened to the biopsy channel of the echoendoscope, and then it is advanced just slightly beyond the scope into the gut lumen. At this point, the stylet is retracted approximately 1 cm. The needle is passed into the lesion. The stylet is replaced into the needle to expel any tissue from normal structures and then is removed completely, and a suction syringe is attached. Sampling is performed with and without suction. The needle is moved into various locations throughout the lesion ("fanning the lesion") to improve sampling. After approximately 20 back-and-forth movements, the suction is turned off, the needle is retracted back into the catheter, and the entire assembly is removed.
Expressing material on slide	A dedicated cytology technician holds the end of the catheter over a labeled glass slide. The needle is advanced approximately 1 cm from the catheter by the endoscopy technician, and a stylet is slowly advanced back into the needle. This produces a controlled passage of drops of material out from the tip. The cytology technician alternately places drops onto a slide and into transport medium. Finally, the needle is flushed with a few milliliters of saline and then air to expel any remaining material into the liquid medium.
Preparing and staining cytologic material	Slides are prepared depending on the amount of material. As rapidly as possible, the drops of aspirated material are spread downward onto the slides by using another clean glass slide. Half of the slides are air dried, and the remaining slides are immediately immersed in 95% ethyl alcohol for later Papanicolaou staining. The air-dried slides are stained with Diff-Quik stain for immediate cytologic evaluation by the pathologist (see later in the chapter). When the procedure is finished, an additional dedicated pass may be placed in transport medium (e.g., Hank's balanced salt solution) and transported to the laboratory, and a cell block is prepared. The material in cell suspension is centrifuged into a pellet, to which thrombin is added. The pellet is resuspended, and the resulting clot is removed, wrapped in lens paper, placed in a tissue cassette, fixed in formalin, and routinely processed for paraffin embedding and H&E or immunostaining. If indicated, material for flow cytometric immunophenotyping or other studies is removed from the medium, and the cell block is prepared. The alcohol-fixed slides are stained with a standard Papanicolaou stain.
Immediate cytologic evaluation	A pathologist, advanced trainee, or experienced cytotechnologist examines air-dried Diff-Quik–stained slides prepared at the site and provides assessment of specimen adequacy. Based on this report, the endoscopist may continue with the same technique or may change needle position to procure more tissue. Immediate cytologic evaluation also helps triage the specimen or obtain additional passes for special studies.

FNA, fine-needle aspiration; H&E, hematoxylin and eosin.

TABLE 23-4

SOME COMMON EUS CYTOLOGIC DIAGNOSES IN SPECIFIC SITES

Site	Cytologic Diagnoses
Lung	Adenocarcinoma, squamous carcinoma, small cell carcinoma, granuloma or infection
Esophagus	Squamous carcinoma, adenocarcinoma, granular cell tumors, leiomyoma or other spindle cell tumors (GIST or neurofibroma)
Stomach	Carcinoma, carcinoid, GIST, MALT lymphoma
Pancreas	Ductal adenocarcinoma, chronic pancreatitis, autoimmune pancreatitis, pancreatic endocrine neoplasm, metastatic carcinoma, intraductal papillary mucinous neoplasm, mucinous cystic neoplasm, solid pseudopapillary tumor
Rectum and perirectal lymph nodes	Metastatic adenocarcinoma or squamous carcinoma, GIST
Liver	Metastatic carcinoma, melanoma, sarcoma, lymphoma, primary hepatocellular tumors

GIST, gastrointestinal stromal tumor; MALT, mucosa-associated lymphoid tissue.

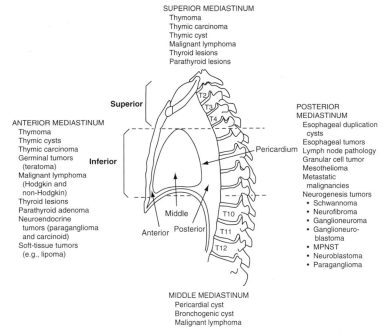

SUPERIOR MEDIASTINUM
Thymoma
Thymic carcinoma
Thymic cyst
Malignant lymphoma
Thyroid lesions
Parathyroid lesions

Superior

POSTERIOR
MEDIASTINUM
Esophageal duplication
  cysts
Esophageal tumors
Lymph node pathology
Granular cell tumor
Mesothelioma
Metastatic
  malignancies
Neurogenesis tumors
 • Schwannoma
 • Neurofibroma
 • Ganglioneuroma
 • Ganglioneuro-
   blastoma
 • MPNST
 • Neuroblastoma
 • Paraganglioma

ANTERIOR MEDIASTINUM
Thymoma
Thymic cysts
Thymic carcinoma
Germinal tumors
  (teratoma)
Malignant lymphoma
  (Hodgkin and
  non-Hodgkin)
Thyroid lesions
Parathyroid adenoma
Neuroendocrine
  tumors (paraganglioma
  and carcinoid)
Soft-tissue tumors
  (e.g., lipoma)

Inferior

Pericardium

Middle

Anterior Posterior

MIDDLE MEDIASTINUM
Pericardial cyst
Bronchogenic cyst
Malignant lymphoma

FIGURE 23-1 Common lesions of the mediastinum. MPNST, malignant peripheral nerve sheath tumor.

dark, nucleus described as an "ink dot" (Figure 23-2). The cytoplasm is orange-pink to blue, depending on the degree of keratin accumulation. Benign, mature squamous cells appear single, unless they are from the deeper layers of the epithelium, in which case they may remain together as large sheets of cells with less keratinization of the cytoplasm. Benign glandular epithelium from the stomach (Figure 23-3), intestine, and pancreas also demonstrates an orderly arrangement of differentiated cells with organ-specific variations. In smears, duodenal epithelium consists of folded or draped sheets of columnar cells, with interspersed goblet cells appearing as clear spaces among the absorptive cells (Figure 23-4). Glandular cells are polarized, with the nucleus present at one end of each cell in the sheet of epithelium. The cytoplasm may be filled with a single mucin droplet (the goblet cell), smaller more finely divided vacuoles, or other secretory products such as zymogen granules. Classically, benign columnar

epithelium has a honeycomb pattern. Changing the microscope plane to focus reveals the hexagonal borders of the apical cytoplasm and polarized, orderly nuclei at the base of the honeycomb sheet. In contrast, benign stromal or mesenchymal cells have elongated nuclei and usually abundant cytoplasm. Occasionally, small vascular structures are visible in smears of benign tissue.

The cells represented in an aspirate of normal tissue are proportionate to their mixture in the organ. For example, benign pancreatic tissue is composed mostly of acini, with relatively few ductal structures (see Figure 23-5) and islets usually represented on FNA smears. A benign reactive lymph node (Figure 23-6) contains a polymorphic mixture of cell types, with large and small lymphocytes, macrophages, and sometimes identifiable germinal centers, whereas lymphoid malignancy is usually monomorphic. In contrast to the order inherent in benign tissue, malignant cells deviate in their

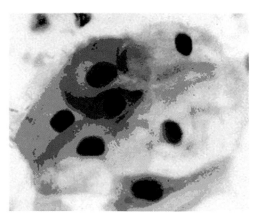

FIGURE 23-2 Sample from the esophageal squamous mucosa showing polygonal cells with abundant hard cytoplasm with hyperchromatic nuclei. Squamous cells also show maturation, as evidenced by keratinization.

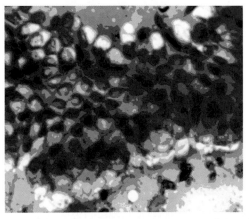

FIGURE 23-3 Smears from the gastric mucosa reveal foveolar cells with cohesive cell groups with minimal overlapping. The cells show a columnar shape with nuclei lined at the base. They also show a round, regular nuclear membrane and inconspicuous nucleoli, if any (Diff-Quik stain; magnification ×20).

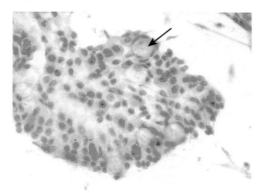

FIGURE 23-4 Smear reveals a cohesive two-dimensional group of epithelial cells with a honeycomb appearance. The group also reveals interspersed goblet cells *(arrow)* consistent with surface duodenal mucosal cells (Papanicolaou stain; magnification ×40).

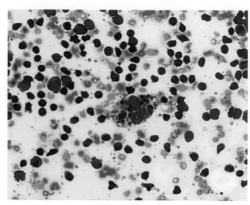

FIGURE 23-6 EUS fine-needle aspiration from a reactive mediastinal lymph node reveals many lymphocytes of varying sizes. Tingible body macrophages are also noted (Diff-Quik stain; magnification ×20).

organization and demonstrate predictable unpredictability in architecture.

Normal epithelial cells exhibit cohesion, whereas malignant epithelial cells are loosely aggregated or single cells. The degree of dyshesion is relative and is an important criterion in the overall assessment of malignancy. In contrast to epithelial cells, some tissue types are normally dyshesive. Unlike carcinomas, which reveal cohesive cell clusters and many single cells, FNA from noncarcinoid tumors and melanoma are usually noted as single cells. An overzealous smearing technique may artificially separate epithelial cells and may lead to overestimation of dyshesion.

Malignant cells also exhibit disorganization of their normal arrangement of polarity. The loss of polarity is a particular diagnostic feature in lesions arising in columnar epithelium. An important EUS FNA example is the diagnosis of atypia or malignancy in mucinous neoplasms. Once the low-power assessment of the general characteristic of the smear has been evaluated for cell types, overall organization, cohesion, and

detailed analysis of the nucleus and cytoplasm allow characterization of a cell as benign or malignant. Specific nuclear features determine malignancy, whereas cytoplasmic features and microarchitecture demonstrate differentiation of the cell.

EUS Fine-Needle Aspiration of Specific Sites

The usefulness of EUS FNA in various organ systems and the associated pitfalls in diagnostic interpretation are discussed in the following sections.

Pancreas

EUS is, in itself, a highly effective modality for detecting, staging, and determining respectability of pancreatic carcinomas. FNA was documented to be as accurate as frozen section diagnosis and is less invasive, faster, and more cost effective for the diagnosis of both resectable as well as nonresectable pancreatic carcinomas. Investigators also showed that EUS FNA is better than percutaneous FNA for obtaining accurate preoperative diagnosis. The objectives of EUS FNA of lesions of the pancreas are to obtain the initial diagnosis of a clinically suspicious malignant neoplasm, to obviate the need for surgery for the purpose of obtaining tissue for diagnosis, and to obtain tissue confirmation of the diagnosis before surgical resection with curative intent or initiating adjuvant chemotherapy. As a result, this modality has now found its rightful place as a preferred technique for obtaining tissue diagnosis and confirmation by the members of the National Comprehensive Cancer Network.

Global Approach to Diagnosis

An algorithmic morphology-based approach to the diagnosis of pancreatic FNA may result in a better diagnostic workup and determine the need for additional ancillary studies to confirm and support the diagnosis (Figure 23-7). What treating clinicians want to know from a cytologist is whether a given lesion is benign or malignant. This determination and the associated differential diagnosis generally rest on the imaging characteristics of the lesion (solid versus cystic pancreatic lesion).

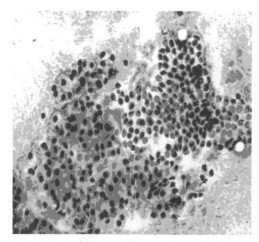

FIGURE 23-5 Smear from EUS fine-needle aspiration of pancreas reveals many acini and ductal cells. Acinar cells show moderate granular and two-toned amphophilic cytoplasm. The nuclei are centrally placed with a round, regular nuclear membrane. In comparison, the smear also reveals ductal epithelial cells. These cells show a cohesive two-dimensional honeycomb group of ductal epithelial cells. These cells reveal clear, well-demarcated cytoplasm (Diff-Quik stain; magnification ×20).

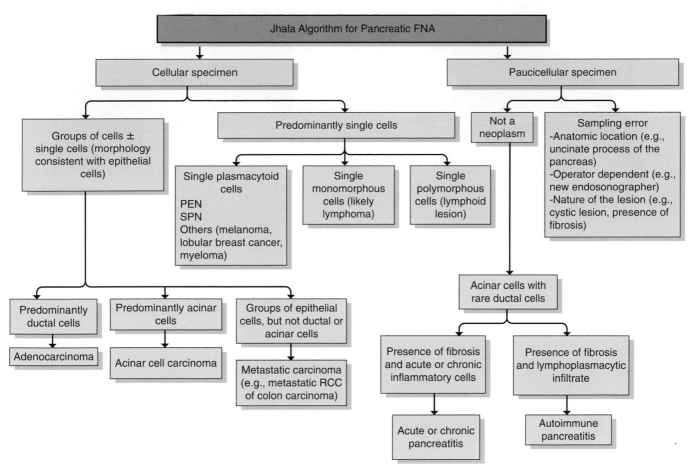

FIGURE 23-7 Morphology-based practical algorithm approach to pancreatic fine-needle aspiration (FNA). PEN, pancreatic endocrine neoplasm; RCC, renal cell carcinoma; SPN, solid pseudopapillary neoplasm.

Table 23-5 demonstrates more common lesions that should be considered in the differential diagnosis of solid pancreatic lesions. When a solid pancreatic mass in an older patient is noted, the major differential diagnosis remains pancreatic adenocarcinoma versus chronic pancreatitis.

Pancreatic Adenocarcinoma and Chronic Pancreatitis

Distinguishing chronic pancreatitis from pancreatic carcinoma is not a diagnostic challenge when cellular features are characteristic. This is more challenging for cytopathologists when a well-differentiated pancreatic adenocarcinoma is aspirated. Diagnostic criteria for pancreatic adenocarcinoma have

been described in the literature, and they include the following: increased cellularity; the predominance of a single cell type; three-dimensional groups (overlapping cells); a "drunken honeycomb" appearance (Figure 23-8); the presence of many pleomorphic single cells (Figure 23-9); tall cells with large nuclei (tombstones); and cells with an increased nuclear-to-cytoplasmic (N/C) ratio, irregular nuclear membrane, coarse and clumped chromatin, macronucleoli, and abnormal mitoses. The presence of abortive glands in a background of tumor-associated necrosis is another feature that may help suggest carcinoma over reactive ductal epithelium.[43] Carcinomas may also show tumor diathesis, mucin production, occasional signet ring cells with mucin vacuoles, bizarre cells, and squamoid cells. Cytologic features of pancreatic carcinoma vary by histologic subtype, including the presence of keratinization in adenosquamous carcinomas and many giant cells in giant cell tumors of the pancreas. In contrast, reactive ductal epithelial cells show many tight cohesive two-dimensional groups of ductal cells with minimal, if any, overlapping. Reactive cells show moderate cytoplasm, well-defined borders, nuclei with a round and regular nuclear membrane, and inconspicuous nucleoli. In some instances, however, nuclear enlargement may be more conspicuous, there may be more single cells, and occasional cytologic atypia may be noted. Chronic pancreatitis may also be characterized by dense fibrous connective tissue and few chronic inflammatory cells (Figure 23-10).

TABLE 23-5

DIFFERENTIAL DIAGNOSIS OF COMMON SOLID PANCREATIC LESIONS

Benign	Malignant
Chronic pancreatitis	Pancreatic carcinoma
Autoimmune pancreatitis	Acinar cell carcinoma
Pancreatic endocrine neoplasm	Pancreatic endocrine neoplasm (well-differentiated endocrine carcinoma)
Acute pancreatitis	
Infections	Metastatic malignancies
	Non-Hodgkin lymphoma

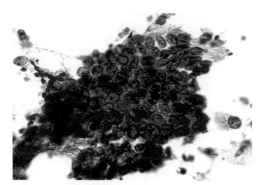

FIGURE 23-8 Smear from a well-differentiated adenocarcinoma of the pancreas reveals a tightly cohesive group of epithelial cells. Cells show mild overlapping with loss of cell polarity. Nuclei show coarse chromatin clumping, nuclear membrane irregularity, and conspicuous nucleus (Papanicolaou stain; magnification ×20).

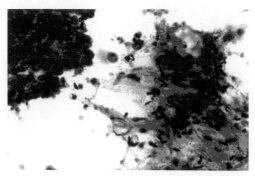

FIGURE 23-10 Smear from chronic pancreatitis. The smear reveals reactive ductal cells with tight cohesive groups, few inflammatory cells, and dense fibrous connective tissue (Papanicolaou stain; magnification ×40).

Pitfalls. A polymorphous cell population as opposed to predominance of cells of one type is a major consideration when evaluating specimens for pancreatic adenocarcinoma. With EUS FNA, the pancreatic mass is approached from the gastrointestinal tract. The approach to the lesion in the pancreas using EUS varies with its topographic location. In addition, in EUS FNA, as with percutaneous FNA, the needle passes through a background of chronic pancreatitis before it reaches the target lesion. This may cause additional cells to be noted on the slide preparations and may give the false impression of a polymorphous cell population. The approaches taken by the endoscopist to lesions in different locations in the pancreas and the cells that may be observed by a cytopathologist are listed in Table 23-6.

Increased cellularity is one of the criteria used to distinguish well-differentiated adenocarcinoma from chronic pancreatitis. The cellularity of a sample is influenced by several factors, including operator technique and the anatomic location of the tumor. Trained operators usually obtain cellular samples from EUS FNA. Some of the possible reasons for the increased cellularity of the samples obtained with EUS FNA include the proximity to the lesion and the better visualization of the lesions. The use of cellularity as a criterion in the differentiation of chronic pancreatitis and well-differentiated

adenocarcinoma should therefore be used with caution, especially when the samples have been obtained using EUS FNA.

Causes of False-Negative Diagnosis. False-negative diagnoses may result from technical difficulties, sampling error, or interpretive errors. For a cytopathologist, offering a diagnosis based on hypocellular samples is a common cause of false diagnosis. A sampling error may result from the technical difficulty associated with reaching the tumor, such as when a tumor is located in the uncinate process. It also is possible that the marked desmoplasia of pancreatic adenocarcinoma may result in an inadequate specimen or an inconclusive diagnosis (atypical or suspicious for malignancy), both of which require further investigations or repeat FNA.

Interpretative causes of false-negative diagnosis may include a tumor with mixed cellularity in which a component of chronic pancreatitis is also noted along with few tumor cells. It is also challenging to make a diagnosis of well-differentiated adenocarcinoma of the pancreas because of subtle morphologic changes. In such instances, the use of biomarkers may further aid in distinguishing reactive ductal epithelium from carcinoma cells. The list of such markers is ever increasing. Investigators have demonstrated that a lack of SMAD4 and clusterin in suspicious cells supports the diagnosis of carcinoma. In addition, mesothelin, p53, and MUC4 expression in suspicious cells further aids in supporting the diagnosis of carcinoma.[44] In an ever-expanding field other markers such as S1OOP, XIAP, fascin and multiprobe FISH have also been investigated.[45–47] In the authors' analysis, an

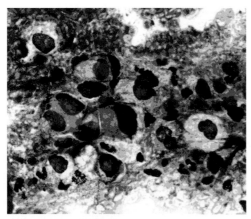

FIGURE 23-9 Pancreatic carcinoma. Smear from a poorly differentiated pancreatic carcinoma reveals many single cells with marked cytologic atypia, including enlarged nuclei, marked nuclear membrane irregularity, and background necrosis (Papanicolaou stain; magnification ×40).

TABLE 23-6

TRANSLUMINAL APPROACH TO PANCREAS AND GASTROINTESTINAL MUCOSAL CELLS

EUS Approach	Lesion in the Pancreas	Contaminating Gastrointestinal Mucosal Cells
Transgastric	Body and tail, occasionally uncinate process	Foveolar cells, parietal cells, chief cells, smooth muscle cells
Transduodenal	Head and uncinate process	Villi, Bruner's glands, and smooth muscle

abnormal pattern is consistently noted when a set of 4 FISH probes were used. This finding shows great promise as an adjunct to morphology in diagnosis of pancreatic carcinoma on limited samples.

Causes of False-Positive Diagnosis. Chronic pancreatitis and autoimmune pancreatitis are the most common reasons for a false-positive diagnosis of malignancy. Some of the cytologic features that may mimic malignancy in chronic pancreatitis are occasional atypical cells, which include enlarged cells, enlarged nuclei with degenerative vacuoles, single cells, and occasional mitosis. Chronic pancreatitis may also be characterized by areas with necrosis, especially in patients with development of early pseudocysts.

Aspirations from autoimmune pancreatitis often show marked stromal reaction with embedded small clusters of epithelial cells. These cells may show features of reactive atypia. However, autoimmune pancreatitis should be suspected if the patient has a history of autoimmune disease, a characteristic EUS image, and an associated increase in lymphoplasmacytic infiltrates. When in doubt, serum or tissue estimations of immunoglobulin G_4 (IgG_4) may further aid in suggesting this diagnosis. This value becomes more informative when elevated IgG_4 levels are interpreted in context of total IgG levels.

The cytologic features of primary pancreatic carcinomas are similar to the features of many other adenocarcinomas that can metastasize to the pancreas. Thus, it is crucial for endosonographers to provide adequate clinical information about any history of prior malignant diseases. It also may happen that a history of prior malignancy is obtained after the EUS FNA sample is procured. In some cases, it becomes important to determine the primary site of origin. Several immunohistochemical stains can reliably suggest possible primary tumor sites. Therefore, some investigators suggested an additional dedicated pass, to make a cell block to aid in performing immunohistochemical stains if and when required.

Pancreatic Neuroendocrine Tumors

Pancreatic neuroendocrine tumors (PNETs) more frequently manifest in the body or tail of the pancreas. They are usually well-demarcated solid lesions, although they may infrequently manifest as cystic lesions as well. Cytologic characteristics of these tumors include moderate to highly cellular smears.[48]

These smears predominantly have single cells with occasional loose cellular aggregates, as well as rosette formation (Figure 23-11A).[49] Neoplastic cells are plasmacytoid without perinuclear huff, small cytoplasmic vacuoles, and the cytoplasm may show neurosecretory granules (see Figure 23-11B).[50] Nuclei show a round, regular nuclear membrane and usually do not reveal conspicuous nucleoli, although exceptions have been noted. Cells may also show marked anisonucleosis. Cytologic features usually cannot distinguish benign from malignant neoplasms. However, increased proliferative activity and necrosis have been associated with malignant lesions.

Major Differential Diagnosis

Solid Pseudopapillary Neoplasm of the Pancreas. These tumors are usually noted in body or tail of the pancreas of young females. A multi-institutional study noted that solid pseudopapillary neoplasms (SPNs) of the pancreas are not infrequently diagnosed as pancreatic neuroendocrine neoplasms (PENs) on EUS FNA samples.[51] In a recent study, Hooper and colleagues noted that when adequate samples were procured by endosonographers, one of the most significant errors in their hands was tumor misclassification, which was most often SPN of the pancreas.[52] Some of the factors that may lead to such misclassification are a result of overlapping morphologic spectrum shared by PNET and SPN. Both tumors may show moderate cellularity, dyscohesive cells, low N/C ratio, and plasmacytoid cells. Some of the features that suggest SPN over PEN include pseudopapillary groups, cytoplasmic hyaline globules, and a chromatic matrix material and nuclei with "coffee bean" appearance (Figure 23-12). We have recently identified that in cases where the morphologic differential diagnosis is between PNET and SPN, detection of large cytoplasmic vacuoles would favor SPNs.[50] Other observers now independently validate this finding.

Cytologic features, however, are not always confirmatory. In such instances, a limited panel of immunohistochemical stains is needed to distinguish PEN from SPN. There are many immunohistochemical stains that have been utilized to characterize immunophenotypic pattern for SPN.[53] Positive staining with chromogranin, synaptophysin, and CD56 stains support a diagnosis of PEN. Infrequently, SPN may also stain for chromogranin. Most SPNs will stain for CD56 and about

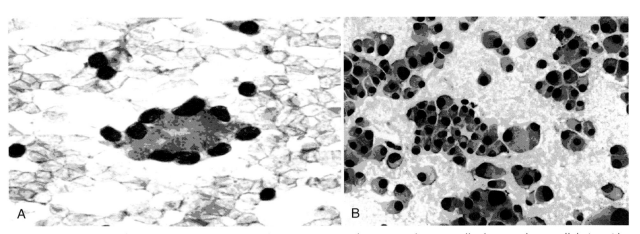

FIGURE 23-11 Pancreatic endocrine neoplasms. **A,** Smears from pancreatic endocrine neoplasms usually show moderate cellularity with rosette formation and many single cells with peripherally placed nuclei (Papanicolaou stain; magnification ×40). **B,** The nuclei reveal evenly dispersed chromatin without conspicuous nucleoli. They also reveal coarse neurosecretory granules (Diff-Quik stain; magnification ×20).

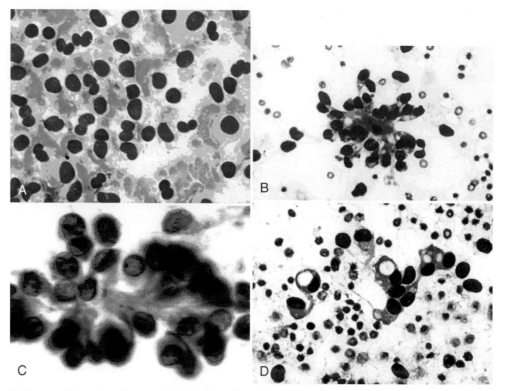

FIGURE 23-12 **A** to **D,** Fine-needle aspirates from a solid pseudopapillary neoplasm of the pancreas show wispy nondescript cytoplasm with nuclei lined away from the stroma. These cells also show (**A**) a preserved nuclear-to-cytoplasmic ratio, plasmacytoid cells and an eosinophilic cytoplasmic globule (Diff-Quik stain; magnification ×20), (**B**) a characteristic metachromatic matrix (Diff-Quik stain; magnification ×20), (**C**) nuclei with a "coffee bean" appearance (Papanicolaou stain; magnification ×40), and (**D**) large cytoplasmic vacuoles (Diff-Quik stain; magnification ×40).

one-third of cases with synaptophysin. We have identified that FNA samples are extremely limited in quantity; a judicious staining with chromogranin, CD10 and E-cadherin, and/or β-catenin will reliably separate SPN from PNET.[54]

Other tumors that may mimic PNET such as acinar cell carcinoma and pancreatoblastoma are out of the scope of this chapter.

Cystic Pancreatic Lesions

Guidelines for performing FNA for cystic lesions and associated morphologic findings are changing, and as a result, not all cysts should be aspirated. As a result, the role of the cytopathologists is also constantly evolving.

The diagnosis of cystic lesions requires a coordinated multispecialty team approach. Cytologists are largely faced with assessment of five major cystic lesions of the pancreas that have characteristic demographic, EUS, and cytologic features. However, taken individually, clinical features, EUS findings, and cytologic features do not provide adequate sensitivity.

It is known that cysts that are lined by mucinous epithelium (intraductal papillary mucinous neoplasm and mucinous cystic neoplasia) can progress to adenocarcinoma of the pancreas. As a result it is important to detect them early and identify dysplasia occurring in these cysts early for early interventions (Figure 23-13).

Intraductal Papillary Mucinous Neoplasia (IPMN). Our understanding has substantially improved because this tumor was first characterized as a separate entity. These tumors can occur within the main duct (main duct IPMN) or within smaller branches of the pancreatic ducts (side branch IPMN or branch duct IPMN). In essence both forms of IPMN develop cysts lined by mucin-secreting epithelium and will communicate with the pancreatic duct. Main duct IPMNs generally are noted in male patients and more often are noted near the head of the pancreas. Pancreatic ducts in such cases are generally dilated and mucin is often noted to ooze out from the ampulla in the second portion of the duodenum. In contrast, branch duct IPMNs do communicate with the main pancreatic ducts but do not result in dilatation of the main pancreatic duct. These lesions are often multicentric and their risk of developing into carcinoma is lower than that of main duct IPMNs. IPMNs, regardless of whether they are main duct or branch duct, are lined by different types of mucin-secreting epithelia (intestinal, pancreaticobiliary, foveolar, and oncocytic) and their risk of progression to carcinoma also varies. International consensus guidelines have been developed to manage patients with IPMN.[55]

When such lesions are aspirated, they characteristically have large papillary epithelial groups with a fibrovascular core lying in pools of mucin (Figure 23-14). The neoplastic cells are columnar or cuboidal and show loss of cell polarity. A few single cells may also be seen. Individual cells may demonstrate a wide range of morphologic changes depending upon the type of epithelium that lines the cyst. It is recognized that sensitivity of cytology is low in distinguishing mucinous form nonmucinous cysts of the pancreas. It is, however, quite clear that cytologic characteristics do help in determining the degree of dysplasia and malignant transformation within neoplastic cysts.[56,57]

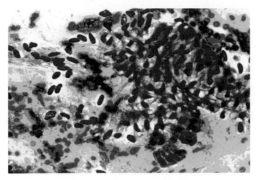

FIGURE 23-13 EUS fine-needle aspiration of the pancreas from a mucinous cyst adenoma reveals cuboidal neoplastic epithelial cells. These cells are in close proximity to the spindled cells representing the ovarian stroma (Papanicolaou stain; magnification ×40).

Causes of False Diagnosis. These tumors are lined by various cell types including gastric foveolar epithelium, colonic epithelium, pancreaticobiliary epithelium, and oncocytic cells with granular eosinophilic cytoplasm. This poses significant challenges of interpretation when there is contamination in samples when a needle traverses either the stomach or the duodenum. Intestinal-type IPMN will be very difficult to characterize when a needle traverses through the duodenum. Similarly, will be difficult to distinguish neoplastic foveolar cells when the needle traverses through the stomach. A close interaction between endosonographers and cytopathologists is of paramount importance to accurately determine the site of lesion as well as which route is used to obtain cells from the pancreas (transduodenal versus transgastric).

It is also important to note the type of mucin. Thick mucin that develops a ferning pattern when air dried is an important clue to being neoplastic mucin as opposed to mucin noted when the gastric mucosa is aspirated.

Mucinous Cystic Neoplasm. These tumors almost exclusively arise in female patients. They also are noted in young patients and are predominantly located in the tail of the pancreas. These tumors do not communicate with the main pancreatic duct. When cells are obtained from the center of the cyst, they reveal only cyst contents as suggested by cell debris, macrophages, and crystals. When the wall is aspirated, these tumors may show cuboidal or columnar mucin-secreting epithelial cells with a preserved N/C ratio. Smears from these tumors reveal elongated stromal cells in close approximation to bland cuboidal or columnar epithelial cells (Figure 23-14). The stromal cells most likely represent ovarian stroma. When these cysts have dysplastic or malignant components, the cells begin to show atypia. Features of atypia include many single cells and hyperchromatic and enlarged nuclei with cell pleomorphism. The nuclei begin to look wrinkled and also may reveal prominent nucleoli.

Causes of False Diagnosis. Paucicellular aspirates: Aspiration from these cysts frequently reveals paucicellular aspirates. In this setting, a definitive diagnosis of neoplastic mucinous cyst cannot be made with certainty. Mucinous cystic neoplasms also frequently reveal sloughed mucosa. Aspiration from such areas may reveal only acellular debris or necrotic debris with inflammatory cells reminiscent of pseudocysts.

Lining cells: When aspirate reveals goblet cells, it becomes a challenge to differentiate these cells from duodenal cells. Knowledge of the point of needle entry is very useful in this setting to avoid false-negative interpretation.

Ancillary Studies That Can Help Distinguish Neoplastic Mucinous Cysts from Nonmucinous Cysts of the Pancreas

Biochemical Estimations. One of the major challenges facing clinical teams is to distinguish between a neoplastic mucinous cyst and a nonmucinous cyst (e.g., pseudocyst). Determining the fluid viscosity is a simple method of distinguishing between the two types of cysts. Fluid viscosity of greater than 1.6 is generally associated with a neoplastic mucinous cyst.[58] Over a period of time, biochemical estimation of carcinoembryonic antigen (CEA) in combination with estimation of amylase levels has emerged as a powerful adjunct to distinguish a neoplastic mucinous cyst from a non-neoplastic cyst. This concept was developed and popularized by robust studies conducted by the cooperative pancreatic cyst study group led by Brugge and colleagues.[7] In this initial study, a CEA level more than 192 ng/dL was associated with a neoplastic mucinous cyst. Later, based on analysis of pooled data from multiple studies it was suggested that a CEA level greater than 800 ng/dL provides a specificity of 98% for a mucinous cyst.[59] A more recent follow-up study on over 800 patients suggest that CEA cyst fluid levels of 110 ng/dL or above will also provide similar sensitivity and specificity.[60] It is also interesting to note that cyst fluid amylase levels in thousands

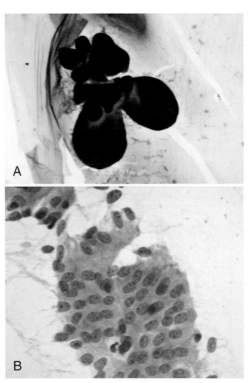

FIGURE 23-14 Intraductal papillary mucinous neoplasm. **A,** Smear from intraductal papillary mucinous neoplasia reveals pool of mucin with a large papillary epithelial group (Papanicolaou stain; magnification ×10). **B,** Higher magnification reveals columnar cells with a preserved nuclear-to-cytoplasmic ratio. The nuclei show a round, regular nuclear membrane with inconspicuous nucleoli (Papanicolaou stain; magnification ×40).

should be viewed in conjunction with CEA levels. A very low CEA level in conjunction with amylase levels in thousands is supportive of a pseudocyst. In comparison, higher CEA levels along with higher amylase levels will be associated with a neoplastic mucinous cyst. Occasionally, lymphoepithelial cysts as well as pseudocysts may be associated with spurious elevations in cyst fluid CEA levels.

Molecular Analysis of Cyst Fluid. The algorithmic approach highlighted in Figure 23-15 is useful for distinguishing common cystic pancreatic lesions. A few studies also demonstrated how molecular analysis of the cysts can help improve the diagnosis of cystic lesions. This analysis used determinations of DNA quality and quantity, loss of heterozygosity of k-*ras* mutation and its amplification, and mutations in seven other loci.[61,62] Based on a set formula, the cysts are categorized into neoplastic versus non-neoplastic cysts. Although the preliminary data are promising, such tests may become cost prohibitive for the help they provide in the management of patients with cystic pancreatic lesions.

Newer Markers. The use of high-throughput technologies has produced novel findings that are specifically associated with IPMN. Recent studies show that mutation in codon 201 of the *GNAS* gene is specifically noted in IPMN but not with any other types of cysts including mucinous cystadenomas. It is also noted by these observers that *GNAS* mutations were present in 66% of IPMNs and that either k-*ras* or *GNAS* mutations could be identified in 96% of these cases.[63] Mutation in *GNAS* is also more frequently noted in intestinal type IPMN. This mutation, however, cannot reliably distinguish the degree of dysplasia noted in these neoplastic cysts.[64] By these studies it becomes clear that mutation in codon 201 of *GNAS* gene along with k-*ras* can reliably distinguish IPMN from other cysts of the pancreas.

Lymph Nodes

EUS FNA for mediastinal and intra-abdominal lymphadenopathy has emerged as a very rapid cost-effective and reliable modality to stage malignancies as well as to detect primary or secondary hematopoietic malignancies.[25,65-69] Most of the studies evaluated the use of EUS FNA for staging of malignancies, including those from the lung, gastrointestinal tract, and pancreas. Determination of nodal metastasis by EUS FNA results in a change in preoperative staging that prevents unnecessary surgeries and a change in management strategies for patients with primary malignant neoplasms of the lung, gastrointestinal tract, and pancreas. EUS FNA of deep-seated lymphadenopathy can also be used to provide a diagnosis of primary lesions, including granulomas, infections, and lymphomas (non-Hodgkin and Hodgkin lymphoma).

Sample Collection

If the clinical information or the rapid interpretation of on-site cytology suggests malignant non-Hodgkin lymphoma, the endoscopist should provide an additional sample for flow cytometric, gene rearrangement, or cytogenetic examination. Generally, these cells should be collected in RPMI 1640 solution for flow cytometric analysis or molecular genetic analysis. Experience suggests that simple Hank's balanced salt solution can also be used as a transport medium to perform flow cytometric evaluation. If the sample has not been collected for flow cytometry, a sample collected for cell block can be stained with immunohistochemical stains for appropriate phenotyping. It is also equally important to understand that transport media do affect further management. A saline-rich medium might affect extraction of DNA and may give false-negative diagnosis. Optimization of sample collection especially for staging of lung cancer is therefore critical. Gene rearrangement studies can also be performed on such samples.

Algorithmic Approach to Interpretation of Lymph Node Aspirates

Using a stepwise methodical approach for lymph node aspirations leads to improved accuracy[66] (Figure 23-16). Earlier reports suggested that FNA was not always useful to test diagnoses of malignant non-Hodgkin lymphoma. This, however, is proved incorrect by several observers. The power of EUS-guided tissue sampling is increasing exponentially. Use of aspirates combined with Tru-Cut biopsies can improve the diagnosis of difficult lesions such as Hodgkin lymphoma.

How to Confirm Lymph Nodes

Lymphoid tissue demonstrates cellular aspirates with many single dyscohesive cells composed of polymorphous lymphoid cells of varying sizes. These cells may have germinal centers with debris containing (tingible body) macrophages. Diff-Quik stain also highlights the presence of cytoplasmic fragments such as lymph glandular bodies (see Figure 23-6).

Differential Diagnosis

When a range of small, medium, and large lymphocytes is noted in a lymph node aspirate in elderly patients from unexplained lymphadenopathy, one must be aware of conditions such as follicular center cell lymphoma and other small lymphocytic lymphomas. A similar pleomorphic cell type with plasma cells and eosinophils should raise suspicion for Hodgkin lymphoma. In such instances, additional samples should be obtained for flow cytometry, cytogenetics, or cell block analysis. Cell block analysis is more useful especially for the diagnosis of Hodgkin lymphoma, in which additional

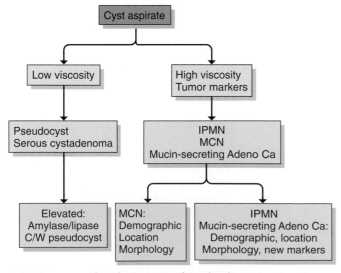

FIGURE 23-15 Algorithmic approach to the diagnosis of cystic pancreatic lesions. Ca, carcinoma; C/W, consistent with; IPMN, intraductal papillary mucinous neoplasia; MCN, mucinous cystic neoplasm.

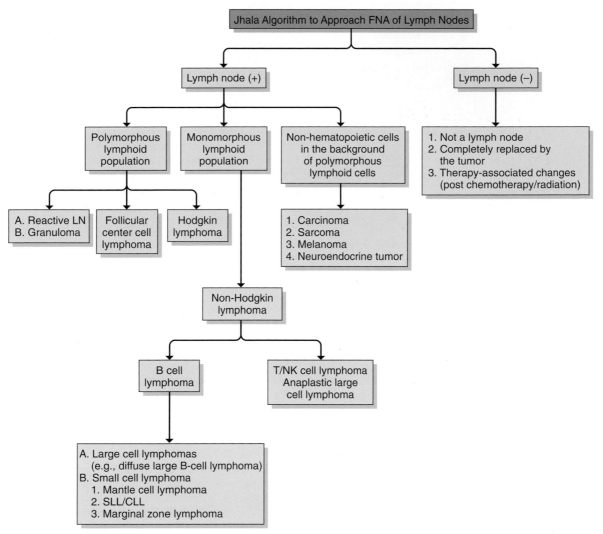

FIGURE 23-16 An algorithmic approach to the interpretation of lymph node aspirates. LN, lymph node; NK, natural killer; SLL/CLL, small lymphocytic lymphoma/chronic lymphocytic lymphoma.

immunohistochemical stains rather than flow cytometry will provide a definitive answer.

Similarly, if lymph node aspirates reveal many polygonal cells that also have reniform nuclei with inconspicuous nucleoli, granuloma should be suspected. Granulomas show aggregates of epithelioid histiocytes (Figure 23-17), with occasional multinucleated giant cells. In such instances, additional studies should be undertaken to determine possible causes.

Monomorphous Lymphoid Population

When a lymph node aspirate reveals a sea of monomorphic lymphoid population (small, intermediate, or large), the strong possibility of lymphoma should be considered, and additional samples should be obtained for ancillary studies.

Pitfalls. Diffuse large B-cell non-Hodgkin lymphomas have fragile cytoplasm and therefore frequently reveal large nuclei stripped of their cytoplasm. These cells also reveal prominent nucleoli that raise the suspicion of a differential diagnosis of melanoma. The cytoplasm with B-cell markers may be sheared while passing through the narrow capillary bore of a flow

cytometer. Thus, it is not uncommon to see that flow cytometry may have a false-negative result.[25] Immunohistochemical stains performed on cell block or gene rearrangement studies may aid in confirming this difficult diagnosis.

Small lymphocytic lymphomas fall on other end of the spectrum. The smears may contain only small, mature lymphocytes. These lesions cannot be distinguished from mature lymphocytes or lymphocyte-predominant Hodgkin lymphoma or other lymphomas with small lymphoid morphology such as mantle cell or marginal zone lymphomas. Therefore in a patient with multiple groups of lymph node enlargement, it is advisable to obtain an additional sample for ancillary studies.

Nonhematopoietic Cells in Background of Lymphoid Cells

When nonhematopoietic cells are noted in lymph node aspirates, the diagnosis is metastatic malignancy unless proved otherwise. These metastases can be from carcinoma, melanoma, or neuroendocrine tumors. The characteristic morphologic features of each entity can distinguish these tumors.

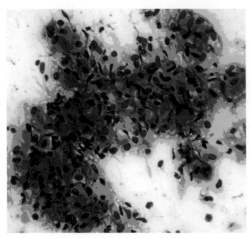

FIGURE 23-17 EUS fine-needle aspiration of mediastinal lymph node. The aspirate reveals aggregates of epithelioid histiocytes characteristic of granulomas (Diff-Quik stain; magnification ×40).

Pitfalls. Although generally it is not difficult to distinguish metastatic malignancies, the diagnosis of small cell carcinomas may pose diagnostic challenges. Tumor cells in small cell carcinomas demonstrate an increased N/C ratio, nuclei that are hyperchromatic, and possibly also nuclear molding. These cells are fragile and reveal stretching of DNA material. They also show frequent apoptosis and absent or inconspicuous nucleoli. Although these features are easily recognizable, poorly prepared smears from lymph nodes may also reveal shearing of cells from overzealous spread. They may show loose aggregates of cells that reveal a low N/C ratio, hyperchromatic nuclei, and inconspicuous nucleoli. In such cases, the pattern of chromatin architecture may help to differentiate the two. Small cell carcinomas reveal a fine, evenly distributed chromatin pattern, whereas lymphocytes may have margination of the chromatin pattern.

One must also not overinterpret benign gastrointestinal tract epithelium noted in a background of lymph node aspirates as diagnostic of metastatic malignancy. When these aspirates are evaluated carefully, up to 60% may show some form of gastrointestinal contamination.

Nonhematopoietic Cells Without the Background of Lymphoid Cells

Rarely, a lesion deemed as a lymph node on EUS imaging turns out to be a tumor nodule. This possibility should be suspected when multiple passes reveal only neoplastic cells, and no lymphoid component is noted. Tumor cells generally fall into one of four categories: (1) carcinoma, in which cells show cohesive groups with single cells; (2) melanoma, in which the cells are mostly single, with mild to moderate cytoplasm that may or may not have pigment; nuclei also reveal intranuclear cytoplasmic inclusions and prominent nucleoli; this tumor not infrequently has double mirror image nuclei; (3) carcinoid tumors, which are well-differentiated neuroendocrine carcinomas that reveal many single plasmacytoid cells with anisonucleosis; the cytoplasm may show neurosecretory granules, and occasionally these tumors also have a spindled appearance giving rise to a biphasic pattern of cells; these tumors may also form rosettes; and (4) sarcoma. In rare instances, patients treated with either chemotherapy

or radiation therapy show transformational changes in lymph nodes; in such cases, they may only show mucinous or myxoid change with few inflammatory cells.[2]

In recent years, EUS FNA samples are increasingly being utilized to characterize underlying molecular background of cells to guide therapies. Increasingly medical oncology teams request such assays, including analysis for EGFr, KRAS, BRAF, EMALK44, and ROS1 mutations, increasing the power of small samples.[70] These targets are increasingly recognized and we should be prepared to look beyond morphology for managing these patients. Many platforms are utilized to detect such molecular alterations. New guidelines for managing lung cancer diagnosis now may require high throughput and very sensitive technologies such as platforms including next generation sequencing of cells to help identify mutations that are not easily identified by standard technologies.

Spleen

FNA of the spleen has proven useful for the detection of malignant non-Hodgkin lymphoma, metastatic carcinoma, sarcoidosis, infectious conditions, and extramedullary hematopoiesis.[71-73] Percutaneous FNA of the spleen is highly specific (100%) and yields an overall accuracy of 84.9% to 88% for needle aspirates. Eloubeidi and colleagues noted that the diagnostic accuracy of splenic FNA can be increased by obtaining samples for flow cytometry.[71] Some investigators suggested, however, that a potential risk for increased bleeding contributes to the lack of use of FNA of the spleen in the United States. Preliminary experience suggested that judicious use of EUS FNA may permit the detection of unsuspected neoplasms, the determination of a preoperative diagnosis of splenic lesions, or both. However, further studies are needed to determine the safety and efficacy of this modality in the detection of splenic lesions.

Gastrointestinal Tract

For cytologic diagnosis, endoscopic brushing is a useful modality for the detection of surface lesions.[1] However, this modality is not useful for the diagnosis of submucosal lesions. EUS with FNA offers the advantages of direct visualization of the mucosal surface and accuracy in determining the extent and size of the submucosal lesion.[74] Therefore EUS permits preoperative determination of the depth of tumor invasion, or T-staging, as well as determination of the N status, and thus provides valuable information concerning the TNM staging of gastrointestinal tract malignancies.[18,74] EUS also has been used to determine the extent of involvement and response to therapy of mucosa-associated lymphoid tissue (MALT) lymphomas of the stomach. Specifically, EUS FNA has shown value in the following areas for cytologic diagnosis.

Detection of Foregut Cysts

One of the major differential diagnoses for a patient with a posterior mediastinal lesion, which may manifest with dysphagia, is a foregut duplication cyst.[75] This category includes esophageal reduplication and bronchogenic cysts.[76] These cysts may be differentiated based on the presence of complete muscle wall, the type of lining epithelium, and results of imaging studies. An esophageal reduplication cyst is a rare

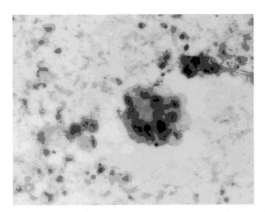

FIGURE 23-18 EUS fine-needle aspiration of an esophageal duplication cyst. The aspirate reveals macrophages, giant cells, and cell debris consistent with the cyst content (Papanicolaou stain; magnification ×40).

developmental anomaly that clinically and radiologically can mimic a neoplasm.

The cytologic features of the cysts show degenerated cell debris and hemosiderin-laden macrophages (Figure 23-18). In addition, these aspirates may also contain detached ciliated cell fragments, which can be demonstrated by both light and electron microscopy. The presence of numerous squamous cells supports the diagnosis of an esophageal reduplication cyst. The presence of numerous goblet cells with an absence of squamous cells supports the diagnosis of a bronchogenic cyst. Cytologic features alone are not pathognomonic for the diagnosis of a foregut cyst, but can be used to rule out malignant neoplasm and can help to support the diagnosis of foregut cyst when cytology is used in conjunction with imaging studies, including EUS findings.[76]

Gastrointestinal Stromal Tumors

GISTs usually are submucosal and cannot be detected by brush sampling or forceps biopsy. EUS with its associated capabilities such as Doppler as well as FNA capability helps to determine the site, size, and extent of the lesion. Underlying molecular typing to detect these tumors characterizes molecular changes that could be utilized to predict

therapeutic response.[77–80] FNA samples from GISTs show hypercellular groups of spindled cells (Figure 23-19A) and, rarely, epithelioid cells. The spindled cells also show blunt-ended nuclei and may have nuclear angulations. The major pitfall associated with EUS FNA of GISTs is the aspiration of muscle cells from the wall of the gastrointestinal tract or smooth muscle tumors. Because the definitive differentiation of GISTs from other spindle cell lesions influences subsequent therapy, every attempt should be made to distinguish among these lesions. A panel of immunohistochemical stains, including primary antibodies against c-kit (CD117) (see Figure 23-19B), CD34, smooth muscle antigen, muscle-specific actin, DOG1, and S-100, may be used to distinguish GISTs from muscle cells, smooth muscle tumors, and rare tumors, such as solitary fibrous tumors of the gastrointestinal tract. Additional c-kit mutational analysis is being investigated to determine utility of EUS FNA as a predictive tool in management for GIST tumors.

Hepatobiliary Tree

Liver

CT and ultrasound scans have been used to detect and guide the collection of FNA samples from hepatic masses. Several studies explored the usefulness of EUS in the diagnosis of hepatic lesions, as well as the ability of EUS to promote early intervention.[81–83] Investigators reported that EUS is able to identify hepatic lesions when a previous CT scan failed to detect a lesion. FNA is used generally to confirm the diagnosis of metastatic tumors or to diagnose primary tumors such as hepatocellular carcinoma and cholangiocarcinoma. Aspirates from hepatocellular carcinomas generally show adequately cellular samples. The neoplastic hepatocytes may be in groups or single cells. Two patterns of morphologic features are characteristic: (1) groups of hepatocytes with overlapping cells that are lined by sinusoids (basketing pattern) (Figure 23-20A); and (2) overlapping cell groups with vessels transgressing these neoplastic cells. Neoplastic hepatocytes may have a range of morphologic features based on their cellular differentiation and histologic subtype. It may be difficult to

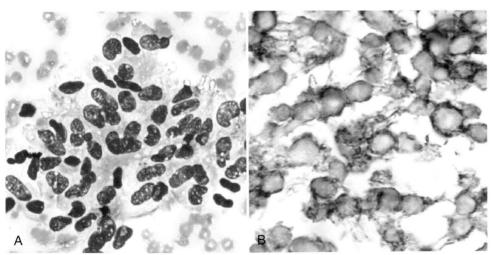

FIGURE 23-19 **A** and **B**, EUS fine-needle aspiration of a gastric submucosal tumor reveals a paucicellular aspirate with many spindled cells suggestive of gastrointestinal tract stromal tumor (GIST). These cells also were stained by CD117 (c-kit), which confirmed the diagnosis of GIST tumor (**A**, Diff-Quik stain; magnification ×40; **B**, immunohistochemical stain; magnification ×40).

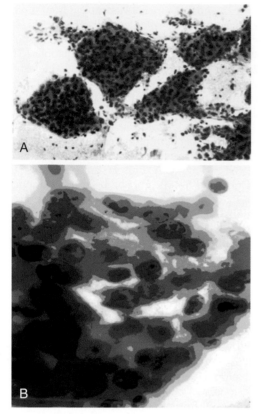

FIGURE 23-20 Hepatocellular carcinoma. **A,** Aspirate from hepatocellular carcinoma shows increased cellularity and reveals groups of hepatocytes with sinusoids around the periphery (basketing pattern) (Papanicolaou stain; magnification ×20). **B,** Individual tumor cells either show no or very little cytoplasm with increased nuclear-to-cytoplasmic ratio. Nuclei reveal irregular nuclear membranes and have prominent nucleoli (Papanicolaou stain; magnification ×40).

distinguish well-differentiated hepatocellular carcinomas from hepatocellular adenoma, focal nodular hyperplasia, or macroregenerative nodules. In such instances, an altered architectural pattern highlighted on reticulin stain on cell block examination may prove to be a valuable adjunct.[84] Moderately or more poorly differentiated tumors may show many single atypical hepatocytes, the presence of bile, or single nuclei stripped of their cytoplasm. These cells also may have clear cytoplasmic vacuoles representing steatosis. Malignant cells show an increased N/C ratio, nuclear membrane irregularity, abnormal mitoses, and prominent nucleoli (see Figure 23-20B). Similarly, EUS FNA has also been useful in the diagnosis of biliary and gallbladder carcinomas.[85,86] This optimistic outlook should be weighed against cautionary notes of potential needle seeding as well as impact on future role of transplantation for patients with cholangiocarcinomas. Potential for such seeding and outcomes have also been highlighted and hence additional studies are needed to further characterize the challenges and opportunities for this procedure.[87]

Adrenal Glands

EUS can detect adrenal gland lesions and can effectively obtain FNA samples from left-sided and some right-sided lesions.[88] This modality is useful for detecting metastatic

malignant neoplasms to the adrenal gland, especially from the lung.[89,90] Samples from normal adrenal glands reveal single cells or small aggregates. The cells usually are uniform; however, anisocytosis sometimes can be noted. The nuclei generally have regular nuclear membranes. Some cells may reveal conspicuous nucleoli. The cytoplasm may be eosinophilic, foamy, or rich in lipids. Because the cytoplasm frequently is disrupted, naked nuclei are often identified, with lipid vacuoles noted in the background.

Summary

EUS is a powerful modality that has forever changed practice patterns related to deep-seated malignant neoplasms. Advances in this technology and rapid evolution of molecular technology platforms and understanding will continue to challenge conventional wisdom in the coming years. Effective use of this technique for patient management, however, requires that cytopathologists form an integral part of the patient management team. Although the diagnostic criteria for a majority of lesions are not affected, endosonographers as well as cytopathologists should be aware of the benefits, limitations, and pitfalls of evaluating samples obtained by EUS-guided FNA.

REFERENCES

1. Jhala N, Jhala D. Gastrointestinal tract cytology: advancing horizons. *Adv Anat Pathol.* 2003;10(5):261-277.
2. Jhala NC, Jhala DN, Chhieng DC, et al. Endoscopic ultrasound-guided fine-needle aspiration. A cytopathologist's perspective. *Am J Clin Pathol.* 2003;120(3):351-367.
3. Varadarajulu S, Hasan MK, Bang JY, et al. Endoscopic ultrasound-guided tissue acquisition. *Dig Endosc.* 2014;26(suppl 1):62-69.
4. Eltoum IA, Alston EA, Roberson J. Trends in pancreatic pathology practice before and after implementation of endoscopic ultrasound-guided fine-needle aspiration: an example of disruptive innovation effect? *Arch Pathol Lab Med.* 2012;136(4):447-453.
5. Yamao K, Sawaki A, Mizuno N, et al. Endoscopic ultrasound-guided fine-needle aspiration biopsy (EUS-FNAB): past, present, and future. *J Gastroenterol.* 2005;40(11):1013-1023.
6. Vazquez-Sequeiros E, Levy MJ, Van Domselaar M, et al. Diagnostic yield and safety of endoscopic ultrasound guided fine needle aspiration of central mediastinal lung masses. *Diagn Ther Endosc.* 2013;2013: 150492.
7. Brugge WR, Lewandrowski K, Lee-Lewandrowski E, et al. Diagnosis of pancreatic cystic neoplasms: a report of the cooperative pancreatic cyst study. *Gastroenterology.* 2004;126(5):1330-1336.
8. Vilmann P, Jacobsen GK, Henriksen FW, Hancke S. Endoscopic ultrasonography with guided fine needle aspiration biopsy in pancreatic disease. *Gastrointest Endosc.* 1992;38(2):172-173.
9. Wiersema MJ, Hawes RH, Tao LC, et al. Endoscopic ultrasonography as an adjunct to fine needle aspiration cytology of the upper and lower gastrointestinal tract. *Gastrointest Endosc.* 1992;38(1):35-39.
10. Varadarajulu S, Jhala NC. Cytopathology: a dying art or something that a gastroenterologist should know? *Gastrointest Endosc.* 2012;76(2): 397-399.
11. Varadarajulu S, Fockens P, Hawes RH. Best practices in endoscopic ultrasound-guided fine-needle aspiration. *Clin Gastroenterol Hepatol.* 2012;10(7):697-703.
12. Eltoum IA, Chhieng DC, Jhala D, et al. Cumulative sum procedure in evaluation of EUS-guided FNA cytology: the learning curve and diagnostic performance beyond sensitivity and specificity. *Cytopathology.* 2007;18(3):143-150.
13. Kida M, Araki M, Miyazawa S, et al. Comparison of diagnostic accuracy of endoscopic ultrasound-guided fine-needle aspiration with 22- and 25-gauge needles in the same patients. *J Interv Gastroenterol.* 2011;1(3): 102-107.
14. Sakamoto H, Kitano M, Komaki T, et al. Prospective comparative study of the EUS guided 25-gauge FNA needle with the 19-gauge Trucut

needle and 22-gauge FNA needle in patients with solid pancreatic masses. *J Gastroenterol Hepatol.* 2009;24(3):384-390.

15. Siddiqui UD, Rossi F, Rosenthal LS, et al. EUS-guided FNA of solid pancreatic masses: a prospective, randomized trial comparing 22-gauge and 25-gauge needles. *Gastrointest Endosc.* 2009;70(6):1093-1097.

16. Bang JY, Hebert-Magee S, Trevino J, et al. Randomized trial comparing the 22-gauge aspiration and 22-gauge biopsy needles for EUS-guided sampling of solid pancreatic mass lesions. *Gastrointest Endosc.* 2012; 76(2):321-327.

17. Affolter KE, Schmidt RL, Matynia AP, et al.. Needle size has only a limited effect on outcomes in EUS-guided fine needle aspiration: a systematic review and meta-analysis. *Dig Dis Sci.* 2013;58(4):1026-1034.

18. Knight CS, Eloubeidi MA, Crowe R, et al. Utility of endoscopic ultrasound-guided fine-needle aspiration in the diagnosis and staging of colorectal carcinoma. *Diagn Cytopathol.* 2011;41(12):1031-1037.

19. Madhoun MF, Wani SB, Rastogi A, et al. The diagnostic accuracy of 22-gauge and 25-gauge needles in endoscopic ultrasound-guided fine needle aspiration of solid pancreatic lesions: a meta-analysis. *Endoscopy.* 2013;45(2):86-92.

20. Lee JH, Stewart J, Ross WA, et al. Blinded prospective comparison of the performance of 22-gauge and 25-gauge needles in endoscopic ultrasound-guided fine needle aspiration of the pancreas and peri-pancreatic lesions. *Dig Dis Sci.* 2009;54(10):2274-2281.

21. Centeno BA, Enkemann SA, Coppola D, et al. Classification of human tumors using gene expression profiles obtained after microarray analysis of fine-needle aspiration biopsy samples. *Cancer.* 2005;105(2): 101-109.

22. Stigt JA, 'tHart NA, Knol AJ, et al. Pyrosequencing analysis of EGFR and KRAS mutations in EUS and EBUS-derived cytologic samples of adenocarcinomas of the lung. *J Thorac Oncol.* 2013;8(8):1012-1018.

23. Kanagal-Shamanna R, Portier BP, Singh RR, et al. Next-generation sequencing-based multi-gene mutation profiling of solid tumors using fine needle aspiration samples: promises and challenges for routine clinical diagnostics. *Modern Pathol.* 2013;27(2):314-327.

24. Deftereos G, Finkelstein SD, Jackson SA, et al. The value of mutational profiling of the cytocentrifugation supernatant fluid from fine-needle aspiration of pancreatic solid mass lesions. *Modern Pathol.* 2013 doi: 10.1038/modpathol.2013.147. [e-pub ahead of print].

25. Nunez AL, Jhala NC, Carroll AJ, et al. Endoscopic ultrasound and endobronchial ultrasound-guided fine-needle aspiration of deep-seated lymphadenopathy: Analysis of 1338 cases. *Cytojournal.* 2012;9:14.

26. Storch I, Jorda M, Thurer R, et al. Advantage of EUS Trucut biopsy combined with fine-needle aspiration without immediate on-site cytopathologic examination. *Gastrointest Endosc.* 2006;64(4):505-511.

27. Varadarajulu S, Bang JY, Hebert-Magee S. Assessment of the technical performance of the flexible 19-gauge EUS-FNA needle. *Gastrointest Endosc.* 2012;76(2):336-343.

28. Bang JY, Ramesh J, Trevino J, et al. Objective assessment of an algorithmic approach to EUS-guided FNA and interventions. *Gastrointest Endosc.* 2013;77(5):739-744.

29. Kate MS, Kamal MM, Bobhate SK, Kher AV. Evaluation of fine needle capillary sampling in superficial and deep-seated lesions. An analysis of 670 cases. *Acta Cytol.* 1998;42(3):679-684.

30. Wallace MB, Kennedy T, Durkalski V, et al. Randomized controlled trial of EUS-guided fine needle aspiration techniques for the detection of malignant lymphadenopathy. *Gastrointest Endosc.* 2001;54(4):441-447.

31. Puri R, Vilmann P, Saftoiu A, et al. Randomized controlled trial of endoscopic ultrasound-guided fine-needle sampling with or without suction for better cytological diagnosis. *Scand J Gastroenterol.* 2009;44(4): 499-504.

32. Weston BR, Bhutani MS. Optimizing diagnostic yield for EUS-guided sampling of solid pancreatic lesions: a technical review. *Gastroenterol Hepatol.* 2013;9(6):352-363.

33. Jhala NC, Jhala D, Eltoum I, et al. Endoscopic ultrasound-guided fine-needle aspiration biopsy: a powerful tool to obtain samples from small lesions. *Cancer.* 2004;102(4):239-246.

34. LeBlanc JK, Ciaccia D, Al-Assi MT, et al. Optimal number of EUS-guided fine needle passes needed to obtain a correct diagnosis. *Gastrointest Endosc.* 2004;59(4):475-481.

35. Bang JY, Magee SH, Ramesh J, et al. Randomized trial comparing fanning with standard technique for endoscopic ultrasound-guided fine-needle aspiration of solid pancreatic mass lesions. *Endoscopy.* 2013;45(6): 445-450.

36. Jhala NC, Eltoum IA, Eloubeidi MA, et al. Providing on-site diagnosis of malignancy on endoscopic-ultrasound-guided fine-needle aspirates: should it be done? *Ann Diagn Pathol.* 2007;11(3):176-181.

37. Klapman JB, Logrono R, Dye CE, Waxman I. Clinical impact of on-site cytopathology interpretation on endoscopic ultrasound-guided fine needle aspiration. *Am J Gastroenterol.* 2003;98(6):1289-1294.

38. Petrone MC, Arcidiacono PG, Carrara S, et al. Does cytotechnician training influence the accuracy of EUS-guided fine-needle aspiration of pancreatic masses? *Dig Liv Dis.* 2012;44(4):311-314.

39. Burlingame OO, Kesse KO, Silverman SG, Cibas ES. On-site adequacy evaluations performed by cytotechnologists: correlation with final interpretations of 5241 image-guided fine-needle aspiration biopsies. *Cancer Cytopathol.* 2012;120(3):177-184.

40. Collins BT. Telepathology in cytopathology: challenges and opportunities. *Acta Cytol.* 2013;57(3):221-232.

41. Marotti JD, Johncox V, Ng D, et al. Implementation of telecytology for immediate assessment of endoscopic ultrasound-guided fine-needle aspirations compared to conventional on-site evaluation: analysis of 240 consecutive cases. *Acta Cytol.* 2012;56(5):548-553.

42. Goyal A, Jhala N, Gupta P. TeleCyP (Telecytopathology): real-time fine-needle aspiration interpretation. *Acta Cytol.* 2012;56(6):669-677.

43. Eloubeidi MA, Jhala D, Chhieng DC, et al. Yield of endoscopic ultrasound-guided fine-needle aspiration biopsy in patients with suspected pancreatic carcinoma. *Cancer.* 2003;99(5):285-292.

44. Jhala N, Jhala D, Vickers SM, et al. Biomarkers in diagnosis of pancreatic carcinoma in fine-needle aspirates. *Am J Clin Pathol.* 2006;126(4): 572-579.

45. Kosarac O, Takei H, Zhai QJ, et al. S100P and XIAP expression in pancreatic ductal adenocarcinoma: potential novel biomarkers as a diagnostic adjunct to fine needle aspiration cytology. *Acta Cytol.* 2011;55(2): 142-148.

46. Dim DC, Jiang F, Qiu Q, et al. The usefulness of S100P, mesothelin, fascin, prostate stem cell antigen, and 14-3-3 sigma in diagnosing pancreatic adenocarcinoma in cytological specimens obtained by endoscopic ultrasound guided fine-needle aspiration. *Diagn Cytopathol.* 2011. doi: 10.1002/dc.21684. [e-pub ahead of print]

47. Reicher S, Boyar FZ, Albitar M, et al. Fluorescence in situ hybridization and K-ras analyses improve diagnostic yield of endoscopic ultrasound-guided fine-needle aspiration of solid pancreatic masses. *Pancreas.* 2011;40(7):1057-1062.

48. Gu M, Ghafari S, Lin F, Ramzy I. Cytological diagnosis of endocrine tumors of the pancreas by endoscopic ultrasound-guided fine-needle aspiration biopsy. *Diagn Cytopathol.* 2005;32(4):204-210.

49. Jhala D, Eloubeidi M, Chhieng DC, et al. Fine needle aspiration biopsy of the islet cell tumor of the pancreas: a comparison between computerized axial tomography and endoscopic ultrasound guided fine needle aspiration biopsy. *Ann Diagn Pathol.* 2002;2:106-112.

50. Jhala N, Siegal GP, Jhala D. Large, clear cytoplasmic vacuolation: an under-recognized cytologic clue to distinguish solid pseudopapillary neoplasms of the pancreas from pancreatic endocrine neoplasms on fine-needle aspiration. *Cancer.* 2008;114(4):249-254.

51. Bardales RH, Centeno B, Mallery JS, et al. Endoscopic ultrasound-guided fine-needle aspiration cytology diagnosis of solid-pseudopapillary tumor of the pancreas: a rare neoplasm of elusive origin but characteristic cytomorphologic features. *Am J Clin Pathol.* 2004;121(5):654-662.

52. Hooper K, Mukhtar F, Li S, Eltoum IA. Diagnostic error assessment and associated harm of endoscopic ultrasound-guided fine-needle aspiration of neuroendocrine neoplasms of the pancreas. *Cancer Cytopathol.* 2013.

53. Liu X, Rauch TM, Siegal GP, Jhala N. Solid-pseudopapillary neoplasm of the pancreas: three cases with a literature review. *Appl Immunohistochem Mol Morphol.* 2006;14(4):445-453.

54. Burford H, Baloch Z, Liu X, et al. E-cadherin/beta-catenin and CD10: a limited immunohistochemical panel to distinguish pancreatic endocrine neoplasm from solid pseudopapillary neoplasm of the pancreas on endoscopic ultrasound-guided fine-needle aspirates of the pancreas. *Am J Clin Pathol.* 2009;132(6):831-839.

55. Tanaka M, Fernandez-del Castillo C, Adsay V, et al. International Consensus Guidelines 2012 for the Management of IPMN and MCN of the Pancreas. *Pancreatology.* 2012;12(3):183-197.

56. Pitman MB, Centeno BA, Daglilar ES, et al. Cytological criteria of high-grade epithelial atypia in the cyst fluid of pancreatic intraductal papillary mucinous neoplasms. *Cancer Cytopathol.* 2014;122(1): 40-47.

57. Genevay M, Mino-Kenudson M, Yaeger K, et al. Cytology adds value to imaging studies for risk assessment of malignancy in pancreatic mucinous cysts. *Ann Surg.* 2011;254(6):977-983.

58. Bhutani MS, Gupta V, Guha S, et al. Pancreatic cyst fluid analysis—a review. *J Gastrointestin Liver Dis.* 2011;20(2):175-180.

59. van der Waaij LA, van Dullemen HM, Porte RJ. Cyst fluid analysis in the differential diagnosis of pancreatic cystic lesions: a pooled analysis. *Gastrointest Endosc.* 2005;62(3):383-389.

60. Cizginer S, Turner BG, Bilge AR, et al. Cyst fluid carcinoembryonic antigen is an accurate diagnostic marker of pancreatic mucinous cysts. *Pancreas.* 2011;40(7):1024-1028.

61. Sreenarasimhaiah J, Lara LF, Jazrawi SF, et al. A comparative analysis of pancreas cyst fluid CEA and histology with DNA mutational analysis in the detection of mucin producing or malignant cysts. *JOP.* 2009;10(2):163-168.

62. Sawhney MS, Devarajan S, O'Farrel P, et al. Comparison of carcinoembryonic antigen and molecular analysis in pancreatic cyst fluid. *Gastrointest Endosc.* 2009;69(6):1106-1110.

63. Wu J, Matthaei H, Maitra A, et al. Recurrent GNAS mutations define an unexpected pathway for pancreatic cyst development. *Sci Transl Med.* 2011;3(92):92ra66.

64. Dal Molin M, Matthaei H, Wu J, et al. Clinicopathological correlates of activating GNAS mutations in intraductal papillary mucinous neoplasm (IPMN) of the pancreas. *Ann Surg Oncol.* 2013;20:3802-3808.

65. Pugh JL, Jhala NC, Eloubeidi MA, et al. Diagnosis of deep-seated lymphoma and leukemia by endoscopic ultrasound-guided fine-needle aspiration biopsy. *Am J Clin Pathol.* 2006;125(5):703-709.

66. Bakdounes K, Jhala N, Jhala D. Diagnostic usefulness and challenges in the diagnosis of mesothelioma by endoscopic ultrasound guided fine needle aspiration. *Diagn Cytopathol.* 2008;36(7):503-507.

67. Srinivasan R, Bhutani MS, Thosani N, et al. Clinical impact of EUS-FNA of mediastinal lymph nodes in patients with known or suspected lung cancer or mediastinal lymph nodes of unknown etiology. *J Gastrointestin Liver Dis.* 2012;21(2):145-152.

68. Coe A, Conway J, Evans J, et al. The yield of EUS-FNA in undiagnosed upper abdominal adenopathy is very high. *J Clin Ultrasound.* 2013;41(4):210-213.

69. Eloubeidi MA, Desmond R, Desai S, et al. Impact of staging transesophageal EUS on treatment and survival in patients with non–small-cell lung cancer. *Gastrointest Endosc.* 2008;67(2):193-198.

70. Fischer AH, Benedict CC, Amrikachi M. Five top stories in cytopathology. *Arch Pathol Lab Med.* 2013;137(7):894-906.

71. Eloubeidi MA, Varadarajulu S, Eltoum I, et al. Transgastric endoscopic ultrasound-guided fine-needle aspiration biopsy and flow cytometry of suspected lymphoma of the spleen. *Endoscopy.* 2006;38(6):617-620.

72. Handa U, Tiwari A, Singhal N, et al. Utility of ultrasound-guided fine-needle aspiration in splenic lesions. *Diagn Cytopathol.* 2013;41(12):1038-1042.

73. Iwashita T, Yasuda I, Tsurumi H, et al. Endoscopic ultrasound-guided fine needle aspiration biopsy for splenic tumor: a case series. *Endoscopy.* 2009;41(2):179-182.

74. Bhutani MS. Endoscopic ultrasound in the diagnosis, staging and management of colorectal tumors. *Gastroenterol Clin North Am.* 2008;37(1):215-227, viii.

75. Faigel DO, Burke A, Ginsberg GG, et al. The role of endoscopic ultrasound in the evaluation and management of foregut duplications. *Gastrointest Endosc.* 1997;45(1):99-103.

76. Napolitano V, Pezzullo AM, Zeppa P, et al. Foregut duplication of the stomach diagnosed by endoscopic ultrasound guided fine-needle aspiration cytology: case report and literature review. *World J Surg Oncol.* 2013;11:33.

77. Ito H, Inoue H, Ryozawa S, et al. Fine-needle aspiration biopsy and endoscopic ultrasound for pretreatment pathological diagnosis of gastric gastrointestinal stromal tumors. *Gastroenterol Res and Pract.* 2012;2012:139083.

78. Gomes AL, Bardales RH, Milanezi F, et al. Molecular analysis of c-Kit and PDGFRA in GISTs diagnosed by EUS. *Am J Clin Pathol.* 2007;127(1):89-96.

79. Gu M, Ghafari S, Nguyen PT, Lin F. Cytologic diagnosis of gastrointestinal stromal tumors of the stomach by endoscopic ultrasound-guided fine-needle aspiration biopsy: cytomorphologic and immunohistochemical study of 12 cases. *Diagn Cytopathol.* 2001;25(6):343-350.

80. Saftoiu A. Endoscopic ultrasound-guided fine needle aspiration biopsy for the molecular diagnosis of gastrointestinal stromal tumors: shifting treatment options. *J Gastrointestin Liver Dis.* 2008;17(2):131-133.

81. Crowe DR, Eloubeidi MA, Chhieng DC, et al. Fine-needle aspiration biopsy of hepatic lesions: computerized tomographic-guided versus endoscopic ultrasound-guided FNA. *Cancer.* 2006;108(3):180-185.

82. Crowe A, Knight CS, Jhala D, Bynon SJ, Jhala NC. Diagnosis of metastatic fibrolamellar hepatocellular carcinoma by endoscopic ultrasound-guided fine needle aspiration. *Cytojournal.* 2011;8:2.

83. tenBerge J, Hoffman BJ, Hawes RH, et al. EUS-guided fine needle aspiration of the liver: indications, yield, and safety based on an international survey of 167 cases. *Gastrointest Endosc.* 2002;55(7):859-862.

84. Wee A. Fine needle aspiration biopsy of hepatocellular carcinoma and hepatocellular nodular lesions: role, controversies and approach to diagnosis. *Cytopathology.* 2011;22(5):287-305.

85. Meara RS, Jhala D, Eloubeidi MA, et al. Endoscopic ultrasound-guided FNA biopsy of bile duct and gallbladder: analysis of 53 cases. *Cytopathology.* 2006;17(1):42-49.

86. Ohshima Y, Yasuda I, Kawakami H, et al. EUS-FNA for suspected malignant biliary strictures after negative endoscopic transpapillary brush cytology and forceps biopsy. *J Gastroenterol.* 2011;46(7):921-928.

87. Levy MJ, Heimbach JK, Gores GJ. Endoscopic ultrasound staging of cholangiocarcinoma. *Curr Opin Gastroenterol.* 2012;28(3):244-252.

88. Jhala NC, Jhala D, Eloubeidi MA, et al. Endoscopic ultrasound-guided fine-needle aspiration biopsy of the adrenal glands: analysis of 24 patients. *Cancer.* 2004;102(5):308-314.

89. Uemura S, Yasuda I, Kato T, et al. Preoperative routine evaluation of bilateral adrenal glands by endoscopic ultrasound and fine-needle aspiration in patients with potentially resectable lung cancer. *Endoscopy.* 2013;45(3):195-201.

90. Bodtger U, Vilmann P, Clementsen P, et al. Clinical impact of endoscopic ultrasound-fine needle aspiration of left adrenal masses in established or suspected lung cancer. *J Thorac Oncol.* 2009;4(12):1485-1489.

SECTION VII

Interventional EUS

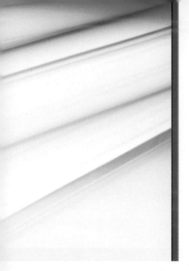

24

EUS-Guided Drainage of Pancreatic Fluid Collections

Stefan Seewald • Tiing Leong Ang • Shyam Varadarajulu • Paul Fockens

Key Points

- EUS-guided drainage is the preferred treatment for symptomatic pancreatic pseudocysts.
- Randomized trials have shown superiority to non–EUS-guided endoscopic transmural drainage and equivalent efficacy as surgical cystogastrostomy.
- The equipment includes a therapeutic linear echoendoscope, a 19-G puncture needle, cystotome, dilators, balloon catheter, 0.035-inch guidewires, double-pigtail stents, and nasocystic drainage catheter.
- The procedure is very safe with clinical success rates exceeding 90%. However, the clinical success rates for walled-off pancreatic necrosis are lower than for pseudocysts.

Pancreatic fluid collections (PFCs) may occur as a result of acute or chronic pancreatitis, surgery, trauma, or neoplasia. With the exception of cyst neoplasia, collections form as a consequence of either a disruption of the pancreatic duct with subsequent leakage or maturation of pancreatic necrosis. A pancreatic pseudocyst is defined as an encapsulated collection of fluid with a well-defined inflammatory wall usually outside the pancreas with minimal or no necrosis. This entity usually occurs more than 4 weeks after onset of interstitial edematous pancreatitis. A walled-off pancreatic necrosis (WON) is a mature, encapsulated collection of pancreatic and/or peripancreatic necrosis that has developed a well-defined inflammatory wall. WON usually occurs more than 4 weeks after onset of necrotizing pancreatitis.[1] The original Atlanta Classification included the term "pancreatic abscess" defined as a "localized collection of purulent material without significant necrotic material."[2] This finding is extremely uncommon, and because the term is confusing and has not been adopted widely, it is now abandoned.[1] Acute PFCs generally do not warrant any intervention because they occur early in the course of the disease, lack a well-defined wall, and are spontaneously reabsorbed within a few weeks after the onset of acute pancreatitis. Symptomatic pseudocysts causing pain and mechanical obstruction of the gastric outlet or biliary system, and infected pseudocysts require drainage. Drainage of infected walled-off necrosis is required for the effective control of sepsis. Drainage is also indicated if the pseudocyst continues to increase in size without resolution after 6 weeks, in order to avoid subsequent development of complications such as hemorrhage, perforation, or secondary infection. A prerequisite for EUS-guided drainage is the presence of a well-defined mature wall. For pseudocysts, a time frame of 4 to 6 weeks

is necessary. The fluid collection must be accessible endoscopically, such as being located within 1 cm of the duodenal or gastric walls; paracolic collections cannot be accessed and would require adjunctive methods such as percutaneous drainage. Coagulopathy, if present, should be corrected.[3] The current therapeutic options include surgery, endoscopy, and percutaneous drainage. Since the first reports of endoscopic drainage of pseudocysts in the 1980s, increasing experience has led to compelling results that support this approach to patient management. Endoscopic ultrasound (EUS)-guided drainage has emerged as the preferred treatment modality for symptomatic pseudocysts. Alternative drainage techniques such as non–EUS-guided endoscopic transmural drainage, percutaneous drainage, and surgical cystogastrostomy are considered second-line options. This chapter reviews the rationale and advantages of EUS guidance, the technique of EUS-guided drainage, and results of key published data.

Current Treatment Approaches and Limitations

Surgical Cystogastrostomy

Open surgical drainage entails the creation of a cystogastrostomy or cystenterostomy. This can be accomplished laparoscopically through an anterior transgastric approach, which requires an anterior gastrotomy for access and a cystogastrostomy creation through the posterior gastric wall, or a posterior approach through the lesser sac.[4] The procedure can also be performed through a lesser sac approach, which is technically easier and is associated with less intraoperative bleeding.[5]

Pancreatic pseudocysts that are not in close proximity to the stomach require the creation of a cystojejunostomy.[6] The cystojejunostomy is sometimes created through a Roux limb of jejunum. Although the technical and treatment success rates for surgery are high, the procedure is associated with a 10% to 30% morbidity rate and a 1% to 5% mortality rate.[7] The technique is invasive, associated with a prolonged hospital stay, and more expensive than the alternatives[8] (Table 24-1).

Percutaneous Drainage

Percutaneous drainage performed under radiologic guidance is less invasive than surgery. Major drawbacks of this technique include the inability to clear solid debris that necessitates surgical rescue in 50% to 60% of patients, the risk of puncture of adjacent viscera, infection, prolonged periods of external drainage, and predisposition to the development of pancreaticocutaneous fistula.[9] It is an important adjunctive therapy when the fluid collection is multifocal and extends to areas not accessible for endoscopic drainage or lacking a mature wall. Percutaneous drainage appears more likely to be successful in patients with normal pancreatic ducts and in patients with strictures but no communication between the duct and the pseudocyst, compared with patients with strictures and duct-cyst communication or those with complete cutoff of the duct. These features predispose patients to long-term pancreaticocutaneous fistula formation.[10]

Non–EUS-Guided Endoscopic Transmural Drainage

Non–EUS-guided endoscopic transmural drainage entails the creation of a fistulous tract between the pseudocyst and the gastric lumen (cystogastrostomy) or duodenal lumen (cystoduodenostomy). After establishing access, a nasocystic catheter or a transluminal stent is placed into the pseudocyst to facilitate drainage. The technical success rate of this approach is between 50% and 60%, and most treatment failures are caused by the lack of endoscopically visible luminal compression.[11,12] The risk of perforation is particularly high when luminal compression is absent.[13-15] Another major complication is hemorrhage, which is encountered in approximately 6% of cases.[13-18] There is also the potential for misdiagnosing a malignant cyst neoplasm or a necrotic collection as a pseudocyst and managing it inappropriately by transmural stenting.[12,19,20]

EUS-Guided Endoscopic Transmural Drainage

EUS, by virtue of its ability to visualize outside the lumen of the gastrointestinal tract, enables drainage of pancreatic pseudocysts that do not cause luminal compression. The technical success rate of EUS for pancreatic pseudocyst drainage has been reported to be greater than 90%, and the complication

---

TABLE 24-1

COMPARISON OF SURGICAL, PERCUTANEOUS, AND ENDOSCOPIC APPROACHES TO PSEUDOCYST MANAGEMENT

Treatment Modality	Advantages	Disadvantages
Surgical cystogastrostomy	1. Effective therapy 2. Salvage therapy following failed endoscopic or percutaneous drainage	1. Invasive 2. High morbidity and 1% to 5% mortality 3. Longer hospital stay 4. Expensive
Percutaneous drainage	1. Less invasive 2. Useful adjunct to endoscopic drainage when pseudocyst is inaccessible by endoscopy 3. Can be undertaken in high-risk patients too sick to undergo surgical or endoscopic drainage	1. Cutaneous infections and local complications such as bleeding 2. Inadequate therapy in the presence of debris 3. Predisposes to pancreaticocutaneous fistula formation
Non–EUS-guided endoscopic drainage	1. Less invasive than surgery and organ-preserving intervention 2. Rescue measure in postoperative pancreatic fluid collections	1. Feasible only if the pseudocyst is adjacent to the gastrointestinal lumen and causes luminal compression 2. May only be a temporizing measure if the underlying anatomic predisposition requires surgical correction 3. Inability to visualize interposed vessels may cause hemorrhage 4. Possibility of perforation because of the relatively "blind" technique 5. Potential for misdiagnosing cyst neoplasms and necrotic collections as pseudocysts. 6. Infection
EUS-guided pseudocyst drainage	1. Ability to access pseudocysts that do not cause luminal compression 2. Distinguish cyst neoplasms and necrotic collections from pseudocysts 3. Real-time puncture minimizes bleeding, perforation risks	1. Limited availability and lack of dedicated accessories 2. Infection 3. Surgery may be required to correct underlying anatomic defects not amenable for endotherapy

TABLE 24-2

	STUDIES EVALUATING THE IMPACT OF EUS ON PATIENTS UNDERGOING PSEUDOCYST DRAINAGE			
Authors (yr)	**Change in Management (%)**	**Alternate Diagnosis (%)**	**Pseudocyst Size Variation Between Time of CT and EUS (%)**	**Other Impact (%)**
Fockens et al[24] (1997)	37.5	6	9	22.5[a]
Varadarajulu et al[12] (2007)	16	8	8	—

CT, computed tomography.

[a]The presence of intervening vessels, normal pancreatic parenchyma, and distance between the pseudocyst and the gut lumen precluded transluminal drainage. In this study, all drainages were undertaken by esophagogastroduodenoscopy following assessment of the pancreatic fluid collection by EUS.

rate is less than 5%.[12,21–23] Apart from issues related to access and safety, performing routine EUS before endoscopic drainage leads to a change in management in 5% to 37% of cases.[24,25] The reason is that EUS establishes an alternate diagnosis of cyst neoplasm in 3% to 5% of cases that were originally misclassified as a pseudocyst by computed tomography (CT)[12,24] (Table 24-2). From a treatment point of view, the differentiation of WON from pseudocyst is very important, and EUS is much more sensitive than CT in making this distinction. Moreover, if a CT scan has not been performed recently, EUS can assess suitability for drainage because pseudocysts tend to resolve or become smaller over time.[12,24,25]

Standard One-Step EUS Technique

When a therapeutic echoendoscope and access to fluoroscopy are available, pancreatic pseudocyst drainage can be performed as a one-step procedure under EUS guidance. The technique is relatively straightforward but requires expertise with therapeutic maneuvers such as guidewire exchange and stent deployment. This section reviews the basic techniques and keys to success for EUS-guided pseudocyst drainage. Accessories for the procedure include the following:

- Therapeutic linear echoendoscope with a working channel 3.7 or 3.8 mm
- 19-G fine-needle aspiration (FNA) needle (lumen of the 22-G needle does not permit a 0.035-inch guidewire)
- 0.025- or 0.035-inch guidewires
- 4.5- or 5-Fr ERCP cannula or Soehendra dilators or an over-the-wire needle-knife catheter or cystotome catheter
- Over-the-wire biliary balloon dilator
- 7-, 8-, 8.5-, or 10-Fr double-pigtail plastic stents.

Noncautery Technique: Graded Dilation Technique (Video 24-1). After excluding the presence of vasculature in the path of the needle by using color Doppler ultrasound, a 19-G FNA needle is used to puncture the pseudocyst under EUS guidance (Figure 24-1A). A 0.035-inch guidewire is introduced through the needle and is coiled within the pseudocyst under fluoroscopic guidance (see Figure 24-1B). The tract is then sequentially dilated under fluoroscopic guidance (see Figure 24-1C) by first passing a 4.5- or 5-Fr endoscopic retrograde cholangiopancreatography (ERCP) cannula over the guidewire (see Figure 24-1D). Another alternative is to use the Soehendra biliary dilators. Further dilation is then undertaken using a 6- to 15-mm over-the-wire biliary balloon dilator (see Figure 24-1E). Following dilation, two 7-, 8-, 8.5-, or 10-Fr double-pigtail stents are deployed within the pseudocyst under fluoroscopic guidance (see Figure 24-1F). Multiple stents and a 7- or 10-Fr nasocystic drainage catheter may have to be deployed in patients with infected PFC for periodic flushing and evacuation of the cyst contents.

Technical Tips: A major advantage of the graded dilation technique is that electrocautery is not used during any step of the procedure. In the largest series reported to date on EUS-guided pseudocyst drainage using the foregoing technique, no major complication such as bleeding or perforation was encountered in any patient.[26] In patients with a thick pseudocyst wall, the ERCP cannula may "bounce off" if it is not aligned properly. It is important that the cannula be in line with the guidewire when it exits the echoendoscope, to penetrate the pseudocyst perpendicularly (see Figures 24-1C and D). Once within the pseudocyst, the cannula should be withdrawn into the echoendoscope, and repeated penetration of the pseudocyst should be attempted, to dilate the transmural tract further.

Cautery Technique: Use of Needle-Knife Technique (Video 24-2). After a guidewire has been coiled within the pseudocyst by using a 19-G FNA needle, the transmural tract is dilated using electrocautery administered through an over-the-wire needle-knife catheter (rather than dilating the tract

Video 24-1. Noncautery technique: graded dilation technique.

Video 24-2. Cautery technique: use of needle-knife technique.

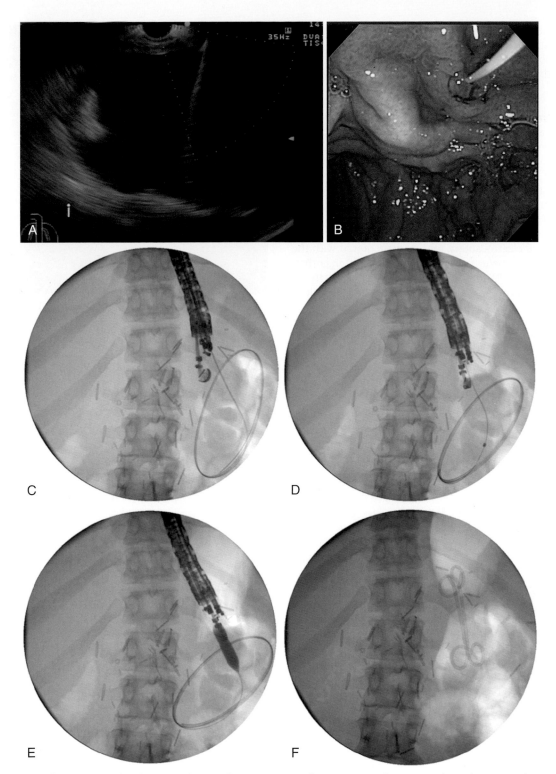

FIGURE 24-1 **A,** Pseudocyst accessed with a 19-G fine-needle aspiration needle. **B,** Passage of a 0.035-inch guidewire into the pseudocyst. Note the edematous gastric mucosa in severe hypoalbuminemia. **C,** Passage of a 0.035-inch guidewire under fluoroscopy. **D,** Passage of a 5-Fr endoscopic retrograde cholangiopancreatography catheter to dilate the transmural tract. **E,** Dilation of the transmural tract with use of a balloon. **F,** Placement of two transmural stents.

with an ERCP cannula). Following access to the pseudocyst, dilation and stenting are performed as outlined earlier. However, the challenge of the technique is the fact that the tip of the needle knife is parallel to the guidewire, such that if not properly oriented and positioned, it may not follow adequately the direction of the inserted guidewire.

Cautery Technique: Use of Cystotome Catheter Technique. After a guidewire has been coiled within the pseudocyst by using a 19-G FNA needle, the transmural tract is dilated using electrocautery administered through the over-the-wire diathermy sheath of a cystotome. Unlike the needle knife, where the tip of the fine needle is parallel to the guidewire, a diathermy ring at the tip completely encloses the guidewire, such that the axis can be maintained correctly during the process of electrocautery. Following access to the pseudocyst, dilation and stenting are performed as outlined earlier.

Cautery Technique: Use of Cystotome. Another alternative includes the use of a dedicated commercially available cystotome.[27] The cystotome is a modified needle-knife papillotome that consists of an inner wire with a needle-knife tip, a 5-Fr inner catheter, and a 10-Fr outer catheter equipped with a diathermy ring at its distal tip. The proximal end of this device includes a handle with connectors for administration of electrocautery. The pancreatic pseudocyst is punctured with the cystotome by using the knife tip of the inner catheter, with administration of electrocautery, and is then entered with the inner catheter. The metal part of the inner catheter is then withdrawn, and a 0.035-inch guidewire is passed through the inner catheter into the cyst cavity. The outer 10-Fr sheath of the cystotome, which is equipped with a diathermy ring, is advanced through the puncture site by using electrocautery. The cystotome is then removed, leaving the guidewire in the cyst cavity. The transmural tract is then dilated followed by stent deployment. The drawback is that the endosonographic view of the cystotome needle tip may not be as clear as an FNA needle.

Technical Tips: An advantage of the needle-knife technique is that it penetrates the pseudocyst wall with relative ease. The main disadvantage of the technique is that perforation was reported as a complication in several series.[11,23,28–30] This is possibly due to the fact that the guidewire is parallel to the needle tip, rather than passing through it, such that the axis of cautery may end up tangential to the axis of the guidewire. Generally, EUS is performed for pseudocyst drainage in patients without luminal compression. Pseudocysts that do not cause luminal compression are usually located in the pancreatic tail region or in atypical locations such as the right upper quadrant. The location of these pseudocysts is such that they are accessed from the gastric cardia or the fundus of the stomach. When a catheter is deployed at these locations, because of the acute angulation of the echoendoscope, the deployed needle-knife points tangentially and leads to an undesirable incision. Maintaining a degree of tension over the guidewire keeps the needle-knife catheter in plane with the guidewire as it exits the echoendoscope and can possibly minimize the risk of perforation. The cautery technique using the diathermy sheath of the cystotome set (when available) following initial 19-G FNA needle puncture would be preferred over the use of the needle knife and would be very useful when puncturing thick cyst walls that preclude insertion of ERCP catheters or Soehendra dilators for tract dilatation.

EUS-Guided Drainage Using the Double Guidewire Technique. Because of the advantage of easily allowing repeat stent placement, the current trend is to insert two guidewires. This "double-wire" approach, in which two guidewires are inserted through the same catheter prior to stent placement, has been used to avoid the need to recannulate the pseudocyst after gaining initial transmural access. Recannulation of the cavity may be potentially difficult due to a tangential axis of puncture and poor visibility from fluids flowing out from the

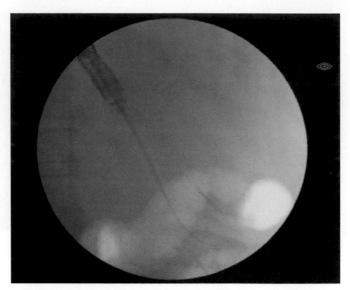

FIGURE 24-2 Insertion of two guidewires simultaneously under fluoroscopic guidance.

pseudocyst. The current most commonly used technique is to insert a second guidewire through an 8.5- to 10-Fr cystotome catheter. In this technique, a 19-G needle is used to puncture the pseudocyst, and a guidewire is inserted. The cystotome catheter is then inserted over the guidewire into the pseudocyst cavity.[31] Other similar approaches include the use of a novel prototype three-layer puncture kit that allowed the simultaneous insertion of two guidewires at the initial puncture,[32] as well as the use of a 10-Fr Soehendra biliary dilator (Figure 24-2),[33] which is inserted into the pseudocyst cavity over the single guidewire inserted at the initial EUS-guided puncture, followed by insertion of a second guidewire (Video 24-3). Sequential transmural stent and drainage catheter placement can then be performed without a loss of access to the pseudocyst cavity. An important technical issue to note is that the working channel of a therapeutic EUS scope is 3.7 mm. With two guidewires of 0.025 to 0.035 inches within the working channel, the diameter of the first transmural stent cannot be 10 Fr because there will be no space. Hence in such a situation, an 8.5-Fr double-pigtail stent is inserted first. Thereafter, one guidewire is removed and then a 10-Fr double-pigtail stent is inserted over the remaining guidewire. To facilitate the insertion of double-pigtail stents, one can apply silicone lubricant over the stent surface. This technique can potentially enable the placement of more guidewires for multiple stent placements.

Video 24-3. Double-wire technique for drainage of pancreatic fluid collections.

Other Technical Variations

Forward-Viewing Echoendoscope

A forward-viewing therapeutic echoendoscope (Olympus, Tokyo, Japan) has been developed, and unlike the conventional echoendoscope, its endoscopic and ultrasonic axes are aligned. It has a narrower ultrasonic view and does not have an elevator. The basic technique of EUS-guided drainage is similar to what was described earlier, the main difference being the axis for puncture and drainage. A multicenter study compared the use of forward-viewing and oblique-viewing linear echoendoscopes for pseudocyst drainage. There was no difference in ease of drainage or procedure safety and efficacy.[34] However, from a practical view point, due to the absence of an elevator and the direction of the insertion axis, situations may arise where it will be potentially difficult to adequately transmit the pressure necessary for stent placement.

Use of Self-Expandable Metallic Stents

As an alternative to standard plastic double-pigtail stents that have a maximum inner diameter of 3.3 mm (10 Fr), recent publications have explored the use of self-expandable metallic stents (SEMS). Enteral SEMS were used initially, but stent migration was a problem with these stents. Specifically designed SEMS for drainage purpose have now been introduced.[35,36] The lumen-apposing stent (AXIOS, Xlumena Inc, Mountain View, California, USA) is a fully covered, 10-mm diameter, nitinol, braided stent with bilateral anchor flanges. When fully expanded, the flange diameter is twice that of the "saddle" section and is designed to hold tissue layers in apposition (Figure 24-3).[35] The stent is delivered constrained

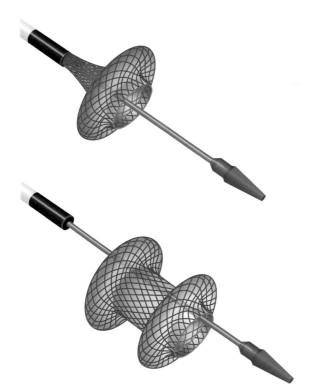

FIGURE 24-3 The lumen-apposing one-step device designed for transluminal drainage of pancreatic fluid collections.

through a 10.5-Fr catheter that is inserted over the guidewire within the pseudocyst cavity. The "NAGI" covered SEMS (Taewoong-Medical Co, Seoul, South Korea) is another specially designed SEMS with a 10-mm diameter in the center and 20-mm ends that can reduce the risk of migration.[36] The potential advantage of SEMS is a larger drainage orifice and the possibility of facilitating repeat entry into the cavity for endoscopic necrosectomy in the context of infected walled-off necrosis. Its potential utility is probably limited to the management of infected walled-off necrosis.[37] However, given the high costs of SEMS the issue of cost effectiveness will need to be addressed. In addition, patients may have underlying pancreatic duct disruption such that once the SEMS is removed the collection may recur, necessitating repeat drainage and reinsertion of plastic stents. In contrast, if EUS-guided drainage is performed using plastic stents, an all-in-one solution would have been provided at the start, with the initial plastic stent draining the fluid collection; the stent's long-term placement would prevent the pseudocyst from reaccumulation.[38]

Keys to Technical Success and Other Considerations

Stent Deployment

When pseudocyst drainages are performed through the cardia or fundus of the stomach and the duodenum, the tip of the echoendoscope is acutely angulated. Deployment of 10-Fr transmural stents at these sites can be technically challenging unless the tip of the echoendoscope can be kept straightened with fluoroscopic guidance (Figure 24-4). This limitation can also be overcome by placement of multiple 7-Fr double-pigtail stents. However, 10-Fr stents should be preferentially deployed if a pseudocyst is infected. Unlike the duodenoscope, which has a 4.2-mm working channel, the working channel of most therapeutic echoendoscopes is only 3.7 mm. When deploying 10-Fr stents, it is important not to have another 0.035-inch guidewire in the biopsy channel because it increases the friction and makes stent deployment very difficult.

Use of the Small Channel Curvilinear Echoendoscope for Pseudocyst Drainage

When a therapeutic echoendoscope is not available, pseudocyst drainage can still be undertaken using a small channel curvilinear echoendoscope by passing a 0.035-inch guidewire into the pseudocyst through a 19-G FNA needle. The echoendoscope is then exchanged over the guidewire for a double-channel gastroscope or duodenoscope, and pseudocyst drainage can be completed successfully.

Bedside EUS for Pseudocyst Drainage

For patients in the intensive care unit who are unstable and deemed too sick to be transported safely to the endoscopy unit, drainage of PFCs can be undertaken at the bedside if a portable fluoroscopy machine is available. This concept was demonstrated in a study of six patients who underwent bedside EUS in the intensive care unit.[39] A pancreatic pseudocyst and a mediastinal abscess were drained successfully in two of these six patients. For convenience, these procedures are easier to perform when the EUS processor is small and can be placed on the endoscopy cart.

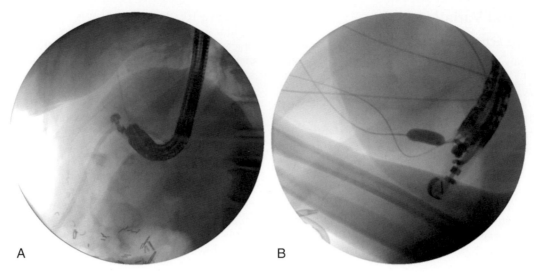

FIGURE 24-4   A, Acute angulation of the echoendoscope at drainage through the gastric fundus. A transpapillary pancreatic stent is seen in the background. **B,** After guidewire passage, the tip of the echoendoscope is straightened for undertaking further endotherapy.

Multiple Pancreatic Pseudocysts

Approximately 10% of patients have pseudocysts at multiple locations, and their management poses a clinical dilemma. These patients are generally managed by surgery or percutaneous drainage. In a study reported in 2008, 6 of 60 patients with PFCs had multiple fluid collections (≥6 cm), and pancreatography revealed complete duct disruption in all 6 cases.[26] With EUS, 15 individual PFCs were drained successfully in these 6 patients with a successful clinical outcome in all 3 patients with pancreatic pseudocysts. Three pseudocysts were drained at three different sites in each of these three patients. Generally, the largest pseudocyst is drained at an index procedure. A repeat procedure is warranted for drainage of other pseudocysts if a patient has persistent symptoms with a noncommunicative fluid collection on follow-up imaging.

Patients with Altered Anatomy

In patients with postsurgical anatomy, identification of focal disorder at EUS can be technically challenging. However, EUS-guided drainage of pancreatic pseudocysts may still be technically feasible because symptomatic pseudocysts usually tend to be large and frequently communicate or extend to other areas in the lesser sac. Reviewing a CT scan before the procedure will provide important information on the landmarks and the best site from which the pseudocyst can be accessed. Caution must be exercised during navigation of the echoendoscope through different limbs because the presence of adhesions can increase the risk for perforation.[26,40,41]

Management of Small Symptomatic Pseudocysts

It is technically not feasible to place transmural stents in patients with pseudocysts that measure 4 cm or less. Therefore symptomatic pseudocysts up to 4 cm in size that communicate with the main pancreatic duct are managed by transpapillary pancreatic stenting. In these patients, after pancreatic stenting, the pseudocyst is aspirated completely by EUS-guided FNA. Despite the lack of published data, observations indicate that these patients experience quicker and better symptom relief.

Advantages

When the requisite accessories and technical expertise are available, EUS enables one-step drainage of pancreatic pseudocysts irrespective of the presence or absence of luminal compression. Because it is a one-step procedure, drainage can be undertaken in a timely manner with minimal discomfort to the patient and less need for additional sedation. Confirmation of diagnosis and therapy can be undertaken in the same setting. The ability to drain the pseudocyst in real time under ultrasound guidance minimizes the risk of complications. Intracystic hemorrhage is a rare but serious complication encountered during FNA of cystic lesions of the pancreas. During EUS, the bleeding manifests as hyperechoic foci within the pseudocyst. Early identification of bleeding at EUS permits timely intervention and thereby minimizes the risk for serious adverse events. During non–EUS-guided endoscopic drainage, if a guidewire is accidentally dislodged after balloon dilation of the transmural tract, it may be difficult to access the pseudocyst again because the luminal compression may have disappeared. This is not a major problem with EUS-guided drainage, because the pseudocyst is well visualized at all times and re-entry to the pseudocyst can be easily accomplished.

Disadvantages

The EUS-guided pseudocyst drainage approach has no major disadvantages. Deployment of 10-Fr stents can sometimes be technically challenging when the tip of the echoendoscope is acutely angulated. This problem can be overcome by straightening the tip of the echoendoscope with the aid of fluoroscopy or by deployment of 7-Fr stents.

Adjunctive Measures

After placement of transmural stents and drainage catheters, further adjunctive measures may be necessary. These measures are the same whether or not EUS guidance was used to obtain initial access of the collection. In the context of an

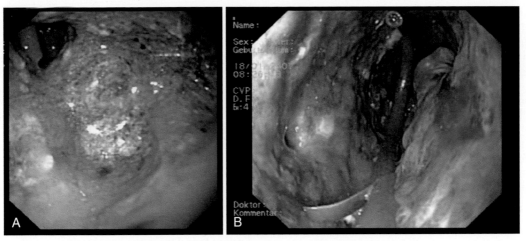

FIGURE 24-5   **A**, Endoscopic image of walled-off pancreatic necrosis. **B.** Endoscopic view of the necrosis cavity post-treatment.

infected pancreatic fluid collection, continuous saline irrigation and drainage with a nasocystic catheter is important until sepsis has resolved.

In the presence of infected pancreatic necrosis, adjunctive endoscopic necrosectomy (Figure 24-5) is essential to improve the treatment success rates.[42–47] This approach is recognized by the soon-to-be published updated International Association of Pancreatology guidelines, which were published as the summary report of a consensus conference. The guidelines also acknowledged the role of minimally invasive techniques as a treatment option.[48] Since the time when the technique was first reported in 2000 as a case report,[42] followed by a case series detailing an aggressive endoscopic approach,[43] outcome data from large multicenter case series are now available.[44–47] Although proven to be effective, there is a risk of significant morbidity and mortality. Hence the extent and aggressiveness of necrosectomy will need to be individualized and weighed against the risks of complications. In fact, complete necrosectomy may not be required in all instances, and flushing and irrigation may be adequate. A multicenter randomized study compared a minimally invasive step-up approach with open necrosectomy and found that a minimally invasive step-up approach reduced the rate of the composite end point of major complications or death among patients with infected necrosis. In fact, in 35% of cases, percutaneous irrigation and drainage alone was sufficient.[49]

Another issue that must be addressed is the presence of pancreatic duct disruption. A good quality magnetic resonance cholangiopancreatography (MRCP), especially with secretin use, may be able to fully visualize the ductal anatomy. ERCP is not required in most instances. Therapeutic ERCP may be needed in the context of pancreatic duct stricture or stones. Duct disruption can be treated by pancreatic duct stenting. If the fistula does not resolve after a prolonged period of pancreatic duct stenting, endoscopic sealing with a topical skin adhesive (e.g., Histoacryl) can be considered.[50] As an alternative to ERCP, long-term transmural stenting has also been reported for treatment of pancreatic duct disruption in order to prevent recurrence of pseudocysts.[38]

Clinical Outcomes of EUS-Guided Drainage

When assessing treatment outcomes, it is important to distinguish between technical success and clinical success. The former refers to successfully achieving access and drainage of the fluid collection, whereas the latter pertains to complete resolution and recovery. This concept is important, because technically one can be successful in terms of placing transmural stents for an infected walled-off necrosis, but this will not lead to resolution of the collection because additional steps such as endoscopic necrosectomy are necessary. When a collection is suitable and accessible, technical success can inevitably be achieved in expert hands. Another point is that when one compares EUS-guided with non–EUS-guided drainage, the difference exists only at the initial stage of attempting to puncture and accessing the fluid collection. All subsequent steps are similar in both approaches.

Pseudocysts and Infected Pseudocysts

For pseudocysts, very high treatment success rates exceeding 90%[22,51,52] and even reaching 100%[53] have been achieved. The term "pancreatic abscess" is no longer recommended based on the new terminology,[1] although prior publications have used this term. It should be regarded as equivalent to an infected pseudocyst. High treatment success rates greater than 90%[29,51] have been reported.[29,51]

Infected Walled-Off Pancreatic Necrosis

The results for clinical resolution are generally poorer than pseudocyst drainage because of the need to remove necrotic debris. In a comparative study, it was reported that the success rate of pseudocyst drainage was 92%, compared to 72% in patients with necrosis.[54] Another study reported the success rate of simple drainage to be as low as 25%.[51] If an aggressive endoscopic approach using endoscopic necrosectomy is adopted, success rates ranging from 75%[45] to 84%[44] and even up to 91%[47] can be achieved based on reported data from large series. Adjunctive surgical and percutaneous drainage may be needed.[20] A recently published randomized controlled trial showed that in patients with infected necrotizing pancreatitis, endoscopic necrosectomy reduced the pro-inflammatory response as well as the composite clinical end point of major complications compared with surgical necrosectomy.[55] The enthusiasm for endoscopic necrosectomy must, however, be tempered by the realization of the procedural risks, as well as the fact that an aggressive approach toward necrosectomy may not be needed in the majority of patients,[49,56] such that even if endoscopic necrosectomy were to be performed, clinical resolution may even be achieved with less extensive debridement.

Comparison of EUS-Guided Drainage with Alternative Drainage Techniques

Surgical versus Percutaneous and Endoscopic Drainage

Vosoghi and colleagues reviewed and compared the results of case series of surgical, percutaneous, and endoscopic drainage of symptomatic pseudocysts.[53] The success rates of surgical, percutaneous, non–EUS-guided transmural drainage, and EUS-guided transmural drainage were 100%, 84%, 90%, and 94%, respectively. Complication rates were higher for surgical (28% to 34%, with 1% to 8.5% mortality) and percutaneous drainage (18%, with 2% mortality) compared with non–EUS-guided (15%, with 0% mortality) and EUS-guided transmural (1.5%, with 0% mortality) drainage.

EUS-Guided Cystogastrostomy versus Surgical Cystogastrostomy

A retrospective study compared the clinical outcomes of EUS-guided cystogastrostomy with surgical cystogastrostomy for the management of patients with uncomplicated pancreatic pseudocysts and performed a cost analysis of each treatment modality.[8] The investigators showed that EUS-guided drainage was similar to surgery in terms of rates of treatment success (100% versus 95%), but it had advantages in terms of shorter hospital stay (mean length of stay, 2.7 versus 6.5 days) and lower costs (Table 24-3). Similar findings were reported in a randomized trial that compared EUS and surgery for pancreatic cystogastrostomy.[57] In this trial, which included 40 randomized patients, no difference was noted in the rates of technical (both cohorts, 100%) and treatment success (95% [EUS] versus 100% [surgery]) and of procedural complications (none in both cohorts). At a median follow-up of 24

months, no difference was reported in rates of pseudocyst recurrence (0% [EUS] versus 5% [surgery]) or repeat interventions (5% in each cohort). At long-term follow-up of 24 months, the physical and mental health scores were significantly better for the endoscopy cohort. Compared to surgery, the median length of postprocedure hospital stay and average costs were also significantly less for EUS-guided cystogastrostomy. The investigators concluded that EUS-guided cystogastrostomy should be the preferred treatment approach for patients with uncomplicated symptomatic pancreatic pseudocysts because the procedure was less costly, was associated with shorter length of hospital stay, yielded better physical and mental health scores, and had long-term clinical outcomes comparable to surgery.

EUS-Guided versus Non–EUS-Guided Endoscopic Drainage

The difference between EUS-guided and non–EUS-guided endoscopic drainage is at the initial step of gaining access to the pancreatic fluid collection. All the subsequent steps are similar (i.e., insertion of guidewires with fluoroscopic guidance, insertion of transmural stents or nasocystic catheters, balloon dilatation of the cystogastrostoma, and endoscopic necrosectomy). Non–EUS-guided endoscopic drainage is a blind procedure, and the presence of endoscopic bulging is a prerequisite. The fluid collection is punctured at the site of maximum endoscopic bulging. There is also a potential risk of hemorrhage from interposed vessels during transmural drainage. On the other hand, with EUS guidance the fluid collection is visualized during the entire puncture process, and endoscopic bulging is not mandatory. One may potentially decrease the bleeding rate by avoiding interposed blood vessels through the use of Doppler ultrasound. EUS can also differentiate a pseudocyst from a cystic tumor and ascertain the nature of a fluid collection and guide the drainage strategy; for instance, a pseudocyst may be treated by placing transmural stents, whereas a necrotic collection requires additional endoscopic debridement. The importance of EUS was highlighted in a case series in which EUS was used to evaluate pseudocysts prior to attempting endoscopic drainage. It was shown that EUS provided essential information that led to a change in management strategy in 37.5% of cases.[24] Another case series showed that EUS could be used to guide pseudocyst drainage in patients with portal hypertension, thereby reducing the bleeding risk.[58]

Direct comparison of EUS-guided and non–EUS-guided endoscopic drainage has been made. Non–EUS-guided transmural drainage was compared with EUS-guided drainage in

TABLE 24-3

STUDIES COMPARING EUS AND SURGERY FOR PANCREATIC PSEUDOCYST DRAINAGE

Authors (study type)	Number of Patients	Technical Success (%)	Treatment Success (%)	Complications	Length of Hospital Stay (days)	Recurrence (%)	Cost (US$)
Varadarajulu[8] (case control)	30	95 vs 100	100 vs 95	None	2.6 vs 6.5	None	9077 vs 14,815
Varadarajulu[57] (randomized trial)[a]	40	100 each cohort	95 vs 100	None	2 vs 6	0 vs 5	7011 vs 15,052

All comparisons are between EUS and surgery, with EUS numbers indicated first.
[a]Quality of life for both mental and physical health scores was superior for endoscopy.

TABLE 24-4

RANDOMIZED TRIALS COMPARING EUS AND NON–EUS ENDOSCOPIC TECHNIQUES FOR PSEUDOCYST DRAINAGE

Authors (yr)	EUS (%)	EGD (%)	p
Technical Success			
Varadarajulu et al[59] (2008)	100	33.3	<0.001
Park et al[60] (2009)	94	72	0.03
Treatment Success			
Varadarajulu et al[59] (2008)	100	87	0.48
Park et al[60] (2009)	89	86	0.6
Complications			
Varadarajulu et al[59] (2008)	0	13	0.48
Park et al[60] (2009)	7	10	0.6

EGD, esophagogastroduodenoscopy.

a study in which patients with pseudocysts with bulging and no obvious portal hypertension underwent conventional transmural drainage, whereas all remaining patients underwent EUS-guided drainage.[24] No significant differences were noted between both groups in terms of efficacy or safety. Indirectly, this study supported the concept that EUS-guided drainage is superior because it can be used to drain pseudocysts not amenable to conventional transmural drainage without any increased risks.

In another study (Table 24-4), the rate of technical success between EUS-guided and non–EUS-guided transmural drainage of pancreatic pseudocysts was directly compared prospectively.[59] All the patients randomized to EUS (n = 14) underwent successful drainage; in contrast, the procedure was technically successful in only 33% randomized to non–EUS-guided drainage (n = 15). The reasons for technical failure were the absence of luminal compression in nine patients and severe bleeding following attempted puncture of the pseudocyst in one patient. All 10 patients subsequently underwent successful drainage of the pseudocyst under EUS guidance. In a similar study, the technical success rate of pseudocyst drainage was higher in patients undergoing EUS-guided drainage compared with those without EUS guidance (94% versus 72%).[60] Several studies reported on the technical feasibility and safety profile of EUS to perform transesophageal drainage of PFCs even in the absence of luminal compression in the esophagus.[61-64]

Technical Proficiency

Currently, in most parts of North America and Asia, dedicated devices to perform EUS-guided drainage are not commercially available. There is no predetermined threshold for the number of procedures that need to be performed under supervision before competency assessment. In the opinion of the authors, an endoscopist skilled in EUS FNA and ERCP should be able to perform the procedure competently. Endoscopists who want to perform pseudocyst drainage but who do not perform ERCPs need to be proficient with use of accessories such as 0.035-inch guidewires, needle-knife catheters, balloon dilators, and double-pigtail stents. In a study that evaluated performance of a single endosonographer, the technical proficiency for performing pseudocyst drainages improved significantly after 25 procedures.[26] The median procedural duration after performing 25 cases decreased from 70 to 25 minutes.

Technical Limitations

It is clear that EUS-guided drainage offers several advantages compared with traditional drainage techniques. However, the EUS procedure has limitations related to the echoendoscope design that result in technical difficulties during endoscopic drainage. An important limitation is that the size of the working channel of a therapeutic linear echoendoscope is 3.7 or 3.8 mm, smaller than that of a therapeutic duodenoscope (4.2 mm). This size limits the suction ability, which is important when copious fluid is draining from the pseudocyst cavity after the initial puncture. Additionally, although placing a 10-Fr stent is not an issue with a linear echoendoscope, one may need to place multiple stents or a nasocystic catheter for irrigation. In these situations, it may be faster and easier to use a double-wire technique. However, the smaller working channels of echoendoscopes limit the use of double-wire techniques in that the size of the first transmural stent inserted must be 8.5 Fr or smaller because of excessive resistance within a 3.7-mm working channel with two guidewires in place. The first stent that is placed cannot be the preferred, larger, 10-Fr size.

Another limitation is the oblique view of current echoendoscopes. This configuration limits the endoscopic view and results in a tangential puncture axis. Puncturing at an angle may hamper successful completion of the procedure because the force that is applied when accessories are introduced through the working channel cannot be fully directed toward the puncture site. The tangential axis also makes subsequent cannulation of the pseudocyst cavity difficult, unless there was prior balloon dilatation of the puncture site or a double-wire technique was used.

A prototype forward-viewing therapeutic echoendoscope developed by Olympus allows a forward axis of needle puncture and insertion of accessories, parallel to the scanning axis. This facilitates forward transmission of force when inserting accessories, stents, and catheters. In a pilot study, all pseudocysts were successfully drained without complications, and some pseudocysts could be punctured only with the forward-viewing scope.[34] The forward-viewing echoendoscope is limited by a 3.7-mm working channel, a lack of elevator, and an ultrasonic view of only 90 degrees.

Endoscopic drainage is feasible only for pseudocysts located around the stomach and duodenum. When pseudocysts involve more distal locations such as the paracolic regions, they are not accessible endoscopically, and other adjunctive measures such as percutaneous or surgical drainage need to be considered.

Complications of EUS-Guided Drainage

The main potential complications of concern are severe bleeding and perforation. To minimize risk, only fluid collections with a mature wall and within 1 cm of gastrointestinal lumen should undergo endoscopic drainage. Any coagulopathy, if present, should be corrected. Patients with pseudocysts undergoing drainage should receive prophylactic antibiotics in order to prevent secondary infection of a sterile collection.[65,66] A review showed that complication rates were higher for surgical (28% to 34%, with 1% to 8.5% mortality) and percutaneous drainage (18%, with 2% mortality), compared to non–EUS-guided (15%, with 0% mortality) and EUS-guided transmural (1.5%, with 0% mortality) drainage.[53] A recent publication specifically examined the frequency of complications during EUS-guided drainage of PFCs in 148 consecutive patients over a 7-year period. Perforation was encountered at the site of transmural stenting in two patients (1.3%). Other complications included bleeding in one patient (0.67%), stent migration in one patient (0.67%), and infection in four patients (2.7%). These could be managed endoscopically except for the perforations that required surgery.[67] Perforation rates of 3% to 4% have been reported in the context

of endoscopic necrosectomy.[3] This risk can be reduced by adhering to key principles such as draining only a collection with a mature wall, performing stepwise balloon dilatation of the cystogastrostoma, using carbon dioxide for insufflation, and performing gentle debridement using saline lavage and aspiration, baskets, soft snares, and retrieval nets.

As stated earlier, effective decompression and drainage of WON yields treatment success in a substantial proportion of patients without the need for direct necrosectomy. In a recently described "multiple transluminal gateway technique" (Video 24-4), several openings were created in the gastric wall for placement of endoprosthesis to effectively drain the necrotic cavity.[68] The opening most proximal in the stomach was used for irrigation via a nasal drainage catheter, and the other openings for drainage of necrotic contents (Figure 24-6). In a study of 60 patients with WON, the multiple transluminal gateway

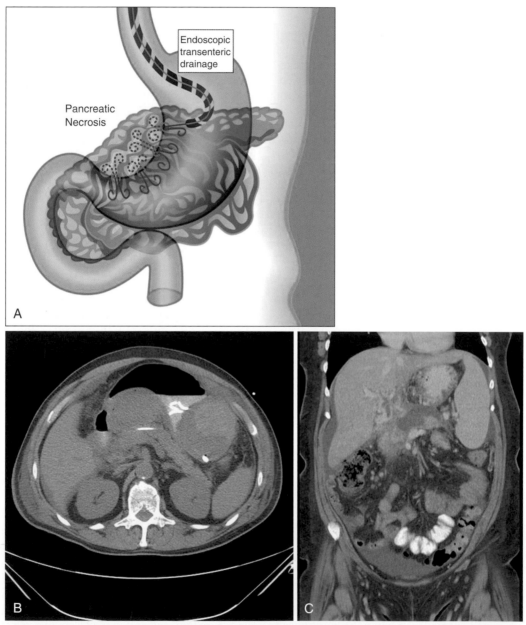

FIGURE 24-6 **A,** Illustration of the multiple transluminal gateway technique for drainage of walled-off pancreatic necrosis. **B,** CT image revealing a large complex walled-off necrosis treated by the multiple transluminal gateway technique. **C,** Effective resolution of the necrosis is observed on follow-up CT.

Video 24-4. Video demonstrating the multiple transluminal gateway technique for drainage of walled-off pancreatic necrosis.

technique yielded a treatment success of 91.7% versus 52.1% for patients treated by conventional drainage techniques. Unlike conventional endoscopic drainage, EUS enables access to the necrotic cavity even after the luminal compression disappears after initial puncture and facilitates effective drainage.

Summary

EUS-guided drainage is an effective and safe technique for the treatment of symptomatic PFCs. To minimize risk and increase efficacy, key principles should be adhered to. In addition, it must be recognized that not all endosonographers have the technical expertise to perform such complex procedures. Apart from the ability to perform linear EUS, a background in ERCP is important, and additional exposure and specific training are required. EUS-guided drainage can also provide an all-in-one solution for patients with pseudocysts due to disconnected pancreatic duct syndrome by draining the collection at initial stent insertion, followed by prevention of recurrence with indwelling stents.

REFERENCES

1. Banks PA, Bollen TL, Dervenis C, Acute Pancreatitis Classification Working Group, et al. Classification of acute pancreatitis—2012: revision of the Atlanta classification and definitions by international consensus. *Gut.* 2013;62:102-111.
2. Bradley EL III. A clinically based classification system for acute pancreatitis. *Arch Surg.* 1993;128:586-590. September 11 through 13, 1992, Summary of the International Symposium on Acute Pancreatitis, Atlanta, GA.
3. Seewald S, Ang TL, Teng KC, Soehendra N. EUS-guided drainage of pancreatic pseudocysts, abscesses and infected necrosis. *Dig Endosc.* 2009;21(suppl 1):S61-S65.
4. Park AE, Heniford BT. Therapeutic laparoscopy of the pancreas. *Ann Surg.* 2002;236:149-158.
5. Davila-Cervantes A, Gomez F, Chan C, et al. Laparoscopic drainage of pancreatic pseudocysts. *Surg Endosc.* 2004;18:1420-1426.
6. Kohler H, Schafmayer A, Ludtke FE, et al. Surgical treatment of pancreatic pseudocysts. *Br J Surg.* 1987;74:813-815.
7. Bhattacharya D, Ammori BJ. Minimally invasive approaches to the management of pancreatic pseudocysts. *Surg Laparosc Endosc Percutan Tech.* 2003;13:141-148.
8. Varadarajulu S, Lopes TL, Wilcox CM. EUS versus surgical cyst-gastrostomy for management of pancreatic pseudocysts. *Gastrointest Endosc.* 2008;68:649-655.
9. Bradley EL 3rd, Howard TJ, van Sonnenberg E, et al. Intervention in necrotizing pancreatitis: an evidence based review of surgical and percutaneous alternatives. *J Gastrointest Surg.* 2008;12:634-639.
10. Adams DB, Anderson MC. Percutaneous catheter drainage compared with internal drainage in the management of pancreatic pseudocyst. *Ann Surg.* 1992;215:571-576.
11. Kahaleh M, Shami VM, Conaway MR, et al. Endoscopic ultrasound drainage of pancreatic pseudocyst: a prospective comparison with conventional endoscopic drainage. *Endoscopy.* 2006;38:355-359.
12. Varadarajulu S, Wilcox CM, Tamhane A, et al. Role of EUS in drainage of peripancreatic fluid collections not amenable for endoscopic transmural drainage. *Gastrointest Endosc.* 2007;66:1107-1119.
13. Bejanin H, Liquory C, Ink O, et al. Endoscopic drainage of pseudocysts of the pancreas: study of 26 cases. *Gastroenterol Clin Biol.* 1993;17:804-810.
14. Smits ME, Rauws EA, Tytgat GN, et al. The efficacy of endoscopic treatment of pancreatic pseudocysts. *Gastrointest Endosc.* 1995;42:202-207.
15. Sharma SS, Bhargawa N, Govil A. Endoscopic management of pancreatic pseudocyst: a long-term follow-up. *Endoscopy.* 2002;34:203-207.
16. Sahel J, Bastid C, Pellat B, et al. Endoscopic cystoduodenostomy of cysts of chronic calcifying pancreatitis: a report of 20 cases. *Pancreas.* 1987;2:447-453.
17. Cremer M, Deviere J, Engelholm L. Endoscopic management of cysts and pseudocysts in chronic pancreatitis: long-term follow-up after 7 years of experience. *Gastrointest Endosc.* 1989;35:1-9.
18. Monkemuller KE, Baron TH, Morgan DE. Transmural drainage of pancreatic fluid collections without electrocautery using the Seldinger technique. *Gastrointest Endosc.* 1998;48:195-200.
19. Baron TH, Thaggard WG, Morgan DE, et al. Endoscopic therapy for organized pancreatic necrosis. *Gastroenterology.* 1996;111:755-764.
20. Papachristou GI, Takahashi N, Chahal P, et al. Per oral endoscopic drainage/debridement of walled-off pancreatic necrosis. *Ann Surg.* 2007;245:943-951.
21. Kruger M, Schneider AS, Manns MP, et al. Endoscopic management of pancreatic pseudocysts or abscesses after an EUS-guided 1-step procedure for initial access. *Gastrointest Endosc.* 2006;63:409-416.
22. Lopes CV, Pesenti C, Bories E, et al. Endoscopic-ultrasound–guided endoscopic transmural drainage of pancreatic pseudocysts and abscesses. *Scand J Gastroenterol.* 2007;42:524-529.
23. Antillon MR, Shah RJ, Stiegmann G, et al. Single-step EUS-guided transmural drainage of simple and complicated pancreatic pseudocysts. *Gastrointest Endosc.* 2006;63:797-803.
24. Fockens P, Johnson TG, van Dullemen HM, et al. Endosonographic imaging of pancreatic pseudocysts before endoscopic transmural drainage. *Gastrointest Endosc.* 1997;46:412-416.
25. Norton ID, Clain JE, Wiersema MJ, et al. Utility of endoscopic ultrasonography in endoscopic drainage of pancreatic pseudocysts in selected patients. *Mayo Clin Proc.* 2001;76:794-798.
26. Varadarajulu S, Tamhane A, Blakely J. Graded dilation technique for EUS-guided drainage of peripancreatic fluid collections: an assessment of outcomes, complications and technical proficiency. *Gastrointest Endosc.* 2008;68:656-666.
27. Cremer M, Deviere J, Baize M, Matos C. New device of endoscopic cystoenterostomy. *Endoscopy.* 1990;22:76-77.
28. Azar RR, Oh YS, Janec EM, et al. Wire-guided pancreatic pseudocyst drainage by using a modified needle knife and therapeutic echoendoscope. *Gastrointest Endosc.* 2006;63:688-692.
29. Giovannini M, Pesenti CH, Rolland AL, et al. Endoscopic ultrasound guided drainage of pancreatic pseudo-cyst and pancreatic abscess using a therapeutic echoendoscope. *Endoscopy.* 2001;33:473-477.
30. Will U, Wegener C, Graf KI, et al. Differential treatment and early outcome in the interventional endoscopic management of pancreatic pseudocysts in 27 patients. *World J Gastroenterol.* 2006;12:4175-4178.
31. Jansen JM, Hanrath A, Rauws EA, et al. Intracystic wire exchange facilitating insertion of multiple stents during endoscopic drainage of pancreatic pseudocysts. *Gastrointest Endosc.* 2007;66:157-161.
32. Seewald S, Thonke F, Ang TL, et al. One-step, simultaneous double-wire technique facilitates pancreatic pseudocyst and abscess drainage (with videos). *Gastrointest Endosc.* 2006;64:805-808.
33. Ang TL, Teo EK, Fock KM. EUS-guided drainage of infected pancreatic pseudocyst: use of a 10F Soehendra dilator to facilitate a double-wire technique for initial transgastric access (with videos). *Gastrointest Endosc.* 2008;68:192-194.
34. Voermans RP, Ponchon T, Schumacher B, et al. Forward-viewing versus oblique-viewing echoendoscopes in transluminal drainage of pancreatic fluid collections: a multicenter, randomized, controlled trial. *Gastrointest Endosc.* 2011;74:1285-1293.
35. Itoi T, Binmoeller KF, Shah J, et al. Clinical evaluation of a novel lumen-apposing metal stent for endosonography-guided pancreatic pseudocyst and gallbladder drainage (with videos). *Gastrointest Endosc.* 2012;75:870-876.
36. Itoi T, Nageshwar Reddy D, Yasuda I. New fully-covered self-expandable metal stent for endoscopic ultrasonography-guided intervention in infectious walled-off pancreatic necrosis (with video). *J Hepatobiliary Pancreat Sci.* 2013;20:403-406.

37. Fabbri C, Luigiano C, Cennamo V, et al. Endoscopic ultrasound-guided transmural drainage of infected pancreatic fluid collections with placement of covered self-expanding metal stents: a case series. *Endoscopy.* 2012;44:429-433.

38. Arvanitakis M, Delhaye M, Bali MA, et al. Pancreatic fluid collections: a randomized controlled trial regarding stent removal after endoscopic transmural drainage. *Gastrointest Endosc.* 2007;65:609-619.

39. Varadarajulu S, Eloubeidi MA, Wilcox CM. The concept of bedside EUS. *Gastrointest Endosc.* 2008;67:1180-1184.

40. Larghi A, Seerden TC, Galasso D, et al. EUS-guided cystojejunostomy for drainage of a pseudocyst in a patient with Billroth II gastrectomy. *Gastrointest Endosc.* 2011;73:169-171.

41. Trevino JM, Varadarajulu S. Endoscopic ultrasound-guided transjejunal drainage of pancreatic pseudocyst. *Pancreas.* 2010;39:419-420.

42. Seifert H, Wehrmann T, Schmitt T, et al. Retroperitoneal endoscopic debridement for infected peripancreatic necrosis. *Lancet.* 2000;356:653-655.

43. Seewald S, Groth S, Omar S, et al. Aggressive endoscopic therapy for pancreatic necrosis and pancreatic abscess: a new safe and effective treatment algorithm (videos). *Gastrointest Endosc.* 2005;62:92-100.

44. Seifert H, Biermer M, Schmitt W, et al. Transluminal endoscopic necrosectomy after acute pancreatitis: a multicentre study with long-term follow-up (the GEPARD Study). *Gut.* 2009;58:1260-1266.

45. Yasuda I, Nakashima M, Iwai T, et al. Japanese multicenter experience of endoscopic necrosectomy for infected walled-off pancreatic necrosis: The JENIPaN study. *Endoscopy.* 2013;45:627-634.

46. Seewald S, Ang TL, Richter H, et al. Long-term results after endoscopic drainage and necrosectomy of symptomatic pancreatic fluid collections. *Dig Endosc.* 2012;24:36-41.

47. Gardner TB, Coelho-Prabhu N, Gordon SR, et al. Direct endoscopic necrosectomy for the treatment of walled-off pancreatic necrosis: results from a multicenter U.S. series. *Gastrointest Endosc.* 2011;73:718-726.

48. Freeman ML, Werner J, van Santvoort HC, et al. International Multidisciplinary Panel of Speakers and Moderators. Interventions for necrotizing pancreatitis: summary of a multidisciplinary consensus conference. *Pancreas.* 2012;41:1176-1194.

49. van Santvoort HC, Besselink MG, Bakker OJ, et al. Dutch Pancreatitis Study Group. A step-up approach or open necrosectomy for necrotizing pancreatitis. *N Engl J Med.* 2010;362:1491-1502.

50. Seewald S, Brand B, Groth S, et al. Endoscopic sealing of pancreatic fistula by using N-butyl-2-cyanoacrylate. *Gastrointest Endosc.* 2004;59:463-470.

51. Hookey LC, Debroux S, Delhaye M, et al. Endoscopic drainage of pancreatic-fluid collections in 116 patients: a comparison of etiologies, drainage techniques, and outcomes. *Gastrointest Endosc.* 2006;63:635-643.

52. Weckman L, Kylanpaa ML, Puolakkainen P, et al. Endoscopic treatment of pancreatic pseudocysts. *Surg Endosc.* 2006;20:603-607.

53. Vosoghi M, Sial S, Garrett B, et al. EUS-guided pancreatic pseudocyst drainage: review and experience at Harbor-UCLA Medical Center. *Medgenmed.* 2002;4:2.

54. Baron TH, Harewood GC, Morgan DE, et al. Outcome differences after endoscopic drainage of pancreatic necrosis, acute pancreatic pseudocysts, and chronic pancreatic pseudocysts. *Gastrointest Endosc.* 2002;56:7-17.

55. Bakker OJ, van Santvoort HC, van Brunschot S, et al. Dutch Pancreatitis Study Group. Endoscopic transgastric vs surgical necrosectomy for infected necrotizing pancreatitis: a randomized trial. *JAMA.* 2012;307:1053-1061.

56. van Santvoort HC, Bakker OJ, Bollen TL, et al. Dutch Pancreatitis Study Group. A conservative and minimally invasive approach to necrotizing pancreatitis improves outcome. *Gastroenterology.* 2011;141:1254-1263.

57. Varadarajulu S, Bang JY, Sutton BS, et al. Equal efficacy of endoscopic and surgical cystogastrostomy for pancreatic pseudocyst drainage in a randomized trial. *Gastroenterology.* 2013;145:583-590.

58. Sriram PV, Kaffes AJ, Rao GV, Reddy DN. Endoscopic ultrasound-guided drainage of pancreatic pseudocysts complicated by portal hypertension or by intervening vessels. *Endoscopy.* 2005;37:231-235.

59. Varadarajulu S, Christein JD, Tamhane A, et al. Prospective randomized trial comparing EUS and conventional endoscopy for transmural drainage of pancreatic pseudocysts. *Gastrointest Endosc.* 2008;68:1102-1111.

60. Park DH, Lee SS, Moon SH, et al. Endoscopic ultrasound-guided versus conventional transmural drainage for pancreatic pseudocysts: a prospective randomized trial. *Endoscopy.* 2009;41:842-848.

61. Gupta R, Munoz JC, Garg P, et al. Mediastinal pancreatic pseudocyst: a case report and review of the literature. *Medgenmed.* 2007;9:8-13.

62. Saftouia A, Cuirea T, Dumitrescu D, et al. Endoscopic ultrasound-guided transesophageal drainage of a mediastinal pancreatic pseudocyst. *Endoscopy.* 2006;38:538-539.

63. Baron TH, Wiersema MJ. EUS-guided transesophageal pancreatic pseudocyst drainage. *Gastrointest Endosc.* 2000;52:545-549.

64. Trevino JM, Christein JD, Varadarajulu S. EUS-guided transesophageal drainage of peripancreatic fluid collections. *Gastrointest Endosc.* 2009;70:793-797.

65. Seewald S, Ang TL, Teng KY, et al. Endoscopic ultrasound-guided drainage of abdominal abscesses and infected necrosis. *Endoscopy.* 2009;41(2):166-174.

66. Seewald S, Ang TL, Kida M, et al. EUS 2008 Working Group. EUS 2008 Working Group document: evaluation of EUS-guided drainage of pancreatic-fluid collections (with video). *Gastrointest Endosc.* 2009;69(2 suppl):S13-S21.

67. Varadarajulu S, Christein JD, Wilcox CM. Frequency of complications during EUS-guided drainage of pancreatic fluid collections in 148 consecutive patients. *J Gastroenterol Hepatol.* 2011;26:1504-1508.

68. Varadarajulu S, Phadnis MA, Christein JD, et al. Multiple transluminal gateway technique for EUS-guided drainage of symptomatic walled-off pancreatic necrosis. *Gastrointest Endosc.* 2011;74:74-80.

25

EUS-Guided Drainage of the Biliary and Pancreatic Ductal Systems

Larissa L. Fujii • Michael J. Levy

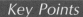

Key Points

- EUS-guided pancreaticobiliary drainage is emerging as an alternative to percutaneous or surgical drainage in patients in whom ERCP fails to access the ducts. Consider EUS-guided main pancreatic duct as the first endoscopic intervention in patients with an anastomotic stricture after pancreaticoduodenectomy due to the higher success rate than ERP.
- A clear understanding of the procedure goals will help to guide equipment selection, including the appropriate needle and guidewire.
- Use of the cystotome or needle knife for tract dilation should only be considered as a rescue technique when other approaches (e.g., dilating balloon, catheter, or cannula) fail due to the perceived risk of cautery-induced injury.
- The suggested algorithmic approach to EUS-guided pancreaticobiliary drainage is to proceed with transpapillary/transanastomotic stent placement (either retrograde or antegrade depending on local expertise) followed by antegrade transluminal stent placement if the other fails. In patients with transluminal stent placement during initial intervention, it is recommended to attempt to traverse the site of obstruction and papilla/anastomosis during subsequent evaluations.
- The need and timing of reintervention after pancreaticobiliary stent placement is unclear based on published reports, but data suggest that patients may benefit from routine stent exchanges, particularly if the prolonged stent duration is required.
- Because EUS-guided pancreaticobiliary drainage is likely the most technically challenging procedure among EUS and ERCP, it should only be performed at tertiary referral centers with experienced endosonographers and available pancreaticobiliary interventional radiologists and surgeons.
- Additional studies are needed to determine the long-term outcomes of EUS-guided pancreaticobiliary drainage.

The role of endoscopic ultrasound (EUS) has evolved over the last three decades with initial use restricted to the evaluation of subepithelial lesions and gastrointestinal luminal cancer staging. The development of linear instruments allowed fine-needle aspiration (FNA) with cytologic evaluation and Tru-Cut biopsy (TCB) with histologic assessment, and thus further expanded the role of EUS.[1,2] Similarly, EUS is used to guide therapeutic interventions including celiac plexus and ganglia blockade and neurolysis,[3–5] pancreatic fluid drainage,[6–9] cholecystenterostomy,[10] and delivery of cytotoxic agents such as chemotherapy, radioactive seeds, and gene therapy.[11,12] In the mid-1990s, the concept of combining therapeutic endoscopic retrograde cholangiopancreatography (ERCP) with interventional EUS technology led to the concept of endoradiosonographic cholangiopancreatography (ERSCP).[13] The continued need to develop less invasive alternatives to surgical and interventional radiological therapies drove the development of EUS-guided methods for biliary and pancreatic intervention. The purpose of this chapter is to review existing data and focus on the EUS techniques for obtaining access and subsequent drainage of biliary and pancreatic ducts.

General Role

ERCP is the method most commonly employed to access the bile duct or main pancreatic duct (MPD) and is routinely performed to obtain diagnostic information and/or provide therapy. Indications for ERCP include evaluation of benign disorders (e.g., inflammatory stricture, stone, congenital ductal anomalies) or malignancy (e.g., cholangiocarcinoma, pancreatic carcinoma). Percutaneous and surgical approaches are available for patients in whom access cannot be achieved via ERCP.[14,15] An emerging alternative to these more invasive and potentially risky interventions is EUS-guided access and drainage. EUS-guided techniques appear ideally suited following failed ERCP, which may occur secondary to a patient's underlying disease (e.g., gastric or duodenal obstruction, disrupted duct), because of the presence of anatomical variants (e.g., duodenal diverticulum), or due to surgically altered anatomy (e.g., Billroth II resection, pancreaticoduodenectomy). EUS approaches are also considered for patients who are poor operative candidates and for persons declining surgical intervention.

Patient Preparation

Although EUS is typically performed in an ambulatory setting, most perform interventional EUS examinations of this nature in a hospital endoscopy unit with fluoroscopic capability and using monitored anesthesia care or general anesthesia. As for diagnostic EUS examinations, the initial evaluation should include a thorough history, physical examination, and review of pertinent medical records to identify factors that influence the need, risks, benefits, alternatives, and timing of EUS and for documenting acquisition of informed consent. Laboratory and radiological studies are ordered as necessary for management of the underlying disorder and sometimes to clarify the anatomy and to help guide planned interventions. Relative contraindications to this procedure include patients with a significant coagulopathy (INR > 1.5) or thrombocytopenia (platelets < 50,000) and those with hemodynamic instability precluding the use of adequate general anesthesia. Antibiotics (e.g., levofloxacin or ciprofloxacin) are routinely administered prior to the procedure.

Equipment and Technical Considerations

EUS is ideally performed with a therapeutic channel linear array echoendoscope to allow use of a broader array of accessories and insertion of large-caliber 10-Fr stents. Smaller caliber diagnostic echoendoscopes may be used to perform rendezvous wire passage or for placement of 7-Fr or smaller stents. Duct access may be achieved with any of the currently available 25-, 22-, or 19-G FNA needles in conjunction with a wide selection of available wires. Prior to use, it is important to verify that the selected FNA needle will allow passage of a particular guidewire. One cannot automatically assume that a needle of a particular gauge, or wire of a particular caliber, can replace a similarly sized needle or wire because of the minor variation that exists in equipment among companies.[16,17] Use of a larger caliber needle offers the ability to use a larger gauge guidewire that may facilitate traversal of stenotic strictures and facilitate passage of other accessories. However, initial duct access may be more difficult when using larger gauge and stiffer needles. A clear understanding of the procedure goals can help guide equipment selection. For instance, it may be reasonable to use a 25-G needle if the intended goal is to obtain only a cholangiogram or pancreatogram. Some also prefer a smaller gauge needle to determine if contrast freely flows into the anastomosed bowel lumen suggesting absence of critical stenosis, thereby potentially obviating the need for therapeutic intervention (e.g., anastomotic dilation and stenting).

Guidewire use largely depends on needle selection. Use of a 0.035-inch guidewire requires selection of a 19-G needle. While these stiffer wires may be more difficult to insert into the bile or pancreatic duct, their use may enable traversal of obstructed segments, facilitating subsequent interventions, and are generally the preferred wire in this setting. An 0.018-inch guidewire may be used with a 19- or 22-G needle. These wires are more flexible and may improve duct access and facilitate traversal of obstructed segments but due to the floppy nature can make subsequent interventions more difficult. Similarly, one may select either Teflon-coated hydrophilic wires and/or angled wires, which may facilitate traversal of narrowed and/or tortuous segments. The selected guidewire is advanced antegrade across the site of stenosis and then the papilla or anastomosis, and then coiled in the small bowel. These steps are performed under fluoroscopic guidance.

Various accessories may be used to create the fistula between the gut lumen (stomach, duodenum, or jejunum) and duct (bile or pancreatic) to facilitate passage of other accessories and/or for dilation of anastomotic strictures. A variety of standard biliary and pancreatic catheter dilators and pneumatic dilators may be used with selection based on the patient's anatomy. No formal comparative trials exist to clarify the relative value of available devices. Equipment use varies among endoscopists and often requires trial and error even within the same patient.

EUS-Guided Access and Therapy of the Biliary Ductal System

Wiersema and colleagues performed the first EUS-guided cholangiogram following an unsuccessful ERCP, demonstrating successful opacification of the biliary tree in 7 of 10 patients.[18] Since then, the practice has gradually evolved, and many technical modifications have been reported. In broad terms, EUS-guided intrahepatic (i.e., hepatogastrostomy) or extrahepatic (i.e., choledochoduodenostomy) drainage is achieved following transluminal access from the stomach or duodenum, respectively.

Indications

The most common indications for EUS-guided biliary access and therapy are following failed endoscopic retrograde cholangiography (ERC) to evaluate and manage:

1. Malignant biliary obstruction (e.g., pancreatic carcinoma or cholangiocarcinoma)
2. Benign biliary obstruction (e.g., inflammatory stricture, stones, congenital ductal anomalies).

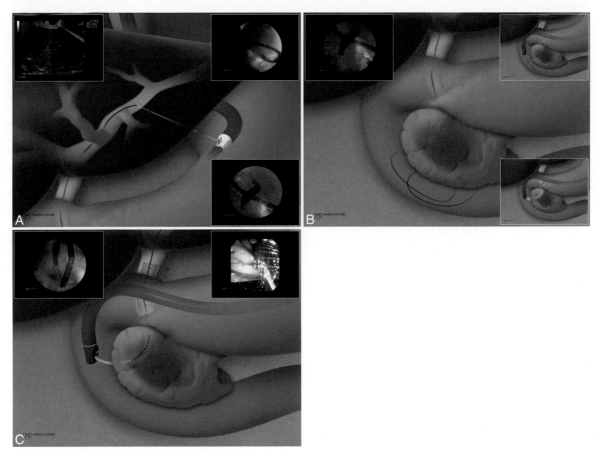

FIGURE 25-1   The technique for intrahepatic biliary access and transpapillary drainage with rendezvous instrumentation and retrograde stent insertion is demonstrated. **A,** Artwork demonstrates the typical site of instrument positioning with needle insertion and wire placement in the bile duct as accessed via a left intrahepatic bile duct branch. EUS demonstrates the typical orientation of a desired intrahepatic bile duct with needle insertion. Fluoroscopy reveals the ideal scope position with resulting cholangiography and initial wire insertion. **B,** The guidewire is passed through the site of obstruction, into the duodenum and coiled in the small bowel as demonstrated in the artwork and fluoroscopic image. The rendezvous portion of the examination follows with guidewire retrieval using a biopsy cable or snare with dilatation if required. **C,** A stent may then be placed in a retrograde fashion using standard techniques.

Technique

Intrahepatic Approach (Hepatogastrostomy) (Figure 25-1; Videos 25-1A–C)

While EUS-guided intrahepatic bile duct drainage will be reviewed first, many of the techniques and principles also apply to the other routes and sites of drainage. Table 25-1 summarizes the types of EUS-guided drainage techniques. In order to access the intrahepatic bile ducts, the echoendoscope must be positioned within the proximal stomach (cardia, fundus, or proximal body) and oriented along the lesser curve

or more posterior position. The liver is scanned to identify a dilated intrahepatic bile duct and the optimal location for needle puncture.

A location is selected that allows the least distance between the transducer and a left intrahepatic bile duct branch and is ideally oriented in a plane that facilitates subsequent therapy. It is important to exclude intervening structures, such as blood vessels and undesired ducts. Once the needle is advanced to the target duct, bile should be aspirated to confirm access and contrast is then injected to fluoroscopically delineate the biliary anatomy. Under fluoroscopic

Video 25-1A. Retrograde intrahepatic transpapillary stent placement.

Video 25-1B. Antegrade intrahepatic transpapillary stent placement.

Video 25-1C. Antegrade intrahepatic transluminal stent placement.

guidance, a guidewire is advanced through the FNA needle, which is passed in an antegrade fashion through the site of obstruction and into the duodenum. The guidewire is advanced further to form loops within the duodenal lumen in order to reduce the risk of wire dislodgement that may occur either during removal of the echoendoscope or when inserting the side-viewing duodenoscope. Passage of the wire across the site of obstruction and into the small bowel allows subsequent transpapillary or transanastomotic stenting.

Once the wire is adequately positioned within the small bowel, the echoendoscope is back-loaded leaving the guidewire in place. The retrograde (rendezvous) portion of the procedure is then performed by passing a side- or forward-viewing endoscope to the papilla or surgical anastomosis (see Video 25-1A). The luminal end of the guidewire is grasped with a snare or biopsy cable and the wire is withdrawn through the endoscope leaving both ends of the guidewire exiting the patient's mouth and under the endoscopist's control. Alternatively, the duodenoscope may be passed over the guidewire, thereby eliminating the need to grasp the guidewire and withdraw through the accessory channel. However, some find this latter approach to be technically challenging and/or believe that this method places

unacceptable tension on the wire and risks injury to the liver parenchyma, bile duct, or duodenum. The ERC (retrograde) portion of the procedure can be performed with a standard side-viewing duodenoscope in patients with unaltered gastroduodenal anatomy. In patients with an afferent jejunal limb or Roux-en-Y reconstruction following pancreaticoduodenectomy, an extended forward-viewing instrument such as a colonoscope is often employed.

Once the selected instrument is properly positioned and guidewire control is achieved, biliary stent insertion and other interventions may be performed in standard fashion. It is often necessary to work over the guidewire until initial dilatation is performed. After dilating the site of obstruction with a catheter or balloon, subsequent interventions may be performed over or alongside the guidewire (if desired), thereby maintaining access with a safety wire. Following dilatation, a cannula can be passed alongside the safety wire, leaving a separate wire within the bile duct, and thereby allowing subsequent stent insertion and duct drainage.

In contrast, with the transpapillary/transanastomotic approach, one may opt to perform the entire examination, including stent insertion, with an echoendoscope alone without a need for the rendezvous portion of the examination (Figure 25-2, see Video 25-1B). For this technique, tract dilatation is required including the gastric wall, hepatic parenchyma, and intrahepatic bile duct wall. Tract dilation can be performed via many approaches, and it is the authors' preference to initially use a dilating balloon, standard cannula, or tapered catheter. Adequate dilatation may require use of several such devices. While some routinely rely on cystotome or needle knife entry, the authors do so only as a rescue technique when other approaches fail due to the perceived risk of cautery-induced injury. Whenever possible, the stent is advanced so that the distal end rests within the small bowel and the proximal end of the stent lies within the stomach, which may optimize duct drainage and diminish the risk of inadvertent stent migration. However, at times it may not be possible to advance the guidewire beyond the site of obstruction and/or papilla (or anastomosis). In this situation, the stent may be inserted so that the distal tip rests within the biliary tree, whereas the proximal end lies within the gastric lumen, sometimes referred to as transluminal or transmural drainage (Figure 25-3, see Video 25-1C). Stents of varying caliber and length have been used. While the authors generally favor pigtail stents, straight stents may be used as well. Extra side holes may be created within the intraductal portion of the stent to facilitate drainage.

Extrahepatic Approach (Choledochoduodenostomy) (Videos 25-2A–B)

Giovannini and colleagues performed the first clinical EUS-guided biliary drainage in a patient with pancreatic adenocarcinoma, via transduodenal access of the extrahepatic bile duct with plastic stent insertion.[19] With this approach, the echoendoscope is advanced to the duodenum where the extrahepatic (either intrapancreatic or suprapancreatic) bile duct can be accessed. The FNA needle is inserted into the extrahepatic bile duct, and a guidewire is advanced in an antegrade direction into the duodenum (Figure 25-4). The procedure is completed in a similar fashion to the transhepatic technique with the stent advanced through the site of obstruction providing transpapillary drainage into the duodenum.

TABLE 25-1	
TYPES OF EUS-GUIDED PANCREATICOBILIARY PROCEDURES	
Type	**Definition**
Location of needle puncture	Intrahepatic bile ducts: Hepatogastrostomy Extrahepatic bile ducts: Choledochoenterostomy Main pancreatic duct: Pancreaticogastrostomy
Approach	Retrograde: Duodenoscope or extended forward-viewing endoscope is inserted with stent placement from the gut lumen through the papilla/anastomosis into the duct (often referred to as a "rendezvous procedure") Antegrade: Entire procedure including stent placement is performed with the echoendoscope and with stent placement from the gut lumen into the duct with or without crossing the obstruction and papilla/anastomosis
Technique	Transpapillary: Stent traverses the papilla Transanastomotic: Stent traverses the surgical anastomosis Transluminal (transmural): Distal end of the stent lies within the duct itself, rather than crossing the papilla or anastomosis; only performed in the antegrade approach

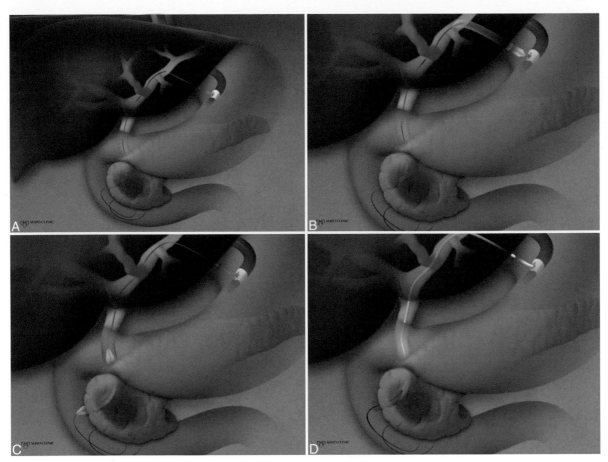

FIGURE 25-2 The technique for intrahepatic biliary access and transpapillary drainage with antegrade stent insertion to the small bowel, performed solely via an echoendoscope, is demonstrated. **A,** EUS is utilized to access a branch of the left intrahepatic bile duct. A guidewire is then passed into the biliary tree and duodenum. **B,** Tract dilatation is required to include the gastric wall, hepatic parenchyma, and intrahepatic bile duct wall. **C,** The site of obstruction is then dilated to facilitate stent insertion. **D,** Plastic or metal stent placement may then be achieved in an antegrade direction, all performed via an echoendoscope under ultrasound and fluoroscopic guidance.

Depending on the orientation of the echoendoscope relative to the biliary anatomy, wire insertion from this position has a tendency for passage proximal into the intrahepatic bile ducts instead of distally through the papilla (or anastomosis). This problem can usually be overcome by altering the scope position and/or by elevator deflection. Alternatively, the guidewire may be further advanced into the intrahepatic biliary tree to induce looping and eventual passage in the alternate direction toward the papilla. Fistula patency is maintained by the indwelling stent, resulting in creation of an endoscopic choledochoduodenostomy with transluminal stenting and decompression of the proximal biliary tree without traversal of the obstructing mass or papilla (Figure 25-5).

Technical Success, Outcomes, and Complications

While the technical success of these procedures can be established, data pertaining to clinical success, therapeutic response, and complications are more difficult to discern from current reports. The paucity of data, study heterogeneity, and overall methodology limit the strengths of any conclusions regarding these techniques. Studies vary greatly in terms of the precise endoscopic procedures performed, the procedural goals, technical and clinical endpoints, definitions of success, duration and extent of follow-up, and overall extent and detail of documentation. While not practical, the lack of controlled,

Video 25-2A. Antegrade extrahepatic transpapillary stent placement.

Video 25-2B. Antegrade extrahepatic transluminal stent placement.

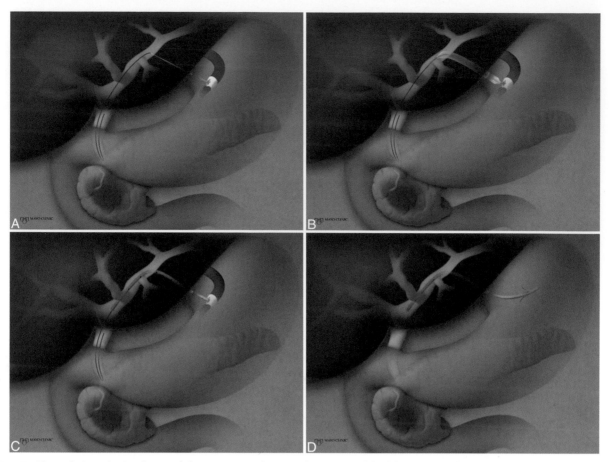

FIGURE 25-3 The technique for intrahepatic biliary access and antegrade stenting of the biliary tree to the stomach, as performed solely with an echoendoscope, is demonstrated. **A,** EUS is utilized to access a branch of the left intrahepatic bile duct followed by guidewire passage into the biliary tree. **B,** Tract dilatation is required to include the gastric wall, hepatic parenchyma, and intrahepatic bile duct wall. **C** and **D,** The stent is advanced so that the distal tip rests within the biliary tree and the proximal end of the stent lies within the stomach.

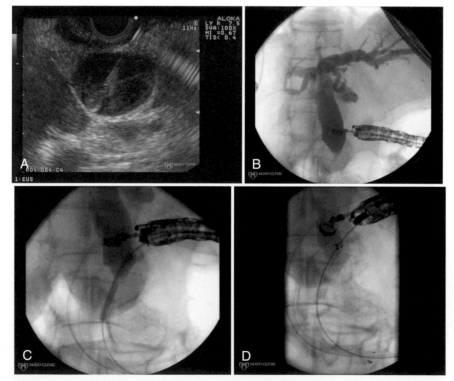

FIGURE 25-4 The technique for extrahepatic biliary access and transpapillary drainage following antegrade stent insertion, performed solely with an echoendoscope, is demonstrated. **A,** EUS-guided needle access into the extrahepatic bile duct allows initial cholangiography to aid needle insertion. **B,** Fluoroscopic imaging reveals a malignant appearing distal biliary stricture in a patient with a duodenal stent placed as therapy for gastric outlet obstruction. **C,** The entire tract is dilated to facilitate stent insertion. **D,** A self-expandable metal stent is deployed in an antegrade manner using EUS and fluoroscopic guidance.

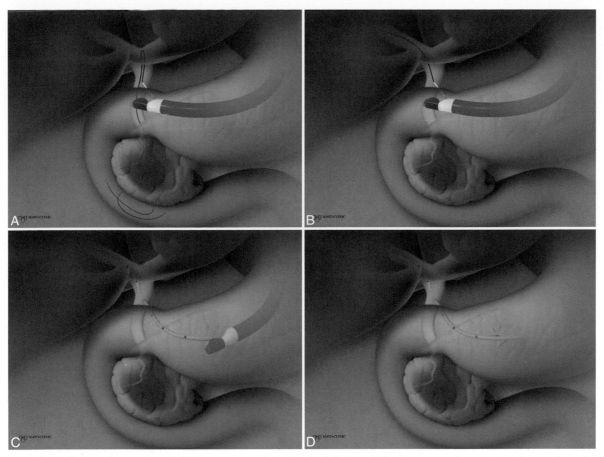

FIGURE 25-5   The technique for extrahepatic biliary access and transluminal drainage following antegrade stent insertion, performed solely with an echoendoscope, is demonstrated. **A,** EUS is utilized to access the extrahepatic bile duct with subsequent cholangiography and needle placement. **B,** The guidewire may be advanced into the intrahepatic bile ducts to provide a straight angle of access and stent delivery. **C** and **D,** The stent is advanced so that the distal tip rests within the biliary tree and the proximal end of the stent lies within the stomach or duodenum.

randomized, comparative data, and absence of blinding further limit our understanding of the utility and role of these techniques. Finally, there is likely reporting and publication bias, thereby impacting these data. Despite the limitations, these studies offer preliminary data suggesting the relative efficacy of EUS-guided biliary access and drainage, but raise concerns regarding their risks.

Evaluating the collective literature to date (2004 to 2013, $n = 297$ patients, excluding case reports and studies focusing only on EUS-guided cholangiography), it appears that EUS-guided intrahepatic biliary access has an 89.6% ($n = 266$) technical success rate and a 25.3% ($n = 75$) complication rate when excluding stent-specific complications (Table 25-2). Reported complications included hemorrhage ($n = 19$), pneumoperitoneum ($n = 16$), bile leak and/or biloma ($n = 15$), cholangitis ($n = 11$), abdominal pain ($n = 4$), multiple adverse events ($n = 2$), ileus ($n = 1$), nausea ($n = 1$), aspiration pneumonia ($n = 1$), and other ($n = 5$). Grouped data for patients undergoing attempted EUS-guided extrahepatic biliary access (2003 to 2013, $n = 416$ patients, excluding case reports and studies focusing only on EUS-guided cholangiography), indicate a 91.3% ($n = 380$) success rate and an 18% ($n = 75$) complication rate (Table 25-3). Reported complications included bile leak or bile peritonitis ($n = 26$), cholangitis ($n = 11$), pneumoperitoneum ($n = 9$), bleeding ($n = 9$),

abdominal pain ($n = 7$), pancreatitis ($n = 4$), multiple adverse events ($n = 4$), cardiopulmonary failure ($n = 2$), other ($n = 2$), and cholecystitis ($n = 1$). One study suggested that the use of a needle knife for fistula dilation was associated with an increased risk of adverse events.[20]

Two large studies that did not differentiate between intrahepatic and extrahepatic bile duct access were not included in the above grouped data. Vila and colleagues reviewed the Spanish experience in a national multicenter study that included 19 hospitals performing a total of 106 EUS-guided biliary drainage procedures.[40] The technical success in this study was lower at 67.2% ($n = 84$) than previous reports, but this may be a reflection of the fact that the study focused on the hospitals' early experience with this procedure. Furthermore, they commented that the multicenter study design may inherently have a lower publication bias, and 44% of the stents were placed across the papilla/anastomosis rather than transluminal. The adverse event rate was 23.2% (including patients with pancreatic duct intervention) with seven bile peritonitis (two deaths), six hemorrhages (one death), five acute pancreatitis, four perforations (two deaths), three cholangitis, two liver hematomas, and one abscess and one pancreatic pseudocyst. Risk factors for complications using logistic regression included male gender (OR 3.8 [95% CI 1.4-10.5]) and technical failure (OR 2.5 [95% CI 1-6.2]). This

TABLE 25-2

HEPATICOGASTROSTOMY (INTRAHEPATIC) STENT PLACEMENT FOR DRAINAGE

Author (year)	Approach	Technical Success	Complications
Kahaleh et al (2004, 2005)[21,22]	TP/TA[a] (n = 24)	29/35	Pneumoperitoneum (n = 3)
Maranki et al (2009)[23]	Transluminal (n = 5)		Bleeding (n = 1)
			Aspiration pneumonia (n = 1)
Bories et al (2007)[24]	Transluminal (n = 10)	10/11	Ileus (n = 1)
			Biloma (n = 1)
			Cholangitis (n = 1)
Will et al (2007)[25]	Transluminal (n = 8)	8/9	Cholangitis (n = 1)
Horaguchi et al (2009)[26]	Transluminal (n = 7)	7/7	None
Park et al (2009, 2010, 2011, 2013)[20,27–29]	TP/TA[a] (n = 17) Transluminal (n = 40)	57/60	Total n = 7 (others NS) Pneumoperitoneum (n = 1) Stent migration, biloma (n = 1)
Iwamuro et al (2010)[30]	Transluminal (n = 2; all with duodenal stents)	2/2	Bile leak, pneumoperitoneum (n = 2)
Nguyen-Tang et al (2010)[31]	TP/TA[a,b] (n = 49)	58/66	Hepatic subcapsular hematoma (n = 1)
Shah et al (2012)[32]	Transluminal (n = 9)		Infection/bacteremia (n = 1)
Belletrutti et al (2011)[33]	Transluminal (n = 2)	2/3	None
Ramirez-Luna et al (2011)[34]	Transluminal (n = 2)	2/2	None
Artifon et al (2012)[35]	TP/TA[a]	132/145	Bleeding (n = 18)
Gupta et al (2013)[36]	Transluminal		Bile leak (n = 14)
			Pneumoperitoneum (n = 11)
			Cholangitis (n = 7)
			Abdominal pain (n = 4)
Iwashita et al (2012)[37]	Retrograde TP/TA (n = 4)	4/9	Pneumoperitoneum (n = 1)
Khashab et al (2012)[38]	TP[a]	2/2	Nausea (n = 1)
Kim et al (2012)[39]	Transluminal (n = 3)	3/4	Stent migration with peritonitis & pneumoperitoneum (n = 1)
Vila et al (2012)[40]	Retrograde TP/TA (n = 32)[b] Transluminal (n = 22)	73/106	Biloma (n = 3) Bleeding (n = 3) Perforation (n = 2) Liver hematoma (n = 2) Abscess (n = 1)
Kawakubo et al (2013)[41]	Retrograde TP/TA (n = 5)	5/5	None
Tonozuka et al (2013)[42]	Transluminal (n = 3; all with duodenal stents)	3/3	Cholangitis (n = 2; unclear if occurred in HG or CD groups)

Excludes case reports and reports only on EUS-guided cholangiography.
CD, choledochoduodenostomy; HG, hepaticogastrostomy; NS, not specified; TP, transpapillary; TA, transanastomotic.
[a]Includes both retrograde and antegrade transpapillary or transanastomotic stent placement.
[b]Combined HG and CD cases as not differentiated in the case series.

emphasizes the importance of patient selection and endoscopist experience to ensure that any attempt at EUS-guided pancreaticobiliary drainage has the highest likelihood of success. Shah and colleagues also reported their results in 66 patients combining the intrahepatic and extrahepatic bile duct access.[32] In this single center study, patients with an accessible or inaccessible papilla using the duodenoscope initially underwent retrograde or antegrade stent placement, respectively. If the initial attempt at stent placement failed, the patient underwent the opposite technique. Transpapillary or transanastomotic stent placement was preferred over transluminal stent placement, which was only used if the site of obstruction could not be traversed by the guidewire. Technical success in the initial attempts were 74% and 81% in the retrograde and antegrade techniques, respectively, which increased to an overall rate of success in 75% and 86% when including the patients that crossed over after an initial failed attempt. Complications occurred in six patients including acute pancreatitis (n = 3), bile leak (n = 1), bacteremia (n = 1), and perforation (n = 1).

In the largest case series to date, Gupta and colleagues reported on 240 patients from six international centers who either failed prior ERC or were deemed to not be a candidate for ERC due to an inaccessible papilla with a duodenoscope.[36] Overall, 56% of patients had a distal obstruction, 44% with a hilar obstruction, and 81% had a malignancy as the cause of their obstruction. The intrahepatic approach was used in 60% and a metal stent was placed in 60% of patients. Technical success was achieved in 87% of subjects with no significant difference between the intrahepatic and extrahepatic approaches (90.4% and 84.3%, respectively; p = 0.15). Malignant biliary obstruction was associated with higher technical success than benign causes (90.2% versus 77.3%; p = 0.02). Complications occurred in 35.6% of intrahepatic and 32.6% of extrahepatic biliary drainage (p = 0.64), with no differences found in benign or malignant disease

TABLE 25-3

CHOLEDOCHODUODENOSTOMY (EXTRAHEPATIC) STENT PLACEMENT FOR DRAINAGE

Author (year)	Approach	Technical Success	Complications
Burmester et al[43] (2003)	Transluminal ($n = 2$)	2/3	Bile peritonitis ($n = 1$)
Kahaleh et al[21,22] (2004, 2005)	TP/TA[a] ($n = 8$)	12/14	Pneumoperitoneum ($n = 1$)
Maranki et al[23] (2009)	Transluminal ($n = 4$)		Bile peritonitis ($n = 1$)
			Abdominal pain ($n = 1$)
Mallery et al[16] (2004)	Retrograde TP/TA ($n = 2$)	2/2	None
Puspok et al[44] (2005)	Retrograde TP/TA ($n = 1$)	4/5	Subacute phlegmonous cholecystitis ($n = 1$)
	Transluminal ($n = 3$)		
Yamao et al[45,46] (2006, 2008)	Transluminal ($n = 5$)	5/5	Pneumoperitoneum ($n = 1$)
Ang et al[47] (2007)	Transluminal ($n = 2$)	2/2	Pneumoperitoneum ($n = 1$)
Itoi et al[48] (2008)	Transluminal ($n = 4$)	4/4	Bleeding, focal peritonitis ($n = 1$)
			Acute cholangitis due to stent clogging ($n = 1$)
Tarantino et al[49] (2008)	Retrograde TP/TA ($n = 3$)	7/7	None
	Transluminal ($n = 4$)		
Brauer et al[50] (2009)	Retrograde TP/TA ($n = 8$)	11/12	Peritonitis ($n = 1$)
	Transluminal ($n = 3$)		Cardiorespiratory failure ($n = 1$)
Hanada et al[51] (2009)	Transluminal ($n = 4$)	4/4	None
Horaguchi et al[26] (2009)	Transluminal ($n = 9$)	9/9	Peritonitis ($n = 1$)
Park et al[20,27,29] (2009, 2011, 2013)	TP/TA[a] ($n = 17$)	39/42	Total $n = 8$ (others NS)
	Transluminal ($n = 22$)		Bile peritonitis ($n = 3$)
			Pneumoperitoneum ($n = 2$)
			Pancreatitis ($n = 1$)
Artifon et al[52] (2010)	Transluminal ($n = 3$; retrograde TP failed in all prior to transluminal stenting)	3/3	None
Eum et al[53] (2010)	Transluminal ($n = 2$)	2/2	None
Iwamuro et al[30] (2010)	Transluminal ($n = 5$; all with duodenal stents)	5/5	Abdominal pain, fever ($n = 1$)
Kim et al[54] (2010)	TP/TA[a]	75/89	Bile leak ($n = 13$)
Artifon et al[35] (2012)	Transluminal		Bleeding ($n = 8$)
Gupta et al[36] (2013)			Cholangitis ($n = 4$)
			Pneumoperitoneum ($n = 1$)
			Abdominal pain ($n = 1$)
Belletrutti et al[33] (2011)	Transluminal ($n = 4$)	4/4	None
Fabbri et al[55] (2011)	Retrograde TP ($n = 3$)	12/15	Pneumoperitoneum ($n = 1$)
	Transluminal ($n = 9$)		
Hara et al[56] (2011)	Transluminal ($n = 17$)	17/18	Peritonitis ($n = 2$)
			Hemobilia ($n = 1$)
Komaki et al[57] (2011)	Retrograde TP ($n = 1$)	15/15	Cholangitis ($n = 4$)
	Transluminal ($n = 14$)		Peritonitis ($n = 2$)
Ramirez-Luna et al[34] (2011)	Transluminal ($n = 8$)	8/9	Biloma ($n = 1$)
Siddiqui et al[58] (2011)	Transluminal ($n = 8$)	8/8	Abdominal pain ($n = 1$)
			Stent migration with duodenal perforation ($n = 1$)
Dhir et al[59] (2012)	Retrograde TP/TA ($n = 57$)	57/58	Abdominal pain from contrast medium leak ($n = 2$)
Iwashita et al[37] (2012)	Retrograde TP/TA ($n = 25$)	25/31	Pancreatitis ($n = 2$)
			Abdominal pain ($n = 1$)
			Sepsis/death ($n = 1$)
Khashab et al[38] (2012)	TP[a] ($n = 5$; 2 through cystic duct)	7/7	Pancreatitis, cholecystitis ($n = 1$)
	Transluminal ($n = 2$)		Abdominal pain ($n = 1$)
Kim et al[39] (2012)	Transluminal ($n = 9$)	9/9	Pneumoperitoneum, peritonitis ($n = 1$)
Nicholson et al[60] (2012)	Transluminal ($n = 5$)	5/5	None
Shah et al[32] (2012)	TP/TA[a,b] ($n = 49$)	58/66	Bile leak ($n = 1$)
	Transluminal ($n = 9$)		Perforation ($n = 1$)
			Pancreatitis ($n = 2$)
Song et al[61] (2012)	Transluminal ($n = 13$)	13/15	Pneumoperitoneum ($n = 2$)
			Cholangitis ($n = 1$)
Vila et al[40] (2012)	Retrograde TP/TA ($n = 32$)[b]	73/106	Biloma ($n = 1$)
	Transluminal ($n = 19$)		Bleeding ($n = 1$)
			Pancreatitis ($n = 1$)
			Cholangitis ($n = 1$)
Kawakubo et al[41] (2013)	Retrograde TP/TA ($n = 9$)	9/9	Bile peritonitis ($n = 1$)
			Pancreatitis ($n = 1$)
Tonozuka et al[42] (2013)	Transluminal ($n = 5$; all with duodenal stents)	5/5	Cholangitis ($n = 2$; unclear if occurred in HG or CD groups)

Excludes case reports and reports only on EUS-guided exchangiography.
CD, choledochoduodenostomy; HG, hepaticogastrostomy; NS, not specified; TP, transpapillary; TA, transanastomotic.
[a]Includes both retrograde and antegrade transpapillary or transanastomotic stent placement.
[b]Combined intrahepatic and extrahepatic cases as not differentiated in the case series.

and the use of metal or plastic stents. A higher incidence of pneumoperitoneum was noted in patients undergoing the intrahepatic route (11 patients versus 1 patient in the extrahepatic group; $p = 0.03$). Although the exact mechanism of the increased risk was unknown, the authors hypothesized that it could be due to the greater dilation required for transgastric access.

In a prospective study comparing EUS-guided choledochoduodenostomy to percutaneous transhepatic drainage, 25 patients with unresectable malignant biliary obstruction were randomized to either EUS-guided transluminal ($n = 13$) or percutaneous ($n = 12$) metal stent placement.[35] Randomization was performed while the patient was still sedated after a failed ERC and/or EUS-guided transpapillary rendezvous attempt. Technical success occurred in all 25 patients, no statistical difference was noted in clinical outcomes including liver enzymes at day 7, quality of life, and cost effectiveness between the two groups. Complications occurred in two patients in the EUS group (bleeding, bile leak) and three patients in the percutaneous group (bile leak and two abscesses). The authors concluded that EUS-guided transluminal drainage may be as effective and safe as standard percutaneous drainage, with the added benefits of its ability to be performed in a single session after failed ERC and lacking the problems associated with an external drain.

Dhir and colleagues compared EUS-guided extrahepatic retrograde transpapillary stent placement and precut papillotomy in patients who failed five cannulation attempts with ERC.[59] Fifty-eight consecutive patients who failed ERC underwent EUS-guided rendezvous between May 2010 and April 2011 and were compared to a historical cohort of 144 patients who underwent precut papillotomy in 2009. Technical success was significantly higher in the EUS cohort (98.3% versus 90.3% in the precut group; $p = 0.03$). The only failure experienced in the EUS group occurred because of the inability to pass the guidewire distal to the obstruction; a transluminal stent placement was not attempted. There was no difference ($p = 0.27$) between complications in those undergoing precut papillotomy (6.9%; four pancreatitis and six bleeding) and EUS (3.4%; two self-limited pericholedochal contrast medium leaks). The authors attributed their high technical success rate to the use of a shorter wire that allowed better steerability and a small biopsy forceps that anchored the wire in the stomach during guidewire exchange. This study was limited by its retrospective nonrandomized design, but suggested that EUS-guided biliary drainage may be a more efficacious and safe technique than precut papillotomy.

As a result of study limitations, the need and timing of reintervention and long-term clinical outcomes cannot be accurately determined based on published reports. However, Yamao and colleagues noted that stents occluded from 4 weeks to 4 months.[45] In a prospective study by Park and colleagues, stent occlusion or migration occurred in 16 of 55 patients (29%).[20] The mean stent patency length was 132 days in EUS-guided hepatogastrostomies and 152 days in EUS-guided choledochoduodenostomies. Reintervention with stent exchange in patients with metal stents was successful 100% of the time compared to 50% in those with plastic stents ($p = 0.36$). Metal stents may have a longer patency than plastic stents. Median duration of stent patency was 99 days for plastic stents in one study[57] and 264 to 272 days for metal stents in other studies.[56,61]

Video 25-3A. Retrograde main pancreatic duct transpapillary stent placement.

EUS-Guided Access and Therapy of the Pancreatic Ductal System

EUS-guided pancreatography was first reported by Harada in 1995 as a case report involving a patient requiring removal of an MPD stone following pancreaticoduodenectomy.[62]

Indications

EUS-guided pancreatic duct access and therapy is most often attempted following failed endoscopic retrograde pancreatography (ERP) in patients with the following:

1. Chronic pancreatitis requiring decompression (secondary to strictures and/or stones)
2. Prior pancreaticoduodenectomy with suspected pancreaticojejunal anastomotic stenosis (manifested by recurrent pancreatitis, pain, steatorrhea, or evaluation of tumor recurrence)
3. Endoscopic snare ampullectomy (when prophylactic stent insertion fails)
4. Main pancreatic duct disruption.

Technique (Videos 25-3A–C)

Most of the aforementioned technical aspects for performing EUS-guided biliary access and therapy also apply to pancreatic interventions. The optimal point of MPD access varies depending on the site of ductal obstruction and is located anywhere from the gastric cardia to the second portion of the duodenum. EUS-guided MPD access can be more difficult than the biliary tree because of the tendency for guidewire passage into and through pancreatic duct side branches. Otherwise, similar to biliary access, the MPD is localized and punctured using EUS guidance. MPD access is confirmed by contrast injection and antegrade pancreatography. A guidewire is then advanced through the EUS FNA needle into the MPD and then duodenum. As with biliary access, fluoroscopy

Video 25-3B. Antegrade main pancreatic duct transpapillary stent placement.

Video 25-3C. Antegrade main pancreatic duct transluminal stent placement.

is used to verify the echoendoscope position, to perform ductography, and to facilitate guidewire passage. Subsequent steps, including fistula enlargement and stent insertion, also proceed in the same manner as noted for the biliary tree. Stent insertion may then be achieved via a rendezvous procedure and retrograde stent placement (Figure 25-6, see Video 25-3A), via an antegrade route utilizing endosonography alone (Figure 25-7, see Video 25-3B), or by transluminal stent drainage of the pancreatic duct to the gastric lumen (Figure 25-8, see Video 25-3C).

The technique has been previously highlighted in the post snare ampullectomy setting with a subsequently inaccessible pancreatic duct requiring stenting.[63] Tessier and colleagues

suggested that a minimum MPD caliber of 6 mm is needed to achieve access.[64] While a larger duct caliber does facilitate access, MPD access has been reported in ducts as small as 0.8 mm.[65] Several technical variations have been described for MPD drainage. The initial approach was reported by Bataille and colleagues who created a pancreaticoenteric fistula with antegrade wire passage to facilitate the subsequent rendezvous with retrograde stent insertion.[66] Subsequently, others provided drainage via creation of a pancreaticogastric fistula with antegrade stent insertion.[32,40,50,65,67–72]

EUS-guided pancreaticoduodenostomy is a more recently described technique employed in patients with either acute or chronic pancreatitis and allows access to the MPD from the duodenal bulb.[69] Săftoiu and colleagues reported combined EUS-assisted rendezvous stenting of the MPD with subsequent transpapillary stenting of the common bile duct for managing pancreatic fluid collections.[73] Other variations have included access and drainage through the minor papilla.[74]

Technical Success, Outcomes, and Complications

Although the results of these studies are encouraging, they too suffer from methodologic shortcomings that limit the strength of the conclusions. Among the 222 reported patients

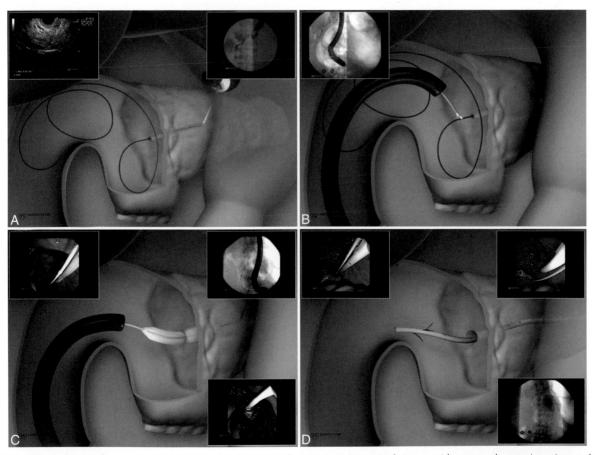

FIGURE 25-6 The technique for pancreatic duct access and transpapillary/transanastomotic drainage with retrograde stent insertion performed via a rendezvous procedure is demonstrated. **A,** EUS imaging reveals the main pancreatic duct with needle advancement, wire placement, and pancreatography. **B,** A side-viewing or forward-viewing instrument is then passed to the small bowel allowing either biopsy cable or snare retraction of the guidewire. **C,** Standard techniques may be used to perform duct cannulation and balloon dilatation in retrograde fashion. **D,** Standard techniques are also used for retrograde stent insertion.

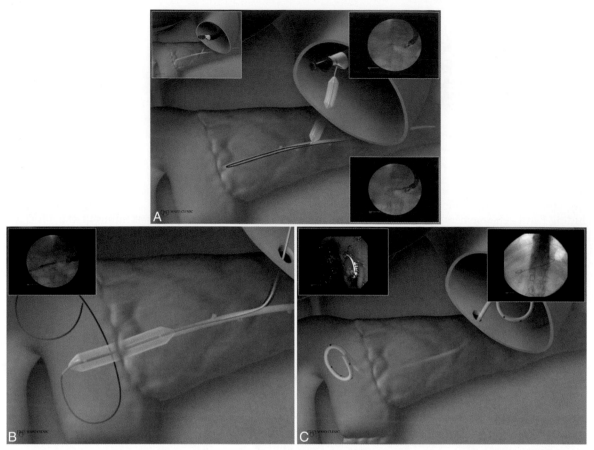

FIGURE 25-7   The technique for pancreatic duct access and transpapillary/transanastomotic drainage following antegrade stent insertion, performed entirely via an echoendoscope, is demonstrated. **A,** EUS imaging reveals the main pancreatic duct with needle advancement, wire placement and pancreatography with balloon dilatation of the gastric wall, pancreatic parenchyma, and pancreatic duct wall. **B,** A guidewire is passed through the site of obstruction or anastomosis followed by balloon dilatation. **C,** A stent is advanced in an antegrade fashion from the gastric lumen, into the pancreatic duct and through the site of obstruction.

(excluding case reports and studies focusing on EUS-guided pancreatogram only), the technical success of EUS-guided MPD intervention was 170 (76.6%) and complications developed in 42 (18.9%) patients (Table 25-4). Complications included abdominal pain ($n = 17$), pancreatitis ($n = 7$), bleeding ($n = 4$), unspecified ($n = 3$), perforation ($n = 2$), peripancreatic abscess ($n = 2$), shaving of the guidewire coating ($n = 2$), and one patient each developed fever, pneumoperitoneum, pseudocyst alone, aneurysm and pseudocyst, and perigastric fluid collection.

In the largest report to date, Fujii and colleagues reviewed their single-center experience in 43 patients undergoing

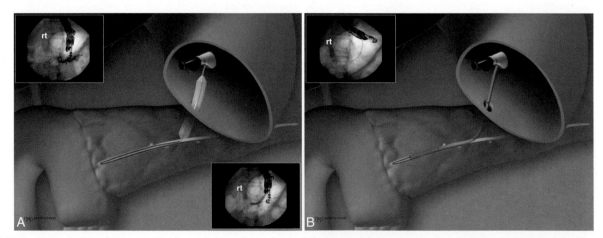

FIGURE 25-8   The technique for pancreatic duct access and transluminal drainage of the pancreatic duct to the gastric lumen following antegrade stent insertion, performed solely with an echoendoscope, is demonstrated. **A,** EUS imaging of the pancreas and main pancreatic duct allows guided needle insertion, wire placement and pancreatography with balloon dilatation of the gastric wall, pancreatic parenchyma, and pancreatic duct wall. **B,** Antegrade stent insertion is performed via the echoendoscope.

TABLE 25-4			
PANCREATIC DUCT STENT PLACEMENT FOR DRAINAGE			
Author (year)	**Approach**	**Technical Success**	**Complications**
Francois et al[67] (2002)	Transluminal ($n = 4$)	4/4	None
Kahaleh et al[68,70] (2003, 2007)	TP/TA[a] ($n = 5$) Transluminal ($n = 5$)	10/12	Bleeding ($n = 1$) Perforation ($n = 1$)
Mallery et al[16] (2004) Kinney et al[75] (2009)	Retrograde TP/TA ($n = 4$)	4/11[b]	Pancreatitis & retroperitoneal air ($n = 1$) Fever ($n = 1$)
Tessier et al[64] (2007)	Transluminal ($n = 33$)	33/36	Bleeding ($n = 1$) Acute pancreatitis ($n = 1$) Unspecified mild complication ($n = 3$)
Will et al[76] (2007)	Retrograde TP/TA ($n = 4$) Transluminal ($n = 5$)	9/12	Abdominal pain ($n = 4$) Bleeding ($n = 1$) Perforation ($n = 1$)
Brauer et al[50] (2009)	Retrograde TP/TA ($n = 3$) Transluminal ($n = 4$)	7/8	None
Barkay et al[77] (2010)	Retrograde TP/TA ($n = 10$)	10/21	Peripancreatic abscess ($n = 1$) Pancreatitis ($n = 1$) Shaving of guidewire coating ($n = 1$)
Ergun et al[71] (2011)	Retrograde TP/TA ($n = 5$) Transluminal ($n = 13$)	18/20	Bleeding ($n = 1$) Perigastric fluid collection ($n = 1$)
Shah et al[32] (2012)	TP/TA[a] ($n = 9$) Transluminal ($n = 10$)	19/22	Pneumoperitoneum ($n = 1$) Pancreatitis ($n = 3$)
Vila et al[40] (2012)	Retrograde TP/TA ($n = 9$) Transluminal ($n = 2$)	11/19	Pseudocyst ($n = 1$)
Fujii et al[65] (2013)	TP/TA[a] ($n = 27$) Transluminal ($n = 5$)	32/43	Pancreatitis ($n = 1$) Peripancreatic abscess ($n = 1$) Shaving of guidewire coating ($n = 1$) Abdominal pain ($n = 13$)
Kurihara et al[72] (2013)	Retrograde TP/TA ($n = 10$) Transluminal ($n = 3$)	13/14	Aneurysm, pseudocyst ($n = 1$)

Excludes case reports and reports only on EUS-guided pancreatography.
NS, not specified; TP, transpapillary; TA, transanastomotic.
[a]Includes both retrograde and antegrade transpapillary/transanastomotic stent placement.
[b]Includes two cases from the 2004 publication that did not have a previous pancreaticoduodenectomy.

attempted EUS-guided pancreatic duct drainage.[65] As compared to most prior studies that focused on patients who failed prior ERP, 14.3% of patients in this report did not have a prior ERP, reflecting a change in our practice that employs EUS-guided MPD drainage as the first endoscopic intervention in patients with anastomotic stricture after pancreaticoduodenectomy due the higher success rate in stent placement. Overall technical success was achieved in 32 patients (74%), with stents placed in the retrograde fashion in 14 patients and antegrade transpapillary/transanastomotic or transluminal route in 13 and 5 patients, respectively. The site of obstruction and papilla/anastomosis was able to be traversed in subsequent procedures in two patients who initially underwent transluminal stent placement. Reasons for failed stent placement included the inability to advance the guidewire into the MPD ($n = 1$) or through the papilla or anastomosis ($n = 8$), inability to adequately dilate the track ($n = 1$), or loss of the guidewire during subsequent duodenoscope advancement ($n = 1$). Five patients (45%) in whom EUS-guided MPD drainage failed required pancreatic surgery. A higher chance of technical failure occurred when the EUS-guided portion was performed on the same day as a failed ERP, likely reflecting anatomic factors, inflammation induced by ERP attempts, or less commitment by the endosonographer in the setting of a

long procedure time. Long-term outcomes (at least 12 months of follow-up) were available for 29 patients (91%) who were successfully stented with complete clinical success defined as symptom resolution occurring in 69.6% and partial symptom resolution in the remaining 30.4%. An initial use of a shorter stent and any structural indication besides a benign anastomotic stricture were associated with complete clinical success on univariate analysis. Although the statistical significance of a shorter stent length may be a type I error, it may also reflect a shorter distance required for drainage. Moderate or severe complications occurred in three patients (5.8%), including acute pancreatitis, peripancreatic abscess treated with EUS-guided transmural drainage, and shaving of the guidewire coating into the retroperitoneum.

As for EUS-guided biliary interventions, the need and timing of reintervention and long-term clinical outcomes cannot be accurately determined based on published data. However, Will and colleagues noted that during the follow-up period that spanned 4 weeks to 3 years, 29% of patients required surgical intervention.[76] Tessier and colleagues reported stent dysfunction in 55% (20 of 36) of patients that required a total of 29 repeat endoscopies.[64] Similarly, Ergun and colleagues reported stent dysfunction in 50% of patients (9 of 18) during a median follow-up of 37 months.[71] Our stent dysfunction occurred in eight patients (25%) with migration in five patients and occlusion in three patients.[65] Although not statistically significant, stent migration occurred less frequently in patients who had a double-pigtail plastic stent placed (rather than straight plastic stents). Stent dysfunction was treated with attempts to place additional stents during the subsequent procedure to provide flow both within and between stents. The rate of stent dysfunction may be lower in our study as we typically scheduled patients to either remove or replace their stent at a median of 90 and 46 days, respectively. Eighteen patients underwent subsequent stent exchanges with a maximum of five stents placed until maximum resolution of the stenosis was achieved. Five patients still have their stent in place at a median of 42.6 months, whereas two patients required stent removal at more than 40 months out from their initial procedure due to symptoms of abdominal pain and recurrent pancreatitis related to the stent. The latter two patients did well after their stent was removed. This data suggest that patients may benefit from routine stent exchange, particularly if they require prolonged stent duration.

Suggested Algorithmic Approach to EUS-Guided Pancreaticobiliary Drainage

Decisions regarding the role of EUS-guided pancreaticobiliary access and drainage within a treatment algorithm must consider numerous factors, including the available expertise of the endoscopist and support staff, interventional radiologist, and surgeon, the success and adverse event profile within a particular center, the procedure indication, clinical status, emergency/urgency of the procedure, examination efficiency, cost, and having informed consent.

Once the decision is made to proceed with EUS-guided pancreaticobiliary drainage, the intent of the procedure should be to achieve transpapillary or transanastomotic drainage as this follows physiologic drainage and allows for potential resolution of the obstruction with recanalization of the ductal lumen. Transpapillary/transanastomotic drainage can be performed either through the retrograde or antegrade approach, which should be guided by the expertise of the performing endoscopist. Many reports used the retrograde route due to the ERCP experience of the endoscopist and available equipment.* We typically prefer antegrade placement of a transpapillary/transanastomotic stent because it typically is a shorter procedure length as it only requires one expert endosonographer to perform the entire procedure without the need to switch scopes. A caveat to performing antegrade stent placement is the creation of a fistula between the stomach/small bowel into the pancreaticobiliary ducts with an increased risk of pancreatic fluid or bile leak, particularly if stent placement is unsuccessful. This risk should be minimized by limiting the degree of balloon dilatation of the tract to the minimal level required for stent advancement, which in the authors' practice usually results in use of a 4- or 6-mm dilating balloon. The authors' approach is the opposite of the one taken by Vila and colleagues who reported a higher rate of technical success

_____

*37,40,41,59,65,71,75

when two endoscopists performed the different aspects of the rendezvous procedure.[40] Therefore, the ultimate decision on the approach should be made by the local expertise of the endoscopists.

Only if transpapillary/transanastomotic stent placement fails, would the authors suggest proceeding with transluminal stent placement. The transluminal technique has a potentially increased risk of stent dislodgement with subsequent pancreatic fluid leak causing pancreatitis or a pseudocyst or bile leak leading to a biloma or bile peritonitis. In patients with a transluminal stent placed during initial intervention, it is recommended to attempt to traverse the site of obstruction and papilla/anastomosis during subsequent procedures.

While EUS-guided pancreaticobiliary drainage is typically performed after failed ERCP, the authors often consider EUS-guided MPD drainage before ERP in patients with a pancreaticoduodenectomy because of the higher reported success rate with this procedure.[75,78–81] The option of EUS guidance should be considered relatively early in a difficult cannulation because same-day ERCP was associated with a higher rate of technical failure.[65]

Technical Challenges and Tips

A number of technical challenges may be faced during attempted EUS-guided pancreaticobiliary access and drainage and maneuvers that may help overcome these difficulties. Risk of inadvertent parenchymal or vascular injection may occur that may be minor in volume or more severe, potentially hindering further interventions. Care should be taken to limit the volume and concentration of the contrast injected, which may reduce the risk and help maintain visualization of targeted areas.

The guidewire often inadvertently passes into ductal side branches, which is prone to occur when there is a nearly perpendicular orientation of the echoendoscope to the desired duct. This problem may be overcome by altering the needle angle of entry and/or by the selection of an alternate wire, for instance a glide wire or angled wire. These maneuvers, along with careful wire manipulation, usually allow access to the desired segment.

Guidewire passage across the papilla, anastomosis, or other site of obstruction may be difficult leading to wire buckling or inadvertent passage into undesired ducts or parenchyma. While gradual retraction and readvancement may suffice, at times the wire will not traverse the site of obstruction despite repeated efforts. Fluoroscopic techniques such as the use of magnification can facilitate wire passage. In addition, it is ideal to utilize a fluoroscopic C-arm, if available, to allow imaging from multiple angles to display the anatomy in various orientations. Insertion of a catheter or balloon into the duct in close proximity to the site of obstruction should be considered. In this position, the catheter or balloon may serve to constrain the guidewire and allow delivery of greater longitudinal force to facilitate wire passage through the site of obstruction. It may also be helpful to select an alternate wire.

Even with a guidewire in place, it may be difficult to pass a catheter or balloon across the gastric or duodenal wall, site of anastomosis, or other site of obstruction. Catheter dilations are associated with an axial dilation force, which may lead to separation of the tissue planes with advancement. Balloon dilators, on the other hand, lead to radial dilation force, which may increase the risk of perforation, leaks, and bleeding.[82] Prolonged pressure with either catheter may allow the device to suddenly pass. Initial dilatation with the needle sheath can aid passage as well. Selection of alternate devices that may traverse otherwise inaccessible strictures may be considered.

One must always be mindful to the risk of wire shaving that occurs when retracting the wire into the needle at an acute angle. The risk is minimized by avoiding acute angles during wire retraction and by gently retracting the guidewire. The authors have also found that when resistance is felt and the wire cannot be removed, withdrawal of the wire and needle in unison allows safe removal.

When attempting to dilate the tract, the balloon may inadvertently pass between the gut wall and target organ, which may be suggested by difficulty when inserting subsequent devices. The risk may be minimized by careful observation using EUS and fluoroscopic guidance.

During biliary access, when one is attempting to pass a guidewire from the left intrahepatic bile duct to the extrahepatic bile duct, the wire is prone to pass instead into the right intrahepatic duct. Fluoroscopy is useful for guiding wire passage. Similarly, use of an alternate guidewire may facilitate duct access as may selection of a left intrahepatic duct that provides an opportune angle for wire passage.

Finally, there tends to be a loss of apposition between the stomach and liver, which predisposes to a biliary leak when one is performing hepaticogastrostomy. Placement of a longer, pigtail stent may diminish this risk as may the placement of transpapillary stents, which is the authors' preference whenever possible.

Physician Experience and Training

EUS-guided pancreaticobiliary access and drainage procedures are likely the most technically complex and challenging to perform among all ERCP and EUS procedures. Endoscopists are well served by having a full skill set that includes advanced ERCP and EUS training because the interventions performed include techniques that have been historically considered with either ERCP or EUS. Therefore performing physicians ideally will receive dedicated training in both disciplines. These procedures may also be performed by teaming two endoscopists with separate EUS and ERCP skills, but doing so complicates scheduling, decreases room efficiency, and has financial impact. As an increasing number of advanced training programs provide dual training and are performing a greater number of these procedures, the availability of adequately trained endoscopists will gradually increase. However, due to the somewhat delayed exposure to this procedure, the procedural complexity, and the relative paucity of cases, few advanced endoscopy trainees will graduate with sufficient skills to allow independent performance of all aforementioned techniques. We encourage graduates to develop their practice in a stepwise manner that is influenced by a particular patient's health and clinical needs, their particular skill set, their practice setting, and available nonendoscopic expertise. Given the complexity and limited need for such procedures in any given center, it may be preferable to limit these exams to one or few fully trained and not partially trained endosonographers/ERCPists.

Summary

EUS often allows access and drainage of the biliary and pancreatic ducts following failed ERCP and can obviate the need for percutaneous and surgical interventions. As a result of the complexity of these procedures, new techniques and equipment are needed. These procedures are likely to be aided by the development of sheer-resistant guidewires and by creation of multistep, combination devices that aid initial access, dilation, and stenting.

These procedures are technically challenging and time and personnel intensive. Caution must be exercised as complications are relatively common and can be severe. In addition, few data and methodological limitations of current reports exist, thereby limiting our understanding of the utility and role of these techniques. Additional data are needed to more accurately define the risks and long-term outcomes before their role can be clarified. Until then, EUS-guided intervention cannot be broadly advocated and must be performed in carefully selected patients managed by a multidisciplinary team of physicians.

REFERENCES

1. Levy MJ, Wiersema MJ. EUS-guided TruCut biopsy. *Gastrointest Endosc.* 2005;62:417-426.
2. Kulesza P, Eltoum IA. Endoscopic ultrasound-guided fine-needle aspiration: sampling, pitfalls, and quality management. *Clin Gastroenterol Hepatol.* 2007;5:1248-1254.
3. Wiersema MJ, Wiersema LM. Endosonography-guided celiac plexus neurolysis. *Gastrointest Endosc.* 1996;44:656-662.
4. Levy MJ, Wiersema MJ. Endoscopic ultrasound-guided pain control for intra-abdominal cancer. *Gastroenterol Clin North Am.* 2006;35: 153-165, x.
5. Levy MJ, Topazian MD, Wiersema MJ, et al. Initial evaluation of the efficacy and safety of endoscopic ultrasound-guided direct ganglia neurolysis and block. *Am J Gastroenterol.* 2008;103:98-103.
6. Seifert H, Dietrich C, Schmitt T, et al. Endoscopic ultrasound-guided one-step transmural drainage of cystic abdominal lesions with a large-channel echo endoscope. *Endoscopy.* 2000;32:255-259.
7. Norton ID, Clain JE, Wiersema MJ, et al. Utility of endoscopic ultrasonography in endoscopic drainage of pancreatic pseudocysts in selected patients. *Mayo Clin Proc.* 2001;76:794-798.
8. Kruger M, Schneider AS, Manns MP, Meier PN. Endoscopic management of pancreatic pseudocysts or abscesses after an EUS-guided 1-step procedure for initial access. *Gastrointest Endosc.* 2006;63:409-416.
9. Lopes CV, Pesenti C, Bories E, et al. Endoscopic ultrasound-guided endoscopic transmural drainage of pancreatic pseudocysts. *Arq Gastroenterol.* 2008;45:17-21.
10. Kwan V, Eisendrath P, Antaki F, et al. EUS-guided cholecystenterostomy: a new technique (with videos). *Gastrointest Endosc.* 2007;66:582-586.
11. Chang KJ, Nguyen PT, Thompson JA, et al. Phase I clinical trial of allogeneic mixed lymphocyte culture (cytoimplant) delivered by endoscopic ultrasound-guided fine-needle injection in patients with advanced pancreatic carcinoma. *Cancer.* 2000;88:1325-1335.
12. Chang KJ. EUS-guided fine needle injection (FNI) and anti-tumor therapy. *Endoscopy.* 2006;38(suppl 1):S88-S93.
13. Erickson RA. EUS-guided pancreaticogastrostomy: invasive endosonography coming of age. *Gastrointest Endosc.* 2007;65:231-232.
14. Voegeli DR, Crummy AB, Weese JL. Percutaneous transhepatic cholangiography, drainage, and biopsy in patients with malignant biliary obstruction. An alternative to surgery. *Am J Surg.* 1985;150:243-247.
15. Oh HC, Lee SK, Lee TY, et al. Analysis of percutaneous transhepatic cholangioscopy-related complications and the risk factors for those complications. *Endoscopy.* 2007;39:731-736.
16. Mallery S, Matlock J, Freeman ML. EUS-guided rendezvous drainage of obstructed biliary and pancreatic ducts: Report of 6 cases. *Gastrointest Endosc.* 2004;59:100-107.
17. Kahaleh M, Hernandez AJ, Tokar J, et al. guided cholangiography: evaluation of a technique in evolution. *Gastrointest Endosc.* 2006;64: 52-59.

18. Wiersema MJ, Sandusky D, Carr R, et al. Endosonography-guided cholangiopancreatography. *Gastrointest Endosc.* 1996;43:102-106.

19. Giovannini M, Moutardier V, Pesenti C, et al. Endoscopic ultrasound-guided bilioduodenal anastomosis: a new technique for biliary drainage. *Endoscopy.* 2001;33:898-900.

20. Park do H, Jang JW, Lee SS, et al. EUS-guided biliary drainage with transluminal stenting after failed ERCP: predictors of adverse events and long-term results. *Gastrointest Endosc.* 2011;74:1276-1284.

21. Kahaleh M, Yoshida C, Kane L, Yeaton P. Interventional EUS cholangiography: a report of five cases. *Gastrointest Endosc.* 2004;60:138-142.

22. Kahaleh M, Wang P, Shami VM, et al. EUS-guided transhepatic cholangiography: report of 6 cases. *Gastrointest Endosc.* 2005;61:307-313.

23. Maranki J, Hernandez AJ, Arslan B, et al. Interventional endoscopic ultrasound-guided cholangiography: long-term experience of an emerging alternative to percutaneous transhepatic cholangiography. *Endoscopy.* 2009;41:532-538.

24. Bories E, Pesenti C, Caillol F, et al. Transgastric endoscopic ultrasonography-guided biliary drainage: results of a pilot study. *Endoscopy.* 2007;39:287-291.

25. Will U, Thieme A, Fueldner F, et al. Treatment of biliary obstruction in selected patients by endoscopic ultrasonography (EUS)-guided transluminal biliary drainage. *Endoscopy.* 2007;39:292-295.

26. Horaguchi J, Fujita N, Noda Y, et al. Endosonography-guided biliary drainage in cases with difficult transpapillary endoscopic biliary drainage. *Dig Endosc.* 2009;21:239-244.

27. Park do H, Koo JE, Oh J, et al. EUS-guided biliary drainage with one-step placement of a fully covered metal stent for malignant biliary obstruction: a prospective feasibility study. *Am J Gastroenterol.* 2009;104:2168-2174.

28. Park do H, Song TJ, Eum J, et al. EUS-guided hepaticogastrostomy with a fully covered metal stent as the biliary diversion technique for an occluded biliary metal stent after a failed ERCP (with videos). *Gastrointest Endosc.* 2010;71:413-419.

29. Park DH, Jeong SU, Lee BU, et al. Prospective evaluation of a treatment algorithm with enhanced guidewire manipulation protocol for EUS-guided biliary drainage after failed ERCP (with videos). *Gastrointest Endosc.* 2013.

30. Iwamuro M, Kawamoto H, Harada R, et al. Combined duodenal stent placement and endoscopic ultrasonography-guided biliary drainage for malignant duodenal obstruction with biliary stricture. *Dig Endosc.* 2010;22:236-240.

31. Nguyen-Tang T, Binmoeller KF, Sanchez-Yague A, Shah JN. Endoscopic ultrasound (EUS)-guided transhepatic anterograde self-expandable metal stent (SEMS) placement across malignant biliary obstruction. *Endoscopy.* 2010;42:232-236.

32. Shah JN, Marson F, Weilert F, et al. Single-operator, single-session EUS-guided anterograde cholangiopancreatography in failed ERCP or inaccessible papilla. *Gastrointest Endosc.* 2012;75:56-64.

33. Belletrutti PJ, DiMaio CJ, Gerdes H, Schattner MA. Endoscopic ultrasound guided biliary drainage in patients with unapproachable ampullae due to malignant duodenal obstruction. *J Gastrointest Cancer.* 2011;42:137-142.

34. Ramirez-Luna MA, Tellez-Avila FI, Giovannini M, et al. Endoscopic ultrasound-guided biliodigestive drainage is a good alternative in patients with unresectable cancer. *Endoscopy.* 2011;43:826-830.

35. Artifon EL, Aparicio D, Paione JB, et al. Biliary drainage in patients with unresectable, malignant obstruction where ERCP fails: endoscopic ultrasonography-guided choledochoduodenostomy versus percutaneous drainage. *J Clin Gastroenterol.* 2012;46:768-774.

36. Gupta K, Perez-Miranda M, Kahaleh M, et al. Endoscopic ultrasound-assisted bile duct access and drainage: multicenter, long-term analysis of approach, outcomes, and complications of a technique in evolution. *J Clin Gastroenterol.* 2013.

37. Iwashita T, Lee JG, Shinoura S, et al. Endoscopic ultrasound-guided rendezvous for biliary access after failed cannulation. *Endoscopy.* 2012;44:60-65.

38. Khashab MA, Fujii LL, Baron TH, et al. EUS-guided biliary drainage for patients with malignant biliary obstruction with an indwelling duodenal stent (with videos). *Gastrointest Endosc.* 2012;76:209-213.

39. Kim TH, Kim SH, Oh HJ, et al. Endoscopic ultrasound-guided biliary drainage with placement of a fully covered metal stent for malignant biliary obstruction. *WJG.* 2012;18:2526-2532.

40. Vila JJ, Perez-Miranda M, Vazquez-Sequeiros E, et al. Initial experience with EUS-guided cholangiopancreatography for biliary and pancreatic duct drainage: a Spanish national survey. *Gastrointest Endosc.* 2012;76:1133-1141.

41. Kawakubo K, Isayama H, Sasahira N, et al. Clinical utility of an endoscopic ultrasound-guided rendezvous technique via various approach routes. *Surg Endosc.* 2013.

42. Tonozuka R, Itoi T, Sofuni A, et al. Endoscopic double stenting for the treatment of malignant biliary and duodenal obstruction due to pancreatic cancer. *Dig Endosc.* 2013;25(suppl 2):100-108.

43. Burmester E, Niehaus J, Leineweber T, Huetteroth T. EUS-cholangio-drainage of the bile duct: report of 4 cases. *Gastrointest Endosc.* 2003;57:246-251.

44. Puspok A, Lomoschitz F, Dejaco C, et al. Endoscopic ultrasound guided therapy of benign and malignant biliary obstruction: a case series. *Am J Gastroenterol.* 2005;100:1743-1747.

45. Yamao K, Sawaki A, Takahashi K, et al. EUS-guided choledochoduodenostomy for palliative biliary drainage in case of papillary obstruction: report of 2 cases. *Gastrointest Endosc.* 2006;64:663-667.

46. Yamao K, Bhatia V, Mizuno N, et al. EUS-guided choledochoduodenostomy for palliative biliary drainage in patients with malignant biliary obstruction: results of long-term follow-up. *Endoscopy.* 2008;40:340-342.

47. Ang TL, Teo EK, Fock KM. EUS-guided transduodenal biliary drainage in unresectable pancreatic cancer with obstructive jaundice. *JOP.* 2007;8:438-443.

48. Itoi T, Itokawa F, Sofuni A, et al. Endoscopic ultrasound-guided choledochoduodenostomy in patients with failed endoscopic retrograde cholangiopancreatography. *WJG.* 2008;14:6078-6082.

49. Tarantino I, Barresi L, Repici A, Traina M. EUS-guided biliary drainage: a case series. *Endoscopy.* 2008;40:336-339.

50. Brauer BC, Chen YK, Fukami N, Shah RJ. Single-operator EUS-guided cholangiopancreatography for difficult pancreaticobiliary access (with video). *Gastrointest Endosc.* 2009;70:471-479.

51. Hanada K, Iiboshi T, Ishii Y. Endoscopic ultrasound-guided choledochoduodenostomy for palliative biliary drainage in cases with inoperable pancreas head carcinoma. *Dig Endosc.* 2009;21(suppl 1):S75-S78.

52. Artifon EL, Takada J, Okawa L, et al. EUS-guided choledochoduodenostomy for biliary drainage in unresectable pancreatic cancer: a case series. *JOP.* 2010;11:597-600.

53. Eum J, Park do H, Ryu CH, et al. EUS-guided biliary drainage with a fully covered metal stent as a novel route for natural orifice transluminal endoscopic biliary interventions: a pilot study (with videos). *Gastrointest Endosc.* 2010;72:1279-1284.

54. Kim YS, Gupta K, Mallery S, et al. Endoscopic ultrasound rendezvous for bile duct access using a transduodenal approach: cumulative experience at a single center. A case series. *Endoscopy.* 2010;42:496-502.

55. Fabbri C, Luigiano C, Fuccio L, et al. EUS-guided biliary drainage with placement of a new partially covered biliary stent for palliation of malignant biliary obstruction: a case series. *Endoscopy.* 2011;43:438-441.

56. Hara K, Yamao K, Niwa Y, et al. Prospective clinical study of EUS-guided choledochoduodenostomy for malignant lower biliary tract obstruction. *Am J Gastroenterol.* 2011;106:1239-1245.

57. Komaki T, Kitano M, Sakamoto H, Kudo M. Endoscopic ultrasonography-guided biliary drainage: evaluation of a choledochoduodenostomy technique. *Pancreatology.* 2011;11(suppl 2):47-51.

58. Siddiqui AA, Sreenarasimhaiah J, Lara LF, et al. Endoscopic ultrasound-guided transduodenal placement of a fully covered metal stent for palliative biliary drainage in patients with malignant biliary obstruction. *Surg Endosc.* 2011;25:549-555.

59. Dhir V, Bhandari S, Bapat M, Maydeo A. Comparison of EUS-guided rendezvous and precut papillotomy techniques for biliary access (with videos). *Gastrointest Endosc.* 2012;75:354-359.

60. Nicholson JA, Johnstone M, Raraty MG, Evans JC. Endoscopic ultrasound-guided choledoco-duodenostomy as an alternative to percutaneous trans-hepatic cholangiography. *HPB.* 2012;14:483-486.

61. Song TJ, Hyun YS, Lee SS, et al. Endoscopic ultrasound-guided choledochoduodenostomies with fully covered self-expandable metallic stents. *WJG.* 2012;18:4435-4440.

62. Harada N, Kouzu T, Arima M, et al. Endoscopic ultrasound-guided pancreatography: a case report. *Endoscopy.* 1995;27:612-615.

63. Keenan J, Mallery S, Freeman ML. EUS rendezvous for pancreatic stent placement during endoscopic snare ampullectomy. *Gastrointest Endosc.* 2007;66:850-853.

64. Tessier G, Bories E, Arvanitakis M, et al. EUS-guided pancreatogastrostomy and pancreatobulbostomy for the treatment of pain in patients with pancreatic ductal dilatation inaccessible for transpapillary endoscopic therapy. *Gastrointest Endosc.* 2007;65:233-241.

65. Fujii LL, Topazian MD, Abu Dayyeh BK, et al. EUS-guided pancreatic duct intervention: outcomes of a single tertiary-care referral center experience. *Gastrointest Endosc.* 2013.

66. Bataille L, Deprez P. A new application for therapeutic EUS: main pancreatic duct drainage with a "pancreatic rendezvous technique". *Gastrointest Endosc.* 2002;55:740-743.

67. Francois E, Kahaleh M, Giovannini M, et al. EUS-guided pancreaticogastrostomy. *Gastrointest Endosc.* 2002;56:128-133.

68. Kahaleh M, Yoshida C, Yeaton P. EUS antegrade pancreatography with gastropancreatic duct stent placement: review of two cases. *Gastrointest Endosc.* 2003;58:919-923.

69. Will U, Meyer F, Manger T, Wanzar I. Endoscopic ultrasound-assisted rendezvous maneuver to achieve pancreatic duct drainage in obstructive chronic pancreatitis. *Endoscopy.* 2005;37:171-173.

70. Kahaleh M, Hernandez AJ, Tokar J, et al. EUS-guided pancreaticogastrostomy: analysis of its efficacy to drain inaccessible pancreatic ducts. *Gastrointest Endosc.* 2007;65:224-230.

71. Ergun M, Aouattah T, Gillain C, et al. Endoscopic ultrasound-guided transluminal drainage of pancreatic duct obstruction: long-term outcome. *Endoscopy.* 2011;43:518-525.

72. Kurihara T, Itoi T, Sofuni A, et al. Endoscopic ultrasonography-guided pancreatic duct drainage after failed endoscopic retrograde cholangiopancreatography in patients with malignant and benign pancreatic duct obstructions. *Dig Endosc.* 2013;25(suppl 2):109-116.

73. Saftoiu A, Dumitrescu D, Stoica M, et al. EUS-assisted rendezvous stenting of the pancreatic duct for chronic calcifying pancreatitis with multiple pseudocysts. *Pancreatology.* 2007;7:74-79.

74. Gleeson FC, Pelaez MC, Petersen BT, Levy MJ. Drainage of an inaccessible main pancreatic duct via EUS-guided transgastric stenting through the minor papilla. *Endoscopy.* 2007;39(suppl 1):E313-E314.

75. Will U, Fueldner F, Thieme AK, et al. Transgastric pancreatography and EUS-guided drainage of the pancreatic duct. *J Hepatobiliary Pancreat Surg.* 2007;14:377-382.

76. Kinney TP, Li R, Gupta K, et al. Therapeutic pancreatic endoscopy after Whipple resection requires rendezvous access. *Endoscopy.* 2009;41:898-901.

77. Barkay O, Sherman S, McHenry L, et al. Assisted endoscopic retrograde pancreatography after failed pancreatic duct cannulation at ERCP. *Gastrointest Endosc.* 2010;71:1166-1173.

78. Chahal P, Baron TH, Topazian MD, et al. Endoscopic retrograde cholangiopancreatography in post-Whipple patients. *Endoscopy.* 2006;38:1241-1245.

79. Farrell J, Carr-Locke D, Garrido T, et al. Endoscopic retrograde cholangiopancreatography after pancreaticoduodenectomy for benign and malignant disease: indications and technical outcomes. *Endoscopy.* 2006;38:1246-1249.

80. Matsushita M, Takakuwa H, Uchida K, et al. Techniques to facilitate ERCP with a conventional endoscope in patients with previous pancreatoduodenectomy. *Endoscopy.* 2009;41:902-906.

81. Kikuyama M, Itoi T, Ota Y, et al. Therapeutic endoscopy for stenotic pancreatodigestive tract anastomosis after pancreatoduodenectomy (with videos). *Gastrointest Endosc.* 2011;73:376-382.

82. Kahaleh M, Artifon EL, Perez-Miranda M, et al. Endoscopic ultrasonography guided biliary drainage: summary of consortium meeting, May 7th, 2011, Chicago. *WJG.* 2013;19:1372-1379.

KEY READING LIST

Fujii LL, Topazian MD, Abu Dayyeh BK, et al. EUS-guided pancreatic duct intervention: outcomes of a single tertiary-care referral center experience. *Gastrointest Endosc.* 2013.

Gupta K, Perez-Miranda M, Kahaleh M, et al. Endoscopic ultrasound-assisted bile duct access and drainage: multicenter, long-term analysis of approach, outcomes, and complications of a technique in evolution. *J clin gastro.* 2013.

Park do H, Jang JW, Lee SS, et al. EUS-guided biliary drainage with transluminal stenting after failed ERCP: predictors of adverse events and long-term results. *Gastrointest Endosc.* 2011;74:1276-1284.

Shah JN, Marson F, Weilert F, et al. Single-operator, single-session EUS-guided anterograde cholangiopancreatography in failed ERCP or inaccessible papilla. *Gastrointest Endosc.* 2012;75:56-64.

Tessier G, Bories E, Arvanitakis M, et al. EUS-guided pancreatogastrostomy and pancreatobulbostomy for the treatment of pain in patients with pancreatic ductal dilatation inaccessible for transpapillary endoscopic therapy. *Gastrointest Endosc.* 2007;65:233-241.

Vila JJ, Perez-Miranda M, Vazquez-Sequeiros E, et al. Initial experience with EUS-guided cholangiopancreatography for biliary and pancreatic duct drainage: a Spanish national survey. *Gastrointest Endosc.* 2012;76:1133-1141.

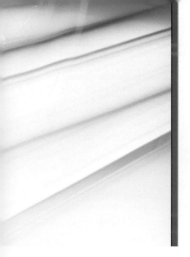

26

EUS-Guided Ablation Therapy and Celiac Plexus Interventions

Abdurrahman Kadayifci • William R. Brugge

Key Points

- In its simplest form, EUS-guided ablative therapy consists of injection of cytotoxic agents into cystic cavities or ganglia to eliminate premalignant epithelium or to produce neurolysis.
- Celiac plexus block or neurolysis is the most common EUS-guided intervention in current practice. Significant pain control is achieved with injection of ethanol in the setting of pancreatic cancer. More modest results are seen in patients with abdominal pain arising from chronic pancreatitis.
- More advanced techniques include the use of photodynamic therapy, brachytherapy, and radiofrequency ablation. Although preliminary data are promising, most of these procedures are still experimental.
- Although many of these EUS-based techniques are designed to be used to ablate or control pancreatic malignancies, some may facilitate the delivery of radiation therapy by placement of radiopaque markers into the tumor.

EUS represents one of the major developments in endoscopy since 1990. Although endoscopic ultrasonography (EUS) was originally designed to assist the endoscopist in the imaging of gastrointestinal malignancies, the procedure has evolved into a means of guiding tissue acquisition from the gastrointestinal tract and adjacent organs. Using fine-needle aspiration (FNA) accessories, interventional EUS is often based on fine-needle injection (FNI) therapy. Developments in interventional EUS have also highlighted a broad range of therapies beyond FNI, including tissue ablation and cancer therapeutics.

Instrumentation

Therapeutic EUS is performed using a linear echoendoscope because of the ability of linear EUS to guide needle placement into structures adjacent to the gastrointestinal tract. Numerous EUS accessories have been introduced that make interventional EUS possible.[1]

The quality of linear instruments has steadily increased in terms of ultrasound image processing, flexibility, and shaft diameter. The availability of a 3.2-mm instrument channel has made it possible to use a broader range of accessories. The enhanced sensitivity of color and flow Doppler in real-time imaging has improved the ability of clinicians to detect small lesions and to avoid vascular structures during injection therapy.

Endoscopic Ultrasound-Guided Radiotherapy

Radiofrequency Ablation

The principle of radiofrequency ablation (RFA) is the induction of thermal injury to the target tissue through the use of electromagnetic energy. In monopolar RFA, the patient is part of a closed-loop circuit that includes an radiofrequency (RF) generator, an electrode needle, and a large dispersive electrode (ground pad). The delivery of electromagnetic energy in tissue results in rapid movement of ions in tissue. The agitation of ions produces frictional heat around an electrode. The tissue destruction depends on both the tissue temperature achieved and the duration of heating. At temperatures between 60°C and 100°C, near immediate protein coagulation is induced. Cells experiencing this extent of thermal damage undergo coagulative necrosis over the course of several days.

The procedural technique used for RFA is based on the EUS guidance of a needle catheter into the target lesion. In RFA of liver and pancreatic lesions, this procedure requires placement of the needle across the gastric or duodenal walls. In contrast, the needle in traditional RFA is placed through the skin and into the liver by using ultrasound or computed tomography (CT) guidance. Because the RF catheter must be precisely directed into the target lesion, the lesion must be

TABLE 26-1

EXAMPLES OF EUS-GUIDED TUMOR ABLATION THERAPY

	Radiofrequency Ablation	TNFerade	Cryotherm (cool-tipped RFA)	Ethanol Injection	Brachytherapy	Paclitaxel (Taxol) Injection
Device used	Needle prongs	FNA needle	Dedicated catheter	FNA needle	FNA needle	19-G needle
Animal model	Swine	N/A	Swine	Swine	Swine	Swine
Mechanism of action	Heat-induced necrosis	Radiation sensitizer	Heat-induced necrosis	Protein denaturation	DNA damage	Cytotoxic
Target lesion	Liver	Pancreatic cancer	Pancreas, liver, spleen	Neuroendocrine tumors, IPMN, celiac ganglia	Pancreatic adenocarcinoma	Cystic lesions
Human studies	None	Yes	IRB protocols	Yes	Yes	Yes
Availability	Research	Research	Clinical trials	Widely	Yes	Widely

FNA, fine-needle aspiration; IPMN, intraductal papillary mucinous neoplasia; IRB, institutional review board; N/A, not applicable; RFA, radiofrequency ablation.

visible by ultrasound or CT. Once the needle has been successfully placed into the tissue mass, the RF current is delivered. During heating of tissue, ultrasound monitoring demonstrates a hyperechoic "cloud" surrounding the tip of the needle. EUS-guided delivery of ablative energy to localized malignant tumors has become increasingly possible through the introduction of commercial devices. EUS-guided RFA was originally described using a modified EUS needle and a commercial RF catheter. RFA resulted in tissue necrosis of an area of 1 to 3 cm surrounding the RF needle catheter (Table 26-1). Focal tissue ablation has been demonstrated using a single RFA 19-G needle placed into the normal porcine pancreas.[2] EUS RFA of the pancreatic body and tail was found to be feasible, effective, and relatively safe in a porcine model using a novel 18-G endoscopic RFA electrode with an ablation zone of 2.3 cm.[3] Recently, a small EUS RFA probe (Habib catheter, Emcision Ltd, London) was used to apply EUS-guided RFA to the head of pancreas in a porcine model.[4] The procedure was well tolerated in five pigs and with minimal amount of pancreatitis. The Habib catheter is a monopolar RFA probe with a working length of 190 cm, 3.6-F (1.2-mm) diameter, and 1-Fr (0.33-mm) wire, compatible with 19- and 22-G FNA needles (Figures 26-1 and 26-2). It is designed to achieve a more limited injury to tissue compared to other RFA devices.

Procedural Technique (Video 26-1)

The echoendoscope is inserted through the esophagus to the stomach and duodenum. After the pancreatic lesion is located, a 19- or 22-G FNA needle is inserted through the working channel of the echoendoscope into the target lesion. The stylet is then removed from the FNA needle and the monopolar Habib catheter is gently advanced through the hollow of the FNA needle. The RFA probe is connected to an electrosurgical RF generator. The wattage and exposure time has not been standardized yet. However, in pilot studies, RF energy was applied for 90 to 120 seconds at the 5- to 25-W setting. The ablation was repeated two to six times in each session in previous clinical studies.[5,6]

Clinical Outcomes

EUS RFA of pancreatic cystic neoplasms (PCN), neuroendocrine tumors (NET), and pancreatic ductal adenocarcinoma (PDAC) was recently described in humans using the Habib EUS RFA catheter in two separate studies by the same

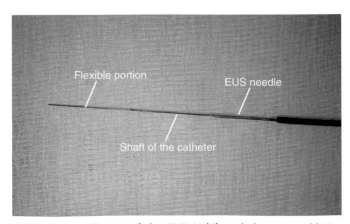

FIGURE 26-1 The tip of the EUS Habib radiofrequency ablation catheter.

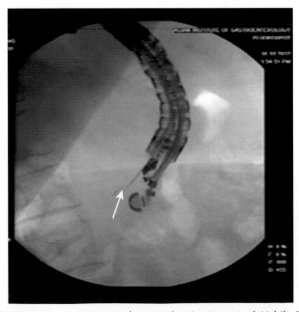

FIGURE 26-2 Fluoroscopy showing the tip (arrow) of Habib EUS radiofrequency ablation catheter.

Video 26-1. Video demonstrating the technique of EUS-guided RFA application to pancreas using Habib catheter.

authors.[5,6] The PDAC study[5] included seven patients with the lesions located in the head of pancreas in five patients and in the body of pancreas in two patients. RF was applied at 5 to 15 W in over 90 seconds and the procedure was completed in all patients. The postprocedure imaging after 3 to 6 months showed a decrease in size of the lesion in two patients, whereas the lesions were unchanged in the rest of the patients. The procedure was well tolerated in all patients and no complication was detected except in one patient with mild pancreatitis that settled with conservative management. The PCN-NET study[6] included eight patients with a neoplastic lesion (six PCN and two NET) located in the head of the pancreas. In the six patients with a PCN, the postprocedure imaging after 3 to 6 months showed complete resolution of the cysts in two patients and a 48.4% reduction in size in three patients. Only one patient had to undergo a second session. Cross-sectional imaging in the two patients with NET demonstrated a change in vascularity and central necrosis after EUS RFA. No episodes of pancreatitis, perforation, or bleeding were reported within 48 hours of the procedure. These initial results suggest that the procedure is technically easy and safe. However, more studies are needed to show especially the effectiveness of the method.

A commercial cool-tipped cryotherm device was designed and tested in an animal model for pancreatic ablation[7] (Figure 26-3). A flexible bipolar ablation probe combining RF and cryotechnology was used to induce foci of complete pancreatic ablation. The heated tip of the probe was cooled with simultaneous cryogenic carbon dioxide (650 psi). EUS-guided cryotherm RFA was also successfully used in the liver and spleen.[8] The size of the tissue ablation was time dependent and correlated with the abnormal tissue echogenicity. In the first human clinical trial, the flexible bipolar ablation probe

was successfully applied under EUS guidance in 16 of 22 (72.8%) patients with advanced pancreatic carcinoma.[9] In six patients, it failed because of excessive resistance of the gastrointestinal wall and of the tumor. Median postablation survival time was 6 months.

Brachytherapy

Brachytherapy in the form of small seeds or beads can also be used for the local control of malignant disease. Solid gastrointestinal malignant tumors often respond to the local administration of radiation therapy, and the risk of recurrence is reduced.[10] Traditionally, radiation therapy was provided intraoperatively, but precise targeting is difficult. CT-guided placement of radiation beads and seeds adjacent to malignant gastrointestinal tumors is reportedly safe and somewhat effective.[11] EUS-guided brachytherapy was described in an animal model of pancreatic cancer.[12] Localized tissue necrosis and fibrosis were achieved in the pancreas, without significant complications. Through an 18-G EUS needle, multiple small radioactive seeds were placed into the pancreatic tissue to provide interstitial brachytherapy.

A pilot study in patients with unresectable stage III and stage IV pancreatic adenocarcinoma demonstrated the feasibility and safety of the procedure with a mean of 22 seeds per patient.[13] Although the tumor response to brachytherapy was modest (33% of the tumors were stabilized), there was a transient clinical benefit in patients (30%) who experienced a reduction in abdominal pain. The mean total implanted activity was 20 mCi, the minimum peripheral dose was 14,000 cGy, and the mean volume of implants was 52 cm[3]. EUS-guided radioactive iodine-125 seed placement into pancreatic cancer was also reported to produce a transient decrease in abdominal pain.[14] In this trial of 22 patients, all patients were successfully implanted with iodine-125 seeds by EUS, with a median of 10 seeds and a maximum of 30 seeds per procedure. The estimated median survival time was 9 months. Partial remission was achieved in three patients (13.6%) during the 4-week period, and disease in 10 patients (45.5%) remained stable. Pain scores dropped from 5.1 to 1.7 1 week after brachytherapy but increased again to 3.5 a month later. The long-term outcome of EUS-guided brachytherapy was prospectively demonstrated in 100 cases of unresectable pancreatic cancer.[15] Gemcitabine-chemotherapy was combined with RFA in 85 patients, 1 week after brachytherapy. The mean follow-up time was 7.8 ± 6.1 months, and the estimated median progress-free survival and overall-survival were 4.5 months and 7.0 months, respectively. Visual Analog Scare (VAS) scores dropped dramatically after 1-week post implantation and were maintained at significantly lower levels until the third month. The cases with postimplantation chemotherapy had a longer median survival as long as 7.8 months, compared with those patients who were untreated (4 months). The outcome of the study suggested EUS-guided iodine-125 seed implantation plus chemotherapy is an effective method to prolong survival of patients with pancreatic cancer.

EUS-Guided Fiducial Placements

Advances in radiation therapy have provided the opportunity for the real-time delivery of radiation using three-dimensional

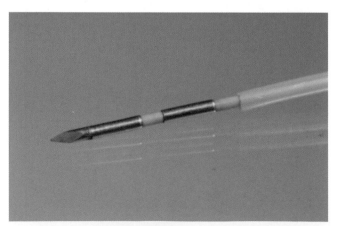

FIGURE 26-3 Cool-tipped radiofrequency catheter designed for EUS.

Video 26-2. Video demonstrating the technique of EUS-guided fiducial placement.

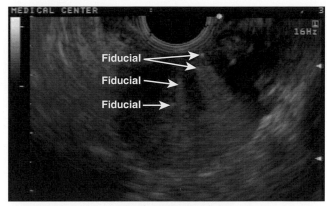

FIGURE 26-5 EUS image demonstrating fiducial placement within a pancreatic mass.

mapping guided by radiopaque markers. Respiratory-dependent movement of the target lesions often results in inappropriate radiation exposure to surrounding tissue. Marking of focal malignancy allows the precise targeting of focused beams of radiation despite respiratory movements.

Although CT scanning is capable of guiding the placement of fiducials in and adjacent to pancreatic malignancy, EUS guidance is probably more precise.[16] These small radiopaque markers are placed into the periphery of a malignant lesion to facilitate better targeting of radiation therapy.

Procedural Technique (Video 26-2)

After identifying the tumor and excluding the presence of intervening vasculature, EUS-guided fiducial placement is undertaken using 19-G FNA needles. Commercially available sterilized gold fiducial markers 3 mm in length and 0.8 mm in diameter are preloaded into the needle by retracting the stylet and manually back-loading the fiducials into the tip of the needle. The tip of the needle is then sealed with bone wax to prevent accidental dislodgment of the fiducials. Smaller fiducials have been developed that enable deployment through 22-G FNA needles. After identifying a target lesion, the tumor is punctured, and the fiducial is deployed by advancing the stylet forward. Resistance can be encountered during deployment of fiducials if the tip of the echoendoscope is deflected. This resistance can be overcome by removing the stylet and applying hydrostatic pressure from a syringe containing sterile water attached to the needle to deposit the markers into the

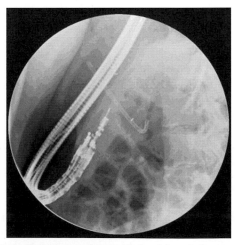

FIGURE 26-4 Fluoroscopy demonstrating fiducial placement within a pancreatic mass.

tumor. Depending on the size of the tumor, four to six fiducials should be deployed into the tumor to provide for ample separation of fiducials in distance, angulation, and plane. Both fluoroscopic and ultrasonographic visualization may be used to enable correct positioning of the fiducials within the tumor mass (Figures 26-4 and 26-5). Although preliminary studies mainly focused on the role of EUS-guided fiducial placement in pancreatic cancer, fiducials can potentially be deployed into any intramural or extramural malignant tumor that can be accessed by EUS.[17]

In a study reported in 2006, fiducials were deployed under EUS guidance in 13 patients with mediastinal or intra-abdominal tumors.[16] All patients were scheduled to undergo Cyberknife stereotactic radiosurgery following fiducial placement. The EUS procedure was technically successful in 11 of 13 (85%) patients. Failures were caused by an inability to advance the echoendoscope into the duodenum in a patient with gastric outlet obstruction and by the presence of an intervening vasculature in another. The investigators used fiducials that were either 3 or 5 mm in length and reported difficulty with deployment of 5-mm fiducials when the tip of the echoendoscope was angulated. This technical difficulty was overcome either by straightening the tip of the echoendoscope during fiducial deployment or by placing 3-mm fiducials instead. The fiducials are readily seen with fluoroscopy as small radiopaque objects within the target tissue (Figure 26-6). One patient in this study developed cholangitis 25 days following the procedure.

A new EUS-guided multifiducial delivery system was tested in a porcine model with a 95.6% success rate. All fiducials were deployed on target quickly, easily, and accurately without adverse events.[18]

EUS-guided gold fiducials were successfully inserted in 50 of 57 (88%) patients with locally advanced unresectable pancreatic adenocarcinoma into or near the tumor by using a 19-G needle.[19] Fluoroscopy was not used in the study and successful placement was determined by CT. The role of prophylactic antibiotics for this procedure and the impact of EUS-guided fiducial placement on patient survival or quality of life are unclear. EUS-guided fiducial placement was used successfully in two patients with small pancreatic neuroendocrine tumors to aid intraoperative localization and parenchymal-sparing pancreatic surgery.[20]

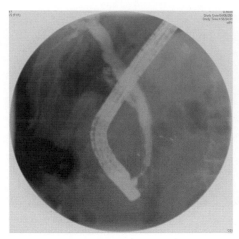

FIGURE 26-6 Multiple fiducials are seen within the tumor mass (with fluoroscopy during endoscopic retrograde cholangiopancreatography) after completion of placement.

Celiac Ganglion Irradiation

EUS-guided direct celiac ganglion irradiation with iodine-125 seeds was applied in 23 patients with unresectable pancreatic carcinoma for the palliation of pain in a recent study.[21] The mean number of seeds implanted in the celiac ganglion per patient was four. Pain relief and analgesic consumption showed no significant changes compared with preoperative values, but six patients (26%) reported pain exacerbation after the procedure. Two weeks later, the VAS score and mean analgesic consumption were significantly less than preoperative values. No procedure-related deaths or major complications were reported.

Other Ablation Methods

The effectiveness and feasibility of EUS-guided laser ablation of the pancreas with an Nd:YAG laser was studied in a porcine model.[22] No technical limitations to the performance of the procedure were noted, and tissue necrosis, localized in the pancreatic parenchyma, was observed in all animals on histologic examination.

Ultrasound-guided microwave and high-frequency ultrasound have also been used to ablate pancreatic tissue. A newly designed high-intensity focused ultrasound (HIFU) transducer that is attached to the EUS scope was developed and successfully targeted.[23] It creates ablation in porcine pancreas and liver.

Endoscopic Ultrasound-Guided Injection Therapies

Fine-Needle Injection of Pancreatic Tumors

EUS-guided ethanol injection has been used in a wide range of studies to ablate pancreatic tissue.[24] In animal studies, the concentration of ethanol injected into the pancreatic parenchyma was associated with a linear dose-response relationship with the amount of tissue ablation. Tissue ablation failed to take place with ethanol injection at concentrations of less than 40%, as well as with saline injection.[25] Another study also

demonstrated that ethanol ablation of pancreatic tissue appears to be remarkably safe and resulted in well-controlled ablation, as evidenced by a decrease in vascular perfusion.[26] It appears that the mechanism of action of ethanol injection therapy is localized tissue ischemia with subsequent necrosis but without widespread pancreatitis. Similar results were achieved with hot saline injection into the pancreas.[27] Injection of different injectable formulated chemotherapeutic agents such as paclitaxel, irinotecan, and 5-fluorouracil into pancreas by EUS FNI have been shown feasible and safe in animal models.[12,28,29] However, no human study has been conducted yet.

EUS-guided ethanol injection therapy has been reported in only a few case studies in patients with a localized malignant tumor (see Table 26-1). EUS-guided ethanol injection was used in a patient with an insulinoma.[30] Although the patient developed abdominal pain requiring hospitalization, there was evidence of successful and durable ablation of the insulinoma. Complete resolution of a pancreatic head insulinoma and all hypoglycemic symptoms was reported in another case.[31] A retrospective study analyzed the results of EUS FNI or intraoperative injection of ethanol in eight patients with pancreas insulinoma.[32] Five of the patients treated with EUS FNI suffered no complications after the procedure. Minor complications (peritumoral bleeding, fluid collection, pancreatitis) were detected in the other three patients treated with intraoperative injection but required no intervention. The treatment was very effective during a median 13-month follow-up period. Five of the patients did not report any hypoglycemia-related symptoms, whereas the other three patients reported only mild symptoms.

Successful ablation of a gastrointestinal stromal cell tumor by EUS-guided transgastric ethanol injection has been reported.[33] Localized ethanol injection was also successful at ablating an adrenal metastasis from lung cancer.[34] A left hepatic metastatic carcinoma located within the hepatic porta was also successfully eradicated with EUS-guided ethanol injection in a patient with pancreatic cancer.[35] Successful EUS-guided alcohol ablation of two metastatic pelvic lymph nodes in a patient with rectal cancer was reported with a local complete resolution and no procedure-related complications.[36] In summary, important advances have been made in applications of EUS-guided ethanol ablation therapy of abdominal malignancies in recent years. However, prospective large trials evaluating the indications and complications are needed before it is recommended for widespread use in clinical practice.

The possibility of providing local control of pancreatic cancer with EUS therapy remains a major challenge. The original report of injection therapy into pancreatic malignancy used a sensitized culture of lymphocytes and established the feasibility and safety of this therapy.[37] In a phase I clinical trial, eight patients with unresectable pancreatic adenocarcinoma underwent EUS-guided FNI of cytoimplants. Escalating doses of cytoimplants (3, 6, or 9 billion cells) were implanted using EUS guidance. The median survival was 13.2 months, with two partial responders and one minor response. Major complications including bone marrow toxicity and hemorrhagic, infectious, renal, or cardiopulmonary toxicity were absent. Low-grade fever was encountered in seven of the eight patients and was symptomatically treated with acetaminophen. Although the study demonstrated the safety of the injection therapy, no large-scale trials have been performed.

The technique of EUS-guided FNI has also been applied to deliver antitumor viral therapy.[38] ONYX-015 (dl1520) is an E1B-55-kDa gene-deleted replication-selective adenovirus that preferentially replicates in malignant cells and causes cell death. Twenty-one patients with locally advanced adenocarcinoma of the pancreas or with metastatic disease, but minimal or absent liver metastases, underwent eight sessions of ONYX-015 delivered by EUS injection into the primary pancreatic tumor over 8 weeks. The final four treatments were given in combination with intravenous gemcitabine (1000 mg/m²). After combination therapy, two patients had partial regressions of the injected tumor, two had minor responses, six had stable disease, and 11 had progressive disease. No clinical pancreatitis occurred despite mild, transient elevations in lipase in a minority of patients. Two patients had sepsis before the institution of prophylactic oral antibiotics. Two patients had duodenal perforations from the rigid endoscope tip. No perforations occurred after the protocol was changed to transgastric injections only. Novel oncolytic viruses have shown promising therapeutic effects for pancreatic cancer in recent experimental studies; however, no trials have been reported with EUS FNI.[39]

Dendritic cells (DCs) are potent antigen-presenting cells that can stimulate T-cell–dependent immune response. They were used in experimental studies as a vaccine therapy against various cancers. In a pilot study, seven patients with advanced pancreatic cancer and refractory to gemcitabine therapy received intratumoral injection of immature DCs by EUS FNI.[40] DCs were administrated on days 1, 8, and 15 of every 28-day cycles as often as possible. All injections were well tolerated without clinical toxicity, but median survival was 9.9 months, similar to previous studies reported for chemotherapy patients. EUS FNI DC therapy combined with gemcitabine in five patients with advanced pancreatic cancer was reported.[41] No serious treatment-related adverse events were observed during the study period, and three of the five patients demonstrated a significant response with a partial response in one patient and long stable disease in two patients. The median survival time was 15.9 months with a promising result. It has been suggested that this combination may have a role in the treatment of pancreatic cancer with a synergistic effect of immunotherapy and chemotherapy.

TNFerade is the newest EUS-guided antitumor therapy that involves a novel gene injection.[42] The attractiveness of this approach is the potential to maximize local antitumor activity and minimize systemic toxicity. TNFerade was constructed as a second-generation (E1-, partial E3-, and E4-deleted) adenovector, expressing the cDNA encoding human tumor necrosis factor (TNF).

In a recent multicenter study, TNFerade was applied to 50 locally advanced pancreatic cancers by EUS (n = 27) or percutaneous injection (n = 23).[43] The study design consisted of a 5-week treatment of weekly intratumoral injections of TNFerade (4 × 10⁹, 4 × 10¹⁰, and 4 × 10¹¹ particle units in 2 mL). TNFerade was combined with continuous intravenous 5-fluorouracil (200 mg/m²/day × 5 days/week) and radiation (50.4 Gy). TNFerade was delivered with a single needle pass at a single site in the tumor for percutaneous approaches (PTAs), whereas up to four injections were given by EUS. The long-term results showed that toxicities potentially related to TNFerade were mild and well tolerated. Compared with two lower-dose cohorts (n = 30), the higher-dose group (n = 11)

was associated with greater locoregional control of treated tumors, longer progression-free survival, a greater proportion of patients with stable or decreasing levels of CA 19-9, a greater percentage (45%) of patients resected, and improved median survival. At the 4 × 10¹¹ dose, four of five patients whose tumors became surgically resectable achieved pathologically negative margins, and three survived more than 24 months. The method of TNFerade biologic administration either by EUS or by the percutaneous route did not influence overall outcome.

The experimental basis of EUS-guided chemotherapy injection into solid pancreatic malignant tumors was based on an investigation using a sustained-released chemotherapy gel.[29] More recently, EUS was used to guide the injection of a temperature-sensitive gel containing paclitaxel (Taxol) into a normal pig pancreas (Figure 26-7). Therapeutic tissue levels of paclitaxel were demonstrated in the pancreatic tissue, as far away as 3 to 5 cm from the site of injection. The diffusion of the paclitaxel into the pancreatic tissue was not associated with evidence of pancreatitis or other toxicities. A similar report demonstrated the safety of EUS-guided injection of a biodegradable polymer containing 5-fluorouracil into the canine pancreas.[12]

Pancreatic Cyst Ablation

EUS-guided pancreatic cyst ablation is based on the principle that injection of a cytotoxic agent into a pancreatic cystic lesion will result in ablation of the cyst epithelium. The close contact between the injected agent and the epithelium results in both immediate and delayed tissue necrosis. The cytotoxic agent remains within the cyst cavity without extravasation into the parenchyma.

Procedural Technique (Video 26-3)

EUS-guided ethanol lavage of pancreatic cystic lesions employs techniques based on FNA of the pancreas. After prophylactic antibiotics are administered, a linear echoendoscope positioned in the duodenum, gastric body, or fundus provides access to pancreatic head, body, or tail, respectively, and guides the use of FNA. The injection of ablative agents into a cystic lesion requires the complete or partial evacuation of the

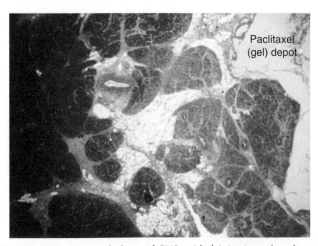

FIGURE 26-7 Histopathology of EUS-guided injection of a chemotherapeutic agent (paclitaxel [Taxol]) into the pancreas.

Video 26-3. Video demonstrating the technique of EUS-guided pancreatic cyst ablation.

fluid contents of the cyst. Although it may be difficult to aspirate the highly viscous fluid of mucinous cysts, it is necessary to provide room for the injected ablative agent. This principle of cyst injection therapy, coupled with a dead space of approximately 0.8 mL in the aspiration needle, limits target cysts to more than 10 mm in diameter. Once the needle is in place within the lumen of the cyst, the ablative agent is injected under ultrasound monitoring. Swirls of aerated liquid are readily observed with ultrasound, and the distribution can be easily determined during the procedure. In many cases, ablative therapy is provided with a lavage of the liquid, such as ethanol, in and out of the cyst over several minutes. Unilocular cysts with a diameter of 1 to 2 cm are easily treated in one or two sessions. Larger and more complex lesions require multiple lavage sessions.[44] The end point of ethanol lavage is elimination of the cyst as evidenced by cross-sectional imaging.

Clinical Outcomes

EUS-guided ethanol injection into pancreatic cystic lesions was originally described using a range of low ethanol concentrations[45] (Table 26-2). In the initial studies, the safety of cyst injection therapy was established first using saline solution, followed by highly dilute ethanol. There was no evidence of clinical pancreatitis with injection of ethanol using concentrations up to 80%. Small numbers of lavaged cystic lesions were resected, and evidence of epithelial ablation with pancreatitis was noted.[45] In a randomized, prospective, multicenter trial, ethanol lavage was found to provide greater rates of complete ablation as compared with saline lavage.[46] The overall CT-defined rate of complete pancreatic cyst ablation was 33.3%. The histology of four resected cysts demonstrated

epithelial ablation ranging from 0% (saline solution alone) to 50% to 100% (one or two ethanol lavages). Although one patient developed transient pancreatitis, approximately 20% of patients from both groups (ethanol and saline) experienced some abdominal pain the day after lavage. Twelve patients with pancreatic cysts that had previously resolved after ethanol lavage were followed up to determine long-term results. The median follow-up was 26 months (range 13 to 39) after initial resolution, and no evidence of cyst recurrence was shown in any patient.[47] Ethanol lavage has been coupled with paclitaxel injection in a large series with a variety of pancreatic cystic lesions.[48] The combination of ethanol and paclitaxel injection resulted in elimination of the cysts, as determined by CT scanning, in 29 of 47 (62%) of patients, in a median follow-up period of 21.7 months (Figure 26-8). On univariate analysis, EUS diameter and original cyst volume predicted resolution. However, the high viscosity of paclitaxel made injection into the cyst difficult. In contrast, ethanol is easily injected and aspirated from the cyst and at times reduces the cyst fluid viscosity, thus aiding in cyst evacuation. The combination of ethanol and paclitaxel is also capable of ablating septated cystic lesions, a much more difficult target for EUS injection therapy.[49] Presumably, the surface area of a septated cyst is quite large, and it is difficult to be certain that the cytotoxic injectant comes in contact with all of the epithelium. Besides all these preliminary studies, the long-term effect of ethanol injection is not yet clear. Thus, it should be used with caution in routine practice. The indication should be limited to selected patients such as those at high risk for surgery.

Celiac Plexus Injections

The principle of celiac injection therapy is based on the ability of EUS to guide injection of cytotoxic agents into the retrogastric space containing the celiac ganglia (Figure 26-9). Presumably, the injected agent, such as ethanol, comes into contact with the ganglia and disrupts the ascending sympathetic ganglia. Histologically, there is evidence of neuronal vacuolization in nerves injected with ethanol.[50] Because the efferent nerves from the pancreas travel with the sympathetic chain, interruption of the celiac ganglia should result in a decreased sense of pain within the pancreas. In the setting of pancreatic cancer, there is evidence of sensory nerve hyperplasia, and this may be the basis for the often observed chronic abdominal pain.

TABLE 26-2				
EUS-GUIDED ABLATION OF PANCREATIC CYSTIC LESIONS				
Authors (year)	**Agent**	**Target**	**Results**	**Complications**
Gan et al[45] (2005)	5%–80% ethanol (diluted with saline)	Pancreatic cystic lesions (EUS guidance)	Resolution of cystic lesion in 8 of 23 patients; resected patients had ablated epithelium	None
Oh et al[48] (2011)	80%–90% ethanol paclitaxel	Pancreatic cystic lesions (EUS guidance)	Resolution of cystic lesion in 29 of 52 patients	Mild pancreatitis and splenic vein obliteration, each occurred in one patient
DeWitt et al[46] (2009)	80% ethanol compared with saline	Pancreatic cystic lesions (EUS guidance)	Resolution of cystic lesion in 12 of 36 patients	Abdominal pain; rare pancreatitis
Oh et al[49] (2009)	80%–90% ethanol paclitaxel	Septated pancreatic cystic lesions	Resolution in 6 of 10 patients	Episode of mild pancreatitis in one patient

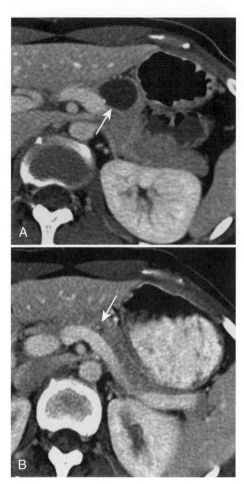

FIGURE 26-8   Pancreatic cyst lavage. Computed tomography scanning before (**A**) and after (**B**) ethanol paclitaxel (Taxol) lavage of a pancreatic cyst *(arrows)*.

Video 26-4. Video demonstrating the technique of EUS-guided celiac plexus neurolysis.

Procedural Technique (Video 26-4)

The technique for EUS-guided celiac plexus neurolysis and block is identical; the only difference is in the substances injected. With a curvilinear array echoendoscope, the region of the celiac plexus is visualized from the lesser curve of the stomach by following the aorta to the origin of the main celiac artery and is traced, using counterclockwise rotation, to its bifurcation into splenic and hepatic arteries, with Doppler control if needed (Figure 26-10). With careful inspection, it is often possible, by using slight rotational movements, even to visualize the celiac ganglia directly (Figure 26-11).

A 22- or 19-G EUS FNA needle is usually used, but in some countries a dedicated 20-G spray needle with multiple side holes is available and allows solutions to spread over a greater area. The needle tip is placed slightly anterior and cephalad to the origin of the celiac artery or directly into the ganglia if these can be identified as discrete structures. Aspiration is first performed to ensure that vascular puncture has not occurred. Bupivacaine is injected first, followed by alcohol (or triamcinolone for block). One of two strategies can be used: injection of the entire solution into the area cephalad of the celiac trunk or injection into the right and left sides of the celiac artery. Patients should be observed for 2 to 4 hours with careful monitoring of pulse, blood pressure, temperature, and pain scores.

Clinical Outcomes

EUS injection therapy has been used clinically since the early 2000s in patients with pain associated with pancreatic diseases. Traditionally, EUS injection therapy was based on

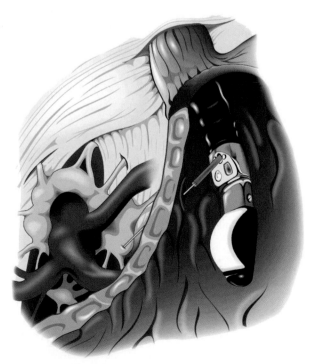

FIGURE 26-9   Illustration of an EUS-guided celiac ganglia injection.

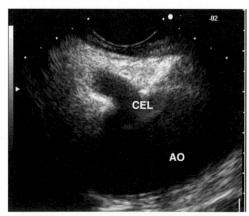

FIGURE 26-10   Celiac plexus neurolysis being undertaken at the space around the celiac artery (CEL). Note the needle at the base of the celiac artery. AO, aorta.

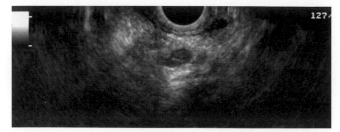

FIGURE 26-11 EUS imaging of a focal round, hypoechoic celiac ganglion.

ethanol-induced celiac ganglion neurolysis for pain relief in pancreatic cancer.[51] The original prospective trial demonstrated a significant reduction in pain scores 2 weeks after EUS celiac plexus injection, an effect that was sustained for 24 weeks when adjusted for morphine use and adjuvant therapy[52] (Table 26-3). Forty-five of the 58 patients (78%) experienced a decline in pain scores after EUS-guided celiac plexus neurolysis. The use of chemotherapy and radiation therapy also aided in the reduction in pain. A meta-analysis of the literature reported that EUS-guided celiac plexus neurolysis was 72.54% effective in managing pain resulting from pancreatic cancer and is a reasonable option for patients with tolerance to narcotic analgesics.[56]

A large retrospective study demonstrated that bilateral celiac neurolysis injection was more effective than central injection in terms of pain reduction.[57] More than 70.4% of patients reported a decrease in pain levels at 7 days, compared with 45.9% of patients receiving a single injection. The most common complication of celiac plexus neurolysis was postprocedural hypotension, at a rate of 3.2%.[58] Occasionally, patients complain of severe abdominal pain after ganglion injection, and the pain may persist.[58] The most serious complication was a single episode of injury to the adrenal artery.

Injection therapy in patients with pain associated with chronic pancreatitis has not been as successful as reported in pain control of pancreatic cancer.[59] The overall rate of response has been approximately 50%, and responses have been transient.[53] Ganglion blockade using local anesthetics rather than permanent chemical neurolysis has generally been the approach in pain control in chronic pancreatitis. LeBlanc and colleagues, in a prospective trial, determined that the average duration of effect of a ganglion block was 1 month, and one injection of bupivacaine and triamcinolone produced the same effect as two injections.[60] Many investigators believe that short-term relief of pain may not be a clinically important effect in the long-term care of patients with chronic pancreatitis.

Developments have focused on the ability of EUS to target celiac ganglia specifically with needle injection therapy.[56] In a retrospective study, 33 patients underwent 36 direct celiac ganglia injections for unresectable pancreatic cancer ($n = 17$) or chronic pancreatitis ($n = 13$) with bupivacaine (0.25%) and alcohol (99%) for neurolysis or methylprednisolone (Depo-Medrol, 80 mg/2 mL) for nerve blockade. Nearly all patients with cancer (94%) reported pain relief. In contrast, patients with chronic pancreatitis experienced lower response rates (80% response rate with alcohol injection and 38% response rate with steroids). Recently, direct celiac ganglia neurolysis after EUS visualization was reported in a large series with pancreatic cancer.[54] Of the 64 patients enrolled in the study, 40 patients (62.5%) with visible celiac ganglia (range 1 to 4) underwent EUS celiac plexus neurolysis with 98% alcohol injection. The 24 patients with unidentified ganglia underwent bilateral injections at the celiac vessel trunk. The response rate, which was defined as at least a two point drop in pain as measured by the visual analog scale in the first week, was 65% in the direct injection group and only 25% in the unidentified group. This yielded a fivefold higher chance of response for those patients with visible ganglia compared with those without and multivariate model showed that visualization of the ganglia was the best predictor of response. This study clearly showed the superiority of targeting celiac ganglia during EUS-guided injection in pancreatic pain control.

In a large, prospective randomized trial, celiac neurolysis provided significant improvement (40% of patients) in severe abdominal pain (for 6 weeks) associated with pancreatic cancer, as compared with a response rate of 14% of patients taking opioids.[61] The effect of early EUS celiac neurolysis was investigated in 96 patients with newly diagnosed, painful, inoperable pancreatic cancer in a randomized, double-blind, controlled trial.[55] Pain relief was greater in the EUS-treated group at 1 month and significantly greater at 3 months. Morphine consumption tended to be lower at 3 months in the neurolysis group. However, there was no difference on quality of life and survival between the groups. Similar to this study, the large trials have failed to demonstrate a significant improvement in quality of life and survival in patients with pancreatic cancer, despite the high rates of response to injection therapy.

TABLE 26-3

PUBLISHED CLINICAL TRIALS OF EUS-GUIDED CELIAC INJECTION THERAPY

Authors (yr)	Patients (n)	Clinical Condition	Neurolysis or Block	Pain Score Change	Major Complications
Gunaratnam et al[52] (2001)	58	Pancreatic cancer	Neurolysis	78% improved	None
Ascunce et al[53] (2011)	64	Pancreatic cancer	Neurolysis	50% improved at first week	None
Wyse et al[54] (2011)	49	Pancreatic cancer	Neurolysis	Significant decrease in mean pain score	None
Levy et al[55] (2008)	33	Pancreatic cancer and chronic pancreatitis	Block and neurolysis	94% improved (cancer); 50% improved (chronic pancreatitis)	None

Summary

EUS-guided injection therapy is based on the accurate placement of ablative agents into various gastrointestinal tissues, including celiac ganglia. Effective tissue ablation has been achieved in the pancreas, pancreatic cystic lesions, and ganglia. Excellent rates of pain control have been observed in patients with pancreatic cancer who were undergoing EUS-guided celiac neurolysis. In the future, local control of malignant tumors will be aided by injection therapy.

REFERENCES

1. Yusuf TE, Tsutaki S, Wagh MS, et al. The EUS hardware store: state of the art technical review of instruments and equipment (with videos). *Gastrointest Endosc.* 2007;66:131-143.
2. Goldberg SN, Mallery S, Gazelle GS, Brugge WR. EUS-guided radiofrequency ablation in the pancreas: results in a porcine model. *Gastrointest Endosc.* 1999;50:392-401.
3. Kim HJ, Seo DW, Hassanuddin A, et al. EUS-guided radiofrequency ablation of the porcine pancreas. *Gastrointest Endosc.* 2012;76:1039-1043.
4. Gaidhane M, Smith I, Ellen K, et al. Endoscopic ultrasound-guided radiofrequency ablation (EUS-RFA) of the pancreas in a porcine model. *Gastroenterol Res Pract.* 2012;2012:431451.
5. Pai M, Yang J, Zhang X, et al. PWE-055 endoscopic ultrasound guided radiofrequency ablation (EUS-RFA) for pancreatic ductal adenocarcinoma. *Gut.* 2013;62:A153.
6. Pai M, Senturk H, Lakhtakia S, et al. 351 endoscopic ultrasound guided radiofrequency ablation (EUS-RFA) for cystic neoplasms and neuroendocrine tumors of the pancreas. *Gastrointest Endosc.* 2013;77:AB143-AB144.
7. Carrara S, Arcidiacono PG, Albarello L, et al. Endoscopic ultrasound-guided application of a new hybrid cryotherm probe in porcine pancreas: a preliminary study. *Endoscopy.* 2008;40:321-326.
8. Carrara S, Arcidiacono PG, Albarello L, et al. Endoscopic ultrasound-guided application of a new internally gas-cooled radiofrequency ablation probe in the liver and spleen of an animal model: a preliminary study. *Endoscopy.* 2008;40:759-763.
9. Arcidiacono PG, Carrara S, Reni M, et al. Feasibility and safety of EUS-guided cryothermal ablation in patients with locally advanced pancreatic cancer. *Gastrointest Endosc.* 2012;76:1142-1151.
10. Skandarajah AR, Lynch AC, Mackay JR, et al. The role of intraoperative radiotherapy in solid tumors. *Ann Surg Oncol.* 2009;16:735-744.
11. Calvo FA, Meirino RM, Orecchia R. Intraoperative radiation therapy part 2. Clinical results. *Crit Rev Oncol Hematol.* 2006;59:116-127.
12. Sun S, Wang S, Ge N, et al. Endoscopic ultrasound-guided interstitial chemotherapy in the pancreas: results in a canine model. *Endoscopy.* 2007;39:530-534.
13. Sun S, Xu H, Xin J, et al. Endoscopic ultrasound-guided interstitial brachytherapy of unresectable pancreatic cancer: results of a pilot trial. *Endoscopy.* 2006;38:399-403.
14. Jin Z, Du Y, Li Z, et al. Endoscopic ultrasonography-guided interstitial implantation of iodine 125-seeds combined with chemotherapy in the treatment of unresectable pancreatic carcinoma: a prospective pilot study. *Endoscopy.* 2008;40:314-320.
15. Jin Z, Du Y, Li Z. Su1575 long-term effect of gemcitabine-combined endoscopic ultrasonography-guided brachytherapy in pancreatic cancer. *Gastrointest Endosc.* 2013;77:AB373.
16. Pishvaian AC, Collins B, Gagnon G, et al. EUS-guided fiducial placement for CyberKnife radiotherapy of mediastinal and abdominal malignancies. *Gastrointest Endosc.* 2006;64:412-417.
17. Yang J, Abdel-Wahab M, Ribeiro A. EUS-guided fiducial placement after radical prostatectomy before targeted radiation therapy for prostate cancer recurrence. *Gastrointest Endosc.* 2011;73:1302-1305.
18. Draganov PV, Chavalitdhamrong D, Wagh MS. Evaluation of a new endoscopic ultrasound-guided multi-fiducial delivery system: a prospective non-survival study in a live porcine model. *Dig Endosc.* 2013.
19. Park WG, Yan BM, Schellenberg D, et al. EUS-guided gold fiducial insertion for image-guided radiation therapy of pancreatic cancer: 50 successful cases without fluoroscopy. *Gastrointest Endosc.* 2010;71:513-518.
20. Law JK, Singh VK, Khashab MA, et al. Endoscopic ultrasound (EUS)-guided fiducial placement allows localization of small neuroendocrine tumors during parenchymal-sparing pancreatic surgery. *Surg Endosc.* 2013;27:3921-3926.
21. Wang KX, Jin ZD, Du YQ, et al. EUS-guided celiac ganglion irradiation with iodine-125 seeds for pain control in pancreatic carcinoma: a prospective pilot study. *Gastrointest Endosc.* 2012;76:945-952.
22. Di Matteo F, Martino M, Rea R, et al. EUS-guided Nd:YAG laser ablation of normal pancreatic tissue: a pilot study in a pig model. *Gastrointest Endosc.* 2010;72:358-363.
23. Hwang JH, Farr N, Morrison K, et al. 876 development of an EUS-guided high-intensity focused ultrasound endoscope. *Gastrointest Endosc.* 2011;73:AB155.
24. Aslanian H, Salem RR, Marginean C, et al. EUS-guided ethanol injection of normal porcine pancreas: a pilot study. *Gastrointest Endosc.* 2005;62:723-727.
25. Matthes K, Mino-Kenudson M, Sahani DV, et al. Concentration-dependent ablation of pancreatic tissue by EUS-guided ethanol injection. *Gastrointest Endosc.* 2007;65:272-277.
26. Giday SA, Magno P, Gabrielson KL, et al. The utility of contrast-enhanced endoscopic ultrasound in monitoring ethanol-induced pancreatic tissue ablation: a pilot study in a porcine model. *Endoscopy.* 2007;39:525-529.
27. Imazu H, Sumiyama K, Ikeda K, et al. A pilot study of EUS-guided hot saline injection for induction of pancreatic tissue necrosis. *Endoscopy.* 2009;41:598-602.
28. Karaca C, Cizginer S, Konuk Y, et al. Feasibility of EUS-guided injection of irinotecan-loaded microspheres into the swine pancreas. *Gastrointest Endosc.* 2011;73:603-606.
29. Matthes K, Mino-Kenudson M, Sahani DV, et al. EUS-guided injection of paclitaxel (OncoGel) provides therapeutic drug concentrations in the porcine pancreas (with video). *Gastrointest Endosc.* 2007;65:448-453.
30. Jurgensen C, Schuppan D, Neser F, et al. EUS-guided alcohol ablation of an insulinoma. *Gastrointest Endosc.* 2006;63:1059-1062.
31. Deprez PH, Claessens A, Borbath I, et al. Successful endoscopic ultrasound-guided ethanol ablation of a sporadic insulinoma. *Acta Gastroenterol Belg.* 2008;71:333-337.
32. Levy MJ, Thompson GB, Topazian MD, et al. EUS-guided ethanol ablation of insulinomas: a new treatment option. *Gastrointest Endosc.* 2012;75:200-206.
33. Gunter E, Lingenfelser T, Eitelbach F, et al. EUS-guided ethanol injection for treatment of a GI stromal tumor. *Gastrointest Endosc.* 2003;57:113-115.
34. Artifon EL, Lucon AM, Sakai P, et al. EUS-guided alcohol ablation of left adrenal metastasis from non–small-cell lung carcinoma. *Gastrointest Endosc.* 2007;66:1201-1205.
35. Hu YH, Tuo XP, Jin ZD, et al. Endoscopic ultrasound (EUS)-guided ethanol injection in hepatic metastatic carcinoma: a case report. *Endoscopy.* 2010;42(suppl 2):E256-E257.
36. DeWitt J, Mohamadnejad M. EUS-guided alcohol ablation of metastatic pelvic lymph nodes after endoscopic resection of polypoid rectal cancer: the need for long-term surveillance. *Gastrointest Endosc.* 2011;74:446-447.
37. Chang KJ, Nguyen PT, Thompson JA, et al. Phase I clinical trial of allogeneic mixed lymphocyte culture (cytoimplant) delivered by endoscopic ultrasound-guided fine-needle injection in patients with advanced pancreatic carcinoma. *Cancer.* 2000;88:1325-1335.
38. Hecht JR, Bedford R, Abbruzzese JL, et al. A phase I/II trial of intratumoral endoscopic ultrasound injection of ONYX-015 with intravenous gemcitabine in unresectable pancreatic carcinoma. *Clin Cancer Res.* 2003;9:555-561.
39. Xu C, Li H, Su C, Li Z. Viral therapy for pancreatic cancer: tackle the bad guys with poison. *Cancer Lett.* 2013;333:1-8.
40. Irisawa A, Takagi T, Kanazawa M, et al. Endoscopic ultrasound-guided fine-needle injection of immature dendritic cells into advanced pancreatic cancer refractory to gemcitabine: a pilot study. *Pancreas.* 2007;35:189-190.
41. Hirooka Y, Itoh A, Kawashima H, et al. A combination therapy of gemcitabine with immunotherapy for patients with inoperable locally advanced pancreatic cancer. *Pancreas.* 2009;38:e69-e74.
42. Chang KJ, Lee JG, Holcombe RF, et al. Endoscopic ultrasound delivery of an antitumor agent to treat a case of pancreatic cancer. *Nat Clin Pract Gastroenterol Hepatol.* 2008;5:107-111.
43. Hecht JR, Farrell JJ, Senzer N, et al. EUS or percutaneously guided intratumoral TNFerade biologic with 5-fluorouracil and radiotherapy for first-line treatment of locally advanced pancreatic cancer: a phase I/II study. *Gastrointest Endosc.* 2012;75:332-338.

44. DiMaio CJ, DeWitt JM, Brugge WR. Ablation of pancreatic cystic lesions: the use of multiple endoscopic ultrasound-guided ethanol lavage sessions. *Pancreas*. 2011;40:664-668.
45. Gan SI, Thompson CC, Lauwers GY, et al. Ethanol lavage of pancreatic cystic lesions: initial pilot study. *Gastrointest Endosc*. 2005;61:746-752.
46. DeWitt J, McGreevy K, Schmidt CM, Brugge WR. EUS-guided ethanol versus saline solution lavage for pancreatic cysts: a randomized, double-blind study. *Gastrointest Endosc*. 2009;70:710-723.
47. DeWitt J, DiMaio CJ, Brugge WR. Long-term follow-up of pancreatic cysts that resolve radiologically after EUS-guided ethanol ablation. *Gastrointest Endosc*. 2010;72:862-866.
48. Oh HC, Seo DW, Song TJ, et al. Endoscopic ultrasonography-guided ethanol lavage with paclitaxel injection treats patients with pancreatic cysts. *Gastroenterology*. 2011;140:172-179.
49. Oh HC, Seo DW, Kim SC, et al. Septated cystic tumors of the pancreas: is it possible to treat them by endoscopic ultrasonography-guided intervention? *Scand J Gastroenterol*. 2009;44:242-247.
50. Vranken JH, Zuurmond WW, Van Kemenade FJ, Dzoljic M. Neurohistopathologic findings after a neurolytic celiac plexus block with alcohol in patients with pancreatic cancer pain. *Acta Anaesthesiol Scand*. 2002;46:827-830.
51. Wiersema MJ, Wiersema LM. Endosonography-guided celiac plexus neurolysis. *Gastrointest Endosc*. 1996;44:656-662.
52. Gunaratnam NT, Sarma AV, Norton ID, Wiersema MJ. A prospective study of EUS-guided celiac plexus neurolysis for pancreatic cancer pain. *Gastrointest Endosc*. 2001;54:316-324.
53. Ascunce G, Ribeiro A, Reis I, et al. EUS visualization and direct celiac ganglia neurolysis predicts better pain relief in patients with pancreatic malignancy (with video). *Gastrointest Endosc*. 2011;73:267-274.
54. Wyse JM, Carone M, Paquin SC, et al. Randomized, double-blind, controlled trial of early endoscopic ultrasound-guided celiac plexus neurolysis to prevent pain progression in patients with newly diagnosed, painful, inoperable pancreatic cancer. *J Clin Oncol*. 2011;29:3541-3546.
55. Levy MJ, Topazian MD, Wiersema MJ, et al. Initial evaluation of the efficacy and safety of endoscopic ultrasound-guided direct ganglia neurolysis and block. *Am J Gastroenterol*. 2008;103:98-103.
56. Kaufman M, Singh G, Das S, et al. Efficacy of endoscopic ultrasound-guided celiac plexus block and celiac plexus neurolysis for managing abdominal pain associated with chronic pancreatitis and pancreatic cancer. *J Clin Gastroenterol*. 2010;44:127-134.
57. Sahai AV, Lemelin V, Lam E, Paquin SC. Central versus bilateral endoscopic ultrasound-guided celiac plexus block or neurolysis: a comparative study of short-term effectiveness. *Am J Gastroenterol*. 2009;104:326-329.
58. O'Toole TM, Schmulewitz N. Complication rates of EUS-guided celiac plexus blockade and neurolysis: results of a large case series. *Endoscopy*. 2009;41:593-597.
59. Puli SR, Reddy JB, Bechtold ML, et al. EUS-guided celiac plexus neurolysis for pain due to chronic pancreatitis or pancreatic cancer pain: a meta-analysis and systematic review. *Dig Dis Sci*. 2009;54:2330-2337.
60. LeBlanc JK, DeWitt J, Johnson C, et al. A prospective randomized trial of 1 versus 2 injections during EUS-guided celiac plexus block for chronic pancreatitis pain. *Gastrointest Endosc*. 2009;69:835-842.
61. Wong GY, Schroeder DR, Carns PE, et al. Effect of neurolytic celiac plexus block on pain relief, quality of life, and survival in patients with unresectable pancreatic cancer: a randomized controlled trial. *JAMA*. 2004;291:1092-1099.

27

EUS-Guided Drainage of Gallbladder, Pelvic Abscess, and Other Therapeutic Interventions

Takao Itoi • Shyam Varadarajulu

Key Points

- EUS facilitates transmural drainage of the gallbladder in symptomatic patients who are at high risk for cholecystectomy and in patients with pelvic fluid collections that are adjacent to the rectum or colonic lumen and within the reach of an echoendoscope.
- The presence of a fluoroscopy unit, therapeutic echoendoscope, accessories such as 19-G needles, ERCP cannula or needle-knife catheters, 0.035-inch guidewires, balloon dilators, dedicated or self-expandable metal stents, double-pigtail plastic stents, and biliary drainage catheters are essential for the procedures.
- Both EUS-guided gallbladder and pelvic abscess drainage are safe procedures with a treatment success rate greater than 90%. Reported complications are mild and can be managed conservatively in most patients.
- EUS-guided hemostasis in gastric varices can be attained with coil embolization and glue injection. While experience is limited, the preliminary data appear promising.
- EUS-guided fiducial placement facilitates better targeting of tumors by radiation therapy and enables intraoperative localization of small pancreatic tumors that can be enucleated without the need for large resection procedures.
- The majority of patients can be discharged home within 2 to 3 days following EUS-guided interventions with optimal clinical outcomes.

The use of the linear array echoendoscope has expanded the realm of therapeutic interventions to include drainage of obstructive biliary ductal system/gallbladder, peripancreatic fluid collections and pelvic abscesses, placement of coils or injection of sclerotic agents in varices, and implantation of chemotherapeutic agents or fiducials in tumors. In this chapter, the technique and outcomes of EUS-guided drainage of gallbladder and pelvic abscesses, its role in the obliteration of gastric varices, and placement of fiducials to facilitate intraoperative tumor localization are reviewed.

EUS-Guided Gallbladder Drainage

Optimal treatment for acute cholecystitis is elective or emergent cholecystectomy.[1] However, percutaneous transhepatic gallbladder drainage (PTGBD) is considered a safe alternative to cholecystectomy, particularly in surgically high-risk patients.[2] Endoscopic nasogallbladder drainage and gallbladder stenting via the transpapillary approach are other alternative methods for the minimally invasive management of acute cholecystitis.[2,3] Recently, there have been several reports of the

successful drainage of gallbladder in high-risk patients under endosonographic guidance.[4,5]

Procedural Technique

Endoscopic ultrasonography-guided gallbladder drainage (EUS GBD) is classified into two types: EUS-guided nasogallbladder drainage (EUS NGD) and EUS-guided gallbladder stenting (EUS GBS).

To access the gallbladder in patients with an intact anatomy, the tip of the curved linear array echoendoscope is usually positioned in the duodenal bulb or the antrum of the stomach in a long-scope position. In contrast, in patients with Billroth I gastrectomy, the gallbladder is identified in a short-scope position from the second portion of the duodenum.

The following procedural steps are then undertaken in sequence (Video 27-1):

1. A 19-G needle is inserted transduodenally or transgastrically into the gallbladder under EUS visualization (Figure 27-1A).

Video 27-1. Video demonstrating the technique of EUS-guided gallbladder drainage.

2. After the stylet is removed, a small amount of bile is aspirated to confirm puncture of the gallbladder. If the gallbladder is not distended, a minimal amount of contrast medium or normal saline may be injected into the gallbladder lumen to induce distension that is critical for performing endotherapy and is otherwise not possible if the gallbladder is contracted.
3. A 450-cm-long, 0.035-inch guidewire is then inserted via the outer sheath of the needle into the gallbladder lumen (Figure 27-1B).
4. The needle tract is then dilated using an over-the-wire electrocautery catheter, an 8-Fr biliary balloon dilator or by passage of 4- to 6-mm papillary balloon dilators.

5. Following dilation, a 5- to 8.5-Fr single-pigtail NGG drainage catheter, 7- to 10-Fr double-pigtail-type plastic stent or a self-expandable metal stent may be deployed into the gallbladder lumen via the stomach or duodenum (Figure 27-1C).

Recently, a dedicated metal stent has been developed for EUS GBS.[4,5] The lumen-apposing stent (AXIOS, Xlumena Inc., Mountain View, California, USA) is fully covered with bilateral anchoring flanges (Figure 27-1D). When fully expanded, the diameter of the flange is approximately twice that of the "saddle." The stent anchors are designed to distribute pressure evenly on the luminal wall and securely anchor the stent thereby preventing migration. The proximal and distal anchor flanges are designed to hold the gallbladder lumen and the stomach or duodenal wall in apposition, thereby preventing leakage between the two nonadherent organs.

Technical and Treatment Outcomes

The first report of EUS-guided gallbladder drainage was published in 2007 by Baron and colleagues, who successfully placed a plastic stent in one patient with no observed complications.[6] Since then, 10 reports have described the

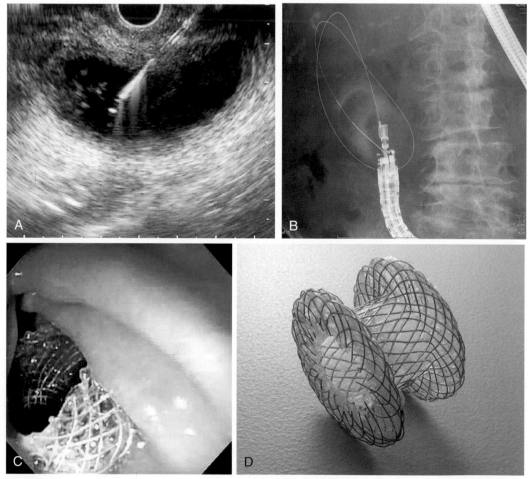

FIGURE 27-1   A, The gallbladder is punctured using a 19-G needle under EUS guidance. B, A 0.035-inch guidewire is coiled within the lumen of the gallbladder. C, Following transmural dilation, a fully covered self-expandable metal stent is deployed for gallbladder drainage. D, A prototype fully covered lumen-apposing stent specially designed for EUS-guided drainage procedures.

TABLE 27-1

PUBLISHED CASE SERIES OF EUS-GUIDED GALLBLADDER DRAINAGE

Author (year)	Number of patients	EUS NGD/ GBS	Approach Route	Technical Success (%)	Treatment Success (%)	Complication (n)
Jang et al[4] (2011)	15	FCSEMS	10TG/5TD	100	100	Pneumoperitoneum (2)
Itoi et al[5] (2012)	5	FCSEMS	1TG/4TD	100	100	None
Baron and Topazian[6] (2007)	1	PS (7F)	TD	100	100	None
Kwan et al[7] (2007)	3	3NGD (5F) (+1PS(8.5F)	1TG/2TD	100	100	Bile leak (1)
Lee et al[8] (2007)	9	NGD (5F)	4TG/5TD	100	100	Pneumoperitoneum (1)
Takasawa et al[9] (2009)	1	PS (7.2F)	TG	100	100	None
Kamata et al[10] (2009)	1	PS (7F)	TG	100	100	None
Song et al[11] (2010)	8	PS (7F)	1TG/7TD	100	100	Bile peritonitis (1), stent migration (1) pneumoperitoneum (1)
Itoi et al[12] (2011)	2	PS (7F)	1TG/1TD	100	100	Bile peritonitis (1)
Jang et al[13] (2012)	30	NGD (5F)	NA	97	100	Pneumoperitoneum (2)
de la Serna-Higuera et al[14] (2013)	13	FCSEMS	12TG/1TD	85	100	Hematoma (1), abdominal pain (1)

EUS, endoscopic ultrasonography; FCSEMS, fully covered self-expandable metal stent; GBS, gallbladder stenting; NA, not available; NGD, nasogallbladder drainage; PS, plastic stent; TD, transduodenal; TD, transduodenal approach; TG, transgastric; TG, transgastric approach.

usefulness of EUS-guided gallbladder drainage in 88 patients[4-14] (Table 27-1) with an overall technical and clinical success rate of 97% and 100% (intention-to-treat analysis, 97%), respectively. Various plastic stents (7 Fr to 8.5 Fr), NGB drainage catheters, and dedicated or fully covered self-expandable metal stents have been used for performing EUS GBD.

Procedure-related complications were encountered in 12 (13.6%) cases of which none were major. Six of twelve complications were self-limited pneumoperitoneum and three were related to bile leak. Relapse of acute cholecystitis due to stent occlusion and inadvertent nasogallbladder catheter removal have been reported as late complications. Although follow-up duration in most series was variable, durable symptom relief was apparent for even up to 9 months in some series.[5]

Comparative outcome data between EUS-guided gallbladder drainage and PTGBD are scant.[13] In a randomized trial that compared EUS GBD and PTGBD, whereas there was no difference in technical feasibility, efficacy, and safety, the postprocedure pain was significantly less in patients undergoing EUS GBD.[13] Also, in the opinion of these authors, relapse of cholecystitis is commonly encountered once the PTGBD catheters are removed, thereby necessitating reinterventions in many patients. On the other hand, due to the presence of an internal conduit that facilitates continuous drainage, EUS GBD procedures are associated with a lower risk of cholecystitis relapse and therefore the need for fewer reinterventions.

Technical Limitations

Some limitations of EUS-guided gallbladder drainage include the following: (1) If the gallbladder wall is thickened and its lumen is not distended, EUS-guided drainage may not be possible due to difficulty with passage of endoscopic accessories; and (2) transmural stenting may not be possible if the

gallbladder is located more than 2 cm further from the gastrointestinal lumen.

EUS-Guided Pelvic Abscess Drainage

Pelvic abscesses can occur after surgery or in patients with medical conditions such as Crohn's disease, diverticulitis, ischemic colitis, sexually transmitted diseases, or septic emboli from endocarditis. Management of a pelvic abscess can be technically challenging because of the need for navigation around the bony pelvis, bowel loops, bladder, reproductive organs in females, prostate in men, rectum, and other neurovascular structures. Historically, these collections necessitated surgery, ultrasound-guided transrectal, or transvaginal intervention, or were drained percutaneously under computed tomography (CT) guidance. Recent advances in the field of interventional EUS have opened a new avenue for management of pelvic abscesses.[15]

Procedural Technique

All patients should undergo a dedicated CT or MRI of the pelvis to define the anatomy and location of the abscess. Abscesses that are multiloculated, measure smaller than 4 cm in size, have immature walls (without a definitive rim), and are located at the level of the dentate line or greater than 2 cm from the EUS transducer should be managed by alternative techniques. It is recommended that patients be administered prophylactic antibiotics prior to the procedure. Patients should undergo local preparation with an enema to assist with optimal visualization and minimize contamination. Laboratory parameters must be checked to ensure that patients are not coagulopathic or thrombocytopenic. It is essential that the procedure take place in a unit equipped with fluoroscopy to guide stent and drain placements within the abscess cavity.

Video 27-2. Video demonstrating the technique for EUS-guided drainage of pelvic abscess.

Also, patients should either void prior to the procedure or have an indwelling Foley catheter to ensure that a distended bladder does not impair visualization of a small fluid collection or that it is not mistaken for an abscess.

The following procedural steps are undertaken in sequence (Video 27-2):

1. First, the abscess must be located using a curved linear array echoendoscope. Once located, intervening vasculature must then be excluded using color Doppler. Under EUS guidance, a 19-G FNA needle is used to puncture the abscess cavity (Figure 27-2A). The stylet is removed and the needle is flushed with saline and aspirated to evacuate as much pus as possible. A sample of purulent material may be sent for gram staining and culture.

2. A standard 0.035-inch guidewire or a stiff-type 0.025-inch guidewire is then passed through the needle and coiled within the abscess cavity (Figure 27-2B). The needle is exchanged over the guidewire for a 5-Fr endoscopic retrograde cholangiopancreatography (ERCP) cannula or a needle-knife catheter to dilate the tract between the rectum and the abscess cavity (Figure 27-2C). The tract is further dilated using an 8-mm over-the-wire biliary balloon dilator (Figure 27-2D).

3. Once the tract is dilated, one or two 7-Fr 4-cm double-pigtail transmural stents are deployed (Figure 27-2E). The decision to place one or more stents is based on the viscosity of the abscess contents: one if the fluid flowed smoothly and more if the contents were thicker.

4. In patients with abscesses that measure 8 cm or more in size and in those abscesses that do not drain well despite placement of transmural stents, an additional transluminal drainage catheter is deployed (Figure 27-2F). The abscess cavity is accessed with a 5-Fr ERCP cannula to pass another 0.035-inch or 0.025-inch guidewire. A 10-Fr, 80-cm single-pigtail drain is deployed over the guidewire. This drain will exit the anus and remain secured to the patient's gluteal region using tape. This drain is then flushed with 30 to 50 mL of normal saline every 4 hours until the aspirate is clear.

5. Follow-up CT should be obtained at 36 to 48 hours to ensure the fluid collection has decreased in size (Figure 27-3). If the size of the abscess cavity is reduced more than

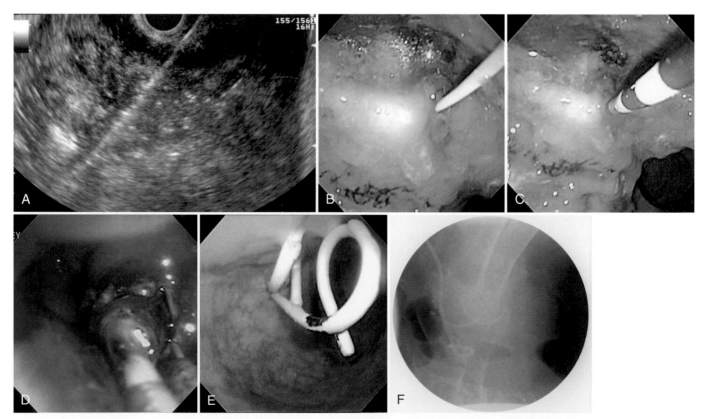

FIGURE 27-2 **A,** A fine-needle aspiration needle is passed into the pelvic abscess under EUS guidance. **B,** A 0.035-inch guidewire is then coiled within the abscess cavity. **C,** The transmural tract is dilated using a 5-Fr endoscopic retrograde cholangiopancreatography cannula. **D,** The transmural tract is then sequentially dilated using an 8-mm balloon dilator. **E,** Two double-pigtail transrectal stents are deployed within the abscess cavity. **F,** A transrectal drainage catheter is seen within the pelvic abscess at fluoroscopy.

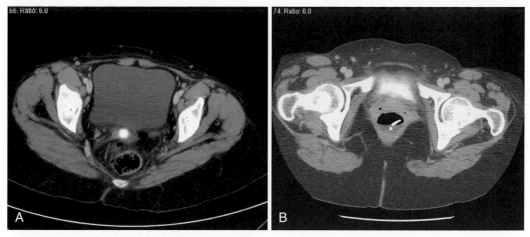

FIGURE 27-3 A, A CT of the pelvic cavity demonstrating an abscess that measures 80 × 60 mm. **B,** After EUS-guided drainage, a follow-up CT at 36 hours demonstrates near complete resolution of the abscess.

50%, the drainage catheter can be removed and the patient discharged home.

6. The remaining stents can continue to assist with drainage and be removed in 2 weeks with sigmoidoscopy as long as a repeat CT of the pelvis shows complete abscess resolution.

Technical and Treatment Outcomes

A total of five studies (Table 27-2) have evaluated the effectiveness of EUS for the treatment of pelvic abscesses.[15–20] In the first report by Giovannini and colleagues, an 8.5- or 10-Fr transrectal stent was deployed for a period of 3 to 6 months and yielded a successful clinical outcome in 8 of 12 patients (75%).[15] Treatment failures were more common in patients with a large abscess that measured more than 8 cm in size. The limitation with transrectal stents is their potential to clog easily, particularly by fecal matter or pus, and when left long-term they can cause perirectal pain or migrate spontaneously. In the second study, this limitation was overcome by placement of a transrectal drainage catheter in four patients.[16] Although the technical and treatment outcomes

were successful, there was the potential for accidental dislodgement of the drainage catheter. Additionally, the need for periodic flushing and aspiration of the drainage catheter mandated a prolonged inpatient hospital stay (median 4 days) for most patients. Therefore a combined technique that included EUS-guided placement of a transrectal drainage catheter and stent for drainage of the pelvic abscess was adopted.[17] The short-term (36 to 48 hours) drainage catheter provided access for continued evacuation of the abscess, whereas the medium-term (2 weeks) stent facilitated maintenance of a patent transmural tract for eventual abscess resolution. This combined therapy demonstrated favorable outcomes for resolution of the abscess in all patients and shortened the postprocedure length of stay to a median of 2 days.

The effectiveness of the above combined approach was then prospectively validated in a cohort of 25 patients with long-term follow-up.[18] The etiology of the abscesses was postsurgical in 68% of patients, perforated diverticulitis or appendicitis in 20%, ischemic colitis, and infective endocarditis and trauma in the remaining 12%. Two of 25 patients had previously failed treatment using percutaneous catheter placements. The mean size of the abscesses was 68.5 mm (range

TABLE 27-2

PUBLISHED CASE SERIES OF EUS-GUIDED DRAINAGE OF PELVIC ABSCESS

Author (year)	Number of Cases	Mean Size (mm)	Drainage Modality	Technical Success (%)	Treatment Success (%)	Complication
Giovannini et al[15] (2003)	12	48.9 × 43.4	Stent	100	88	None
Varadarajulu and Drelichman[16] (2007)	4	68 × 72	Drainage catheter	100	75	None
Trevino et al[17] (2008)	4	93 × 61	Drainage catheter and stent	100	100	None
Varadarajulu and Drelichman[18] (2009)	25	68.5 × 52.4	Drainage catheter and stent	100	96	None
Ramesh et al[19] (2013)	11TC/27TR[a]	75/70[b]	Drainage catheter and stent	100	70/96[a]	None

Studies that involved only abscess aspiration and case reports are not included.
[a]Transcolonic (TC)/transrectal (TR) drainage.
[b]Mean of largest diameter of pelvic abscess.

40 to 96 mm). The authors placed transrectal stents in all patients and an additional drainage catheter in 10 patients whose abscesses measured 80 mm or more. The procedures were technically successful in all patients with a treatment success rate of 96%, and no complications were encountered. Seventy-six percent of the abscesses were drained via the transrectal route and others via the left colon. In this study, two of 25 patients who were critically ill in the intensive care unit underwent EUS-guided drainage at bedside. The mean and median procedural duration was 23 and 14 minutes, respectively. The median duration of postprocedure hospital stay was only 2 days.

One study, which compared the outcomes between transcolonic and transrectal drainage of pelvic abscesses in 38 patients, observed that there was no difference in rates of technical success, treatment success, or complications between both techniques.[19] However, when evaluated by etiology, treatment success for diverticular abscess was significantly lower when compared with other causes (25% versus 97%, $p = 0.002$).

Current data suggest that the time to resolution of pelvic abscess is approximately 8 days with percutaneous techniques. Unlike ultrasound or CT, EUS by facilitating deployment of transluminal stents enables early discharge of patients from the hospital, usually within 2 to 3 days, and does not impair patient mobility. Also, the procedures can be performed within 30 minutes and yields optimal clinical outcome in most patients. Unlike percutaneous catheters that can predispose to fistula formation, transluminal stenting does not seem to pose long-term complications. The technique is effective not only for the management of postsurgical fluid collections but also those secondary to medical illnesses. While most percutaneous procedures require transport to the radiology unit, EUS-guided drainage can be undertaken at bedside if the patient is critically ill. Also, whereas most pelvic fluid collections are either inflammatory or infectious in nature, some may represent another etiology such as a perirectal cyst. EUS can accurately establish an alternative diagnosis in these patients and facilitate appropriate management.

Technical Limitations

Some limitations of the EUS-guided technique include the following: (1) Transmural stenting may not be possible if an abscess is located greater than 2 cm from the gastrointestinal lumen; and (2) with the current limited maneuverability of the curvilinear array echoendoscopes, accessing abscesses that are located more proximally is difficult.

EUS-Guided Glue Injection and Coil Placements

EUS-guided vascular treatment has been introduced as a novel technique for the elective or emergent management of gastric varices.[20,21] Cyanoacrylate glues have been traditionally injected for the treatment of gastric varices. More recently, intravariceal stainless steel coils are being deployed before glue injection.[22,23] It is believed that the intravariceal deployment of a coil before glue injection may minimize the risk of glue embolization. In addition to gastric varices, coil and/or

Video 27-3. Video demonstrating the technique of EUS-guided variceal obliteration by placement of a gastric coil.

glues have been successfully applied for the treatment of rectal varices[24] and ectopic anastomotic varices.[25]

Procedural Technique

The following procedural steps (Video 27-3) are undertaken in sequence:[26]

1. The gastric fundus is filled with water to aid visualization of the varices.
2. A coil size is selected based on the diameter of the varix to be treated.
3. The varix is punctured with a saline-primed 19- or 22-G FNA needle (depending on the size of coil to be delivered). Intravariceal position can be confirmed by either blood aspiration or by injection of saline solution that will produce a flow of bubbles.
4. The coil is loaded into the needle and advanced by using a stylet or the stiff end of a guidewire.
5. Coil deployment within the varix is visualized in a curvilinear echogenic pattern at EUS.
6. Coil deployment is immediately followed by injection of 1 mL of undiluted acrylate glue over 45 to 60 seconds. The glue produces intense echogenicity and shadowing as it fills the varix lumen (Figure 27-4).
7. The needle is flushed with 1 mL of saline solution to clear glue in the "dead space" and is then withdrawn into the sheath. The FNA needle is then removed.
8. Several minutes are allowed for complete glue polymerization. Varix obliteration is confirmed with color Doppler flow.
9. Alternatively, the treated varix can be blunt "palpated" with a closed forceps under endoscopic guidance. An obliterated varix will be hard on palpation.

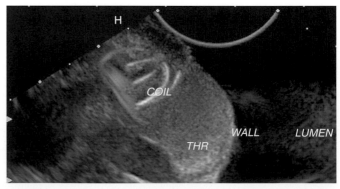

FIGURE 27-4 The presence of a coil that was placed under EUS guidance within a gastric varix.

TABLE 27-3

PUBLISHED CASE SERIES OF EUS-GUIDED VASCULAR THERAPY FOR GASTRIC VARICES

Author (year)	Number of Cases	Injection/ Coil	Echoendoscope	Needle (Gauge)	Approach Route	Technical Success (%)	Treatment Success (%)	Complication
Romero-Castro et al[20] (2007)	5	CYA/–	OVCLA	22	TG	100	100	None
Gonzalez et al[21] (2012)	3	2CYA/–, 1PD/–	OVCLA	19	TG	100	100	None
Binmoeller et al[22] (2011)	30	30CYA/+	28FVCLA/ 2OVCLA	19	TE	100	100	None
Romero-Castro et al[23] (2010)	4	CYA/+	OVCLA	19	TG	100	100	None

+, coil placement; –, no coil placement; CYA, cyanoacrylate; OVCLA, oblique-view curved linear array; PD, polidocanol; FVCLA, forward-view curved linear array; TG, transgastric approach; TE, transesophageal approach.

Technical and Treatment Outcomes

Four case series have reported on EUS-guided variceal obliteration (Table 27-3).[20–23] Glue alone and glue in combination with coil embolization were used in either of the two series. Except for one case series in which a forward-view echoendoscope was used,[22] the oblique-view echoendoscope was used in the remainder of the cases.[20,21,23] The access routes were via the esophagus or the stomach and the 19-G needle was used more commonly. The transesophageal access to gastric varices enables injection in a straight position and is unencumbered by the presence of gastric contents. In addition, by avoiding puncture across the gastric mucosa, often thinned out by large varices, "back-bleeding" into the gastric lumen after needle removal can be prevented. Regardless of the route of access, technical success was 100% in all series and without complications. During the follow-up period, no rebleeding was reported in any of the series.

Technical Limitations

Some limitations of the EUS-guided vascular technique include the following: (1) limited access to the varices via either approaches due to difficult echoendoscope positioning or patient anatomy; and (2) local complications such as bleeding and embolic incidents induced by injection therapy.

EUS-Guided Fiducial Placement for Intraoperative Tumor Localization

Fiducials are implantable radiographic markers that have been used for many years to mark soft tissue in radiology. Recently, the placement of fiducials under EUS guidance has been used as a minimally invasive technique to localize mediastinal and pancreatic cancers before stereotactic body radiotherapy (SBRT).[27–34] Also, the technique has been adopted to facilitate intraoperative localization of small neuroendocrine tumors in patients undergoing enucleation or other resection procedures.[35,36] Patients with these small tumors are ideal candidates for pancreatic tissue sparing procedures such as enucleation that allow for greater preservation of viable parenchyma and function than more extensive resection procedures. However, these small lesions can be difficult to palpate

at the time of surgery and hence fiducials may be helpful to facilitate intraoperative localization.

Procedural Technique

After administration of prophylactic antibiotics, the following steps are undertaken in sequence (Video 27-4):

1. After retracting the stylet of a 19- or 22-G needle by a few millimeters, a fiducial is back-loaded into the needle lumen using a sterile technique.
2. The needle tip is then inserted into sterile bone wax that seals the lumen of the needle to prevent unintended fiducial loss during needle insertion.
3. The FNA needle is advanced into the tumor under EUS guidance, and the fiducial is deployed by advancing the stylet or guidewire (Figure 27-5A,B).
4. The EUS needle is withdrawn, and the procedure is repeated to place a second fiducial. At laparoscopy, the fiducials are identified using cross-table fluoroscopy (Figure 27-5C,D).

Technical and Treatment Outcomes

The first report of EUS-guided fiducial marker placement was published in 2006 by Pishvaian and colleagues, who successfully deployed fiducial markers in six of seven patients with pancreatic cancer who underwent radiation therapy.[31] Later, Varadarajulu and colleagues confirmed the feasibility and safety of EUS-guided fiducial marker placement for the delivery of intensity-modulated radiotherapy (IMRT).[32] Two recent reports have described the utility of fiducials for

Video 27-4. Video demonstrating the technique of EUS-guided fiducial placement.

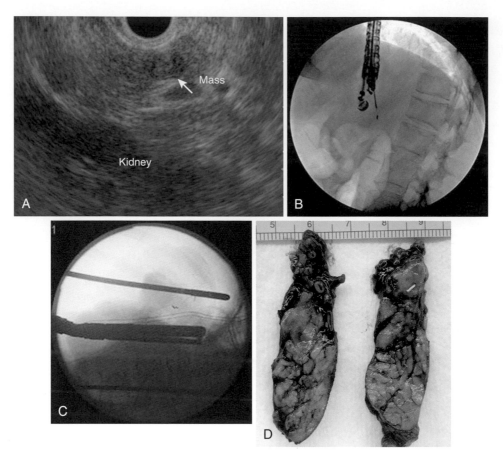

FIGURE 27-5 **A,** At EUS, a small neuroendocrine tumor is identified in the body of the pancreas. **B,** Using EUS guidance, a fiducial is deployed within the tumor as observed on fluoroscopy. **C,** The fiducial is identified intraoperatively using cross-table fluoroscopy. **D,** The fiducial is seen within the substance of the tumor in the resected specimen.

fluoroscopy-aided intraoperative localization of small pancreatic tumors.[35,36] In both reports, the fiducials could be placed successfully without complications and with good operative outcomes.

Technical Limitations

Some limitations of the procedure include the following: (1) Fiducial placement may not always be possible in patients with small tumors in the head or uncinate regions of the pancreas; and (2) radiation therapy may cause dislodgement of the fiducials, the consequences of which are unclear.

The therapeutic applications of endosonography continue to expand. With more innovations in echoendoscope design and the development of dedicated accessories, indications will emerge, and one can expect the exponential growth of interventional EUS procedures.

REFERENCES

1. Miura F, Takada T, Strasberg SM, et al. TG13 flowchart for management of acute cholangitis and cholecystitis. *J Hepatobiliary Pancreat Sci.* 2013;20:47-54.
2. Tsuyuguchi T, Itoi T, Takada T, et al. TG13 indications and techniques for gallbladder drainage in acute cholecystitis (with videos). *J Hepatobiliary Pancreat Sci.* 2013;20:81-88.
3. Itoi T, Coelho-Prabhu N, Baron TH. Endoscopic gallbladder drainage for management of acute cholecystitis. *Gastrointest Endosc.* 2010;71: 1038-1045.
4. Jang JW MD, Lee SS, Park DH, et al. Feasibility and safety of EUS-guided transgastric/transduodenal gallbladder drainage with single-step placement of a modified covered self-expandable metal stent in patients unsuitable for cholecystectomy. *Gastrointest Endosc.* 2011;74: 176-181.
5. Itoi T, Binmoeller KF, Shah J, et al. Clinical evaluation of a novel lumen-apposing metal stent for endosonography-guided pancreatic pseudocyst and gallbladder drainage (with videos). *Gastrointest Endosc.* 2012;75: 870-876.
6. Baron TH, Topazian MD. Endoscopic transduodenal drainage of the gallbladder: implications for endoluminal treatment of gallbladder disease. *Gastrointest Endosc.* 2007;65:735-737.
7. Kwan V, Eisendrath P, Antaki F, et al. EUS-guided cholecystoenterostomy: a new technique (with videos). *Gastrointest Endosc.* 2007;66: 582-586.
8. Lee SS, Park DH, Hwang CY, et al. EUS-guided transmural cholecystostomy as rescue management for acute cholecystitis in elderly or high-risk patients: a prospective feasibility study. *Gastrointest Endosc.* 2007;66: 1008-1012.
9. Takasawa O, Fujita N, Noda Y, et al. Endosonography-guided gallbladder drainage for acute cholecystitis following covered metal stent deployment. *Dig Endosc.* 2009;21:43-47.
10. Kamata K, Kitano M, Komaki T, et al. Transgastric endoscopic ultrasound (EUS)-guided gallbladder drainage for acute cholecystitis. *Endoscopy.* 2009;41(suppl 2):E315-E316.
11. Song TJ, Park do H, Eum JB, et al. EUS-guided cholecystoenterostomy with single-step placement of a 7-F double-pigtail plastic stent in patients who are unsuitable for cholecystectomy: a pilot study (with video). *Gastrointest Endosc.* 2010;71:634-640.
12. Itoi T, Itokawa F, Kurihara T. Endoscopic ultrasonography-guided gallbladder drainage: actual technical presentations and review of the literature (with videos). *J Hepatobiliary Pancreat Sci.* 2011;18: 282-286.

13. Jang JW, Lee SS, Song TJ, et al. Endoscopic ultrasound-guided transmural and percutaneous transhepatic gallbladder drainage are comparable for acute cholecystitis. *Gastroenterology*. 2012;142:805-811.

14. de la Serna-Higuera C, Pérez-Miranda M, Gil-Simón P, et al. EUS-guided transenteric gallbladder drainage with a new fistula-forming, lumen-apposing metal stent. *Gastrointest Endosc*. 2013;77:303-308.

15. Giovannini M, Bories E, Moutardier V, et al. Drainage of deep pelvic abscesses using therapeutic echo endoscopy. *Endoscopy*. 2003;35:511-514.

16. Varadarajulu S, Drelichman ER. EUS-guided drainage of pelvic abscess. *Gastrointest Endosc*. 2007;66:372-376.

17. Trevino J, Drelichman ER, Varadarajulu S. Modified technique for EUS-guided drainage of pelvic abscess. *Gastrointest Endosc*. 2008;68:1215-1219.

18. Varadarajulu S, Drelichman ER. Effectiveness of EUS in drainage of pelvic abscesses in 25 consecutive patients. *Gastrointest Endosc*. 2009;70:1121-1127.

19. Ramesh J, Bang JY, Trevinoa J, et al. Comparison of outcomes between endoscopic ultrasound-guided transcolonic and transrectal drainage of abdominopelvic abscesses. *J Gastroenterol Hepatol*. 2013;28:620-625.

20. Romero-Castro R, Pellicer-Bautista FJ, Jimenez-Saenz M, et al. EUS-guided injection of cyanoacrylate in perforating feeding veins in gastric varices: results in 5 cases. *Gastrointest Endosc*. 2007;66:402-407.

21. Gonzalez JM, Giacino C, Pioche M, et al. Endoscopic ultrasound-guided vascular therapy: is it safe and effective? *Endoscopy*. 2012;44:539-542.

22. Binmoeller KF, Weilert F, Shah JN, et al. EUS-guided transesophageal treatment of gastric fundal varices with combined coiling and cyanoacrylate glue injection (with videos). *Gastrointest Endosc*. 2011;74:1019-1025.

23. Romero-Castro R, Pellicer-Bautista FJ, Giovannini M, et al. Endoscopic ultrasound (EUS)-guided coil embolization therapy in gastric varices. *Endoscopy*. 2010;42:E35-E36.

24. Weilert F, Shah JN, Marson FP, et al. EUS-guided coil and glue for bleeding rectal varix. *Gastrointest Endosc*. 2012;76:915-916.

25. Levy ML, Wong Kee Song LM, Kendrick ML, et al. EUS-guided coil embolization for refractory ectopic variceal bleeding (with videos). *Gastrointest Endosc*. 2008;67:572-574.

26. Cameron R, Binmoeller KF. Cyanoacrylate applications in the GI tract. *Gastrointest Endosc*. 2013;77:846-857.

27. Park WG, Yan BM, Schellenberg D, et al. EUS-guided gold fiducial insertion for image-guided radiation therapy of pancreatic cancer: 50 successful cases without fluoroscopy. *Gastrointest Endosc*. 2010;71:513-518.

28. Sanders MK, Moser AJ, Khalid A, et al. EUS-guided fiducial placement for stereotactic body radiotherapy in locally advanced and recurrent pancreatic cancer. *Gastrointest Endosc*. 2010;71:1178-1184.

29. Ammar T, Cote GA, Creach KM, et al. Fiducial placement for stereotactic radiation by using EUS: feasibility when using a marker compatible with a standard 22-gauge needle. *Gastrointest Endosc*. 2010;71:630-633.

30. DiMaio CJ, Nagula S, Goodman KA, et al. EUS-guided fiducial placement for image-guided radiation therapy in GI malignancies by using a 22-gauge needle (with videos). *Gastrointest Endosc*. 2010;71:1204-1210.

31. Pishvaian AC, Collins B, Gagnon G, et al. EUS-guided fiducial placement for CyberKnife radiotherapy of mediastinal and abdominal malignancies. *Gastrointest Endosc*. 2006;64:412-417.

32. Varadarajulu S, Trevino JM, Shen S, et al. The use of endoscopic ultrasound-guided gold markers in image-guided radiation therapy of pancreatic cancers: a case series. *Endoscopy*. 2010;42:423-425.

33. Owens DJ, Savides TJ. EUS placement of metal fiducials by using a backloaded technique with bone wax seal. *Gastrointest Endosc*. 2009;69:972-973.

34. Khashab MA, Kim KJ, Tryggestad EJ, et al. Comparative analysis of traditional and coiled fiducials implanted during EUS for pancreatic cancer patients receiving stereotactic body radiation therapy. *Gastrointest Endosc*. 2012;76:962-971.

35. Ramesh J, Porterfield J, Varadarajulu S. Endoscopic ultrasound-guided gold fiducial marker placement for intraoperative identification of insulinoma. *Endoscopy*. 2012;44(suppl 2):E327-E328. UCTN.

36. Law JK, Singh VK, Khashab MA, et al. Endoscopic ultrasound (EUS)-guided fiducial placement allows localization of small neuroendocrine tumors during parenchymal-sparing pancreatic surgery. *Surg Endosc*. 2013;27:3921-3926.

Video Appendix

Index